Advances in Gastrointestinal and Liver Disease: From Physiological Mechanisms to Clinical Practice

Editors

Davide Giuseppe Ribaldone
Gian Paolo Caviglia

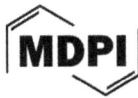

Basel • Beijing • Wuhan • Barcelona • Belgrade • Novi Sad • Cluj • Manchester

Editors
Davide Giuseppe Ribaldone
University of Turin
Turin
Italy

Gian Paolo Caviglia
University of Turin
Turin
Italy

Editorial Office
MDPI
St. Alban-Anlage 66
4052 Basel, Switzerland

This is a reprint of articles from the Special Issue published online in the open access journal *Journal of Clinical Medicine* (ISSN 2077-0383) (available at: https://www.mdpi.com/journal/jcm/special_issues/Advances_in_Gastrointestinal_and_Liver_Disease).

For citation purposes, cite each article independently as indicated on the article page online and as indicated below:

Lastname, A.A.; Lastname, B.B. Article Title. *Journal Name* **Year**, *Volume Number*, Page Range.

ISBN 978-3-7258-0129-9 (Hbk)
ISBN 978-3-7258-0130-5 (PDF)
doi.org/10.3390/books978-3-7258-0130-5

© 2024 by the authors. Articles in this book are Open Access and distributed under the Creative Commons Attribution (CC BY) license. The book as a whole is distributed by MDPI under the terms and conditions of the Creative Commons Attribution-NonCommercial-NoDerivs (CC BY-NC-ND) license.

Contents

About the Editors . . . . **ix**

Gian Paolo Caviglia and Davide Giuseppe Ribaldone
Special Issue "Advances in Gastrointestinal and Liver Disease: From Physiological Mechanisms to Clinical Practice"
Reprinted from: *J. Clin. Med.* **2022**, *11*, 2797, doi:10.3390/jcm11102797 . . . . **1**

Kei Moriya, Norihisa Nishimura, Tadashi Namisaki, Hiroaki Takaya, Yasuhiko Sawada, Hideto Kawaratani, et al.
Zinc Administration and Improved Serum Markers of Hepatic Fibrosis in Patients with Autoimmune Hepatitis
Reprinted from: *J. Clin. Med.* **2021**, *10*, 2465, doi:10.3390/jcm10112465 . . . . **4**

Reiner Wiest, Thomas S. Weiss, Lusine Danielyan and Christa Buechler
Serum Amyloid Beta42 Is Not Eliminated by the Cirrhotic Liver: A Pilot Study
Reprinted from: *J. Clin. Med.* **2021**, *10*, 2669, doi:10.3390/jcm10122669 . . . . **19**

Sylwia Fabiszewska, Edyta Derda, Edyta Szymanska, Marcin Osiecki and Jaroslaw Kierkus
Safety and Effectiveness of Vedolizumab for the Treatment of Pediatric Patients with Very Early Onset Inflammatory Bowel Diseases
Reprinted from: *J. Clin. Med.* **2021**, *10*, 2997, doi:10.3390/jcm10132997 . . . . **32**

Gian Paolo Caviglia, Giorgio Martini, Angelo Armandi, Chiara Rosso, Marta Vernero, Elisabetta Bugianesi, et al.
Risk Factors of Urothelial Cancer in Inflammatory Bowel Disease
Reprinted from: *J. Clin. Med.* **2021**, *10*, 3257, doi:10.3390/jcm10153257 . . . . **39**

Jung Wan Choe, Jae Min Lee, Jong Jin Hyun and Hong Sik Lee
Analysis on Microbial Profiles & Components of Bile in Patients with Recurrent CBD Stones after Endoscopic CBD Stone Removal: A Preliminary Study
Reprinted from: *J. Clin. Med.* **2021**, *10*, 3303, doi:10.3390/jcm10153303 . . . . **48**

Gian Paolo Caviglia, Yulia Troshina, Enrico Garro, Marcantonio Gesualdo, Serena Aneli, Giovanni Birolo, et al.
Usefulness of a Hepatitis B Surface Antigen-Based Model for the Prediction of Functional Cure in Patients with Chronic Hepatitis B Virus Infection Treated with Nucleos(t)ide Analogues: A Real-World Study
Reprinted from: *J. Clin. Med.* **2021**, *10*, 3308, doi:10.3390/jcm10153308 . . . . **58**

Amir Mari, Fadi Abu Baker, Rinaldo Pellicano and Tawfik Khoury
Diagnosis and Management of Achalasia: Updates of the Last Two Years
Reprinted from: *J. Clin. Med.* **2021**, *10*, 3607, doi:10.3390/jcm10163607 . . . . **69**

Antonio Gidaro, Roberto Manetti, Alessandro Palmerio Delitala, Emanuele Salvi, Luigi Bergamaschini, Gianpaolo Vidili and Roberto Castelli
Prothrombotic and Inflammatory Markers in Elderly Patients with Non-Alcoholic Hepatic Liver Disease before and after Weight Loss: A Pilot Study
Reprinted from: *J. Clin. Med.* **2021**, *10*, 4906, doi:10.3390/jcm10214906 . . . . **80**

Lorenzo Onorato, Mariantonietta Pisaturo, Clarissa Camaioni, Pierantonio Grimaldi, Alessio Vinicio Codella, Federica Calò and Nicola Coppola
Risk and Prevention of Hepatitis B Virus Reactivation during Immunosuppression for Non-Oncological Diseases
Reprinted from: *J. Clin. Med.* **2021**, *10*, 5201, doi:10.3390/jcm10215201 . . . . **90**

Ko Miura, Tadayuki Oshima, Akio Tamura, Ken Hara, Takuya Okugawa,
Masashi Fukushima, et al.
Gastric Xanthoma Is Related to the Rapid Growth of Gastric Cancer
Reprinted from: *J. Clin. Med.* 2021, 10, 5704, doi:10.3390/jcm10235704 107

Shuzo Kohno, Masahiro Ikegami, Toru Ikegami, Hiroaki Aoki, Masaichi Ogawa,
Fumiaki Yano and Ken Eto
Risk Factors Associated with the Development of Metastases in Patients with
Gastroenteropancreatic Neuroendocrine Tumors: A Retrospective Analysis
Reprinted from: *J. Clin. Med.* 2022, 11, 60, doi:10.3390/jcm11010060 116

Angelo Armandi, Chiara Rosso, Aurora Nicolosi, Gian Paolo Caviglia, Maria Lorena Abate,
Antonella Olivero, et al.
Crosstalk between Irisin Levels, Liver Fibrogenesis and Liver Damage in Non-Obese,
Non-Diabetic Individuals with Non-Alcoholic Fatty Liver Disease
Reprinted from: *J. Clin. Med.* 2022, 10, 635, doi:10.3390/jcm11030635 126

Dimitri Poddighe, Micol Romano, Kuanysh Dossybayeva, Diyora Abdukhakimova,
Dinara Galiyeva and Erkan Demirkaya
Celiac Disease in Juvenile Idiopathic Arthritis and Other Pediatric Rheumatic Disorders
Reprinted from: *J. Clin. Med.* 2022, 11, 1089, doi:10.3390/jcm11041089 134

Maxime Pichon, Bernard Freche and Christophe Burucoa
New Strategy for the Detection and Treatment of *Helicobacter pylori* Infections in Primary Care
Guided by a Non-Invasive PCR in Stool: Protocol of the French HepyPrim Study
Reprinted from: *J. Clin. Med.* 2022, 11, 1151, doi:10.3390/jcm11051151 144

Marcin Kosmalski, Sylwia Ziółkowska, Piotr Czarny, Janusz Szemraj and Tadeusz Pietras
The Coexistence of Nonalcoholic Fatty Liver Disease and Type 2 Diabetes Mellitus
Reprinted from: *J. Clin. Med.* 2022, 11, 1375, doi:10.3390/jcm11051375 154

Jan-Paul Gundlach, Jannik Kerber, Alexander Hendricks, Alexander Bernsmeier,
Christine Halske, Christian Röder, et al.
Paracrine Interaction of Cholangiocellular Carcinoma with Cancer-Associated Fibroblasts and
Schwann Cells Impact Cell Migration
Reprinted from: *J. Clin. Med.* 2022, 11, 2785, doi:10.3390/jcm11102785 178

Chao-Feng Chang, Wu-Chien Chien, Chi-Hsiang Chung, Hsuan-Hwai Lin, Tien-Yu Huang,
Peng-Jen Chen, et al.
The Clinical Dilemma of Esophagogastroduodenoscopy for Gastrointestinal Bleeding in
Cardiovascular Disease Patients: A Nationwide-Based Retrospective Study
Reprinted from: *J. Clin. Med.* 2022, 11, 3765, doi:10.3390/jcm11133765 195

Shou-Wu Lee, Sheng-Shun Yang, Han-Chung Lien, Yen-Chun Peng, Chun-Fang Tung
and Teng-Yu Lee
The Combining of Tyrosine Kinase Inhibitors and Immune Checkpoint Inhibitors as First-Line
Treatment for Advanced Stage Hepatocellular Carcinoma
Reprinted from: *J. Clin. Med.* 2022, 11, 4874, doi:10.3390/jcm11164874 205

Gian Paolo Caviglia, Chiara Angela Mineo, Chiara Rosso, Angelo Armandi,
Marco Astegiano, Gabriella Canavese, et al.
Predictive Factors of Surgical Recurrence in Patients with Crohn's Disease on Long-Term
Follow-Up: A Focus on Histology
Reprinted from: *J. Clin. Med.* 2022, 11, 5043, doi:10.3390/jcm11175043 214

Riccardo Fornaro, Giovanni Clemente Actis, Gian Paolo Caviglia, Demis Pitoni and Davide Giuseppe Ribaldone
Inflammatory Bowel Disease: Role of Vagus Nerve Stimulation
Reprinted from: *J. Clin. Med.* **2022**, *11*, 5690, doi:10.3390/jcm11195690 . . . . **222**

Kang He, Shanshan Xu, Lijing Shen, Xiaosong Chen, Qiang Xia and Yongbing Qian
Ruxolitinib as Adjunctive Therapy for Hemophagocytic LymPhohistiocytosis after Liver Transplantation: A Case Report and Literature Review
Reprinted from: *J. Clin. Med.* **2022**, *11*, 6308, doi:10.3390/jcm11216308 . . . . **232**

Soo Yeun Lim, Dong Il Chung, Hye Jeong Jeong, Hyun Jeong Jeon, So Jeong Yoon, Hongbeom Kim, et al.
Clinical Outcome of Resected Non-Ampullary Duodenal Adenocarcinoma: A Single Center Experience
Reprinted from: *J. Clin. Med.* **2023**, *12*, 210, doi:10.3390/jcm12010210 . . . . **244**

Gian Paolo Caviglia, Angela Garrone, Chiara Bertolino, Riccardo Vanni, Elisabetta Bretto, Anxhela Poshnjari, et al.
Epidemiology of Inflammatory Bowel Diseases: A Population Study in a Healthcare District of North-West Italy
Reprinted from: *J. Clin. Med.* **2023**, *12*, 641, doi:10.3390/jcm12020641 . . . . **255**

Giuseppe Losurdo, Natale Lino Bruno Caccavo, Giuseppe Indellicati, Francesca Celiberto, Enzo Ierardi, Michele Barone and Alfredo Di Leo
Effect of Long-Term Proton Pump Inhibitor Use on Blood Vitamins and Minerals: A Primary Care Setting Study
Reprinted from: *J. Clin. Med.* **2023**, *12*, 2910, doi:10.3390/jcm12082910 . . . . **263**

About the Editors

Davide Giuseppe Ribaldone

Davide Giuseppe Ribaldone graduated in Medicine and Surgery in 2011, specialized in Gastroenterology in 2017 at the University of Turin, obtained a Doctoral degree in Bioengineering and Medical-Surgical Science in 2022 (Polytechnic University of Turin), and obtained a degree in Telecommunication Engineering in 2005 at the Polytechnic University of Turin. Davide Giuseppe Ribaldone is an Associate Professor at the Department of Medical Sciences, a gastroenterologist consultant, and head of the IBD clinic at "A.O.U. Città della Salute e della Scienza di Torino"—"Molinette" hospital.

Gian Paolo Caviglia

Gian Paolo Caviglia received his M.Sc. from the University of Turin, Italy, in 2009, and his PhD in Medical Physiopathology in 2016. Until 2021, he was a Postdoc at the Unit of Gastroenterology of the Department of Medical Sciences, University of Turin. In January 2022, he achieved the position of Assistant Professor at the same institution.

His research covers multiple aspects of hepatology and gastroenterology, with a special interest in the study of new biomarkers and non-invasive tools for the diagnosis and prognosis of liver diseases.

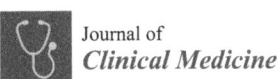

Editorial

Special Issue "Advances in Gastrointestinal and Liver Disease: From Physiological Mechanisms to Clinical Practice"

Gian Paolo Caviglia and Davide Giuseppe Ribaldone *

Division of Gastroenterology, Department of Medical Sciences, University of Torino, 10124 Torino, Italy; gianpaolo.caviglia@unito.it
* Correspondence: davidegiuseppe.ribaldone@unito.it; Tel.: +39-011-6333710

Citation: Caviglia, G.P.; Ribaldone, D.G. Special Issue "Advances in Gastrointestinal and Liver Disease: From Physiological Mechanisms to Clinical Practice". *J. Clin. Med.* **2022**, *11*, 2797. https://doi.org/10.3390/jcm11102797

Received: 11 May 2022
Accepted: 14 May 2022
Published: 16 May 2022

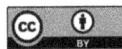

Copyright: © 2022 by the authors. Licensee MDPI, Basel, Switzerland. This article is an open access article distributed under the terms and conditions of the Creative Commons Attribution (CC BY) license (https://creativecommons.org/licenses/by/4.0/).

It is an exciting time for gastroenterology and hepatology. New drugs have entered the market and changed the natural course of several diseases (in particular, hepatitis C and inflammatory bowel disease, IBD), and others are expected in a few years (for example, nonalcoholic fatty liver disease, NAFLD) [1]. Although the identification of the cause of most chronic dysimmune diseases is far from the goal, the daily research that is born in laboratories brings into clinical practice new mechanisms of action and biomarkers useful for personalizing patient management [2,3].

In the next few lines, we want to summarize the most important breakthroughs in the field of gastroenterology and hepatology in the last years.

Hepatis C virus (HCV) treatment is the most important revolution of the past eight years. Before the introduction of direct acting antivirals (DAA), the efficacy and tolerability of interferon-based regimes was far from satisfactory [4]. In 2014, the FDA approved the first all-DAA regimen with sofosbuvir/ledipasvir and sofosbuvir/simeprevir after three clinical trials indicated that DAAs could be administered on their own for HCV genotype 1 treatment with sustained virological response (SVR) rates of 94–99% and significantly fewer adverse effects [5]. The target to eliminate HCV by 2030 no longer appears to be a dream, at least in some countries [6]. Currently under development are a number of new antivirals that target the distinct stages of the HBV life cycle. The goal of these medications, similar to HCV infection, is to cure the infection completely, rather than only inhibiting it. The ultimate goal should be infection control (functional cure) or eradication (complete cure) [7]. Pegylated interferon is the only treatment for chronic hepatitis D (CHD) that has been suggested by professional societies (but not licensed by Drug Regulatory Agencies); it has poor efficacy, and valid CHD treatment has remained an unmet medical need [8]. The goal of current therapeutic attempts is to deprive the HDV of the HBsAg functions that are essential to its life cycle. Three therapy options are currently being tested. Because the HBsAg enters hepatocytes via the sodium taurocholate cotransporting polypeptide (NTCP) on the cell membrane, medications that block the NTCP may prevent the HDV from entering the cells. Because the construction of the HDV virions needs the farnesylation of the large HD antigen by the host, interference with this cellular process could cause the viral assembly to be disrupted. Because the HDV must encapsidate in the HBsAg coat before being released into the bloodstream, nucleic acid polymers (NAPs) that appear to block the formation of subviral HBsAg particles may prevent the HDV from being released into the bloodstream [4].

Regarding IBD, unfortunately a specific cause has not yet been discovered and genetic, environment, immune system, permeability, and microbiome are the main actors described as the cause [9]. Translational research is the key to the basic research of bedside applications. Only in the last 5 years have three new mechanisms of action entered the market: anti-integrin α1β4 with vedolizumab, anti-IL12/23 with ustekinumab, and anti-JAK with tofacitinib. In the next few years several new drugs are expected: anti-IL23, S1P1 regulators, and the more selective anti-JAK [10]. Although we are far from definitively healing these patients, we can try to significantly improve their quality of life, bringing it closer to that of people who do not suffer from these diseases.

In gastrointestinal endoscopy, technology advancement is expressing its maximum potential. The application of artificial intelligence, new techniques, such as submucosal dissection, full thickness resections, and others, are now a reality and we are only at the beginning of the noninvasive treatment of several diseases that once required surgical resection [11].

In this Special Issue, entitled "Advances in Gastrointestinal and Liver disease: From Physiological Mechanisms to Clinical Practice" we welcome frontier papers about novelties in the field of translational research and the clinical management of gastrointestinal and hepatological diseases.

Several papers have already been published in the Special Issue. The etiology of NALD is not yet fully understood and there is a lack of noninvasive biomarkers enabling the differentiation of liver disease severity. Armandi and colleagues conducted a retrospective, cross-sectional investigation to explore the mechanistic involvement of the myokine irisin in a population of biopsy-established NAFLD in the absence of severe metabolic diseases (obesity and type 2 diabetes mellitus) [12]. They discovered that people with severe fibrosis had considerably greater irisin levels. They also discovered a link between circulating irisin and the new collagen remodeling markers PRO-C3 and PRO-C6. The findings point to a synergistic link between irisin and liver fibrogenesis, the hepatic response to inflammatory damage. This supports the idea that irisin is a marker for a more severe phenotype of liver disease, as evidenced by the higher irisin levels found in those with advanced fibrosis. Still, regarding NAFLD, according to research by Gidaro et al., patients with NAFLD have higher levels of C-reactive protein, fibrinogen, PAI-1, von Willebrand factors, and F VII, all of which are linked to an increased risk of thrombosis [13]. Despite having been overtaken by NAFLD in the developed world, HBV infection is a serious health concern [14]. The findings of Caviglia et al. demonstrated that measuring baseline serum HBsAg and the extent to which HBsAg dropped throughout therapy with third-generation nucleot(s)ide analogs can help select chronic HBV patients who are more likely to achieve functional cure [15].

IBD in children is becoming more common around the world and the onset age is getting younger [16], as a consequence, innovative medicinal strategies are essential. The first study on vedolizumab treatment in children with very early onset IBD was published by Fabiszewska et al., and it demonstrated the safety and effectiveness of this anti-integrin agent in the studied group: a clinical response after induction therapy with three doses of vedolizumab was observed in more than 40% of patients [17].

Neuroendocrine tumors (NETs) are diverse malignancies that emerge from systemic endocrine and nerve cells and have a wide range of pathological and clinical features. Their prevalence has been rising [18]. Lymph node metastases can be surgically removed, which can improve prognosis; however, other metastases, which are generally not suggested for surgery, are difficult to remove, underscoring the importance of preoperative diagnosis. In the study of Kohno et al., according to the 2019 WHO classification, factors connected to gastroenteropancreatic-NET metastases were studied. Tumor grade and vascular invasion were revealed to be the most relevant factors. Venous invasion was found to be more strongly associated with metastasis than lymphatic invasion, suggesting that pathological investigation of lymphatic invasion may be difficult.

As the Guest Editors, we are looking forward for other original studies and accomplished reviews regarding recent innovation in gastroenterology and hepatology.

Funding: This paper received no external funding.

Conflicts of Interest: The authors declare no conflict of interest.

References

1. Losurdo, G.; Gravina, A.G.; Maroni, L.; Gabrieletto, E.M.; Ianiro, G.; Ferrarese, A.; Visintin, A.; Frazzoni, L.; Pellegatta, G.; Sessa, A.; et al. Future challenges in gastroenterology and hepatology, between innovations and unmet needs: A SIGE Young Editorial Board's perspective. *Dig. Liver Dis.* **2022**, *54*, 583–597. [CrossRef] [PubMed]
2. Caviglia, G.P.; Armandi, A.; Rosso, C.; Gaia, S.; Aneli, S.; Rolle, E.; Abate, M.L.; Olivero, A.; Nicolosi, A.; Guariglia, M.; et al. Biomarkers of Oncogenesis, Adipose Tissue Dysfunction and Systemic Inflammation for the Detection of Hepatocellular Carcinoma in Patients with Nonalcoholic Fatty Liver Disease. *Cancers* **2021**, *13*, 2305. [CrossRef] [PubMed]
3. Caviglia, G.P.; Rosso, C.; Stalla, F.; Rizzo, M.; Massano, A.; Abate, M.L.; Olivero, A.; Armandi, A.; Vanni, E.; Younes, R.; et al. On-Treatment Decrease of Serum Interleukin-6 as a Predictor of Clinical Response to Biologic Therapy in Patients with Inflammatory Bowel Diseases. *J. Clin. Med.* **2020**, *9*, 800. [CrossRef] [PubMed]
4. Saracco, G.M.; Marzano, A.; Rizzetto, M. Therapy of Chronic Viral Hepatitis: The Light at the End of the Tunnel? *Biomedicines* **2022**, *10*, 534. [CrossRef] [PubMed]
5. Basyte-Bacevice, V.; Kupcinskas, J. Evolution and Revolution of Hepatitis C Management: From Non-A, Non-B Hepatitis Toward Global Elimination. *Dig. Dis.* **2020**, *38*, 137–142. [CrossRef] [PubMed]
6. Isfordink, C.J.; van Dijk, M.; Brakenhoff, S.M.; Kracht, P.A.M.; Arends, J.E.; de Knegt, R.J.; van der Valk, M.; Drenth, J.P.H. Hepatitis C Elimination in the Netherlands (CELINE): How nationwide retrieval of lost to follow-up hepatitis C patients contributes to micro-elimination. *Eur. J. Intern. Med.* **2022**. [CrossRef] [PubMed]
7. Cornberg, M.; Lok, A.S.F.; Terrault, N.A.; Zoulim, F.; Berg, T.; Brunetto, M.R.; Buchholz, S.; Buti, M.; Chan, H.L.Y.; Chang, K.M.; et al. Guidance for design and endpoints of clinical trials in chronic hepatitis B—Report from the 2019 EASL-AASLD HBV Treatment Endpoints Conference. *J. Hepatol.* **2020**, *72*, 539–557. [CrossRef] [PubMed]
8. Caviglia, G.P.; Rizzetto, M. Treatment of hepatitis D: An unmet medical need. *Clin. Microbiol. Infect.* **2020**, *26*, 824–827. [CrossRef] [PubMed]
9. Fiocchi, C. Inflammatory Bowel Disease: Complexity and Variability Need Integration. *Front. Med.* **2018**, *5*, 75. [CrossRef] [PubMed]
10. D'Amico, F.; Peyrin-Biroulet, L.; Danese, S.; Fiorino, G. New drugs in the pipeline for the treatment of inflammatory bowel diseases: What is coming? *Curr. Opin. Pharmacol.* **2020**, *55*, 141–150. [CrossRef] [PubMed]
11. Li, J.W.; Wang, L.M.; Ang, T.L. Artificial intelligence-assisted colonoscopy: A narrative review of current data and clinical applications. *Singap. Med. J.* **2022**, *63*, 118–124. [CrossRef] [PubMed]
12. Armandi, A.; Rosso, C.; Nicolosi, A.; Caviglia, G.P.; Abate, M.L.; Olivero, A.; D'amato, D.; Vernero, M.; Gaggini, M.; Saracco, G.M.; et al. Crosstalk between Irisin Levels, Liver Fibrogenesis and Liver Damage in Non-Obese, Non-Diabetic Individuals with Non-Alcoholic Fatty Liver Disease. *J. Clin. Med.* **2022**, *11*, 635. [CrossRef] [PubMed]
13. Gidaro, A.; Manetti, R.; Delitala, A.P.; Salvi, E.; Bergamaschini, L.; Vidili, G.; Castelli, R. Prothrombotic and Inflammatory Markers in Elderly Patients with Non-Alcoholic Hepatic Liver Disease before and after Weight Loss: A Pilot Study. *J. Clin. Med.* **2021**, *10*, 4906. [CrossRef] [PubMed]
14. Seto, W.K.; Lo, Y.R.; Pawlotsky, J.M.; Yuen, M.F. Chronic hepatitis B virus infection. *Lancet* **2018**, *392*, 2313–2324. [CrossRef]
15. Caviglia, G.P.; Troshina, Y.; Garro, E.; Gesualdo, M.; Aneli, S.; Birolo, G.; Pittaluga, F.; Cavallo, R.; Saracco, G.M.; Ciancio, A. Usefulness of a Hepatitis B Surface Antigen-Based Model for the Prediction of Functional Cure in Patients with Chronic Hepatitis B Virus Infection Treated with Nucleos(t)ide Analogues: A Real-World Study. *J. Clin. Med.* **2021**, *10*, 3308. [CrossRef] [PubMed]
16. Gasparetto, M.; Guariso, G. Highlights in IBD Epidemiology and Its Natural History in the Paediatric Age. *Gastroenterol. Res. Pract.* **2013**, *2013*, 829040. [CrossRef] [PubMed]
17. Fabiszewska, S.; Derda, E.; Szymanska, E.; Osiecki, M.; Kierkus, J. Safety and Effectiveness of Vedolizumab for the Treatment of Pediatric Patients with Very Early Onset Inflammatory Bowel Diseases. *J. Clin. Med.* **2021**, *10*, 2997. [CrossRef] [PubMed]
18. Das, S.; Dasari, A. Epidemiology, Incidence, and Prevalence of Neuroendocrine Neoplasms: Are There Global Differences? *Curr. Oncol. Rep.* **2021**, *23*, 43. [CrossRef] [PubMed]

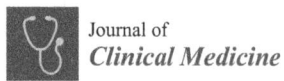

Journal of
Clinical Medicine

Article

Zinc Administration and Improved Serum Markers of Hepatic Fibrosis in Patients with Autoimmune Hepatitis

Kei Moriya [1,*], Norihisa Nishimura [1], Tadashi Namisaki [1], Hiroaki Takaya [1], Yasuhiko Sawada [1], Hideto Kawaratani [1], Kosuke Kaji [1], Naotaka Shimozato [1], Shinya Sato [1], Masanori Furukawa [2], Akitoshi Douhara [1], Takemi Akahane [1], Akira Mitoro [1], Junichi Yamao [2] and Hitoshi Yoshiji [1]

[1] Department of Gastroenterology and Hepatology, Nara Medical University, 840 Shijo-cho, Kashihara, Nara 634-8522, Japan; nishimuran@naramed-u.ac.jp (N.N.); tadashin@naramed-u.ac.jp (T.N.); htky@naramed-u.ac.jp (H.T.); yasuhiko@naramed-u.ac.jp (Y.S.); kawara@naramed-u.ac.jp (H.K.); kajik@naramed-u.ac.jp (K.K.); shimozato@naramed-u.ac.jp (N.S.); shinyasato@naramed-u.ac.jp (S.S.); aki-do@hotmail.co.jp (A.D.); stakemi@naramed-u.ac.jp (T.A.); mitoroak@naramed-u.ac.jp (A.M.); yoshijih@naramed-u.ac.jp (H.Y.)
[2] Department of Endoscopy, Nara Medical University, 840 Shijo-cho, Kashihara, Nara 634-8522, Japan; furukawa@naramed-u.ac.jp (M.F.); juny3126@naramed-u.ac.jp (J.Y.)
* Correspondence: moriyak@naramed-u.ac.jp; Tel.: +81-744-22-3051; Fax: +81-744-24-7122

Citation: Moriya, K.; Nishimura, N.; Namisaki, T.; Takaya, H.; Sawada, Y.; Kawaratani, H.; Kaji, K.; Shimozato, N.; Sato, S.; Furukawa, M.; et al. Zinc Administration and Improved Serum Markers of Hepatic Fibrosis in Patients with Autoimmune Hepatitis. *J. Clin. Med.* **2021**, *10*, 2465. https://doi.org/10.3390/jcm10112465

Academic Editor: Davide Giuseppe Ribaldone

Received: 27 April 2021
Accepted: 31 May 2021
Published: 2 June 2021

Publisher's Note: MDPI stays neutral with regard to jurisdictional claims in published maps and institutional affiliations.

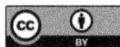

Copyright: © 2021 by the authors. Licensee MDPI, Basel, Switzerland. This article is an open access article distributed under the terms and conditions of the Creative Commons Attribution (CC BY) license (https://creativecommons.org/licenses/by/4.0/).

Abstract: Aim: The aim of the present study is to investigate the effect of long-term zinc supplementation, which is important for the activation of various enzymes that contribute to antioxidant and antifibrotic activities, on the improvement of serum fibrotic markers in patients with autoimmune hepatitis (AIH). Methods: A total of 38 patients with AIH under regular treatment at our hospital who provided their consent for being treated with polaprezinc (75 mg twice daily) were included and classified into 2 groups: the patients with zinc elevation ($n = 27$) and the patients without zinc elevation ($n = 11$). Serum biomarker of fibrosis, protein expression levels of matrix metalloproteinases (MMPs), and their inhibitors (TIMPs) were evaluated. Results: A significant difference was found between the variability of serum procollagen type III and collagen type IV-7S between the 2 groups before and after zinc administration for more than 24 months ($p = 0.043$ and $p = 0.049$). In the patients with zinc elevation, no significant changes were found in collagenase (MMP-1 and MMP-13) before and after zinc administration, whereas a significant increase in the expression of gelatinase (MMP-2 and MMP-9) was found after administration ($p = 0.021$ and $p = 0.005$). As for the relative ratio of MMPs to TIMPs, only MMP-9 to TIMP-1 showed a significant increase ($p = 0.004$). Conclusions: Long-term treatment with polaprezinc has been demonstrated to safely improve serum fibrosis indices through increases in MMP-2/-9 and MMP-9/TIMP-1 and is expected to be well combined with direct antifibrotic therapies such as molecularly targeted agents.

Keywords: autoimmune hepatitis; liver fibrosis; matrix metalloproteinase; serum zinc

1. Introduction

An increasing trend of prevalence of autoimmune hepatitis (AIH) was found according to the nationwide epidemiologic survey [1]. However, the etiology of AIH still remains largely unknown, and no therapeutic agents that can "cure" this disease have been developed [2]. For a tentative treatment, as indicated in the current clinical practice guidelines of the European Association for the Study of the Liver and the American Association for the Study of Liver Diseases, corticosteroid is definitely the first-line treatment and is recommended for a patient with AIH [3,4]. Although in a multi-center prospective cohort study, Yoshizawa et al. reported that long-term outcomes of patients with AIH were comparable with those of the general population; almost all of the patients were intensively treated with prednisolone [5]. Long-term use of prednisolone has been widely known to be associated with various kinds of adverse effects with a high occurrence ratio including the increased susceptibility to infection such as *Pneumocystis jirovecii* and coronavirus disease 2019 [6–8].

In such a situation, clinicians sometimes encounter a case of AIH whose transaminase level remains within the normal limit, but its histological finding reveals mild active hepatitis. Dhaliwal et al. [9] reported that patients with AIH were supposed to have a relatively poor prognosis. Similar to other kinds of chronic liver disease such as nonalcoholic steatohepatitis and viral hepatitis [10,11], the progression of fibrosis is an important factor to predict the long-term prognosis in patients with chronic liver disease, including AIH [12–14]. In this point, keeping the pathological activity of AIH as quiet as possible and inhibiting its fibrosis as definitely as possible are the most important actions for patients with AIH to reach good prognosis.

Next to iron, zinc is the second largest mineral element stored in the human body and has a pivotal role as a micronutrient for antioxidant, antiinflammatory, and antiapoptotic effects [15,16]. Zinc also plays an important role as a cofactor of some enzymes involved in collagen synthesis [17,18]. Collagenase is a zinc metalloenzyme and zinc deficiency causes a decline in the activity of collagenase that results in liver fibrosis [19]. Zhou et al. reported that zinc has cytoprotective activities that protect hepatocytes from oxidative stress. In an animal model, zinc deficiency enhanced sensitivity to drug-induced hepatotoxicity and zinc supplementation suppressed the collagen synthesis in hepatic stellate cells (HSCs) [20,21]. Polaprezinc, composed of elemental zinc and L-carnosine, is known to have an effect of tissue repair, active oxygen removal, and anti-inflammatory properties, and has been available in clinical use for peptic ulcer in Japan. This prospective clinical study aimed to elucidate the inhibitory effect of polaprezinc on the progression of fibrosis in patients with AIH non-invasively through molecular mechanisms. To the end, we evaluated the changes of serum fibrosis indices before and after the zinc administration.

2. Methods

2.1. Patients

Of the 79 patients with histologically diagnosed AIH based on the revised diagnostic scoring system of the International Autoimmune Hepatitis Group (IAIHG) in 1999 and continuous treatment at the Nara Medical University Hospital, 49 patients were enrolled in this prospective study between September 2015 and March 2017 with written informed consent from each individual. The inclusion criteria were as follows: (i) patients who have successfully achieved clinical remission of AIH (in which serum levels of transaminase continuously stayed within normal limits for at least six months), and (ii) with continuous administration of polaprezinc for over two years. The exclusion criteria were as follows: (i) positive for hepatitis C virus (HCV), hepatitis B virus (HBV), and/or human immunodeficiency virus (HIV); (ii) with some liver disease; (iii) under the administration of hepatotoxic drugs; and (iv) with decompensated cirrhosis, severe cytopenia, renal failure, heart failure, and pregnant or lactating women. For zinc administration, polaprezinc (75 mg twice daily) was prescribed to study participants. In addition, we excluded 11 patients who took polaprezinc for <24 months after the study enrollment. All of them discontinued polaprezinc within a year (mean ± standard deviation (SD), 4.9 ± 3.6 months) because of their intentions without any serious reason or discontinuation of medical maintenance owing to reasons such as moving (Supplementary Table S1). A patient quit polaprezinc because of his mild diarrhea, but he quickly recovered after that. Finally, the remaining 38 patients who successfully took polaprezinc for >24 months were divided into two groups: the patients with zinc elevation and the patients without zinc elevation (Figure 1).

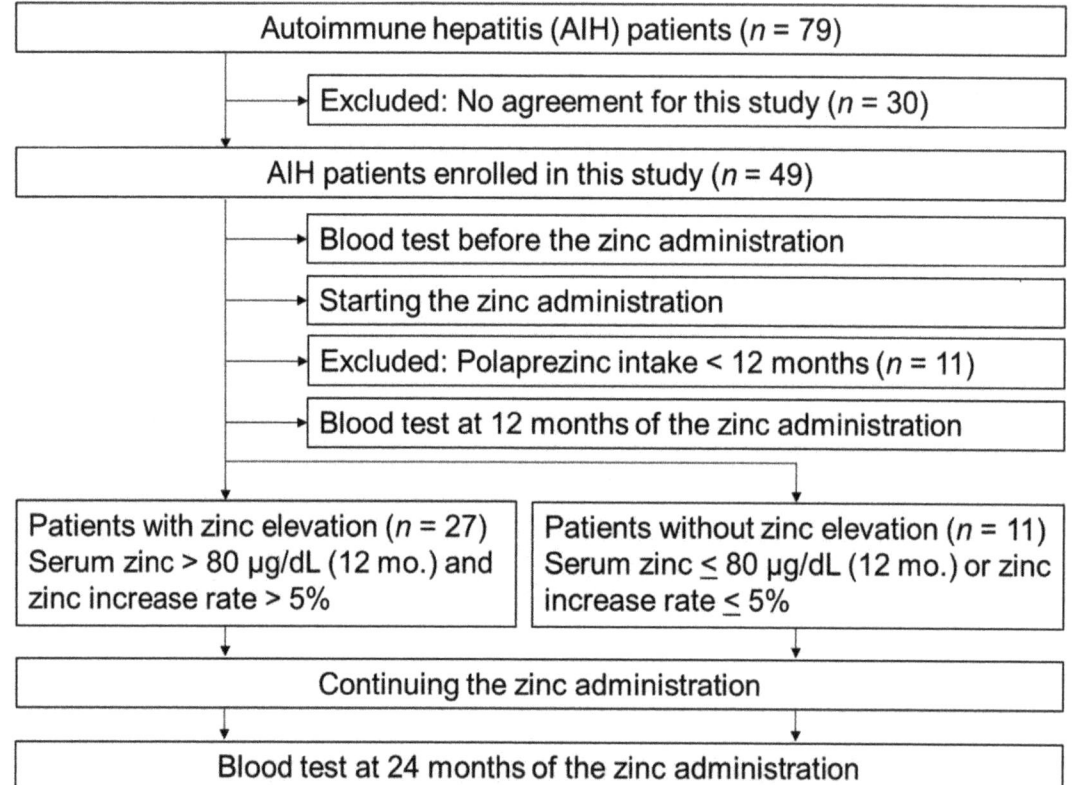

Figure 1. Patient flowchart. A total of 49 patients with AIH were initially included in analysis, 11 of whom were excluded because they withdrew polaprezinc intake within 12 months; 38 patients treated with polaprezinc for >24 months were enrolled and were divided into two groups based on serum zinc level and its increase rate.

The patients with zinc elevation ($n = 27$) were those whose serum zinc level at 12 months after the beginning of administration was >80 μg/dL (the normal lower limit in Japan) and was also increased to >5% during this period. The patients without zinc elevation ($n = 11$) were those whose serum zinc level after the supplementation was either ≤80 μg/dL or increased to ≤5% during this period.

2.2. Laboratory Assessments

All patients underwent a routine laboratory assessment in the hospital, which included complete blood count, a general biochemistry test, and coagulation test. Serum levels of procollagen type III, type IV collagen 7S, and hyaluronic acid were measured by external clinical examination facilities with chemiluminescent immunoassay, chemiluminescent enzyme immunoassay, and latex immunoagglutination assay, respectively. Serum levels of human matrix metalloproteinase-1 (MMP-1), metalloproteinase-2 (MMP-2), metalloproteinase-9 (MMP-9), and metalloproteinase-13 (MMP-13) were measured using the following enzyme-linked immunosorbent assay (ELISA) kits: human MMP-1 ELISA kit #ELH-MMP1 (RayBio®, Norcross, GA, USA), human MMP-2 ELISA kit #KE00077, human MMP-9 ELISA kit #KE00164, and human MMP-13 ELISA kit #KE00078 (Proteintech®, Rosemont, IL, USA). Serum levels of the inhibitor of MMPs, TIMP-1, and TIMP-2 were measured using the following ELISA kits according to the manufacturer's instructions: human TIMP-1 ELISA kit #DTM100 and human TIMP-2 ELISA kit #DTM200 (R&D Systems®, Minneapolis, MN, USA).

2.3. Histological Assessments

The biopsy samples were stained using hematoxylin/eosin and Azan methods. Liver fibrosis was staged based on the METAVIR score (F0, no fibrosis; F1, portal fibrosis without septa; F2, portal fibrosis with few septa; F3, numerous septa without cirrhosis; F4, cirrhosis). F0 to F2 was considered as non-fibrosis to mild fibrosis, whereas F3 to F4 was considered as advanced fibrosis.

2.4. Statistical Analyses and Ethical Issues

The numerical variables were expressed as mean ± SD. The chi-square test, Mann-Whitney U test, and Wilcoxon signed-rank test were used to compare patient characteristics between the groups. Correlation was assessed by using Spearman's rank correlation coefficients. $p < 0.05$ was considered statistically significant. JMP version 14.3 software (SAS Institute Inc., Cary, NC, USA) was used for statistical analyses.

This study was approved by the Ethics Committee of the Nara Medical University Hospital (approval #15-003) and was conducted according to the ethical principles in the Japanese ethical guidelines for epidemiologic research (https://www.mhlw.go.jp/stf/seisakunitsuite/bunya/hokabunya/kenkyujigyou/i-kenkyu/index.html (accessed on 1 December 2020)). This study was conducted according to the Declaration of Helsinki. This study protocol was registered as a clinical trial (UMIN000022959, https://upload.umin.ac.jp/ (accessed on 13 June 2016)), and a written informed consent was obtained from all patients.

3. Results

The clinical profiles of patients in each group before starting zinc supplementation are presented in Table 1. No significant differences were found in age, sex, body weights, and the degree of hepatic fibrosis. There were no significant differences in the basal serum levels of zinc, procollagen III and collagen IV-7S. All study participants were well treated with ursodeoxycholic acids and/or prednisolone, and their transaminase levels were within the normal range. Although the hepatitis activities of patients in both groups were modest, their serum zinc levels seemed to be insufficient.

Before zinc supplementation, serum albumin levels, which generally predict the overall survival of patients with liver diseases [22], correlated with serum zinc levels of patients with AIH in this study ($p < 0.05$) (Figure 2A). Serum zinc levels also inversely correlated with some liver fibrotic markers, such as serum procollagen type III, collagen type IV-7S, and hyaluronic acid ($p < 0.05$) (Figure 2B–D, respectively).

Table 1. Clinical profiles of patients with autoimmune hepatitis before zinc supplementation.

	Patients with Zinc Elevation (n = 27)			Patients without Zinc Elevation (n = 11)			p
Age (years)	65.0	±	11.0	69.2	±	13.9	0.38
Sex							1.00
Male	7.4	%	(2)	9.1	%	(1)	
Female	92.6	%	(25)	90.9	%	(10)	
Body Weights (kg)	54.0	±	9.8	53.0	±	10.1	0.79
Body Mass Index (kg/m^2)	23.0	±	3.8	23.5	±	4.2	0.74
Fibrosis							0.81
F0	3.7	%	(1)	0.0	%	(0)	
F1	44.4	%	(12)	54.5	%	(6)	
F2	29.6	%	(8)	27.3	%	(3)	
F3	14.8	%	(4)	9.1	%	(1)	
F4 (Liver Cirrhosis)	7.4	%	(2)	9.1	%	(1)	
AIH type 1	100	%	(27)	100.0	%	(11)	1.00
AIH type 2	0	%	(0)	0.0	%	(0)	1.00
Morbidity periods (years)	4	±	3.4	5.3	±	3.1	0.30
Blood test							
Zinc (μg/dL)	70.8	±	10.9	74.4	±	13.0	0.44
AST (U/L)	24.6	±	9.2	29.4	±	13.6	0.31
ALT (U/L)	18.1	±	10.1	20.3	±	9.5	0.54
ALP (U/L)	233	±	100	308	±	152	0.15
gamma GT (U/L)	38.9	±	61.2	69.5	±	109	0.40
Total bilirubin (mg/dL)	0.79	±	0.45	0.85	±	0.29	0.65
Albumin (g/dL)	4.16	±	0.26	4.11	±	0.27	0.59
HDL-cholesterol (mg/dL)	67.6	±	22.1	71.3	±	19.5	0.61
Ferritin (ng/mL)	84.4	±	95.6	97.7	±	77.1	0.66
Copper (μg/dL)	121.8	±	27.7	130.3	±	23.1	0.38
IgG (mg/dL)	1389	±	327	1495	±	488	0.52
Hyaluronic acid (ng/mL)	92.2	±	78.2	168	±	187	0.25
Pro-collagen type III (ng/mL)	0.65	±	0.30	0.55	±	0.17	0.25
Type IV collagen 7S (ng/mL)	5.45	±	3.13	4.09	±	1.24	0.08
Platelets (/μL)	19.6	±	5.7	18.9	±	5.4	0.72
Prothrombin time (%)	95.4	±	19.7	96.6	±	16.6	0.84
Treatments							
PSL populations (%)	51.9	%	(14)	36.4	%	(4)	0.48
PSL dose (mg)	5.8	±	1.8	6.3	±	1.9	0.48
UDCA populations (%)	88.9	%	(24)	90.9	%	(10)	1.00
UDCA dose (mg)	600	±	177	630	±	95	0.53
Azathioprine populations (%)	11.0	%	(3)	9.1	%	(1)	0.85
Azathioprine dose (mg)	100	±	0	100	±	0	1.00

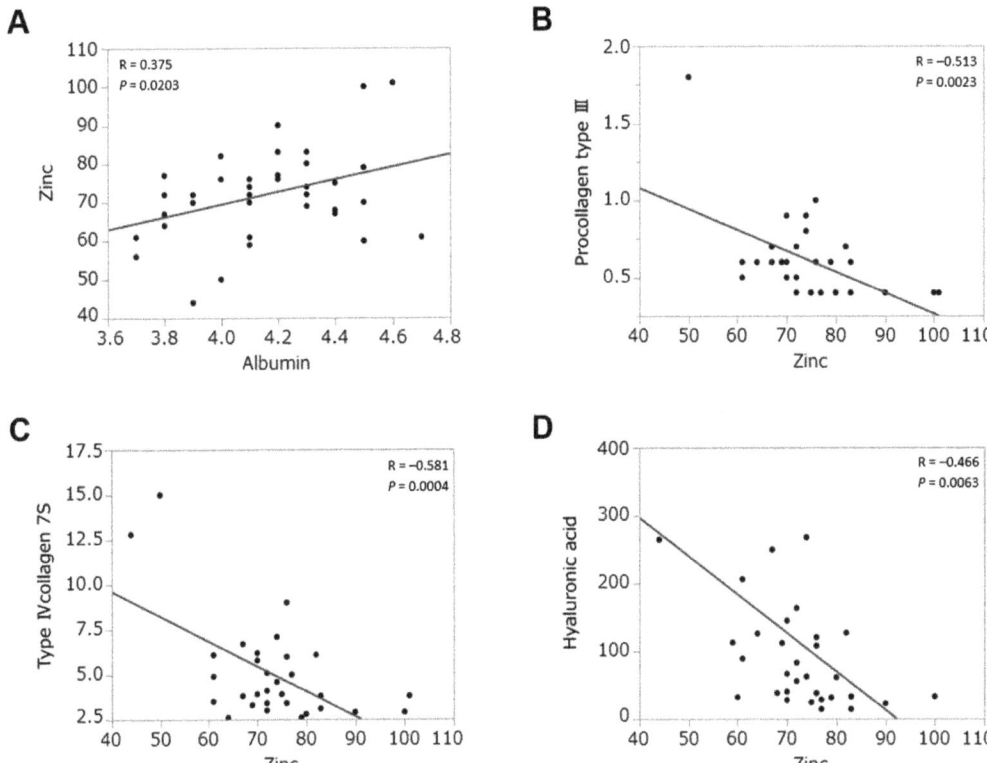

Figure 2. Relations between basal serum zinc level and biochemical markers. (**A**) Relation between zinc and albumin ($p = 0.020$). (**B**) Relation between zinc and procollagen type III ($p = 0.002$). (**C**) Relation between zinc and collagen type IV-7S ($p < 0.001$). (**D**) Relation between zinc and hyaluronic acid ($p = 0.006$).

Serum zinc concentration was increased to >50% at 12 or 24 months after continuous zinc supplementation in the patients with zinc elevation (before, 70.8 ± 10.9 µg/dL; 12 months, 109.9 ± 35.5 µg/dL ($p < 0.001$); 24 months, 105.1 ± 38.0 µg/dL ($p < 0.001$)) (Table 2). The serum ferritin levels (before, 84.4 ± 95.6 ng/mL; 12 months, 56.8 ± 50.8 ng/mL ($p = 0.19$); 24 months, 54.3 ± 42.0 ng/mL ($p = 0.20$)) in the patients with zinc elevation and their serum copper levels (before, 121.8 ± 27.7 µg/dL; 12 months, 107.8 ± 17.7 µg/dL ($p = 0.34$) 24 months, 113.8 ± 20.6 µg/dL ($p = 0.25$)) were not affected and no clinical adverse event such as anemia and neuropathy was observed in this study (Table 2). Although there was no change in the transaminase levels during the entire observation period, the serum levels of procollagen type III and collagen type IV-7S indicated a tendency to decrease at 12 months after zinc supplementation ($p = 0.06$ and $p = 0.07$, respectively). In contrast, in the patients without zinc elevation, serum zinc concentration continuously remained at the baseline level through the course, although their transaminase and the other biliary enzyme levels never changed (Supplementary Table S2). To our surprise, the levels of serum procollagen type III and collagen type IV-7S indicated a gradient increase, but there was no significance because of the small number of cases.

Table 2. Clinical parameters of the patients with zinc elevation before and after zinc supplementation.

Patients with Zinc Elevation (n = 27)	Before Mean		SD	After 12 Months Mean		SD	p	After 24 Months Mean		SD	p
Zinc (µg/dL)	70.8	±	10.9	109.9	±	35.5	<0.001	105.1	±	38.0	<0.001
AST (U/L)	24.6	±	9.2	24.4	±	11.1	0.93	27.2	±	17.8	0.51
ALT (U/L)	18.1	±	10.1	17.0	±	9.3	0.67	19.0	±	13.4	0.79
ALP (U/L)	232.8	±	100.0	275.2	±	279.8	0.46	242.8	±	86.4	0.70
Gamma GT (U/L)	38.9	±	61.2	52.4	±	140.5	0.65	32.3	±	42.0	0.65
Total bilirubin (mg/dL)	0.79	±	0.45	0.78	±	0.42	0.93	0.81	±	0.47	0.88
Albumin (g/dL)	4.16	±	0.26	4.22	±	0.23	0.41	4.21	±	0.18	0.48
HDL-cholesterol (mg/dL)	67.6	±	22.1	64.8	±	19.0	0.63	67.9	±	19.9	0.95
Ferritin (ng/mL)	84.4	±	95.6	56.8	±	50.8	0.19	54.3	±	42.0	0.20
Copper (µg/dL)	121.8	±	27.7	107.8	±	17.7	0.34	113.8	±	20.6	0.25
IgG (mg/dL)	1388.7	±	327.3	1359.3	±	279.5	0.72	1351.8	±	351.7	0.71
Hyaluronic acid (ng/mL)	92.2	±	78.2	65.3	±	53.8	0.16	91.1	±	73.3	0.97
Pro-collagen type III (ng/mL)	0.65	±	0.30	0.52	±	0.16	0.06	0.49	±	0.15	0.06
Type IV collagen 7S (ng/mL)	5.45	±	3.13	4.12	±	1.68	0.07	4.30	±	1.23	0.15
Platelets (/µL)	19.6	±	5.7	20.4	±	5.7	0.61	20.8	±	5.8	0.45
Prothrombin time (%)	95.4	±	19.7	98.7	±	13.4	0.47	95.1	±	13.9	0.96

Based on these findings, we compared the changes of procollagen type III level in the patients with zinc elevation and the patients without zinc elevation at 12 months and 24 months after zinc supplementation. There were significant differences between the patients with zinc elevation and the patients without zinc elevation in terms of the difference in serum procollagen III level at 24 months after zinc supplementation ($p = 0.043$) (Figure 3A). Moreover, in terms of serum collagen type IV-7S level, significant differences between the patients with zinc elevation and the patients without zinc elevation were also found at 12 months and 24 months after zinc supplementation ($p = 0.050$ and $p = 0.049$, respectively) (Figure 3B).

Finally, we also investigated the protein levels of serum collagenase (MMP-1 and MMP-13), gelatinase A (MMP-2), and gelatinase B (MMP-9). In addition, the serum levels of the inhibitor of MMPs, such as TIMP-1 and TIMP-2, were also examined. In the patients with zinc elevation, the levels of these gelatinases were significantly increased after zinc supplementation for >24 months, whereas those of collagenase were not (Figure 4A). The serum level of TIMP-2 was significantly augmented after zinc supplementation, but no significant change was found in TIMP-1 level (Figure 4B). In terms of the ratio of each MMP and its related inhibitor, MMP-9/TIMP-1 was significantly up-regulated. However, there were no significant changes in other ratios, such as MMP-1/TIMP-1, MMP-13/TIMP-1, and MMP-2/TIMP-2 (Figure 4C).

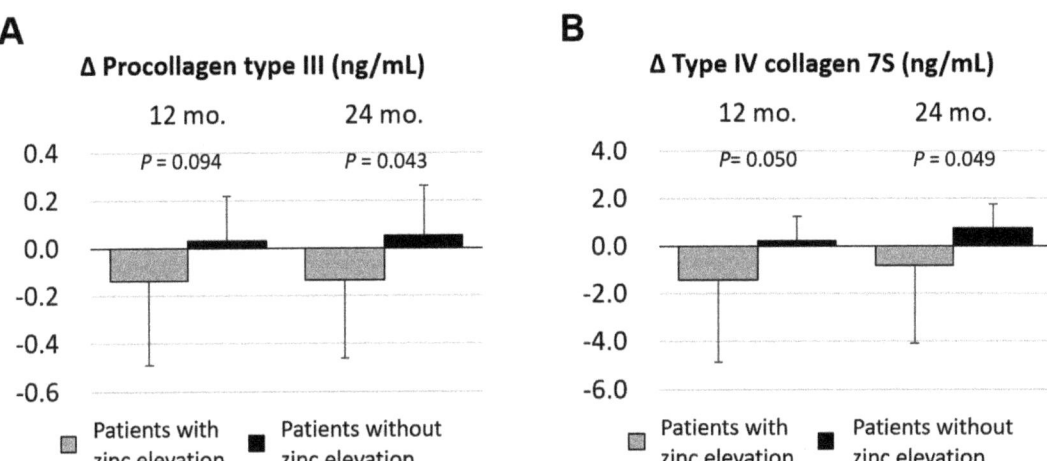

Figure 3. Longitudinal changes of serum fibrotic markers beyond zinc supplementation. (**A**) Changes of serum procollagen type III level after zinc administration of 12 and 24 months ($p = 0.094$ and $p = 0.043$). (**B**) Changes of serum collagen type IV-7S after zinc administration of 12 and 24 months ($p = 0.050$ and $p = 0.049$).

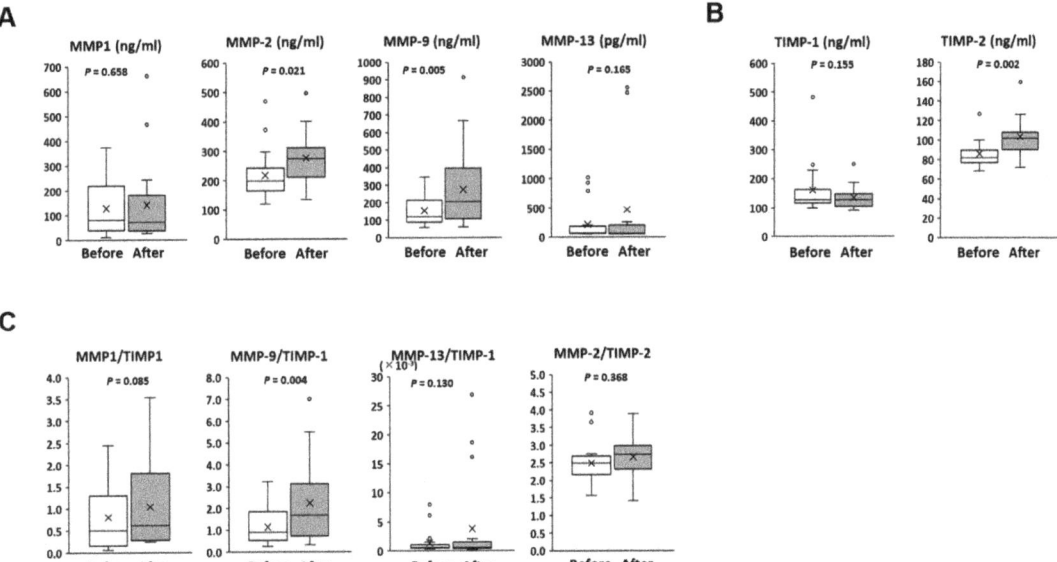

Figure 4. Longitudinal changes of serum matrix metalloproteinase (MMP) and its inhibitor (TIMP) in the patients with zinc elevation. (**A**) Longitudinal changes of serum collagenases level (MMP-1 and MMP-13) and gelatinase level (MMP-2 and MMP-9). (**B**) Longitudinal changes of serum inhibitor of MMP (TIMP-1 and TIMP-2). (**C**) Relative ratios of each MMP and its inhibitor.

4. Discussion

Therapeutic strategies for liver fibrosis include indirect approaches such as the use of nucleic acid analogs and direct-acting antiviral agents, which are first and foremost aimed at eliminating disease factors. In contrast, recent experiments using cell lineage tracing technology and reporter mice have shown that HSCs play a much larger role in collagen production than myeloid cells and myofibroblasts, regardless of the type of liver fibrosis [23–25]. Therefore, in recent years, direct antifibrotic drugs, such as molecularly targeted drugs, small-molecule compounds, antibody drugs, and nucleic acid drugs, have been developed, many of which exert their antifibrotic effects by acting on molecular mechanisms closely related to liver fibrosis, such as inhibition of HSC activation [26–28], inhibition of the response cascade after HSC activation [29,30], or induction of apoptosis of activated HSC [31–37]. These include research and development targeting intrinsic interferons [34,35], but zinc was recently reported to specifically inhibit proinflammatory cytokines and IFNλ3 signaling to improve fibrosis [38]. In their study, Read et al. found that elevated zinc levels in liver tissue induced metallothionein expression and suppressed IFNλ3 expression, resulting in the attenuation of gene expression of interferon-stimulated genes and inflammatory cytokines, thereby suppressing antiviral activity and its immune response and ultimately negatively regulating liver fibrosis.

Zinc is essential for the maintenance of life activities and is an essential trace element, although its content in the body is only 2–3 g [39]. The fact that 10% of proteins encoded in the human genome contain a zinc-binding motif means that a very large number of proteins bind to zinc [40], which suggests the importance of zinc's signaling function inside and outside the cell [41]. In fact, there have been several reports of improvement in liver function with the administration of zinc products, mainly in patients with chronic hepatitis C and cirrhosis [42–46]. Regarding the association between serum zinc concentrations and long-term prognosis in patients with chronic liver disease, in a multicenter, long-term observational study of cirrhotic patients (mean follow-up period, 3 years), Shigefuku et al. found that low serum zinc concentrations (<55 µg/dL) at enrollment were an independent risk factor for liver carcinogenesis [47].

Liver fibrosis is a common pathological process characterized by an accumulation of the extracellular matrix (ECM), which is a kind of tissue remodeling triggered by a consequence of an imbalance between the enhanced ECM synthesis and reduced degradation of connective tissue proteins reflecting the dysregulation of several pathways, including MMPs and tissue inhibitors of MMPs (TIMPs) [48]. MMPs are a large family of zinc-dependent enzymes that degrade the components of ECM [49], whereas TIMPs are specific endogenous inhibitors that bind to MMPs and block them from ECM components. The most potent MMPs are collagenases such as MMP-1, MMP-8, and MMP-13 [50], and the activity of MMPs is highly regulated by the level of gene expression, activation of latent pro-MMPs to active enzymes [51], and TIMPs that form stable, noncovalent complexes with active MMPs [52].

Furthermore, MMPs are known as representative zinc-containing enzymes, and there are strong expectations regarding the effect of zinc preparations on fibrinolysis. The inhibition of hepatic fibrosis by zinc administration would be based on its effects of MMPs involved in collagen synthesis and degradation and its ability to control the function of procollagen and collagen-producing hepatic stellate cells by inhibiting oxidative stress, inflammation, and apoptosis in the liver. Apart from research reagents, the available zinc-containing preparations are currently limited to zinc acetate and polaprezinc. Although there have been some reports on the sedative or prognostic effects of continuous administration of these products [42–46], studies on their effects on the inhibition of hepatic fibrosis have been limited to basic studies, mainly in rodents [53–55], and there have been few reports on the changes in the expression of MMPs or TIMPs in particular. In this regard, in a small but prospective pilot study in a small number of patients with highly advanced chronic liver disease, Takahashi et al. [56] found no significant change in MMPs but a significant decrease in TIMP-1 after polaprezinc administration, suggesting that the decrease in TIMP-1 might be important in the improvement of fibrosis. In contrast, our results indicated a significant increase in MMP-2 and MMP-9 after polaprezinc treatment. In addition, TIMP-2 showed a significant increase after zinc administration, whereas TIMP-1 did not change with significance. Subsequently, MMP-9/TIMP-1 was also significantly increased, whereas MMP-2/TIMP-2 was not affected. Based on these results, not only the increase in MMPs but also the increase in MMP-9/TIMP-1 can be responsible for the improvement of fibrosis. The reason for the significant increase in MMP-2 and MMP-9 after zinc administration in our study is that the disease activity of AIH has already been in clinical remission by corticosteroids and or ursodeoxycholic acid, and the transaminases of the subject patients remained within the normal range during the entire observation period. In this aspect, during the maintenance of remission, MMPs were relatively lower (closer to those of healthy individuals) than during the active phase of the disease, which may facilitate confirmation of the increase in MMPs after zinc administration, which may be a major difference between our study and the other previous studies, which were conducted in patients with viral active hepatitis or liver cirrhosis and in animal models with drug-induced liver injury.

In a family of MMPs, Latronico et al. [57] reported that serum production levels of MMP-2 and MMP-9 were definitely higher than the other MMPs such as MMP-1, MMP-3, MMP-8, and MMP-10, and their levels significantly increased in patients with hepatitis compared with healthy subjects. In that study, serum TIMP-1 levels were correlated with liver stiffness, which reflected the degree of fibrosis, and the result was compatible with the other previous report [58]. Giannelli G et al. [59] reported that the ratio of serum MMP-2/TIMP-2 was definitely lower in cirrhotic patients than healthy subjects, whereas serum MMP-2 levels in cirrhotic patients were similar to those of healthy subjects. In contrast, Watanabe et al. [60] reported that serum MMP-2 levels increased in parallel with the progression of chronic liver disease, and there was a positive correlation between the collagen type IV and MMP-2 levels. Subsequently, an imbalance between MMP-2 and the TIMP-2 might be also responsible for the degradation of ECM components (Figure 5A). In terms of the increase of TIMP-2 after zinc administration in our study, we believe that this is probably an equilibrium response (positive feedback) associated with an increased level of MMP-2, which has a binding affinity with TIMP-2. That is, even though both MMP-2 and TIMP-2 were increased after zinc administration, if MMP-2/TIMP-2 was not decreased, it would be acceptable that the vector in the direction of fibrosis was pointing to amelioration (Figure 5B).

Regarding the safety of zinc preparations, the permissible maximum dose of oral zinc intake for a short period was reported to be approximately 170 mg per day in healthy adult subjects, and this was almost equivalent to 10 times volume of the average intake. In this study, patients took 150 mg of polaprezinc (containing 34 mg of elemental zinc) every day. In contrast, there have been reports of copper deficiency with the long-term administration of polaprezinc and zinc acetate [61–63], as well as reports that caution should be exercised when using zinc acetate rather than polaprezinc [64]. In this study involving polaprezinc, there were no cases of serum copper below baseline levels and no adverse physical findings, such as anemia or neurological symptoms, were observed, including in preexcluded subjects because of their insufficiency of taking polaprezinc. According to the medical guidelines on zinc deficiency [65], many cases of serum copper levels of <10 µg/dL and serum zinc levels of 190–250 µg/dL at the onset of copper deficiency were common; hence, copper deficiency should be noted when serum copper levels are 20–30 µg/dL and serum zinc levels are >200 µg/dL. In addition, although rare, zinc administration can cause inhibition of iron absorption in the intestinal tract, leading to iron deficiency, and therefore, iron deficiency should be noted in the same way as copper [66].

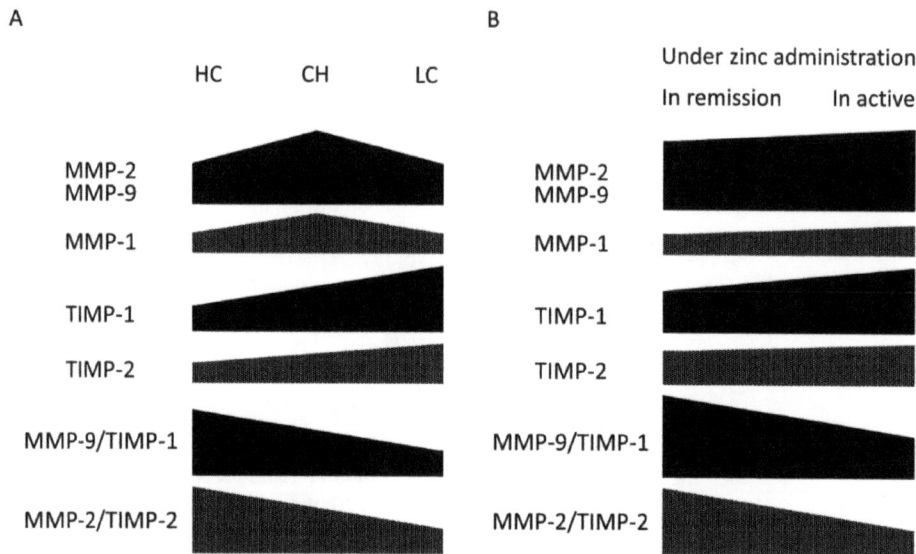

Figure 5. Scheme of the serum levels of matrix metalloproteinase (MMP) and its inhibitor (TIMP) in the course of liver disease progression and mechanistical working-hypothesis of the changes in MMP and TIMP levels under zinc administration. (**A**) Serum levels of MMPs and TIMPs in healthy carriers (HC), patients with chronic hepatitis (CH), and patients with liver cirrhosis (LC). (**B**) Serum levels of MMPs and TIMPs in patients with chronic liver disease in remission and in active phase.

This study has some limitations: (1) a relatively small number of patients were enrolled in this single-center study, (2) tissue sampling by liver biopsy after zinc administration is not sufficiently available and is poorly supported by histopathology, (3) there are relatively few cases of advanced fibrosis, and (4) the study was limited to Japanese patients with AIH, who are generally considered to have a good prednisolone response. Certainly, notwithstanding these limitations, it is significant that our results demonstrate that long-term continuous treatment with zinc preparations for >2 years improves fibrotic markers through increases in MMPs and MMP/TIMPs and that it is safe. Azathioprine, which, along with prednisolone, is the first-line drug for AIH, has a chelating effect that binds metals, and is excreted in the urine after binding to zinc in the body. Considering the metabolism of azathioprine, the possibility of zinc deficiency owing to increased urinary zinc excretion in long-term treatment cannot be ruled out. In this context, it may be worthwhile to use zinc in combination with AIH treatment.

In conclusion, long-term zinc administration for AIH could be a safe and effective antifibrotic treatment. In addition, a zinc acetate preparation with a higher zinc content than polaprezinc has recently been approved for insurance use in Japan, and it is expected to be combined with direct antifibrotic drugs such as molecularly targeted drugs, small-molecule compounds, antibody drugs, and nucleic acid drugs that are currently being developed.

Supplementary Materials: The following are available online at https://www.mdpi.com/article/10.3390/jcm10112465/s1. Supplementary Table S1: Clinical profiles of the drop out patients, Supplementary Table S2: Clinical parameters of the patients without zinc elevation before and after zinc supplementation

Author Contributions: Concept and design: K.M. and H.Y.; Clinical data collection: N.N., H.T., Y.S., H.K., K.K., N.S., S.S., M.F., A.D., A.M., and J.Y.; Writing of article: K.M.; Data analysis: K.M. and T.N.; Supervision: T.A., H.Y. All authors have read and agreed to the published version of the manuscript.

Funding: This research received no external funding.

Institutional Review Board Statement: The study was conducted according to the guidelines of the Declaration of Helsinki, and approved by the Ethics Committee of the Nara Medical University Hospital (protocol code #15-003).

Informed Consent Statement: Informed consent was obtained from all subjects involved in the study.

Data Availability Statement: The datasets used and/or analyzed during the current study are available from the corresponding author on reasonable request.

Acknowledgments: We thank Hiroshi Fukui for his kind and appropriate advice for completing this article.

Conflicts of Interest: The authors declare no conflict of interest.

Abbreviations

AIH	autoimmune hepatitis
ALT	alanine aminotransferase
MMP	matrix metalloproteinase
PBC	primary biliary cirrhosis
TIMP	tissue inhibitor of matrix metalloproteinase
TGF-β	transforming growth factor-β

References

1. Tanaka, A.; Mori, M.; Matsumoto, K.; Ohira, H.; Tazuma, S.; Takikawa, H. Increase Trend in the Prevalence and male-to-female Ratio of Primary Biliary Cholangitis, Autoimmune Hepatitis, and Primary Sclerosing Cholangitis in Japan. *Hepatol. Res.* **2019**, *49*, 881–889. [CrossRef] [PubMed]
2. Tanaka, A. Emerging Novel Treatments for Autoimmune Liver Diseases. *Hepatol. Res.* **2019**, *49*, 489–499. [CrossRef]
3. European Association for the Study of the Liver. EASL Clinical Practice Guidelines: Autoimmune hepatitis. *J. Hepatol.* **2015**, *63*, 971–1004. [CrossRef] [PubMed]
4. Manns, M.P.; Czaja, A.J.; Gorham, J.D.; Krawitt, E.L.; Mieli-Vergani, G.; Vergani, D.; Vierling, J.M. Diagnosis and management of autoimmune hepatitis. *Hepatology* **2010**, *51*, 2193–2213. [CrossRef] [PubMed]
5. Yoshizawa, K.; Matsumoto, A.; Ichijo, T.; Umemura, T.; Joshita, S.; Komatsu, M.; Tanaka, N.; Tanaka, E.; Ota, M.; Katsuyama, Y.; et al. Long-term outcome of Japanese patients with type 1 Autoimmune hepatitis. *Hepatology* **2012**, *56*, 668–676. [CrossRef] [PubMed]
6. Chew, L.-C.; Maceda-Galang, L.M.; Tan, Y.K.; Chakraborty, B.; Thumboo, J. Pneumocystis Jirovecii Pneumonia in Patients With Autoimmune Disease on High-Dose Glucocorticoid. *J. Clin. Rheumatol.* **2015**, *21*, 72–75. [CrossRef]
7. Brenner, E.J.; Ungaro, R.C.; Gearry, R.B.; Kaplan, G.G.; Kissous-Hunt, M.; Lewis, J.D.; Ng, S.C.; Rahier, J.-F.; Reinisch, W.; Ruemmele, F.M.; et al. Corticosteroids, but not TNF antagonists, are associated with adverse COVID-19 outcomes in patients with inflammatory bowel diseases: Results from an international registry. *Gastroenterology* **2020**, *159*, 481–491. [CrossRef]
8. Consani Fernández, S.A.; Díaz Cuña, C.L.; Fernández Rey, L.; Rostán Sellanes, S.; Maciel Oleggini, G.; Facal Castro, J.A. Infections in systemic autoimmune diseases. *Reumatol. Clin.* **2020**, in press.
9. Dhaliwal, H.K.; Hoeroldt, B.; Dube, A.K.; McFarlane, E.; Underwood, J.C.; Karajeh, M.A.; Gleeson, D. Long-Term Prognostic Significance of Persisting Histological Activity Despite Biochemical Remission in Autoimmune Hepatitis. *Am. J. Gastroenterol.* **2015**, *110*, 993–999. [CrossRef]
10. Angulo, P.; Kleiner, D.E.; Dam-Larsen, S.; Adams, L.A.; Björnsson, E.S.; Charatcharoenwitthaya, P.; Mills, P.R.; Keach, J.C.; Lafferty, H.D.; Stahler, A.; et al. Liver fibrosis, but no other histologic features, is associated with long-term outcomes of patients With nonalcoholic fatty liver disease. *Gastroenterology* **2015**, *149*, 389–397. [CrossRef]
11. Niederau, C.; Lange, S.; Heintges, T.; Erhardt, A.; Buschkamp, M.; Hürter, D.; Nawrocki, M.; Kruska, L.; Hensel, F.; Petry, W.; et al. Prognosis of chronic hepatitis C: Results of a large, prospective cohort study. *Hepatology* **1998**, *28*, 1687–1695. [CrossRef] [PubMed]
12. Werner, M.; Wallerstedt, S.; Lindgren, S.; Almer, S.; Björnsson, E.; Bergquist, A.; Prytz, H.; Sandberg-Gertzén, H.; Hultcrantz, R.; Sangfelt, P.; et al. Characteristics and long-term outcome of patients with autoimmune hepatitis related to the initial treatment response. *Scand. J. Gastroenterol.* **2010**, *45*, 457–467. [CrossRef] [PubMed]
13. Hoeroldt, B.; McFarlane, E.; Dube, A.; Basumani, P.; Karajeh, M.; Campbell, M.J.; Gleeson, D. Long-term outcomes of patients with autoimmune hepatitis managed at a nontransplant center. *Gastroenterology* **2011**, *140*, 1980–1989. [CrossRef] [PubMed]
14. Danielsson Borssén, Å.; Marschall, H.U.; Bergquist, A.; Rorsman, F.; Weiland, O.; Kechagias, S.; Nyhlin, N.; Verbaan, H.; Nilsson, E.; Werner, M. Epidemiology and causes of death in a Swedish cohort of patients with autoimmune hepatitis. *Scand. J. Gastroenterol.* **2017**, *52*, 1022–1028. [CrossRef]

15. Powell, S.R. The antioxidant properties of zinc. *J. Nutr.* **2000**, *130* (Suppl. S5), 1447S–1454S. [CrossRef]
16. Stamoulis, I.; Kouraklis, G.; Theocharis, S. Zinc and the liver: An active interaction. *Dig. Dis. Sci.* **2007**, *52*, 1595–1612. [CrossRef] [PubMed]
17. Rojkind, M.; Giambrone, M.-A.; Biempica, L. Collagen Types in Normal and Cirrhotic Liver. *Gastroenterology* **1979**, *76*, 710–719. [CrossRef]
18. Anttinen, H.; Ryhänen, L.; Puistola, U.; Arranto, A.; Oikarinen, A. Decrease in Liver Collagen Accumulation in Carbon Tetrachloride-Injured and Normal Growing Rats Upon Administration of Zinc. *Gastroenterology* **1984**, *86*, 532–539. [CrossRef]
19. Seltzer, J.L.; Jeffrey, J.J.; Eisen, A.Z. Evidence for Mammalian Collagenases As Zinc Ion Metalloenzymes. *Biochim. Biophys. Acta Enzym.* **1977**, *485*, 179–187. [CrossRef]
20. Yuasa, J.; Mitsui, A.; Kawai, T. Emission from a tetrazine derivative complexed with zinc ion in aqueous solution: A unique water-soluble fluorophore. *Chem. Commun.* **2011**, *47*, 5807–5809. [CrossRef]
21. Kojima-Yuasa, A.; Ohkita, T.; Yukami, K.; Ichikawa, H.; Takami, N.; Nakatani, T.; Kennedy, D.O.; Nishiguchi, S.; Matsui-Yuasa, I. Involvement of Intracellular Glutathione in Zinc Deficiency-Induced Activation of Hepatic Stellate Cells. *Chem. Interactions* **2003**, *146*, 89–99. [CrossRef]
22. D'Amico, G.; Garcia-Tsao, G.; Pagliaro, L. Natural History and Prognostic Indicators of Survival in Cirrhosis: A Systematic Review of 118 Studies. *J. Hepatol.* **2006**, *44*, 217–231. [CrossRef]
23. Kisseleva, T.; Uchinami, H.; Feirt, N.; Quintana-Bustamante, O.; Segovia, J.C.; Schwabe, R.F.; Brenner, D. Bone Marrow-Derived Fibrocytes Participate in Pathogenesis of Liver Fibrosis. *J. Hepatol.* **2006**, *45*, 429–438. [CrossRef] [PubMed]
24. Higashiyama, R.; Moro, T.; Nakao, S.; Mikami, K.; Fukumitsu, H.; Ueda, Y.; Ikeda, K.; Adachi, E.; Bou–Gharios, G.; Okazaki, I.; et al. Negligible Contribution of Bone Marrow-Derived Cells to Collagen Production During Hepatic Fibrogenesis in Mice. *Gastroenterology* **2009**, *137*, 1459–1466. [CrossRef]
25. Mederacke, I.; Hsu, C.C.; Troeger, J.S.; Huebener, P.; Mu, X.; Dapito, D.H.; Pradere, J.-P.; Schwabe, R.F. Fate Tracing Reveals Hepatic Stellate Cells As Dominant Contributors to Liver Fibrosis Independent of Its Aetiology. *Nat. Commun.* **2013**, *4*, 2823. [CrossRef]
26. Jia, H.; Aw, W.; Saito, K.; Hanate, M.; Hasebe, Y.; Kato, H. Eggshell Membrane Ameliorates Hepatic Fibrogenesis in Human C3A Cells and Rats through Changes in PPARγ-Endothelin 1 Signaling. *Sci. Rep.* **2014**, *4*, 7473. [CrossRef]
27. Kim, S.-Y.; Cho, B.H.; Kim, U.-H. CD38-mediated Ca2+ signaling contributes to angiotensin II-induced activation of hepatic stellate cells: Attenuation of hepatic fibrosis by CD38 ablation. *J. Biol. Chem.* **2010**, *285*, 576–582. [CrossRef]
28. Lu, D.-H.; Guo, X.-Y.; Qin, S.-Y.; Luo, W.; Huang, X.-L.; Chen, M.; Wang, J.-X.; Ma, S.-J.; Yang, X.-W.; Jiang, H.-X. Interleukin-22 Ameliorates Liver Fibrogenesis by Attenuating Hepatic Stellate Cell Activation and Downregulating the Levels of Inflammatory Cytokines. *World J. Gastroenterol.* **2015**, *21*, 1531–1545. [CrossRef]
29. Pines, M. Halofuginone for fibrosis, regeneration and cancer in the gastrointestinal tract. *World J. Gastroenterol.* **2014**, *20*, 14778–14786. [CrossRef] [PubMed]
30. Adorini, L.; Pruzanski, M.; Shapiro, D. Farnesoid X Receptor Targeting to Treat Nonalcoholic Steatohepatitis. *Drug Discov. Today* **2012**, *17*, 988–997. [CrossRef] [PubMed]
31. Chávez, E.; Castro-Sánchez, L.; Shibayama, M.; Tsutsumi, V.; Moreno, M.G.; Muriel, P. Sulfasalazine prevents the increase in TGF-β, COX-2, nuclear NFkappaB translocation and fibrosis in CCl4-induced liver cirrhosis in the rat. *Hum. Exp. Toxicol.* **2012**, *31*, 913–920. [CrossRef] [PubMed]
32. Crespo, I.; San-Miguel, B.; Fernández, A.; de Urbina, J.O.; González-Gallego, J.; Tuñón, M.J. Melatonin Limits the Expression of Profibrogenic Genes and Ameliorates the Progression of Hepatic Fibrosis in Mice. *Transl. Res.* **2015**, *165*, 346–357. [CrossRef]
33. Wei, Y.; Kang, X.-L.; Wang, X. The Peripheral Cannabinoid Receptor 1 Antagonist VD60 Efficiently Inhibits Carbon Tetrachloride-Intoxicated Hepatic Fibrosis Progression. *Exp. Biol. Med.* **2014**, *239*, 183–192. [CrossRef] [PubMed]
34. Muhanna, N.; Abu Tair, L.; Doron, S.; Amer, J.; Azzeh, M.; Mahamid, M.; Friedman, S.; Safadi, R. Amelioration of Hepatic Fibrosis by NK Cell Activation. *Gut* **2010**, *60*, 90–98. [CrossRef]
35. Glässner, A.; Eisenhardt, M.; Kokordelis, P.; Kramer, B.; Wolter, F.; Nischalke, H.D.; Boesecke, C.; Sauerbruch, T.; Rockstroh, J.K.; Spengler, U.; et al. Impaired CD4+ T Cell Stimulation of NK Cell Anti-Fibrotic Activity May Contribute to Accelerated Liver Fibrosis Progression in HIV/HCV Patients. *J. Hepatol.* **2013**, *59*, 427–433. [CrossRef] [PubMed]
36. Ido, A.; Moriuchi, A.; Numata, M.; Murayama, T.; Teramukai, S.; Marusawa, H.; Yamaji, N.; Setoyama, H.; Kim, I.-D.; Chiba, T.; et al. Safety and Pharmacokinetics of Recombinant Human Hepatocyte Growth Factor (rh-HGF) in Patients With Fulminant Hepatitis: A Phase I/II Clinical Trial, Following Preclinical Studies to Ensure Safety. *J. Transl. Med.* **2011**, *9*, 55. [CrossRef]
37. Bohanon, F.J.; Wang, X.; Graham, B.M.; Ding, C.; Ding, Y.; Radhakrishnan, G.L.; Rastellini, C.; Zhou, J.; Radhakrishnan, R.S. Enhanced Effects of Novel Oridonin Analog CYD0682 for Hepatic Fibrosis. *J. Surg. Res.* **2015**, *199*, 441–449. [CrossRef] [PubMed]
38. Read, S.A.; O'Connor, K.S.; Suppiah, V.; Ahlenstiel, C.; Obeid, S.; Cook, K.; Cunningham, A.; Douglas, M.W.; Hogg, P.J.; Booth, D.; et al. Zinc Is a Potent and Specific Inhibitor of IFN-λ3 Signalling. *Nat. Commun.* **2017**, *8*, 15245. [CrossRef]
39. Hara, T.; Takeda, T.-A.; Takagishi, T.; Fukue, K.; Kambe, T.; Fukada, T. Physiological Roles of Zinc Transporters: Molecular and Genetic Importance in Zinc Homeostasis. *J. Physiol. Sci.* **2017**, *67*, 283–301. [CrossRef]
40. Andreini, C.; Banci, L.; Bertini, I.; Rosato, A. Counting the zinc-proteins encoded in the human genome. *J. Proteome Res.* **2006**, *5*, 196–201. [CrossRef]

41. Fukada, T.; Yamasaki, S.; Nishida, K.; Murakami, M.; Hirano, T. Zinc homeostasis and signaling in health and diseases: Zinc signaling. *J. Biol. Inorg. Chem.* **2011**, *16*, 1123–1134. [CrossRef] [PubMed]
42. Hosui, A.; Kimura, E.; Abe, S.; Tanimoto, T.; Onishi, K.; Kusumoto, Y.; Sueyoshi, Y.; Matsumoto, K.; Hirao, M.; Yamada, T.; et al. Long-Term Zinc Supplementation Improves Liver Function and Decreases the Risk of Developing Hepatocellular Carcinoma. *Nutrients* **2018**, *10*, 1955. [CrossRef] [PubMed]
43. Matsumura, H.; Nirei, K.; Nakamura, H.; Arakawa, Y.; Higuchi, T.; Hayashi, J.; Yamagami, H.; Matsuoka, S.; Ogawa, M.; Nakajima, N.; et al. Zinc Supplementation Therapy Improves the Outcome of Patients With Chronic Hepatitis C. *J. Clin. Biochem. Nutr.* **2012**, *51*, 178–184. [CrossRef] [PubMed]
44. Matsuoka, S.; Matsumura, H.; Nakamura, H.; Oshiro, S.; Arakawa, Y.; Hayashi, J.; Sekine, N.; Nirei, K.; Yamagami, H.; Ogawa, M.; et al. Zinc Supplementation Improves the Outcome of Chronic Hepatitis C and Liver Cirrhosis. *J. Clin. Biochem. Nutr.* **2009**, *45*, 292–303. [CrossRef]
45. Murakami, Y.; Koyabu, T.; Kawashima, A.; Kakibuchi, N.; Kawakami, T.; Takaguchi, K.; Kita, K.; Okita, M. Zinc Supplementation Prevents the Increase of Transaminase in Chronic Hepatitis C Patients During Combination Therapy With Pegylated Interferon Alpha-2b and Ribavirin. *J. Nutr. Sci. Vitaminol.* **2007**, *53*, 213–218. [CrossRef]
46. Himoto, T.; Hosomi, N.; Nakai, S.; Deguchi, A.; Kinekawa, F.; Matsuki, M.; Yachida, M.; Masaki, T.; Kurokochi, K.; Watanabe, S.; et al. Efficacy of Zinc Administration in Patients With Hepatitis C Virus-Related Chronic Liver Disease. *Scand. J. Gastroenterol.* **2007**, *42*, 1078–1087. [CrossRef]
47. Shigefuku, R.; Iwasa, M.; Katayama, K.; Eguchi, A.; Kawaguchi, T.; Shiraishi, K.; Ito, T.; Suzuki, K.; Koreeda, C.; Ohtake, T.; et al. Hypozincemia Is Associated With Human Hepatocarcinogenesis in Hepatitis C virus-related Liver Cirrhosis. *Hepatol. Res.* **2019**, *49*, 1127–1135. [CrossRef]
48. Iredale, J.P.; Thompson, A.; Henderson, N.C. Extracellular Matrix Degradation in Liver Fibrosis: Biochemistry and Regulation. *Biochim. Biophys. Acta Mol. Basis Dis.* **2013**, *1832*, 876–883. [CrossRef]
49. Visse, R.; Nagase, H. Matrix metalloproteinases and tissue inhibitors of metalloproteinases: Structure, function, and biochemistry. *Circ. Res.* **2003**, *92*, 827–839. [CrossRef]
50. Duarte, S.; Baber, J.; Fujii, T.; Coito, A.J. Matrix metalloproteinases in liver injury, repair and fibrosis. *Matrix Biol.* **2015**, *44–46*, 147–156. [CrossRef]
51. Vandooren, J.; van den Steen, P.E.; Opdenakker, G. Biochemistry and molecular biology of gelatinase B or matrix metalloproteinase-9 (MMP-9): The next decade. *Crit. Rev. Biochem. Mol. Biol.* **2013**, *48*, 222–272. [CrossRef] [PubMed]
52. Arpino, V.; Brock, M.; Gill, S.E. The Role of TIMPs in Regulation of Extracellular Matrix Proteolysis. *Matrix Biol.* **2015**, *44–46*, 247–254. [CrossRef] [PubMed]
53. Ye, J.; Zhang, Z.; Zhu, L.; Lu, M.; Li, Y.; Zhou, J.; Lu, X.; Du, Q. Polaprezinc Inhibits Liver Fibrosis and Proliferation in Hepatocellular Carcinoma. *Mol. Med. Rep.* **2017**, *16*, 5523–5528. [CrossRef] [PubMed]
54. Kono, T.; Asama, T.; Chisato, N.; Ebisawa, Y.; Okayama, T.; Imai, K.; Karasaki, H.; Furukawa, H.; Yoneda, M. Polaprezinc Prevents Ongoing Thioacetamide-Induced Liver Fibrosis in Rats. *Life Sci.* **2012**, *90*, 122–130. [CrossRef]
55. Sugino, H.; Kumagai, N.; Watanabe, S.; Toda, K.; Takeuchi, O.; Tsunematsu, S.; Morinaga, S.; Tsuchimoto, K. Polaprezinc Attenuates Liver Fibrosis in a Mouse Model of Non-Alcoholic Steatohepatitis. *J. Gastroenterol. Hepatol.* **2008**, *23*, 1909–1916. [CrossRef]
56. Takahashi, M.; Saito, H.; Higashimoto, M.; Hibi, T. Possible Inhibitory Effect of Oral Zinc Supplementation on Hepatic Fibrosis through Downregulation of TIMP-1: A Pilot Study. *Hepatol. Res.* **2007**, *37*, 405–409. [CrossRef]
57. Latronico, T.; Mascia, C.; Pati, I.; Zuccala, P.; Mengoni, F.; Marocco, R.; Tieghi, T.; Belvisi, V.; Lichtner, M.; Vullo, V.; et al. Liver Fibrosis in HCV Monoinfected and HIV/HCV Coinfected Patients: Dysregulation of Matrix Metalloproteinases (MMPs) and Their Tissue Inhibitors TIMPs and Effect of HCV Protease Inhibitors. *Int. J. Mol. Sci.* **2016**, *17*, 455. [CrossRef]
58. Kasahara, A.; Hayashi, N.; Mochizuki, K.; Oshita, M.; Katayama, K.; Kato, M.; Masuzawa, M.; Yoshihara, H.; Naito, M.; Miyamoto, T.; et al. Circulating Matrix Metalloproteinase-2 and Tissue Inhibitor of Metalloproteinase-1 As Serum Markers of Fibrosis in Patients With Chronic Hepatitis C: Relationship to Interferon Reponse. *J. Hepatol.* **1997**, *26*, 574–583. [CrossRef]
59. Giannelli, G.; Bergamini, C.; Marinosci, F.; Fransvea, E.; Quaranta, M.; Lupo, L.; Schiraldi, O.; Antonaci, S. Clinical Role of MMP-2/TIMP-2 Imbalance in Hepatocellular Carcinoma. *Int. J. Cancer* **2002**, *97*, 425–431. [CrossRef]
60. Watanabe, N.; Nishizaki, Y.; Kojima, S.-I.; Takashimizu, S.; Nagata, N.; Kagawa, T.; Shiraishi, K.; Mine, T.; Matsuzaki, S. Clinical Significance of Serum Matrix Metalloproteinases and Tissue Inhibitors of Metalloproteinases in Chronic Liver Disease. *Tokai J. Exp. Clin. Med.* **2006**, *31*, 96–101.
61. Kadoya, H.; Uchida, A.; Kashihara, N. A case of copper deficiency-induced pancytopenia with maintenance hemodialysis outpatient treated with polaprezinc. *Ther Apher. Dial.* **2016**, *20*, 422–423. [CrossRef]
62. Ozeki, I.; Nakajima, T.; Suii, H.; Tatsumi, R.; Yamaguchi, M.; Arakawa, T.; Kuwata, Y.; Toyota, J.; Karino, Y. Evaluation of Treatment With Zinc Acetate Hydrate in Patients With Liver Cirrhosis Complicated by Zinc Deficiency. *Hepatol. Res.* **2019**, *50*, 488–501. [CrossRef]

63. Katayama, K.; Hosui, A.; Sakai, Y.; Itou, M.; Matsuzaki, Y.; Takamori, Y.; Hosho, K.; Tsuru, T.; Takikawa, Y.; Michitaka, K.; et al. Effects of Zinc Acetate on Serum Zinc Concentrations in Chronic Liver Diseases: A Multicenter, Double-Blind, Randomized, Placebo-Controlled Trial and a Dose Adjustment Trial. *Biol. Trace Element Res.* **2019**, *195*, 71–81. [CrossRef] [PubMed]
64. Okamoto, T.; Hatakeyama, S.; Konishi, S.; Okita, K.; Tanaka, Y.; Imanishi, K.; Takashima, T.; Saitoh, F.; Suzuki, T.; Ohyama, C. Comparison of Zinc Acetate Hydrate and Polaprezinc for Zinc Deficiency in Patients on Maintenance Hemodialysis: A single-center, open-label, Prospective Randomized Study. *Ther. Apher. Dial.* **2020**, *24*, 568–577. [CrossRef]
65. Kodama, H.; Tanaka, M.; Naito, Y.; Katayama, K.; Moriyama, M. Japan's Practical Guidelines for Zinc Deficiency With a Particular Focus on Taste Disorders, Inflammatory Bowel Disease, and Liver Cirrhosis. *Int. J. Mol. Sci.* **2020**, *21*, 2941. [CrossRef] [PubMed]
66. Crofton, R.W.; Gvozdanovic, D.; Gvozdanovic, S.; Khin, C.C.; Brunt, P.W.; Mowat, N.A.; Aggett, P.J. Inorganic Zinc and the Intestinal Absorption of Ferrous Iron. *Am. J. Clin. Nutr.* **1989**, *50*, 141–144. [CrossRef] [PubMed]

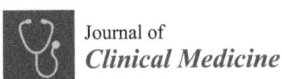

Article

Serum Amyloid Beta42 Is Not Eliminated by the Cirrhotic Liver: A Pilot Study

Reiner Wiest [1], Thomas S. Weiss [2], Lusine Danielyan [3] and Christa Buechler [4],*

[1] Department of Visceral Surgery and Medicine, University Inselspital, 3010 Bern, Switzerland; reiner.wiest@insel.ch
[2] Children's University Hospital (KUNO), Regensburg University Hospital, 93053 Regensburg, Germany; thomas.weiss@klinik.uni-regensburg.de
[3] Department of Clinical Pharmacology, Institute of Clinical and Experimental Pharmacology and Toxicology, University Hospital of Tuebingen, 72074 Tuebingen, Germany; lusine.danielyan@med.uni-tuebingen.de
[4] Department of Internal Medicine I, Regensburg University Hospital, 93053 Regensburg, Germany
* Correspondence: christa.buechler@klinik.uni-regensburg.de; Tel.: +49-94-1944-7009

Abstract: Amyloid-beta (Aβ) deposition in the brain is the main pathological hallmark of Alzheimer disease. Peripheral clearance of Aβ may possibly also lower brain levels. Recent evidence suggested that hepatic clearance of Aβ42 is impaired in liver cirrhosis. To further test this hypothesis, serum Aβ42 was measured by ELISA in portal venous serum (PVS), systemic venous serum (SVS), and hepatic venous serum (HVS) of 20 patients with liver cirrhosis. Mean Aβ42 level was 24.7 ± 20.4 pg/mL in PVS, 21.2 ± 16.7 pg/mL in HVS, and 19.2 ± 11.7 pg/mL in SVS. Similar levels in the three blood compartments suggested that the cirrhotic liver does not clear Aβ42. Aβ42 was neither associated with the model of end-stage liver disease score nor the Child–Pugh score. Patients with abnormal creatinine or bilirubin levels or prolonged prothrombin time did not display higher Aβ42 levels. Patients with massive ascites and patients with large varices had serum Aβ42 levels similar to patients without these complications. Serum Aβ42 was negatively associated with connective tissue growth factor levels ($r = -0.580$, $p = 0.007$) and a protective role of Aβ42 in fibrogenesis was already described. Diabetic patients with liver cirrhosis had higher Aβ42 levels ($p = 0.069$ for PVS, $p = 0.047$ for HVS and $p = 0.181$ for SVS), which is in accordance with previous reports. Present analysis showed that the cirrhotic liver does not eliminate Aβ42. Further studies are needed to explore the association of liver cirrhosis, Aβ42 levels, and cognitive dysfunction.

Keywords: portal vein; MELD score; bilirubin; ascites; hepatic clearance; liver cirrhosis

Citation: Wiest, R.; Weiss, T.S.; Danielyan, L.; Buechler, C. Serum Amyloid Beta42 Is Not Eliminated by the Cirrhotic Liver: A Pilot Study. *J. Clin. Med.* **2021**, *10*, 2669. https://doi.org/10.3390/jcm10122669

Academic Editors: Davide Giuseppe Ribaldone and Gian Paolo Caviglia

Received: 14 May 2021
Accepted: 16 June 2021
Published: 17 June 2021

Publisher's Note: MDPI stays neutral with regard to jurisdictional claims in published maps and institutional affiliations.

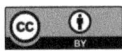

Copyright: © 2021 by the authors. Licensee MDPI, Basel, Switzerland. This article is an open access article distributed under the terms and conditions of the Creative Commons Attribution (CC BY) license (https://creativecommons.org/licenses/by/4.0/).

1. Introduction

Amyloid-beta (Aβ) peptides of variable length are produced by proteolysis of amyloid precursor protein (APP). The two most common isoforms of Aβ are 40 and 42 amino acid peptides [1]. Cerebral accumulation of these Aβ peptides is a characteristic feature of Alzheimer disease [2]. Cell surface Low Density Lipoprotein Receptor-related Protein 1 (LRP1) and soluble LRP1 enhance the clearance of brain and circulating Aβ. In brain, LRP1 is involved in the transport of Aβ across the blood–brain barrier. LRP1 also mediates APP internalization and processing, and thereby contributes to Aβ generation [3]. LRP1 downregulation in brain microvessels of Alzheimer patients correlated with Aβ deposition in the brain [4]. To clarify the in vivo effect of LRP1 on Aβ production/clearance, mice expressing a mutant LRP1 protein, with impaired endocytosis and transcytosis activity, were crossed with a mouse model for Alzheimer disease (which were transgenic mice expressing mutant human APP with both the Swedish (K670N/M671L) and London (V717I) mutations) [3]. Mutant LRP1 finally led to reduced Aβ levels in cerebrospinal fluid and brain interstitial fluid and lower plaque burden [3]. This study provided evidence for a more prominent role of LRP1 in Aβ synthesis than degradation [3].

Recent evidence showed that the kidney, the skin, the gastrointestinal tract, and the liver contribute to peripheral Aβ clearance [5]. Aβ was detected in urine of humans, mice, and rabbits [6]. In a mouse model for Alzheimer disease (APP/Presenilin 1 mice expressing human mutant presenilin 1 and a chimeric mouse/human amyloid precursor protein (Mo/HuAPP695swe)) unilateral nephrectomy increased plasma and brain Aβ deposition and reduced Aβ in urine [6]. Whereas the molecules involved in renal clearance of Aβ have not been defined yet, hepatocytes express LRP1, which mediates Aβ uptake. Rat hepatocytes were shown to degrade these peptides or to excrete Aβ into the bile [7]. Detection of Aβ deposits in the human skin and intestine suggested that these tissues also contribute to peripheral clearance [8]. The exact pathways involved are still unknown [7]. Peripheral monocytes and tissue-resident macrophages eliminate Aβ peptides. Thus, tissue-resident macrophages may contribute to Aβ elimination not only in the skin and small intestine but also in tissues such as the liver [7]. Uptake and degradation of Aβ peptides by peripheral blood monocytes was, indeed, impaired in Alzheimer disease patients and this may also apply for tissue-resident phagocytes [9].

A separate study showed that Aβ levels in axillary lymph nodes of Alzheimer transgenic mice were as high as its brain concentrations and assumed that brain-derived Aβ40 and Aβ42 are cleared by lymphoid tissues. The mice used in this study expressed a human isoform of APP with the Swedish mutation, which causes high levels of Aβ and early onset of Alzheimer disease. Interestingly, Aβ40 and Aβ42 levels in the liver and kidney of these mice were hardly detectable [10].

Hepatic catabolism of Aβ42 was demonstrated in mice, and about 60% of the radio-labeled Aβ peptides accumulated in the liver [11]. Aβ42 protein levels were reduced in human and rodent cirrhotic liver tissues, and plasma Aβ42 levels were high in patients with liver cirrhosis. This may argue for a role of the liver in peptide clearing but may also mean that hepatic release of Aβ peptides is increased in cirrhosis [12,13]. Plasma Aβ42 positively correlated with bilirubin and aspartate aminotransferase (AST) levels and was negatively correlated with albumin, indicating an association between liver function and systemic levels of Aβ42 [12].

Impaired hepatic removal of blood Aβ42 can explain high plasma Aβ42 levels in patients with liver cirrhosis [12]. This may also contribute to low Aβ levels in the cirrhotic liver [12,13]. In the healthy human liver V-PLEX® analysis detected 2.5–7.5 pg/mL Aβ42 levels, which declined about 10 fold in the cirrhotic liver [13]. Of note, hepatic Aβ protein was also low in Alzheimer disease. Aβ42 protein analyzed by ELISA in postmortem liver lysates of controls was 6.4–20.6 ng/g and was as low as 0–2.6 ng/g in the liver of patients with Alzheimer disease [14]. Studies on systemic Aβ42 levels in patients with Alzheimer disease have had mixed results [15]. Whether low hepatic levels are thus, indeed, linked to high systemic concentrations of Aβ42 has not been finally clarified [13,15].

It is important to note that Aβ42 exerts protective functions in the liver. Uptake of Aβ42 peptides by murine hepatic stellate cells suppressed the expression of fibrotic proteins such as transforming growth factor beta (TGFbeta) [13]. TGFbeta strongly contributes to tissue fibrosis and is an excellent inducer of connective tissue growth factor (CTGF) in hepatocytes. Serum CTGF is increased in patients with liver cirrhosis and is related to liver fibrosis [16–18].

Aβ further induced endothelial nitric oxide (NO) synthase in human SV40 immortalized hepatic sinusoidal endothelial cells [13]. NO is a vasodilatory molecule and its bioavailability is reduced in sinusoidal endothelial cells of the cirrhotic liver. This, indeed, contributes to increased intrahepatic vascular resistance and portal hypertension, which is one of the key factors responsible for the development of complications of liver cirrhosis such as varices and ascites [19–21]. Arginine and asymmetric dimethylarginine (ADMA) regulate endothelial function. ADMA is an endogenous inhibitor of NO synthase, whereas arginine can enhance production of NO [21,22]. Plasma levels of ADMA were higher in patients with decompensated than compensated liver cirrhosis, whereas arginine levels did not change [22,23].

There is some evidence that patients with chronic liver diseases have an increased risk for Alzheimer disease [24]. Non-alcoholic fatty liver disease (NAFLD) is a common disorder and may progress to liver cirrhosis and hepatocellular carcinoma [25]. NAFLD induced Alzheimer disease in wild-type mice and in mice carrying the Swedish APP protein and the Δe9 presenilin 1 mutation but lacking mouse APP protein [26]. Neuronal apoptosis, brain inflammation, and β-amyloid plaques were increased, whereas brain expression of LRP1 was reduced in both mouse groups when fed a high-fat diet to induce NAFLD [26]. Dyslipidemia and insulin resistance are characteristics of NAFLD, and abnormal lipid metabolism, as well as type 2 diabetes, increased the risk to develop Alzheimer disease [24]. A longitudinal cohort study identified higher brain Aβ levels in cognitively normal subjects who had abnormal triglyceride levels 20 years ago [27]. High low-density lipoprotein and low high-density lipoprotein levels were linked with higher cerebral Aβ in a cohort of patients with no or mild cognitive impairment [28]. Hypercholesterinemia, oxidative stress, and hyperinsulinemia impair Aβ clearance in type 2 diabetes patients, who have a higher risk of developing Alzheimer disease [7].

Analysis of protein levels in portal venous serum (PVS), hepatic venous serum (HVS), and systemic venous serum (SVS) gives some information about hepatic clearance and synthesis of different proteins and metabolites [29]. The liver can produce and eliminate metabolites and, thus, levels in peripheral blood might not represent the concentrations in portal or hepatic venous blood [29]. Different concentrations of metabolites in these blood compartments can also provide some information about their production in certain tissues. High synthesis of, e.g., cytokines in the gut or visceral adipose tissues may increase the concentration in the portal vein relative to the systemic blood [29,30]. In case that the production of the cytokine is induced in the liver, levels may be higher in the hepatic than the portal vein [29]. PVS and HVS are not available from healthy persons for ethical issues but can be collected from patients with liver cirrhosis during implantation of a transjugular intrahepatic portosystemic shunt. In these blood samples IL-6 levels were higher in PVS than HVS, demonstrating that IL-6 is cleared by the liver [31]. Impaired liver function was thus associated with higher levels of serum IL-6 [31]. IL-6 is an acute phase protein and regulates liver regeneration and metabolism. Permanently high IL-6 is, nevertheless, detrimental to liver health [32].

An increase of sCD163, which is almost exclusively produced by macrophages, from the portal to the hepatic vein showed that liver macrophages released this protein [33,34]. Plasma levels of sCD163 were positively related to the severity of liver disease in patients with liver cirrhosis and indicate activation of Kupffer cells in these patients [33,34].

Resistin in humans is also mainly released by macrophages, and serum levels were induced in liver cirrhosis. Resistin concentrations did, however, not differ between SVS, HVS, and PVS, suggesting that higher serum levels in liver cirrhosis are not a marker of Kupffer cell activation and may be related to the dysfunction of monocytes/macrophages in liver cirrhosis [35].

Chemerin is abundantly expressed in the liver and levels were higher in the hepatic than the portal vein [36–38]. Serum chemerin is a marker for hepatic dysfunction and was low in patients with liver cirrhosis [39,40].

Visfatin is an inflammatory and pro-fibrotic protein, and levels were higher in HVS and PVS when compared to SVS. Whether serum visfatin is changed in patients with liver cirrhosis or is related to liver disease severity has not been finally clarified [35].

Chronic inflammation contributes to the pathogenesis of Alzheimer disease and liver cirrhosis and, thereby, may link liver diseases with cognitive impairment [24,35]. C-reactive protein (CRP) is a routine laboratory marker for inflammation but was not increased in serum of patients with Alzheimer disease [41]. CRP is an acute phase protein synthesized by the liver. Patients with liver cirrhosis have higher systemic CRP. A relationship to the severity of the liver disease did not exist [42].

Here, HVS, PVS, and SVS of patients with liver cirrhosis were used to measure Aβ42. Only a little serum was available, and either Aβ40 or Aβ42 could be analyzed. Regarding that systemic Aβ42 is more strongly related to cognitive status [43], and that both peptides were comparably changed in plasma and liver of patients with liver cirrhosis [12,13], Aβ42 was determined.

It was hypothesized that serum Aβ42 is lower in HVS than PVS because of hepatic extraction. Clearance of Aβ42 by the liver may also contribute to lower serum levels. Moreover, it was postulated that Aβ42 levels increase in patients with more severe liver disease because of impaired removal by the injured liver.

2. Materials and Methods

2.1. Transjugular Intrahepatic Portosystemic Shunt (TIPS)

Twenty patients with clinically diagnosed liver cirrhosis were included in the study. Etiology of liver disease was alcoholic in 18 and hepatitis C infection in two patients. Patients were treated by TIPS implantation due to complications of liver cirrhosis. This procedure has been described earlier, and TIPS was inserted in the fasted state [44]. During this intervention, samples of the hepatic vein (HVS), of the portal vein (PVS), and of a peripheral vein (SVS) were obtained. Medication and alcohol consumption of the patients were not documented. Patients had not been drinking any alcohol at the time the blood samples were drawn.

Standard laboratory values (such as alanine aminotransferase (ALT), aspartate aminotransferase (AST), or albumin) were measured by the Institute for Clinical Chemistry and Laboratory Medicine at our hospital. The study complied with the Declaration of Helsinki. All patients gave written, informed consent and the study was approved by the ethical committee of the University Hospital of Regensburg.

G*Power3.1.6 analysis using the values of plasma Aβ42 in patients with cirrhosis (excluding patients with hepatitis B virus) and healthy controls published by Wang et al. [12] indicated that seven patients per group are enough to identify higher Aβ42 in patients with liver cirrhosis with an alpha error of 0.05 and a power of 0.80. More patients may be necessary to differentiate those with compensated and decompensated cirrhosis (because the difference in Aβ42 levels may be smaller in comparison to healthy controls) but there was no study having analyzed Aβ42 levels in serum of these patients so far and the number of patients needed could not be calculated.

2.2. ELISA

Human Amyloid β (aa1-42) Immunoassay was from R&D Systems (Wiesbaden, Nordenstadt, Germany). Serum was used undiluted. All of the blood samples were analyzed at one day in parallel. Therefore, inter-assay coefficient of variation (CV) could not be calculated. Intra-assay CV for samples with Aβ42 < 10 pg/mL was 12.4%, for samples with Aβ42 < 20 pg/mL was 12.3%, for samples with Aβ42 < 30 pg/mL was 8.1%, and for samples with Aβ42 < 100 pg/mL was 7.2%. The lowest value of the standard curve was 7.8 pg/mL, and almost all serum levels were greater. Median levels of Aβ42 were, indeed, about 20 pg/mL and were nearly three-fold higher than the lowest standard. Therefore, 50% of the analyzed sera had Aβ42 levels above the concentration of the second standard (15.6 pg/mL).

Interleukin (IL)-6, connective tissue growth factor (CTGF), chemerin, resistin, visfatin, arginine, and asymmetric dimethylarginine (ADMA) were already measured in patients with liver cirrhosis, and results were published [16,22,31,36,45].

Standards and samples were measured in duplicate, and the means were used for statistical analyses.

2.3. Statistics

Data are shown as box plots (median value, range of the values, the first and the third quartile—circles or stars outside the boxes indicate outliers). Shapiro–Wilk test showed that Aβ42 and chemerin were not normally distributed in the different blood compartments. Statistical differences were, therefore, calculated by non-parametric tests, namely the Mann–

Whitney U Test, the Kruskal–Wallis Test, the Wilcoxon Test, or Friedman test (IBM SPSS Statistics 26.0). IL-6 was normally distributed, and paired *t*-test was used for calculation. Spearman correlations were analyzed by the IBM SPSS Statistics software.

3. Results

3.1. Aβ42 in Different Blood Compartments of Patients with Liver Cirrhosis

Serum of 20 patients suffering from clinically diagnosed liver cirrhosis was available for this study. Patients' characteristics are given in Table 1.

Table 1. Patient demographics and laboratory parameters (median values and ranges are shown).

	Cirrhosis Patients
Number	20
Sex (female/male)	7/13
MELD score	9 (6–21)
Age (years)	52 (40–81)
Child-Pugh score A/B/C/	6/6/8
C-reactive protein (mg/L)	9.9 (1.0–53.5)
Albumin (g/L)	32.9 (1.6–42.7)
Bilirubin (mg/dL)	1.2 (0.5–4.6)
Quick prothrombin time (%)	71 (28–100)
Aspartate aminotransferase (U/L)	40 (11–82)
Alanine aminotransferase (U/L)	33 (2–68)
Creatinine (mg/dL)	1.1 (0.5–4.5)
Ascites: no or little/modest or massive	8/12
Varices: no or small/large	7/13
Diabetes no/yes	12/8

MELD: Model for end-stage liver disease.

Aβ42 levels were similar in SVS, HVS, and PVS (Friedman test; Figure 1A). A concern is that there were too few patients to identify any differences between the blood compartments. The number of patients was, indeed, too small to confirm higher levels of chemerin in HVS than PVS [36] (Friedman test; Figure 1B). In the current cohort, IL-6 was significantly higher in PVS than HVS, as was reported earlier. The recently described rise of IL-6 in SVS relative to HVS was also identified [31] (paired *t*-test; Figure 1C).

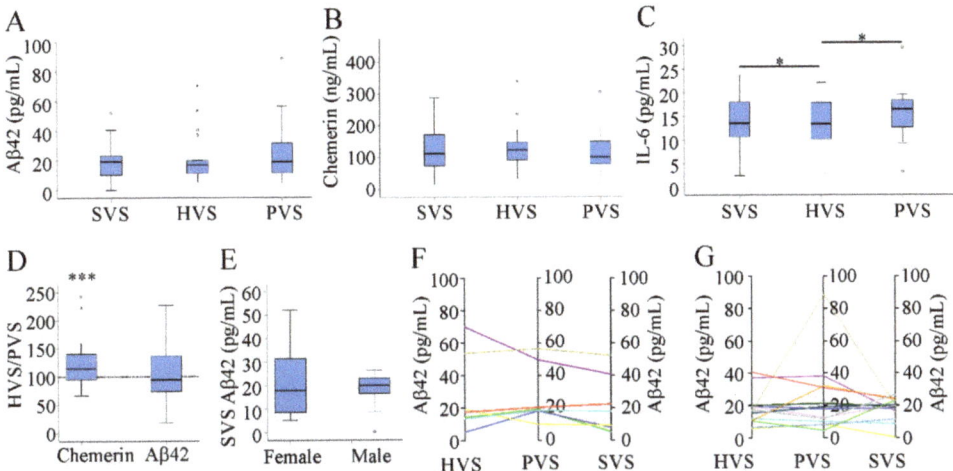

Figure 1. Aβ42, chemerin, and IL-6 in serum of patients with liver cirrhosis. (**A**) Aβ42, (**B**) chemerin, and (**C**) IL-6 in systemic venous (SVS), hepatic venous (HVS), and portal venous (PVS) serum of patients with liver cirrhosis. (**D**) HVS/PVS ratio of chemerin and Aβ42 in %. The dotted line is the 100% value. (**E**) SVS Aβ42 in females and males. (**F**) Aβ42 in HVS, PVS, and SVS of female and (**G**) male patients. * $p < 0.05$, *** $p < 0.001$.

Small effects can be more easily identified when looking at the respective ratios. The mean of the chemerin HVS/PVS ratio was 123%, whereas the Aβ42 HVS/PVS ratio was 103%. The chemerin HVS/PVS ratio was increased relative to the value of 100%, which indicated that the ratio did not change (Wilcoxon Test; Figure 1D).

Aβ42 levels in SVS, HVS, and PVS did not differ between male and female patients (Mann–Whitney U Test; Figure 1E–G). Aβ42 levels in HVS, PVS, and SVS of the individual patients showed that levels of most patients were similar in the three blood compartments (Figure 1F,G).

It has to be noted that systemic Aβ42 levels did not correlate with patients' ages ($r = 0.312$, $p = 0.181$). Median Aβ42 level in SVS of the two patients infected with hepatitis C virus was 16.1 pg/mL and was 19.7 pg/mL in the patients with alcoholic cirrhosis, suggesting that serum Aβ42 was not changed much by hepatitis C infection.

In general, there is a very good correlation between the metabolite concentrations in SVS, HVS, and PVS [29]. This was the case for chemerin and IL-6 levels in the current cohort (Table 2). Correlations for Aβ42 in SVS, PVS, and HVS were also significant. The correlation coefficients were, however, smaller (Spearman correlations; Table 2). A correlation coefficient of 0.838 for PVS and HVS chemerin corresponded to a coefficient of determination (R^2) of 0.702, suggesting that about 70% of HVS chemerin can be explained by its PVS levels. R^2 for PVS and HVS Aβ42 was 0.347, and about 65% of the variability in HVS must be related to other factors than the Aβ42 PVS levels [46].

Table 2. Spearman correlation coefficients and *p*-values (in brackets) for chemerin, IL-6, and Aβ42 levels in the blood compartments.

	HVS Aβ42	PVS Aβ42
SVS Aβ42	0.541 (0.014)	0.463 (0.040)
HVS Aβ42		0.589 (0.006)
	HVS Chemerin	PVS Chemerin
SVS Chemerin	0.811 (<0.001)	0.912 (<0.001)
HVS Chemerin		0.838 (<0.001)
	HVS IL-6	PVS IL-6
SVS IL-6	0.950 (<0.001)	0.689 (0.001)
HVS IL-6		0.726 (<0.001)

HVS: Hepatic venous serum; IL-6: Interleukin-6; PVS: Portal venous serum; SVS: Systemic venous serum.

3.2. Aβ42 in Relation to Scores and Measures of Liver Function

The calculation of the Child–Pugh score uses bilirubin, albumin, international normalized ratio (INR), ascites, and encephalopathy. The model for end-stage liver disease (MELD) score is calculated from bilirubin, INR, and creatinine [47]. Levels of Aβ42 were similar in patients with Child–Pugh scores A, B, and C (Kruskal–Wallis Test; Figure 2A). The median MELD score was 9, and Aβ42 did not differ between patients with a MELD score below or equal to 9 and patients with a MELD score above this median value (Mann–Whitney U Test; Figure 2B). Classification of patients according to normal and abnormal bilirubin levels, creatinine levels, or Quick prothrombin time did not reveal any differences in Aβ42 levels between the groups (Mann–Whitney U Test; Figure 2C–E). Accordingly, Aβ42 in serum did not correlate with serum albumin (Spearman correlation, Figure 2F).

3.3. Aβ42 in Patients with Disturbed Glucose Metabolism

Type 2 diabetes increases the risk for Alzheimer disease [24,48]. In our cohort, diabetic patients had higher Aβ42 serum levels in comparison to the non-diabetic patients. This effect was significant in HVS ($p = 0.047$) but not in PVS ($p = 0.069$) and SVS ($p = 0.181$) (Mann–Whitney U Test; Figure 3A). HVS/PVS Aβ42 ratio (Mann–Whitney U Test; $p = 0.910$) did not differ between diabetic and non-diabetic patients.

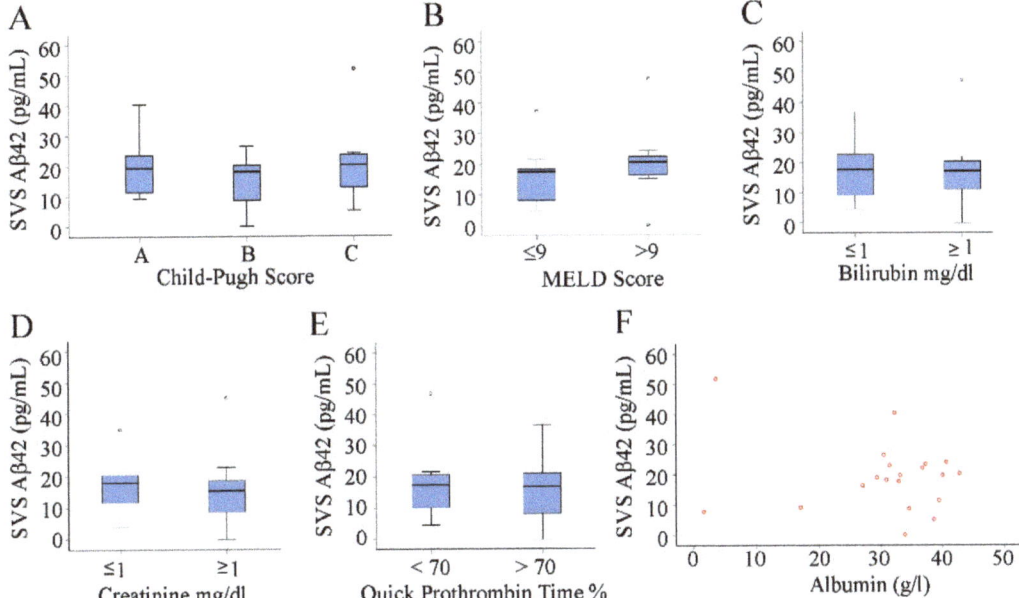

Figure 2. Aβ42 in relation to liver function. Aβ42 in serum of patients with liver cirrhosis stratified for (**A**) the Child–Pugh score (A = six patients, B = six patients, and C = eight patients) or (**B**) the median MELD score (nine patients had a MELD above 9 and 11 patients a MELD score ≤9). (**C**) Aβ42 serum levels in patients with a bilirubin value below (eight patients) or above (12 patients) the upper normal value (1 mg/dL). (**D**) Aβ42 serum levels in patients with creatinine levels below (eight patients) or above (12 patients) the upper normal value (1 mg/dL). (**E**) Aβ42 serum levels in patients with a normal (<70%, 10 patients) or a prolonged (>70%, 10 patients) Quick prothrombin time. (**F**) Spearman analysis showed that Aβ42 serum levels did not correlate with albumin in the 20 patients.

3.4. Association of Aβ42 Levels with Markers of Inflammation, Endothelial Function, and Fibrosis

Systemic inflammation contributes to Alzheimer disease [49,50]. However, serum Aβ42 was not correlated with CRP (Table 3). Resistin, chemerin, IL-6, and visfatin were all described to be associated with inflammation [35,51–53], but serum Aβ42 did not correlate with any of these molecules (Spearman correlation; Table 3).

There was evidence that Aβ42 induced endothelial NO synthase production in the liver [13]. Serum arginine and ADMA are markers of endothelial function and were already measured in the serum of those patients [22,23,54]. Serum Aβ42 did not correlate with arginine and/or ADMA levels (Spearman correlation; Table 3).

Recent studies showed anti-fibrotic effects of Aβ42 [13]. CTGF was identified as a serum marker of ongoing fibrosis [17] and negatively correlated with SVS Aβ42 (Spearman correlation; Table 3, Figure 3B). HVS ($r = -0.253$, $p = 0.283$) or PVS ($r = 0.038$, $p = 0.875$) levels of these proteins were not correlated. Of note, HVS/PVS Aβ42 ratio negatively correlated with CTGF in PVS ($r = -0.541$, $p = 0.014$), HVS ($r = -0.451$, $p = 0.046$), and SVS ($r = -0.489$, $p = 0.029$).

3.5. Aβ42 in Patients with Ascites and Varices

Increased splanchnic and reduced hepatic NO production in liver cirrhosis contribute to portal hypertension [21]. Aβ42 did not correlate with the hepatic venous pressure gradient (Spearman correlation; $r = 0.217$, $p = 0.358$ for SVS; $r = -0.77$, $p = 0.747$ for HVS; $r = -0.311$, $p = 0.182$ for PVS). Esophageal varices and ascites are common complications of portal hypertension [55]. Systemic Aβ42 was similar in patients with modest/massive ascites in comparison to patients with no/little ascites (Mann–Whitney U Test; Figure 3C).

Serum Aβ42 did also not change in patients with large varices in relation to patients with no/small varices (Mann–Whitney U Test; Figure 3D).

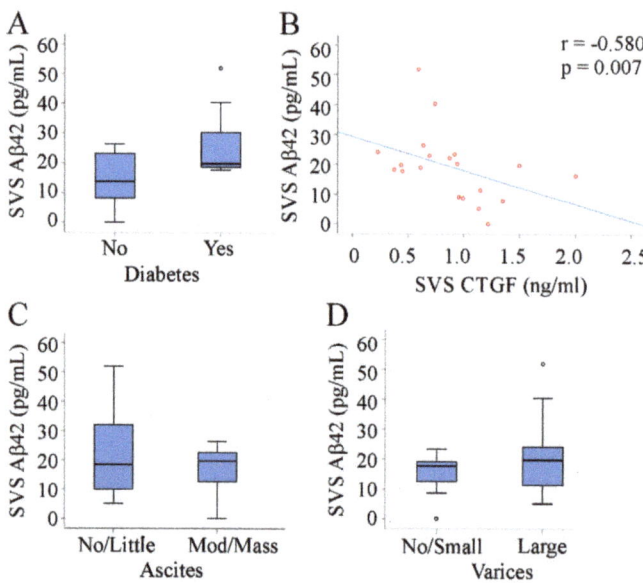

Figure 3. Association of Aβ42 serum levels with diabetes, ascites, and varices. (**A**) SVS Aβ42 serum levels in 8 patients with and 12 patients without diabetes. (**B**) Correlation of SVS Aβ42 with serum CTGF. (**C**) SVS Aβ42 serum levels in eight patients with no/little and 12 patients with moderate/massive ascites. (**D**) SVS Aβ42 serum levels in seven patients with no/small and 13 patients with large varices.

Table 3. Spearman correlation coefficients (r) and *p*-values (*p*) for the association of systemic Aβ42 with inflammatory markers, proteins with a role in nitric oxide production, and connective tissue growth factor (CTGF).

	CRP	Resistin	Chemerin	IL-6	Visfatin	Arginine	ADMA	CTGF
r	0.390	−0.011	−0.290	0.262	0.040	−0.251	−0.036	−0.580
p	0.089	0.965	0.214	0.531	0.867	0.286	0.880	0.007

ADMA: Asymmetric dimethylarginine; CTGF: Connective tissue growth factor; CRP: C-reactive protein; IL-6: Interleukin 6.

4. Discussion

This study showed that serum Aβ42 levels were similar in portal, hepatic, and systemic serum and were not related to measures of liver function in patients with liver cirrhosis.

Impaired elimination of Aβ has been proposed to contribute to elevated serum and brain levels, and thereby progresses in Alzheimer disease [24,56]. Recent studies suggested a role of the liver for Aβ degradation and removal [24]. Labeled Aβ42 peptides were, indeed, taken up by the liver and excreted in bile [11]. This finding gives, however, no information about the final levels of Aβ42 in the hepatic vein considering that the liver generates and degrades Aβ [13]. PVS and HVS Aβ42 levels were similar in the patients with liver cirrhosis. This suggests that the cirrhotic liver does not eliminate portal-venous Aβ42. It is, however, possible that Aβ42 is taken up by the cirrhotic liver for excretion but is also released from this organ into the circulation. APP mRNA and the enzymes for Aβ production are expressed in the liver [13]. Comparable Aβ42 levels in PVS and HVS are achieved when removal and production rates are similar. PVS and HVS levels of most cytokines and chemokines analyzed so far were highly correlated [16,22,31,36,45]. This also applied to chemerin and IL-6 levels in the small study cohort analyzed herein. Correlations of Aβ42 in SVS, PVS, and HVS were smaller and, thus, Aβ42 levels may be more extensively modified when passing the liver.

Whatever the underlying mechanisms are, the present findings indicated that levels of Aβ42 were not significantly reduced when passing the cirrhotic liver. Impaired liver function is associated with a diminished elimination of cytokines such as IL-6, and, accordingly, IL-6 levels increased with higher Child–Pugh score [31,57]. Aβ42 levels did not change in patients with worse liver function as assessed by the MELD score, the Child–Pugh score, and laboratory measures of liver disease severity. This illustrated that serum Aβ42 levels are not correlated with residual liver function in patients with cirrhosis.

It may well be that the healthy liver contributes to Aβ42 elimination. It is, however, difficult to obtain HVS and PVS blood from liver healthy donors. Wang et al. showed increased plasma Aβ42 levels in patients with liver cirrhosis in comparison to healthy controls [12]. This indeed suggests a function of the healthy liver in the regulation of plasma Aβ42 levels. The control group in that study was healthy subjects, and non-cirrhotic patients with chronic liver diseases were not included in the analysis by Wang et al. [12]. Patients infected with hepatitis B had about four-fold higher Aβ42 levels than non-infected patients. This shows that hepatitis B infection has a much greater effect on systemic Aβ42 levels than suffering from liver cirrhosis [12]. Current preliminary analysis suggested that hepatitis C infection (only two patients) was not associated with very high Aβ42 serum levels, but this needs further analysis.

It may well be that hepatic Aβ42 release is enhanced in patients with liver cirrhosis, and this may also reduce levels in the liver tissues and increase systemic concentrations of this peptide [12,13].

In an experimental murine NAFLD model, plasma Aβ42 even declined, and analysis of hepatic pathways involved in Aβ synthesis, catabolism, and clearance revealed that all of them were reduced in NAFLD [58]. Beta-secretase 1 was, however, found induced in the liver of db/db mice, which have a mutated leptin receptor and liver steatosis [59]. In human liver cirrhosis, beta-secretase 1 and neprilysin, which efficiently degrades the Aβ peptides, were suppressed, suggesting that production and degradation pathways were downregulated [13]. Chronic liver diseases may thus be associated with a dysregulation of Aβ production and removal. Major causes of liver cirrhosis are NAFLD, viral infection, and alcohol abuse [60]. Whether disease etiology may affect the hepatic production or clearance of Aβ42 was not studied so far. Data about expression of hepatic enzymes involved in Aβ42 metabolism and hepatic and systemic Aβ42 in patients stratified for etiology of liver cirrhosis are missing.

Aβ42 levels were about three fold higher in the cirrhosis patients studied by Wang et al. in comparison to our cohort. About 30% of their patients had chronic hepatitis B (HBV) [12]. Plasma Aβ42 levels in the non-HBV patients with liver cirrhosis were about 28 pg/mL, and this is comparable to the SVS Aβ42 levels (20 pg/mL) identified in our study where mostly patients with alcoholic cirrhosis were included.

The study by Wang et al. described associations of plasma Aβ42 with bilirubin, albumin, and AST concentrations [12]. The correlation analyses included data of non-HBV and HBV patients with liver cirrhosis and healthy controls, and analysis has to be done separately in these three different cohorts [12]. Positive associations of Aβ42 with markers of liver injury such as bilirubin and AST can also be explained by higher hepatic release of Aβ42 from the damaged liver, and a more detailed analysis is needed to characterize the pathways contributing to increased systemic Aβ42 in liver cirrhosis.

Higher age is a risk factor for liver cirrhosis and Alzheimer disease [2,35]. Aβ42 levels were, however, not correlated with age in the current cohort. A very modest negative association of plasma Aβ42 and age was described in cognitively normal subjects [61]. A second analysis showed a relatively weak positive correlation of plasma Aβ42 level and age [62]. These opposing reports suggest that correlations of Aβ42 level and age are weak and seem to be cohort specific.

Liver cirrhosis is often associated with chronic inflammation, and various cytokines were found induced in serum of these patients [35]. Plasma Aβ42 levels were, however, not correlated with IL-1β, IL-6, TNF, and IFN-γ in the study by Wang et al. [12]. In accordance with these findings, serum Aβ42 did not correlate with inflammatory proteins such as IL-6 and CRP in the current cohort. Therefore, it is unlikely that acute phase proteins or inflammatory proteins contribute to increased serum Aβ42.

There is evidence that Aβ42 is increased in obesity and diabetes. Obese mice had elevated plasma Aβ42 levels [63]. In diabetic patients, plasma Aβ42 levels were higher than in non-diabetic controls [63]. Of note, in the patients with liver cirrhosis studied herein, Aβ42 was significantly induced in HVS of diabetic patients with liver cirrhosis. HVS/PVS Aβ42 ratio did not differ between the diabetic and non-diabetic patients excluding that hepatic production was grossly induced in these patients.

Aβ42 was also shown to impair endothelium-dependent and -independent vasodilation and was associated with a lower NO bioavailability [63]. In the aorta of control and high-fat diet-fed mice, Aβ42 reduced phosphorylated endothelial NO synthase protein. On the other hand, it was shown that Aβ42 increased endothelial NO synthase protein in human liver sinusoidal endothelial cells [13]. It is well known that NO is a key factor in the hemodynamic abnormalities of liver cirrhosis. The reduced production of endothelial NO in the liver and its overproduction in the systemic and splanchnic vasculature are key factors for portal hypertension [21]. Common complications of portal hypertension are ascites and varices [19]. Aβ42 levels were not changed in patients with ascites or varices and did not correlate with the hepatic venous pressure gradient, serum arginine (NO precursor), or ADMA (NO synthase inhibitor) levels. Considering the complex regulation of NO synthesis and the multiple mediators that contribute to portal hypertension [21], this, however, does not exclude a role for Aβ42 in the regulation of splanchnic and hepatic NO production.

An interesting finding was the negative association of serum CTGF with Aβ42 levels. Serum CTGF was highest in patients with ongoing fibrogenesis [17]. Transforming growth factor β (TGF-β) is a strong inducer of hepatocyte CTGF synthesis [18]. Aβ42 reduces TGF-β in hepatic stellate cells [13], and this effect may contribute to the negative correlation of CTGF and Aβ42. HVS/PVS Aβ42 ratio was negatively correlated with CTGF in the three blood compartments, assuming a protective role of this peptide in liver cirrhosis.

The main limitation of this study is that only 20 patients were included. Thus, it was not possible to prove small differences. The use of an ELISA, instead of a highly sensitive technique such as the Single Molecule Array (Simoa)® Aβ42 Advantage Kit, is a further limitation of this study. As mentioned above, Aβ42 levels detected in serum of our study cohort were comparable to the levels described in a previous analysis [12]. Moreover, the ELISA used herein was already applied for analysis of serum Aβ42 in a human study cohort [64]. Because of the low levels of Aβ42, serum had to be used undiluted and the specificity of the commercially available ELISA was not thoroughly checked. Medication and alcohol consumption of the patients were not documented and possible effects on serum Aβ42 could not be evaluated. The study strength is that portal vein, hepatic vein, and systemic blood of relatively well-characterized patients were used for analysis of Aβ42.

The present analysis showed that there is no net effect of the cirrhotic liver on Aβ42 levels in the circulation. Further studies are needed to explore the association of Aβ42 levels, ongoing fibrogenesis, and cognitive dysfunction in patients with liver cirrhosis.

Author Contributions: Formal analysis, C.B.; resources, R.W.; writing—original draft preparation, C.B.; conceptualization, writing, review, and editing, T.S.W., L.D., R.W., and C.B. All authors have read and agreed to the published version of the manuscript.

Funding: This research received no external funding.

Institutional Review Board Statement: The study was conducted according to the guidelines of the Declaration of Helsinki and approved by the Institutional Review Board of the University Hospital Regensburg (protocol code 4/99 and date of approval 20 April 1999).

Informed Consent Statement: Written informed consent was obtained from all subjects involved in the study.

Data Availability Statement: The data presented in this study are available on request from the corresponding author.

Acknowledgments: The technical support of Elena Underberg is greatly appreciated.

Conflicts of Interest: The authors declare no conflict of interest.

References

1. De Nazareth, A.M. Type 2 diabetes mellitus in the pathophysiology of Alzheimer's disease. *Dement. Neuropsychol.* **2017**, *11*, 105–113. [CrossRef] [PubMed]
2. Jellinger, K.A.; Janetzky, B.; Attems, J.; Kienzl, E. Biomarkers for early diagnosis of Alzheimer disease: 'ALZheimer ASsociated gene'—A new blood biomarker? *J. Cell. Mol. Med.* **2008**, *12*, 1094–1117. [CrossRef]
3. Van Gool, B.; Storck, S.; Reekmans, S.M.; Lechat, B.; Gordts, P.L.S.M.; Pradier, L.; Pietrzik, C.U.; Roebroek, A.J.M. LRP1 Has a Predominant Role in Production over Clearance of Aβ in a Mouse Model of Alzheimer's Disease. *Mol. Neurobiol.* **2019**, *56*, 7234–7245. [CrossRef] [PubMed]
4. Shibata, M.; Yamada, S.; Kumar, S.R.; Calero, M.; Bading, J.; Frangione, B.; Holtzman, D.M.; Miller, C.A.; Strickland, D.K.; Ghiso, J.; et al. Clearance of Alzheimer's amyloid-β1-40 peptide from brain by LDL receptor–related protein-1 at the blood-brain barrier. *J. Clin. Investig.* **2000**, *106*, 1489–1499. [CrossRef] [PubMed]
5. Xiang, Y.; Bu, X.-L.; Liu, Y.-H.; Zhu, C.; Shen, L.-L.; Jiao, S.-S.; Zhu, X.-Y.; Giunta, B.; Tan, J.; Song, W.-H.; et al. Physiological amyloid-beta clearance in the periphery and its therapeutic potential for Alzheimer's disease. *Acta Neuropathol.* **2015**, *130*, 487–499. [CrossRef] [PubMed]
6. Tian, D.-Y.; Cheng, Y.; Zhuang, Z.-Q.; He, C.-Y.; Pan, Q.-G.; Tang, M.-Z.; Hu, X.-L.; Shen, Y.-Y.; Wang, Y.-R.; Chen, S.-H.; et al. Physiological clearance of amyloid-beta by the kidney and its therapeutic potential for Alzheimer's disease. *Mol. Psychiatry* **2021**, 1–9. [CrossRef]
7. Cheng, Y.; Tian, D.-Y.; Wang, Y.-J. Peripheral clearance of brain-derived Aβ in Alzheimer's disease: Pathophysiology and therapeutic perspectives. *Transl. Neurodegener.* **2020**, *9*, 1–11. [CrossRef] [PubMed]
8. Joachim, C.L.; Mori, H.; Selkoe, D.J. Amyloid β-protein deposition in tissues other than brain in Alzheimer's disease. *Nat. Cell Biol.* **1989**, *341*, 226–230. [CrossRef]
9. Chen, S.-H.; Tian, D.-Y.; Shen, Y.-Y.; Cheng, Y.; Fan, D.-Y.; Sun, H.-L.; He, C.-Y.; Sun, P.-Y.; Bu, X.-L.; Zeng, F.; et al. Amyloid-beta uptake by blood monocytes is reduced with ageing and Alzheimer's disease. *Transl. Psychiatry* **2020**, *10*, 1–11. [CrossRef]
10. Pappolla, M.; Sambamurti, K.; Vidal, R.; Pacheco-Quinto, J.; Poeggeler, B.; Matsubara, E. Evidence for lymphatic Aβ clearance in Alzheimer's transgenic mice. *Neurobiol. Dis.* **2014**, *71*, 215–219. [CrossRef]
11. Ghiso, J.; Shayo, M.; Calero, M.; Ng, D.; Tomidokoro, Y.; Gandy, S.; Rostagno, A.; Frangione, B. Systemic Catabolism of Alzheimer's Aβ40 and Aβ42. *J. Biol. Chem.* **2004**, *279*, 45897–45908. [CrossRef]
12. Wang, Y.-R.; Wang, Q.-H.; Zhang, T.; Liu, Y.-H.; Yao, X.-Q.; Zeng, F.; Li, J.; Zhou, F.-Y.; Wang, L.; Yan, J.-C.; et al. Associations Between Hepatic Functions and Plasma Amyloid-Beta Levels—Implications for the Capacity of Liver in Peripheral Amyloid-Beta Clearance. *Mol. Neurobiol.* **2017**, *54*, 2338–2344. [CrossRef]
13. Buniatian, G.H.; Weiskirchen, R.; Weiss, T.S.; Schwinghammer, U.; Fritz, M.; Seferyan, T.; Proksch, B.; Glaser, M.; Lourhmati, A.; Buadze, M.; et al. Antifibrotic Effects of Amyloid-Beta and Its Loss in Cirrhotic Liver. *Cells* **2020**, *9*, 452. [CrossRef]
14. Roher, A.E.; Esh, C.L.; Kokjohn, T.A.; Castaño, E.M.; Van Vickle, G.D.; Kalback, W.M.; Patton, R.L.; Luehrs, D.C.; Daugs, I.D.; Kuo, Y.-M.; et al. Amyloid beta peptides in human plasma and tissues and their significance for Alzheimer's disease. *Alzheimer's Dement.* **2009**, *5*, 18–29. [CrossRef]
15. Molinuevo, J.L.; Ayton, S.; Batrla, R.; Bednar, M.M.; Bittner, T.; Cummings, J.; Fagan, A.M.; Hampel, H.; Mielke, M.; Mikulskis, A.; et al. Current state of Alzheimer's fluid biomarkers. *Acta Neuropathol.* **2018**, *136*, 821–853. [CrossRef]
16. Bauer, S.; Eisinger, K.; Wiest, R.; Karrasch, T.; Scherer, M.N.; Farkas, S.; Aslanidis, C.; Buechler, C. Connective tissue growth factor level is increased in patients with liver cirrhosis but is not associated with complications or extent of liver injury. *Regul. Pept.* **2012**, *179*, 10–14. [CrossRef]
17. Gressner, A.M.; Yagmur, E.; Lahme, B.; Gressner, O.; Stanzel, S. Connective Tissue Growth Factor in Serum as a New Candidate Test for Assessment of Hepatic Fibrosis. *Clin. Chem.* **2006**, *52*, 1815–1817. [CrossRef] [PubMed]
18. Gressner, O.A.; Lahme, B.; Demirci, I.; Gressner, A.M.; Weiskirchen, R. Differential effects of TGF-β on connective tissue growth factor (CTGF/CCN2) expression in hepatic stellate cells and hepatocytes. *J. Hepatol.* **2007**, *47*, 699–710. [CrossRef] [PubMed]
19. Laleman, W.; Landeghem, L.; Wilmer, A.; Fevery, J.; Nevens, F. Portal hypertension: From pathophysiology to clinical practice. *Liver Int.* **2005**, *25*, 1079–1090. [CrossRef] [PubMed]

20. Siramolpiwat, S. Transjugular intrahepatic portosystemic shunts and portal hypertension-related complications. *World J. Gastroenterol.* **2014**, *20*, 16996–17010. [CrossRef] [PubMed]
21. Wiest, R.; Groszmann, R.J. The paradox of nitric oxide in cirrhosis and portal hypertension: Too much, not enough. *Hepatology* **2002**, *35*, 478–491. [CrossRef]
22. Eisinger, K.; Krautbauer, S.; Wiest, R.; Karrasch, T.; Hader, Y.; Scherer, M.N.; Farkas, S.; Aslanidis, C.; Buechler, C. Portal vein omentin is increased in patients with liver cirrhosis but is not associated with complications of portal hypertension. *Eur. J. Clin. Investig.* **2013**, *43*, 926–932. [CrossRef]
23. Lluch, P.; Torondel, B.; Medina, P.; Segarra, G.; Del Olmo, J.A.; Serra, M.A.; Rodrigo, J.M. Plasma concentrations of nitric oxide and asymmetric dimethylarginine in human alcoholic cirrhosis. *J. Hepatol.* **2004**, *41*, 55–59. [CrossRef]
24. Estrada, L.D.; Ahumada, P.; Cabrera, D.; Arab, J.P. Liver Dysfunction as a Novel Player in Alzheimer's Progression: Looking Outside the Brain. *Front. Aging Neurosci.* **2019**, *11*, 174. [CrossRef]
25. Buechler, C.; Wanninger, J.; Neumeier, M. Adiponectin, a key adipokine in obesity related liver diseases. *World J. Gastroenterol.* **2011**, *17*, 2801–2811. [CrossRef] [PubMed]
26. Kim, D.-G.; Krenz, A.; Toussaint, L.E.; Maurer, K.J.; Robinson, S.-A.; Yan, A.; Torres, L.; Bynoe, M.S. Non-alcoholic fatty liver disease induces signs of Alzheimer's disease (AD) in wild-type mice and accelerates pathological signs of AD in an AD model. *J. Neuroinflamm.* **2016**, *13*, 1–18. [CrossRef] [PubMed]
27. Nägga, K.; Gustavsson, A.-M.; Stomrud, E.; Lindqvist, D.; Van Westen, D.; Blennow, K.; Zetterberg, H.; Melander, O.; Hansson, O. Increased midlife triglycerides predict brain β-amyloid and tau pathology 20 years later. *Neurology* **2017**, *90*, e73–e81. [CrossRef] [PubMed]
28. Reed, B.; Villeneuve, S.; Mack, W.; DeCarli, C.; Chui, H.C.; Jagust, W. Associations Between Serum Cholesterol Levels and Cerebral Amyloidosis. *JAMA Neurol.* **2014**, *71*, 195–200. [CrossRef]
29. Verlinden, W.; Francque, S.; Vonghia, L. Peripheral Venous, Portal Venous, Hepatic Venous, and Arterial and Intrahepatic Cytokine Levels as Biomarkers and Functional Correlations. In *Biomarkers in Liver Disease. Biomarkers in Disease: Methods, Discoveries and Applications*; Patel, V., Preedy, V., Eds.; Springer: Dordrecht, The Netherlands, 2017. [CrossRef]
30. Fontana, L.; Eagon, J.C.; Trujillo, M.E.; Scherer, P.E.; Klein, S. Visceral Fat Adipokine Secretion Is Associated with Systemic Inflammation in Obese Humans. *Diabetes* **2007**, *56*, 1010–1013. [CrossRef]
31. Wiest, R.; Weigert, J.; Wanninger, J.; Neumeier, M.; Bauer, S.; Schmidhofer, S.; Farkas, S.; Scherer, M.N.; Schäffler, A.; Schölmerich, J. Impaired hepatic removal of interleukin-6 in patients with liver cirrhosis. *Cytokine* **2011**, *53*, 178–183. [CrossRef]
32. Schmidt-Arras, D.; Rose-John, S. IL-6 pathway in the liver: From physiopathology to therapy. *J. Hepatol.* **2016**, *64*, 1403–1415. [CrossRef] [PubMed]
33. Buechler, C.; Eisinger, K.; Krautbauer, S. Diagnostic and prognostic potential of the macrophage specific receptor CD163 in inflammatory diseases. *Inflamm. Allergy Drug Targets* **2013**, *12*, 391–402. [CrossRef]
34. Holland-Fischer, P.; Gronbaek, H.; Sandahl, T.D.; Moestrup, S.K.; Riggio, O.; Ridola, L.; Aagaard, N.K.; Møller, H.J.; Vilstrup, H. Kupffer cells are activated in cirrhotic portal hypertension and not normalised by TIPS. *Gut* **2011**, *60*, 1389–1393. [CrossRef]
35. Buechler, C.; Haberl, E.M.; Rein-Fischboeck, L.; Aslanidis, C. Adipokines in Liver Cirrhosis. *Int. J. Mol. Sci.* **2017**, *18*, 1392. [CrossRef]
36. Eisinger, K.; Krautbauer, S.; Wiest, R.; Weiss, T.S.; Buechler, C. Reduced serum chemerin in patients with more severe liver cirrhosis. *Exp. Mol. Pathol.* **2015**, *98*, 208–213. [CrossRef]
37. Krautbauer, S.; Wanninger, J.; Eisinger, K.; Hader, Y.; Beck, M.; Kopp, A.; Schmid, A.; Weiss, T.S.; Dorn, C.; Buechler, C. Chemerin is highly expressed in hepatocytes and is induced in non-alcoholic steatohepatitis liver. *Exp. Mol. Pathol.* **2013**, *95*, 199–205. [CrossRef] [PubMed]
38. Buechler, C.; Feder, S.; Haberl, E.M.; Aslanidis, C. Chemerin Isoforms and Activity in Obesity. *Int. J. Mol. Sci.* **2019**, *20*, 1128. [CrossRef]
39. Horn, P.; Von Loeffelholz, C.; Forkert, F.; Stengel, S.; Reuken, P.; Aschenbach, R.; Stallmach, A.; Bruns, T. Low circulating chemerin levels correlate with hepatic dysfunction and increased mortality in decompensated liver cirrhosis. *Sci. Rep.* **2018**, *8*, 1–9. [CrossRef]
40. Peschel, G.; Grimm, J.; Gülow, K.; Müller, M.; Buechler, C.; Weigand, K. Chemerin Is a Valuable Biomarker in Patients with HCV Infection and Correlates with Liver Injury. *Diagnostics* **2020**, *10*, 974. [CrossRef]
41. Gong, C.; Wei, D.; Wang, Y.; Ma, J.; Yuan, C.; Zhang, W.; Yu, G.; Zhao, Y. A Meta-Analysis of C-Reactive Protein in Patients With Alzheimer's Disease. *Am. J. Alzheimer's Dis. Dement.* **2016**, *31*, 194–200. [CrossRef] [PubMed]
42. Pieri, G.; Agarwal, B.; Burroughs, A.K. C-reactive protein and bacterial infection in cirrhosis. *Ann. Gastroenterol.* **2014**, *27*, 113–120.
43. Hanon, O.; Vidal, J.-S.; Lehmann, S.; Bombois, S.; Allinquant, B.; Tréluyer, J.-M.; Gelé, P.; Delmaire, C.; Blanc, F.; Mangin, J.-F.; et al. Plasma amyloid levels within the Alzheimer's process and correlations with central biomarkers. *Alzheimer's Dement.* **2018**, *14*, 858–868. [CrossRef]
44. Roessle, M.; Gerbes, A.L. TIPS for the treatment of refractory ascites, hepatorenal syndrome and hepatic hydrothorax: A critical update. *Gut* **2010**, *59*, 988–1000. [CrossRef]
45. Wiest, R.; Moleda, L.; Farkas, S.; Scherer, M.; Kopp, A.; Wönckhaus, U.; Büchler, C.; Schölmerich, J.; Schäffler, A. Splanchnic concentrations and postprandial release of visceral adipokines. *Metabolism* **2010**, *59*, 664–670. [CrossRef] [PubMed]

46. Schober, P.; Boer, C.; Schwarte, L.A. Correlation Coefficients: Appropriate use and interpretation. *Anesth. Analg.* **2018**, *126*, 1763–1768. [CrossRef] [PubMed]
47. Angermayr, B.; Cejna, M.; Karnel, F.; Gschwantler, M.; Koenig, F.; Pidlich, J.; Mendel, H.; Pichler, L.; Wichlas, M.; Kreil, A.; et al. Child-Pugh versus MELD score in predicting survival in patients undergoing transjugular intrahepatic portosystemic shunt. *Gut* **2003**, *52*, 879–885. [CrossRef]
48. Ott, A.; Stolk, R.; Van Harskamp, F.; Pols, H.A.P.; Hofman, A.; Breteler, M.M. Diabetes mellitus and the risk of dementia: The Rotterdam Study. *Neurology* **1999**, *53*, 1937. [CrossRef] [PubMed]
49. Locascio, J.J.; Fukumoto, H.; Yap, L.; Bottiglieri, T.; Growdon, J.H.; Hyman, B.T.; Irizarry, M.C. Plasma Amyloid β-Protein and C-reactive Protein in Relation to the Rate of Progression of Alzheimer Disease. *Arch. Neurol.* **2008**, *65*, 776–785. [CrossRef]
50. Tejera, D.; Mercan, D.; Sanchez-Caro, J.M.; Hanan, M.; Greenberg, D.; Soreq, H.; Latz, E.; Golenbock, D.; Heneka, M.T. Systemic inflammation impairs microglial Aβ clearance through NLRP 3 inflammasome. *EMBO J.* **2019**, *38*, e101064. [CrossRef]
51. Genc, H.; Dogru, T.; Kara, M.; Tapan, S.; Ercin, C.N.; Acikel, C.; Karslioglu, Y.; Bagci, S. Association of plasma visfatin with hepatic and systemic inflammation in nonalcoholic fatty liver disease. *Ann. Hepatol.* **2013**, *12*, 380–387. [CrossRef]
52. Tilg, H. The Role of Cytokines in Non-Alcoholic Fatty Liver Disease. *Dig. Dis.* **2010**, *28*, 179–185. [CrossRef]
53. Bertolani, C.; Sancho-Bru, P.; Failli, P.; Bataller, R.; Aleffi, S.; DeFranco, R.; Mazzinghi, B.; Romagnani, P.; Milani, S.; Ginés, P.; et al. Resistin as an Intrahepatic Cytokine: Overexpression during Chronic Injury and Induction of Proinflammatory Actions in Hepatic Stellate Cells. *Am. J. Pathol.* **2006**, *169*, 2042–2053. [CrossRef]
54. Siroen, M.P.C.; Wiest, R.; Richir, M.C.; Teerlink, T.; Rauwerda, J.A.; Drescher, F.T.; Zorger, N.; Leeuwen, P.A.M.V. Transjugular intrahepatic portosystemic shunt-placement increases arginine/asymmetric dimethylarginine ratio in cirrhotic patients. *World J. Gastroenterol.* **2008**, *14*, 7214–7219. [CrossRef]
55. Iwakiri, Y. Endothelial dysfunction in the regulation of cirrhosis and portal hypertension. *Liver Int.* **2011**, *32*, 199–213. [CrossRef]
56. Maarouf, C.L.; Walker, J.E.; Sue, L.I.; Dugger, B.N.; Beach, T.G.; Serrano, G.E. Impaired hepatic amyloid-beta degradation in Alzheimer's disease. *PLoS ONE* **2018**, *13*, e0203659. [CrossRef]
57. Porowski, D.; Wirkowska, A.; Hryniewiecka, E.; Wyzgał, J.; Pacholczyk, M.; Pączek, L. Liver Failure Impairs the Intrahepatic Elimination of Interleukin-6, Tumor Necrosis Factor-Alpha, Hepatocyte Growth Factor, and Transforming Growth Factor-Beta. *BioMed Res. Int.* **2015**, *2015*, 1–7. [CrossRef]
58. Pinçon, A.; De Montgolfier, O.; Akkoyunlu, N.; Daneault, C.; Pouliot, P.; Villeneuve, L.; Lesage, F.; Levy, B.I.; Thorin-Trescases, N.; Thorin, É.; et al. Non-Alcoholic Fatty Liver Disease, and the Underlying Altered Fatty Acid Metabolism, Reveals Brain Hypoperfusion and Contributes to the Cognitive Decline in APP/PS1 Mice. *Metabolites* **2019**, *9*, 104. [CrossRef]
59. Meakin, P.J.; Mezzapesa, A.; Benabou, E.; Haas, M.E.; Bonardo, B.; Grino, M.; Brunel, J.-M.; Desbois-Mouthon, C.; Biddinger, S.B.; Govers, R.; et al. The beta secretase BACE1 regulates the expression of insulin receptor in the liver. *Nat. Commun.* **2018**, *9*, 1–14. [CrossRef]
60. Buechler, C.; Aslanidis, C. Role of lipids in pathophysiology, diagnosis and therapy of hepatocellular carcinoma. *Biochim. Biophys. Acta (BBA) Mol. Cell Biol. Lipids* **2020**, *1865*, 158658. [CrossRef]
61. Lue, L.-F.; Pai, M.-C.; Chen, T.-F.; Hu, C.-J.; Huang, L.-K.; Lin, W.-C.; Wu, C.-C.; Jeng, J.-S.; Blennow, K.; Sabbagh, M.N.; et al. Age-Dependent Relationship Between Plasma Aβ40 and Aβ42 and Total Tau Levels in Cognitively Normal Subjects. *Front. Aging Neurosci.* **2019**, *11*, 222. [CrossRef]
62. Mayeux, R.; Honig, L.S.; Tang, M.-X.; Manly, J.; Stern, Y.; Schupf, N.; Mehta, P.D. Plasma A 40 and A 42 and Alzheimer's disease: Relation to age, mortality, and risk. *Neurology* **2003**, *61*, 1185–1190. [CrossRef]
63. Meakin, P.J.; Coull, B.M.; Tuharska, Z.; McCaffery, C.; Akoumianakis, I.; Antoniades, C.; Brown, J.; Griffin, K.J.; Platt, F.; Ozber, C.H.; et al. Elevated circulating amyloid concentrations in obesity and diabetes promote vascular dysfunction. *J. Clin. Investig.* **2020**, *130*, 4104–4117. [CrossRef]
64. Ma, F.; Wu, T.; Zhao, J.; Song, A.; Liu, H.; Xu, W.; Huang, G. Folic acid supplementation improves cognitive function by reducing the levels of peripheral inflammatory cytokines in elderly Chinese subjects with MCI. *Sci. Rep.* **2016**, *6*, 37486. [CrossRef]

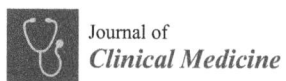

Article

Safety and Effectiveness of Vedolizumab for the Treatment of Pediatric Patients with Very Early Onset Inflammatory Bowel Diseases

Sylwia Fabiszewska, Edyta Derda, Edyta Szymanska *, Marcin Osiecki and Jaroslaw Kierkus

Department of Gastroenterology, Hepatology, Feeding Disorders and Pediatrics,
The Children's Memorial Health Institute, 04-730 Warsaw, Poland; s.fabiszewska@ipczd.pl (S.F.);
e.derda@ipczd.pl (E.D.); m.osiecki@ipczd.pl (M.O.); j.kierkus@ipczd.pl (J.K.)
* Correspondence: edyta.szymanska@onet.com.pl or edyta.szymanska@ipczd.pl

Citation: Fabiszewska, S.; Derda, E.; Szymanska, E.; Osiecki, M.; Kierkus, J. Safety and Effectiveness of Vedolizumab for the Treatment of Pediatric Patients with Very Early Onset Inflammatory Bowel Diseases. *J. Clin. Med.* **2021**, *10*, 2997. https://doi.org/10.3390/jcm10132997

Academic Editors: Gian Paolo Caviglia and Davide Giuseppe Ribaldone

Received: 27 April 2021
Accepted: 1 July 2021
Published: 5 July 2021

Publisher's Note: MDPI stays neutral with regard to jurisdictional claims in published maps and institutional affiliations.

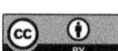

Copyright: © 2021 by the authors. Licensee MDPI, Basel, Switzerland. This article is an open access article distributed under the terms and conditions of the Creative Commons Attribution (CC BY) license (https://creativecommons.org/licenses/by/4.0/).

Abstract: Background: Vedolizumab (vedo) is effective for induction and maintenance of remission in adults with inflammatory bowel disease (IBD). Pediatric data are still limited, especially for the youngest children with very early onset disease (VEO-IBD). The aim of this study was to assess the safety and efficacy of vedo in VEO-IBD. **Methods:** We performed a retrospective review of pediatric IBD patients with VEO-IBD (defined as aged <6 years) receiving vedo. Data on demographics, disease behavior, activity, and previous treatments/surgeries were collected. Disease activity was assessed using the pediatric Crohn's disease (CD) activity index (PCDAI) for CD or pediatric ulcerative colitis (UC) activity index (PUCAI) for UC. Primary outcome was clinical response after induction therapy with vedolizumab (4th dose week). It was defined as a decrease in PCDAI of at least 12.5 points between baseline and 4th dose week for CD, and a decrease in PUCAI of at least 20 points between baseline and this time for UC. Descriptive statistics were performed to analyze the data. **Results:** The study included 16 patients with VEO-IBD who have received vedo: 4/16 (25%) with CD, and 12/16 (75%) with UC at the median age of diagnosis 33.7 months (6.6 months–4.5 years). Median age at vedo initiation was 6.5 years (2.2–16.5 years). Among the analyzed individuals, 56.25% had failed more than one anti-tumor necrosis factor (TNF) alfa agent. Clinical response at 4th dose week was observed in 9/16 (56.3%) patients: mean baseline PCDAI score was 34.4 ± 1.9 and 10.6 ± 1.8 after induction therapy with vedo, while PUCAI score was 26 ± 6 vs. 18 ± 8, respectively. There was improvement in patients' nutritional state: at baseline 2/16 (12.5%) children had body mass index (BMI) below 1 percentile and no child had such BMI after induction therapy with vedo. No infusion reactions or serious adverse events/infections were reported. **Conclusion:** Vedolizumab is safe and effective in the medical management of pediatric patients with VEO-IBD.

Keywords: premedication; infusion reaction; infliximab; inflammatory bowel disease

1. Introduction

The incidence of pediatric inflammatory bowel disease (IBD) is increasing worldwide, and the age of onset has become younger [?]. Very early onset IBD (VEO-IBD) is defined as disease diagnosis under the age of 6 years, and it represents a unique subset of IBD patients [?]. Some of VEO-IBD patients present with immunodeficiency and have genetic causes of their disease which means that loss of function genetic mutations involving immune and/or cytokines pathways lead to development of intestinal inflammation [?].

Most of these young patients present with a highly severe course of IBD and thus require more aggressive treatment due to the failure to both conventional and biological therapies [?].

Therefore, novel medical strategies are absolutely necessary, particularly for this specific group of VEO-IBD.

Monoclonal antibodies against tumor necrosis factor alpha (TNFα), such as infliximab (IFX) or adalimumab (ADA), are safe and effective in induction and maintenance of remission in moderate to severe pediatric Crohn's disease (CD) and ulcerative colitis (UC) patients [? ?]. However, up to one-third of patients are primary non-responders to TNFα antagonist therapy and about 20% of primary responders may develop loss of response per year [? ?]. Moreover, patients who fail one TNFα antagonist are less likely to respond to a second agent, and even those with sustained response may need to discontinue therapy because of infusion reactions or other adverse effects [?].

Vedolizumab (vedo) is a humanized anti-α4β7 integrin, immunoglobulin G1 monoclonal antibody. It may be an alternative for patients with severe IBD who have failed treatment with a TNFα antagonist [?]. This biological agent downregulates intestinal inflammation by specifically inhibiting intestinal T-lymphocyte migration into the tissue. Therefore, its mechanism of action is restricted to the gastrointestinal tract, which potentially decreases the risks of systemic immunosuppression that leads to increased infection rate and malignancies observed in other IBD therapies [?].

Results from adult studies (GEMINI 1 and GEMINI 2 trials) have demonstrated the safety and effectiveness of vedo in induction and maintenance of remission in both UC and CD, with slightly better clinical outcomes in UC [? ?].

Data on vedo treatment in pediatric IBD population is still lacking and, so far, there has been no study performed on patients with VEO-IBD.

Due to the mechanism of action indicating the superior safety profile of this anti-integrin therapy, vedo seems to be a promising biological agent in pediatric IBD and is certainly worth further evaluation, especially in the group of youngest patients.

The aim of this study was to evaluate safety and efficacy of vedo in the treatment of pediatric patients with VEO-IBD.

2. Patients and Methods

This is a single-center retrospective observational cohort study of 16 children under the age of 6 years at diagnosis of IBD (both CD and UC) with a severe course of the disease refractory to both standard therapies and anti-TNF-alfa treatment. In this group, vedo was introduced at any age as a "rescue therapy". Drug's doses were either 150 mg or 300 mg depending on patient's weight, and the infusions' schedule was: 0, 2, and 6 weeks of induction therapy followed by a maintenance phase at 8-week intervals.

Data on demographics, disease behavior, activity, and previous treatments/surgeries were collected from patients' medical charts. Disease activity was assessed using the pediatric Crohn's disease activity index (PCDAI) for CD or pediatric ulcerative colitis activity index (PUCAI) for UC. Mucosal healing (MH) was assessed using fecal calprotectin (FCP) which was measured with enzyme-linked immunosorbent assay (ELISA) test kits and normal values were <50 µg/g.

The primary outcome of the study was:

- Clinical response after induction therapy with vedo (4th dose week) defined as a decrease in PCDAI of at least 12.5 points between baseline and 4th dose week for CD, and for UC a decrease in PUCAI of at least 20 points between baseline and this time.

The secondary outcomes included:

- Clinical remission after induction phase (4th dose week) and maintenance phase (10th dose week) of vedo defined as PCDAI ≤ 10 points for CD or PUCAI ≤ 10 points for UC.
- Improvement in patients' nutritional status after induction and maintenance treatment with vedo assessed by body mass index (BMI) score.
- Improvement in laboratory parameters after induction and maintenance treatment with vedo.
- FCP was used as a surrogate marker of MH—a statistically significant decrease in FCP level between baseline and after vedo commencement was considered as MH.

To analyze the data, descriptive statistics based on intension to treat (ITT) analysis were performed.

All legal guardians provided written informed consent for the treatment with vedo.

Vedolizumab is approved in Poland for adult patients with IBD. It is used it for children as a rescue therapy and thus an agreement of the National Consultant of Pediatric Gastroenterology is obligatory.

The study meets the standards of Helsinki and the National Consultant on Pediatric Gastroenterology agreed to administer the drug.

3. Results

3.1. Patients' Characteristics

Sixteen patients with IBD were included in the study: 4/16 (25%) with CD, and 12/16 (75%) with UC. Median age at disease diagnosis was 33.7 months (6.6 months–4.5 years). Median age at vedo initiation was 6.5 years (2.2–16.5 years). Among these individuals 15/16 (93.75%) had previously received infliximab (IFX), 9/16 (56.25%) had been treated with adalimumab (ADA), and 4/16 (25%) had had an exposure to other biologic therapies, 1/16 (6.25%) was biologic-naive. The most common reason for discontinuation of anti-TNF-alfa therapy was primary non-response: IFX—9/15 participants (60%), ADA—6/9 (66.7%). At baseline 8/16 (50%) patients received concomitant therapy with systemic steroids and 9/16 (56,3%) with immunosuppression (IMM)—either azathioprine (5 patients—AZA) or methotrexate (4 patients—MTX). After induction therapy 6/14 (42,9%) children continued steroids and 8/14 (57,1%) IMM (4 patients—MTX, 4 patients—AZA) (Table S1).

3.2. Outcomes

The response at the 4th dose week (induction phase) was observed in 9/16 (56.3%): 6 with UC and 3 with CD. Additionally, in UC group at 4th dose week 3 patients achieved clinical remission and 4 patients fulfill the criteria of clinical response and clinical remission. In CD group at 4th dose week 1 patient achieved clinical remission and 1 patient fulfilled the criteria of clinical response and clinical remission. Two patients did not respond to vedo therapy and therefore they did not continue the treatment. The mean PCDAI score at initiation of vedo therapy for the CD patients was 34.4 ± 1.9, while the mean PUCAI for children with UC was 26 ± 6. Overall, there was a significant decrease in both clinical indexes from baseline to each follow-up visit, at 4th and 10th dose week: PCDAI—18.1 ± 6.8, 10.6 ± 1.8, and PUCAI—18 ± 8, 17 ± 7, respectively (Figure S1). Four patients with UC had PUCAI = 0 after induction treatment with vedo.

Six patients (37.5%) either did not respond or lost response to vedo: 2 patients did not respond to induction therapy, and 4 children lost response—after the 4th, 8th, 9th and 10th doses of vedo, respectively.

All patients improved their nutritional status: 2/16 individuals (12.5%) had BMI <1 percentile at baseline and none at 4th dose week. Thirteen (81.25%) children had median baseline BMI score at 40th percentile, while all of them achieved this BMI score after induction therapy with vedo (Table S2).

Overall, there was an improvement in laboratory parameters: mean baseline hemoglobin level was 10.5 g/dL and 11.8 g/dL after 3 doses of vedo, and mean serum albumin was 38.5 g/L vs. 42.9 g/L respectively. A decrease in inflammatory markers was reported: mean ESR at week 0 was 29 mm/h vs. 18 mm/h after induction therapy (Table S2).

During our study, 8/16 (50%) patients were tested for FCP (Figure S2). Unfortunately, due to the small sample size we cannot draw any clear conclusions on the impact of vedo treatment on FCP levels.

Three patients still required surgery during vedo therapy: 2 patients underwent total colectomy and 1 had subtotal resection of the intestine (Table S3).

3.3. Safety

Generally, vedo therapy was safe and well-tolerated by our patients. No infusion reactions or serious adverse events (AEs)/infections were reported during the whole treatment. After induction phase only one patient (1/16–6.3%) developed infection of the upper respiratory tract, however we do not know whether it was related to vedo. After nine doses of vedo, 2 patients (12.5%) complained about arthralgia (Table S2).

4. Discussion

In this first study on vedo treatment in children with VEO-IBD we have demonstrated the safety and effectiveness of this anti-integrin agent in the studied group—clinical response after induction therapy with three doses of vedo was observed in more than 40% of patients. Our results are comparable to the outcomes reported so far for the older pediatric patients, which is very satisfactory regarding more severe course of VEO-IBD and thus worse response to treatment.

In the retrospective multi-center study of the pediatric IBD Porto Group of European Society of Pediatric Gastroenterology, Hepatology and Nutrition (ESPGHAN) demonstrating experience with vedo in pediatric population, the remission rate at week 14 was 37% in UC, and 14% in CD, while by last follow-up it was 39% in UC and 24% in CD respectively. However, children in this group were much older than our patients—their mean age at vedo commencement was 14.5 ± 2.8 years, while it was 7.24 years in our cohort. Alike our patients, all of those children were previously treated with anti-TNF-alfa agent (28% primary failure, 53% secondary failure) [?]. However, 17% children still required surgery, including a colectomy for UC. An interesting observation was that concomitant immunomodulatory therapy did not affect remission rate [42% vs. 35%; $p = 0.35$ at Week 22]. In this study, only 3 of 16 children who underwent endoscopic evaluation had MH after treatment (19%). What is most important, only three minor drug-related AEs were observed [?].

In our study 3 patient required surgery and 2 of them underwent toral colectomy. Concomitant treatment with either systemic steroids or IMM was continued in 3/9 (33.33%) children at 4th dose visit, and 6/9 (66.7%) of participants at the 10th dose week. This observation is consistent with the PORTO group results. Due to the very young age of study participants, we decided to assess MH using a non-invasive biomarker, FCP, not an endoscopy which requires general anesthesia and is more stressful for children. The reason for this was that FCP has been proven to correlate best with endoscopic improvement (better than clinical indexes) and, therefore, is considered to be the marker of MH and has been used as such in [?]. Alike in the PORTO group study, significant improvement of the intestinal permeability was not achieved during vedo treatment in our patients, which demonstrates that deeper remission requires more time than clinical and laboratory improvements. Moreover, data published so far show that full effect of vedo is observed between 6 and even 14 weeks of treatment, which indicates that MH may be achieved later than with other biologics.

Nonetheless, it is important to underline that VEO-IBD is characterized by a more severe course than typical pediatric disease and, therefore, the outcomes of medical management may be worse [?]. Similarly in the Porto Group study, vedo was safe and well-tolerated by our patients—during the whole therapy only one child (1/16–6.3%) developed infection of the upper respiratory tract, and 2 patients (12.5%) complained about arthralgia. However, we do not know whether these AEs were related to vedo.

Another multi-center study published in 2016 showing experience with vedo in pediatric IBD has proven its effectiveness and safety in this population [?]. In this trial which included 58% CD and 42% UC patients with median age at vedo initiation of 14.9 (range 7–17) years, week 14 remission rates for UC and CD were 76% and 42%, respectively. In this cohort 90% of patients had failed more than 1 anti-TNF agent. Among anti–TNF-naive patients 80% of them experienced week 14 remission. At week 22, anti–TNF-naive patients had higher remission rates than TNF-exposed patients (100% versus 45%, $p = 0.04$). There were no infusion reactions or serious AEs [?].

These outcomes confirm two major observations from adults' trials—vedo is more effective in UC and anti-TNF-alfa naïve patients have better response to this anti-integrin agent, which is also consistent with results of our study. This may be partially explained by the fact that anti-TNF agents downregulate MadCAM-1 expression which may be the reason that CD patients with previous anti-TNF exposure in the GEMINI studies required a longer duration of vedo treatment to achieve remission [? ? ?].

In the study by Conrad et al. evaluating outcomes of vedo therapy in severe pediatric IBD including 21 subjects, 16 with CD, clinical response was observed in 6/19 (31.6%) of the patients at week 6 and in 11/19 (57.9%) by week 22. There were no infusion reactions. Vedolizumab was discontinued in 2 patients because of severe colitis, requiring surgical intervention [?]. These response rates are comparable to our results.

Standard dosing of vedo in adult patients is 300 mg per infusion, and no specific guidelines exist for pediatric dosing. Children, smaller in size and weight, may require an individualized dose. Our patients received either 150 mg or 300 mg doses of vedo depending on their body mass—due to the younger age of participants in our study than in other pediatric trials, and thus lower body mass, we had to adjust dosing and lower it in the youngest children.

Recent pharmacokinetic data have demonstrated significant correlation between higher vedo drug levels and clinical response in IBD patients which may suggest that, alike with IFX, shortening infusion interval from 8 to 4 weeks should lead to an improved effect [? ? ?].

In our study intervals between vedo infusions were standard—all patients have received the drug every 8 weeks during the maintenance phase.

A very important issue is the drug's safety. Although GEMINI 1 revealed no difference in AE rates between vedo and placebo, [?] GEMINI 2 demonstrated a higher incidence of nasopharyngitis with vedo than with placebo [12.3% vs. 8%]. [?] The adult US VICTORY study of 212 patients reported enteric infections (5 per 100 patient-year follow-up [PYF]), sinopulmonary infections [4.4 per 100 PYF] and arthralgia [3.1 per 100 PYF], among other less common AEs [?]. Other cohorts report infections from 0% to 25%, nasopharyngitis 0–23%, arthralgia 2–20%, and one report of anaphylaxis and rash [? ? ?].

In our study no AEs or serious infections were reported, only minor medical events have been observed and their rate was low—3/16 (18.8%) patients had either respiratory tract infection (1/3) or arthralgia (2/3) during the whole therapy. Therefore, vedo seems to be very safe in children, even the youngest ones.

The limitation of our study is its retrospective design and relatively small cohort. Also, not all patients before and after vedo commencement had their FCP assessed which made it difficult to draw proper conclusions. However, it is still the only study that includes not only pediatric and early onset but also VEO-IBD patients.

To summarize, VEO-IBD group that was analyzed in our study is a unique subset of pediatric IBD patients. It is characterized by more severe course and aggressive behavior with a high treatment failure rate to both conventional and biologic therapies. In the majority of our patients, vedo was applied as a rescue therapy. Therefore, response and remission rates may be lower than in older/adult patients.

5. Conclusions

Vedolizumab is safe and effective for the treatment of VEO-IBD. This anti-integrin therapy provides improvement in patients' nutritional state and in their laboratory parameters. However, achievement of MH may require more time than with other biologics due to the drug's delayed full effect.

Supplementary Materials: The following are available online at https://www.mdpi.com/article/10.3390/jcm10132997/s1 Table S1. Baseline characteristics of the study group. Table S2. Patient's characteristics after vedolizumab initiation compering to baseline. Table S3. Relationship between vedolizumab and surgery in 3 patients who underwent surgery. Figure S1. Patients' disease clinical activity (PCDAI for CD and PUCAI for UC) between baseline and after vedolizumab commencement (4th and 10th week dose). Figure S2. Values of fecal calprotectin for 8 patients tested for this marker before and after vedolizumab commencement.

Author Contributions: E.S.: conceptualization, writing; S.F.: data collection; E.D.: data collection; M.O.: data editing; J.K.: supervision. All authors have read and agreed to the published version of the manuscript.

Funding: This research received no external funding.

Institutional Review Board Statement: The study was conducted according to the guidelines of the Declaration of Helsinki.

Informed Consent Statement: Not applicable.

Data Availability Statement: Not applicable.

Conflicts of Interest: The authors declare no conflict of interest.

References

1. Gasparetto, M.; Guariso, G. Highlights in IBD Epidemiology and Its Natural History in the Paediatric Age. *Gastroenterol. Res. Pr.* **2013**, *2013*, 829040. [CrossRef] [PubMed]
2. Moran, C.J. Very early onset inflammatory bowel disease. *Semin. Pediatr. Surg.* **2017**, *26*, 356–359. [CrossRef]
3. Moazzami, B.; Moazzami, K.; Rezaei, N. Early onset inflammatory bowel disease: Manifestations, genetics and diagnosis. *Turk. J. Pediatr.* **2019**, *61*, 637–647. [CrossRef]
4. Crowley, E.; Muise, A. Inflammatory Bowel Disease: What Very Early Onset Disease Teaches Us. *Gastroenterol. Clin. N. Am.* **2018**, *47*, 755–772. [CrossRef]
5. Hyams, J.S.; Crandall, W.; Kugathasan, S.; Griffiths, A.; Olson, A.; Johanns, J.; Liu, G.; Travers, S.; Heuschkel, R.; Markowitz, J.; et al. Induction and maintenance infliximab therapy for the treatment of moderate-to-severe Crohn's disease in children. *Gastroenterology* **2007**, *132*, 863–873. [CrossRef]
6. Hyams, J.S.; Lerer, T.; Griffiths, A.; Pfefferkorn, M.; Stephens, M.; Evans, J.; Otley, A.; Carvalho, R.; Mack, D.; Bousvaros, A.; et al. Outcome Following Infliximab Therapy in Children with Ulcerative Colitis. *Am. J. Gastroenterol.* **2010**, *105*, 1430–1436. [CrossRef] [PubMed]
7. Gisbert, J.P.; Marin, A.C.; McNicholl, A.G.; Chaparro, M. Systematic review with meta-analysis: The efficacy of a second anti-TNF in patients with inflammatory bowel disease whose previous anti-TNF treatment has failed. *Aliment. Pharmacol. Ther.* **2015**, *41*, 613–623. [CrossRef] [PubMed]
8. Gisbert, J.P.; Panes, J. Loss of response and requirement of infliximab dose intensification in Crohn's disease: A review. *Am. J. Gastroenterol.* **2009**, *104*, 760–767. [CrossRef]
9. Sands, B.E.; Feagan, B.G.; Rutgeerts, P.; Colombel, J.-F.; Sandborn, W.J.; Sy, R.; D'Haens, G.; Ben-Horin, S.; Xu, J.; Rosario, M.; et al. Effects of Vedolizumab Induction Therapy for Patients with Crohn's Disease in Whom Tumor Necrosis Factor Antagonist Treatment Failed. *Gastroenterology* **2014**, *147*, 618–627.e3. [CrossRef]
10. Mosli, M.H.; MacDonald, J.K.; Bickston, S.J.; Behm, B.W.; Tsoulis, D.J.; Cheng, J.; Khanna, R.; Feagan, B.G. Vedolizumab for induction and maintenance of remission in ulcerative colitis: A Cochrane systematic review and meta-analysis. *Inflamm. Bowel Dis.* **2015**, *21*, 1151–1159. [CrossRef] [PubMed]
11. Feagan, B.G.; Rutgeerts, P.; Sands, B.E.; Hanauer, S.; Colombel, J.-F.; Sandborn, W.J.; Van Assche, G.; Axler, J.; Kim, H.-J.; Danese, S.; et al. Vedolizumab as Induction and Maintenance Therapy for Ulcerative Colitis. *N. Engl. J. Med.* **2013**, *369*, 699–710. [CrossRef]
12. Sandborn, W.J.; Feagan, B.G.; Rutgeerts, P.; Hanauer, S.; Colombel, J.-F.; Sands, B.E.; Lukas, M.; Fedorak, R.; Lee, S.; Bressler, B.; et al. Vedolizumab as Induction and Maintenance Therapy for Crohn's Disease. *N. Engl. J. Med.* **2013**, *369*, 711–721. [CrossRef]
13. Ledder, O.; Assa, A.; Levine, A.; Escher, J.C.; De Ridder, L.; Ruemmele, F.; Shah, N.; Shaoul, R.; Wolters, V.M.; Rodrigues, A.; et al. Vedolizumab in Paediatric Inflammatory Bowel Disease: A Retrospective Multi-Centre Experience From the Paediatric IBD Porto Group of ESPGHAN. *J. Crohns Colitis* **2017**, *11*, 1230–1237. [CrossRef] [PubMed]
14. Kostas, A.; Siakavellas, S.I.; Kosmidis, C.; Takou, A.; Nikou, J.; Maropoulos, G.; Vlachogiannakos, J.; Papatheodoridis, G.V.; Papaconstantinou, I.; Bamias, G. Fecal calprotectin measurement is a marker of short-term clinical outcome and presence of mucosal healing in patients with inflammatory bowel disease. *World J. Gastroenterol.* **2017**, *23*, 7387–7396. [CrossRef]
15. Shim, J.O. Recent Advance in Very Early Onset Inflammatory Bowel Disease. *Pediatr. Gastroenterol. Hepatol. Nutr.* **2019**, *22*, 41–49. [CrossRef] [PubMed]

16. Singh, N.; Rabizadeh, S.; Jossen, J.; Pittman, N.; Check, M.; Hashemi, G.; Phan, B.L.; Hyams, J.S.; Dubinsky, M.C. Multi-Center Experience of Vedolizumab Effectiveness in Pediatric Inflammatory Bowel Disease. *Inflamm. Bowel Dis.* **2016**, *22*, 2121–2126. [CrossRef]
17. Biancheri, P.; Di Sabatino, A.; Rovedatti, L.; Giuffrida, P.; Calarota, S.A.; Vetrano, S.; Vidali, F.; Pasini, A.; Danese, S.; Corazza, G.R.; et al. Effect of tumor necrosis factor-alpha blockade on mucosal addressin cell-adhesion molecule-1 in Crohn's disease. *Inflamm. Bowel Dis.* **2013**, *19*, 259–264. [CrossRef] [PubMed]
18. Conrad, M.A.; Stein, R.E.; Maxwell, E.C.; Albenberg, L.; Baldassano, R.N.; Dawany, N.; Grossman, A.B.; Mamula, P.; Piccoli, D.A.; Kelsen, J.R. Vedolizumab Therapy in Severe Pediatric Inflammatory Bowel Disease. *Inflamm. Bowel Dis.* **2016**, *22*, 2425–2431. [CrossRef]
19. Yarur, A.; Bruss, A.; Jain, A.; Kondragunta2, V.; Hester, K.; Luna, T.; Agrawal, D.; Patel, A.; Fox, C.; Werner, S.; et al. Higher vedolizumab levels are associated with deep remission in patients with Crohn's disease and ulcerative colitis on maintenance therapy with vedolizumab. In Proceedings of the European Crohn's and Colitis Organisation 2017 Annual Meeting, Barcelona, Spain, 15–18 February 2017.
20. Schulze, H.; Esters, P.; Hartmann, F.; Stein, J.; Christ, C.; Zorn, M.; Dignass, A. A prospective cohort study to assess the relevance of Vedolizumab drug level monitoring in IBD patients. In Proceedings of the European Crohn's and Colitis Organisation 2017 Annual Meeting, Barcelona, Spain, 15–18 February 2017.
21. Williet, N.; Paul, S.; Del Tedesco, E.; Phelip, J.M.; Roblin, X. Serum vedolizumab assay at week 6 predicts sustained clinical remission and lack of recourse to optimisation in inflammatory bowel disease. In Proceedings of the European Crohn's and Colitis Organisation 2016 Annual Meeting, Amsterdam, The Netherlands, 16–19 March 2016.
22. Dulai, P.S.; Singh, S.; Jiang, X.; Peerani, F.; Narula, N.; Chaudrey, K.; Whitehead, D.; Hudesman, D.; Lukin, D.; Swaminath, A.; et al. The real-world effectiveness and safety of vedolizumab for moderate-severe Crohn's disease: Results from the US VICTORY consortium. *Am. J. Gastroenterol.* **2016**, *111*, 1147–1155. [CrossRef] [PubMed]
23. Vivio, E.E.; Kanuri, N.D.; Gilbertsen, J.J.; Monroe, K.; Dey, N.; Chen, C.-H.; Gutierrez, A.M.; Ciorba, M.A. Vedolizumab Effectiveness and Safety Over the First Year of Use in an IBD Clinical Practice. *J. Crohns Colitis* **2015**, *10*, 402–409. [CrossRef]
24. Baumgart, D.C.; Bokemeyer, B.; Drabik, A.; Stallmach, A.; Schreiber, S. Vedolizumab Germany Consortium. Vedolizumab induction therapy for inflammatory bowel disease in clinical practice—A nationwide consecutive German cohort study. *Aliment. Pharmacol. Ther.* **2016**, *10*, 1090–1102. [CrossRef] [PubMed]
25. Shelton, E.; Allegretti, J.R.; Stevens, B.; Lucci, M.; Khalili, H.; Nguyen, D.D.; Sauk, J.; Giallourakis, C.; Garber, J.; Hamilton, M.J.; et al. Efficacy of vedolizumab as induction therapy in refractory IBD patients: A multicenter cohort. *Inflamm. Bowel Dis.* **2015**, *21*, 2879–2885. [CrossRef] [PubMed]

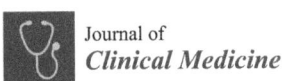

Journal of Clinical Medicine

Article
Risk Factors of Urothelial Cancer in Inflammatory Bowel Disease

Gian Paolo Caviglia [1], Giorgio Martini [1], Angelo Armandi [1,*], Chiara Rosso [1], Marta Vernero [2], Elisabetta Bugianesi [1], Marco Astegiano [3], Giorgio Maria Saracco [1] and Davide Giuseppe Ribaldone [1,*]

[1] Department of Medical Sciences, Division of Gastroenterology, University of Torino, 10126 Torino, Italy; gianpaolo.caviglia@unito.it (G.P.C.); giorgiomartini96@gmail.com (G.M.); chiara.rosso@unito.it (C.R.); elisabetta.bugianesi@unito.it (E.B.); giorgiomaria.saracco@unito.it (G.M.S.)
[2] Department of Internal Medicine, San Matteo Hospital, 27100 Pavia, Italy; martavernero@gmail.com
[3] Department of General and Specialist Medicine, Gastroenterologia-U, Città della Salute e della Scienza di Torino, C.so Bramante 88, 10126 Turin, Italy; mastegiano@cittadellasalute.to.it
* Correspondence: angelo.armandi@unito.it (A.A.); davidegiuseppe.ribaldone@unito.it (D.G.R.); Tel.: +39-011-6333-918 (D.G.R.)

Abstract: Extraintestinal cancers are important complications in patients with inflammatory bowel disease (IBD). A limited number of publications are available regarding the association between IBD and urothelial cancer. The primary outcome of our study was the comparison of the prevalence of urothelial cancer in patients with IBD with respect to the prevalence in the general population. Secondary outcomes were the assessment of risk factors for the onset of urothelial cancer in IBD. In a retrospective study we examined the medical records of all patients with a confirmed diagnosis of IBD followed in our clinic between 1978 and 2021. For each of the patients with identified urothelial cancer, more than ten patients without cancer were analyzed. Furthermore, 5739 patients with IBD were analyzed and 24 patients diagnosed with urothelial cancer were identified. The incidence of urothelial cancer, compared with the incidence in the general population, was not significantly different (0.42% vs. 0.42%; $p = 0.98$). Twenty-three cases were then compared (1 case was discarded due to lack of follow-up data) against 250 controls. During the multivariate analysis, smoking (odds ratio, OR = 8.15; 95% confidence interval, CI = 1.76–37.63; $p = 0.007$) and male sex (OR = 4.04; 95% CI = 1.29–12.66; $p = 0.016$) were found as risk factors. In conclusion, patients with IBD have a similar risk of developing urothelial cancer compared to the general population, but males with a history of smoking are at increased risk.

Keywords: Crohn's disease; ulcerative colitis; malignant; neoplasm; urinary; bladder; ureter; urethra; urothelium

1. Introduction

Inflammatory bowel diseases (IBD) are a heterogeneous group of immune-mediated diseases of unknown etiology that can affect the digestive tract in a variable manner. Traditionally they are grouped into two entities, Crohn's disease (CD) and ulcerative colitis (UC), whose differential diagnosis is based on clinical, histological, laboratory, and endoscopic data. A third entity, unclassified IBD (IBD-U), represents a temporary diagnosis until there are sufficient elements to define whether it is CD or UC [1].

Regarding risk factors, smoking has different effects on IBD. In CD, smoking worsens the course of the disease, leads to a reduced response to medical therapy, and an increased risk of exacerbations and complications, with a more aggressive disease profile and increased surgery rate. The role of smoking in the onset of the disease is unclear, but the higher incidence of CD among smokers would seem to suggest that smoking is part of the events underlying the pathogenesis of the disease; nicotine and its derivatives can directly influence the immune responses of the mucosa, the composition of the microbiome, the production of pro-inflammatory cytokines, the tone of smooth muscle, and intestinal permeability, acting at the vascular level causing coagulation [2]. The use of tobacco, on the other hand, seems to protect against UC and reduce its severity, although it does not seem to improve the natural history of the disease. On the contrary, ex-smokers have a higher risk of developing the disease, which, in these cases, is often more extensive and more refractory to therapy than the disease in individuals who have never smoked [3].

A link between IBD and extraintestinal cancers has been observed in people with IBD [4]. Though the mechanism behind IBD and oncogenesis is unknown, it has been observed that inflammation not only acts as the host's response to malignant tumors, but also triggers carcinogenesis [5]. Furthermore, immunosuppressive medicines, which are commonly used to treat IBD, are thought to be linked to an increased risk of malignancies such as non-Hodgkin lymphoma, acute myeloid leukaemias, non-melanoma skin cancers, and urinary tract cancers [6].

Tumors of urothelial tissue are neoplasms that develop at the level of the transitional epithelium (the tissue that comes into contact with urine and covers the urinary tract from the renal calyxes to the urethra). The bladder is the most frequent site but tumors of the transitional epithelium may also be present in the following areas: renal calyxes, ureters, and urethra. Bladder cancer accounts for 3% of cancers diagnosed globally and is particularly prevalent in the Western world [7]. Tobacco is the best known of the factors favoring the development of bladder cancer, in particular active cigarette smoking is responsible respectively for 60% and 30% of all urothelial carcinomas in males and females [8].

Only a limited number of publications are available in the literature regarding the possible association between urothelial cancer and IBD with conflicting results [9,10], as well as regarding the possible role of azathioprine as a risk factor [11,12].

The aim of our study was to evaluate the frequency of urothelial cancer in a large series of patients with IBD and to search for possible risk factors, including medications.

2. Materials and Methods

We retrospectively reviewed the medical records of all patients with IBD followed in the gastroenterology clinic between 1978 and 2021, with the aim of assessing the frequency of urothelial cancer and comparing it with that of the general population of the same country. Patients were included in the "IBD cohort" (Ethics Committee Approval No. 0056924).

Inclusion criteria were:
- all patients with a confirmed diagnosis of IBD according to the indications of the European Crohn's and Colitis Organization (ECCO) [13];
- minimum age of 16, with no upper age limits.

Exclusion criterion was:
- lack of data on the presence of tumor comorbidities.

The primary outcome was the comparison of the frequency of urothelial cancer in our population with respect to the data available from the AIOM (Italian Association of Medical Oncology) guidelines for the general Italian population [14].

For each of the patients with identified urothelial cancer (cases), more than ten IBD patients who did not develop urothelial cancer (controls) were randomly selected (alphabetically) from the medical records of all patients with IBD followed in the gastroenterology clinic between 1978 and 2021.

The secondary outcomes were the assessment of risk factors for the onset of urothelial cancer in patients with IBD.

The risk factors assessed with a univariate analysis were:
- categorical variables: sex, smoking habit, type of IBD, treatment with mesalazine, treatment with thiopurine, treatment with anti-tumor necrosis factor (TNF), treatment with anti-integrins, and surgical treatment for intestinal disease;

- continuous variables: age at diagnosis of IBD, duration of treatment with mesalamine, duration of treatment with thiopurine, duration of treatment with anti-TNF, and duration of treatment with anti-integrins.

Statistical Analysis

The normal distribution of continuous variables was assessed using the D'Agostino–Pearson test. Continuous variables not normally distributed were reported as median and interquartile range (IQR), continuous variables normally distributed were reported as mean ± standard deviation (SD). Categorical variables were reported as numbers and percentages. The Mann–Whitney test and the chi-square test were used to compare continuous and categorical variables, respectively. Multivariate analysis (logistic regression) was then carried out by inserting the variables of clinical interest. A p-value of less than 0.05 was considered statistically significant. All statistical analyses were performed using MedCalc v.18.9.1 (MedCalc Software Ltd., Ostend, Belgium).

3. Results

In the first phase, we analyzed 5739 patients followed in our clinic from 1978 to 2021, with a confirmed diagnosis of IBD and with available data on the presence of any comorbid tumors; of these, 24 received a diagnosis of urothelial neoplasia (0.42%). Specifically, 20 patients (83.3%) had a bladder tumor, 3 patients (12.5%) had a ureteral tumor, 1 patient (4.2%) had no precise location available, no patient had a tumor in the urethral or kidney pelvis. From the point of view of tumor typing, the information present was partially incomplete and some histological information regarding the tumor was missing. According to the data in our possession, from the point of view of tumor grading, 9 (23.1%) tumors were infiltrating (6 tumors were pTa, 3 were pT1), and 1 (4.4%) tumor was infiltrating (pT3). From the point of view of tumor staging, 2 (8.7%) tumors were G1, 7 (30.4%) tumors were G2, and 2 (8.7%) tumors were G3. Comparing the frequency of urothelial cancer in our patients affected by IBD with that of the whole Italian population, it was no different: 0.42% in both groups ($p = 0.98$).

One patient diagnosed with urothelial cancer was excluded from the second phase (case-control study) due to lack of follow-up data; 250 randomly selected control patients were analyzed. The mean age at diagnosis of urothelial cancer in the 23 patients was 61.3 ± 13.0 years. In 6 cases (26%) the diagnosis of urothelial cancer preceded the diagnosis of IBD (all active smokers), and in 17 cases (74%) it was subsequent. In the 17 patients in whom the diagnosis of urothelial cancer was subsequent to that of IBD, 8.0 ± 10.1 years elapsed between the diagnosis of IBD and the diagnosis of urothelial neoplasia.

The risk factors for developing urothelial cancer are shown in Table 1.

The frequency of urothelial cancer by gender is shown in Figure 1.

Figure 2 shows smoking habits in the 2 groups.

The age comparison at diagnosis of IBD in the 2 groups is shown in Figure 3.

No patient diagnosed with urothelial cancer received anti-integrin treatment.

In multivariate analysis, the factors that were statistically associated with the development of urothelial cancer in the patient with IBD were male sex (odds ratio, OR = 4.04; 95% confidence interval, CI = 1.29–12.66, $p = 0.016$) and a history of cigarette smoking (OR = 8.15, 95% CI = 1.76–37.63, $p = 0.007$). Diagnosis of CD (OR = 1.49, 95% CI = 0.53–4.19, $p = 0.44$), treatment with mesalamine (OR = 0.33, 95% CI = 0.056–1.93, $p = 0.22$), and treatment with thiopurines (OR = 0.57, 95% CI = 0.19–1.69, $p = 0.40$) were not risk factors.

Table 1. Comparison of cases and controls.

Risk Factors	Cases (n = 23)	Controls (n = 250)	p Value
Sex			p = 0.005
Males	19 (82.6%)	131 (52.4%)	
Females	4 (17.4%)	119 (47.6%)	
Smoking habit			p = 0.009
Active smokers	7 (33%)	56 (22.5%)	
Former smokers	12 (57%)	84 (33.7%)	
Never smokers	2 (9.5%)	109 (43.8%)	
IBD type			p = 0.19
Crohn's disease	17 (73.9%)	154 (61.1%)	
Ulcerative colitis	5 (21.7%)	93 (37.2%)	
IBD-U	1 (4.4%)	3 (1.2%)	
Age at diagnosis of IBD			p < 0.0001
Year (median, IQR)	56.0, 40.0–64.8	32.0, 22.0–44.0	
Mesalazine			p = 0.02
Yes	19 (82.6%)	237 (94.8%)	
No	4 (17.4%)	13 (5.2%)	
Duration mesalazine			p = 0.053
Months (median, IQR)	48.0, 8.25–188.25	88.5, 48.00–179.00	
Thiopurine			p = 0.38
Yes	5 (21.7%)	76 (30.4%)	
No	18 (78.3%)	174 (69.9%)	
Duration thiopurine			p = 0.79
Months (median, IQR)	40.00, 18.25–60.00	31, 6.00–82.00	
Anti-TNF			p = 0.012
Yes	1 (4.3%)	71 (28.4%)	
No	22 (95.7%)	179 (71.6%)	
Surgical resection			p = 0.69
Yes	8 (34.8%)	77 (30.8%)	
No	15 (65.2%)	173 (69.2%)	

IBD-U = inflammatory bowel disease unclassified; IQR = interquartile range; TNF = tumor necrosis factor.

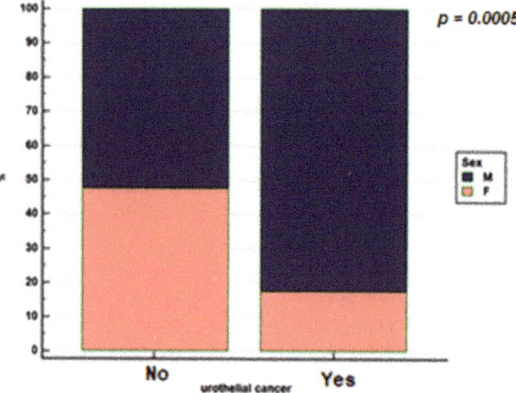

Figure 1. Distribution by gender in the population with IBD with urothelial cancer and without urothelial cancer.

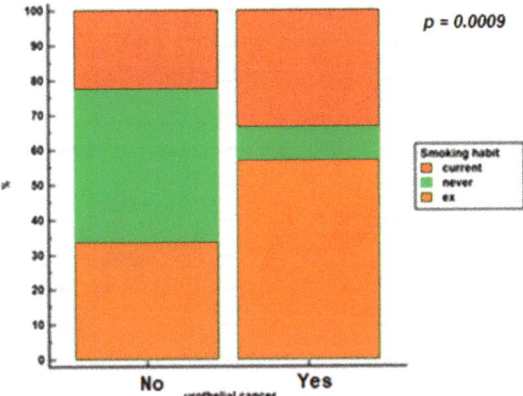

Figure 2. Smoking habits in patients with IBD based on whether or not they have developed urothelial cancer.

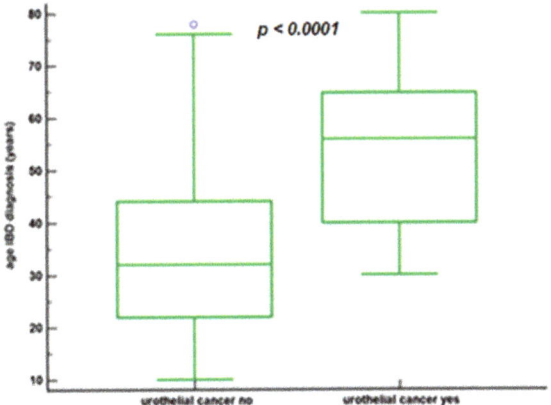

Figure 3. Age at diagnosis of IBD based on whether or not urothelial cancer has developed.

4. Discussion

Malignant tumors, both gastrointestinal and extraintestinal, are known long-term complications in patients with IBD; in fact, the latter have a long-term risk of cancer that is 30% higher for gastrointestinal cancers and 10% for extraintestinal cancers compared to the general population. This could be a consequence of both chronic inflammation and the consequent important use of immunosuppressive drugs to control inflammation [15,16]. While colon cancer is likely to be associated with the inflammatory state caused by intestinal disease, regarding extraintestinal cancers the cause of the increased risk is not well-known. Studies have found a correlation between IBD and an increased risk of a limited number of extraintestinal cancers, such as hematological cancers and lung cancer [4,17,18]. Furthermore, patients with IBD appear to have a slightly higher risk of cancers from the prostate, skin, liver, and biliary system [19,20]. The underlying mechanisms are not clear since tumor etiology is more often multifactorial.

On the other hand, the possibility that chronic intestinal inflammation can be associated with tumors at the urothelial level is widely discussed in the literature. Studies on this are few and show different results. In particular, the study by Madanchi et al. [16] and the study by Algaba et al. [21] are single-center cohort studies and have shown a statistically significant increase in urothelial cancer in patients with IBD. However, the first study evaluates 1026 patients, while the second 590, thus introducing a possible bias linked to the small size of the selected patient cohort. In fact, these results seem isolated, while there are more publications that do not find any association between the two diseases in question [10,15,17,22–27].

In our study, comparing the frequency of urothelial cancer in the population with IBD with that of the Italian population, we observed that a diagnosis of IBD is not a risk factor for the development of urothelial neoplasm ($p = 0.98$). This data takes on an important value since the relevant sample of 5739 patients on which the analysis was carried out makes our study the largest performed on a population of patients belonging to the same center. However, a statistically significant increased risk of tumor was found in patients diagnosed with IBD in men (OR = 4.04; 95% CI = 1.29–12.66) and in patients with a history of cigarette smoking (OR = 8.15; 95% CI = 1.76–37.63). Regarding the risk of urothelial cancer in association with smoking, the study by Algaba et al. [21] found an increased risk of urothelial cancer in smoking IBD patients, while no association was found in the study by Madachi et al. [16].

Regarding the risk of urothelial cancer in association with CD, the study by Kappelman et al. [15] found no increased risk (standardized incidence ratio, SIR = 1.2, 95% CI = 0.8–1.6). Conversely, in the study by Pedersen et al., there was a significant association between CD and urothelial cancer (SIR = 2.03, 95% CI = 1.14–3.63) [4]. In our study, despite a higher prevalence of smoking history in the CD population, the diagnosis of urothelial cancer was not statistically significantly increased.

Important is the finding in our study of an increased frequency of urothelial cancer in male patients with IBD. This figure is in line with that of the general population: an increased incidence of urothelial cancer in men is known (24,000 new diagnoses in men against 5700 diagnoses in women, in 2019) [7]. This is mainly explained by the different incidence of risk factors in the male population, mainly with regard to smoking and occupational exposure to carcinogens [8,28].

Some studies also reported that long-term use of immunosuppressive drugs, particularly thiopurines, in patients with IBD may increase the risk of cancer [4,15,29]. Immunosuppressive drugs, which are widely used for IBD treatment, are thought to be responsible for a small increased risk of extraintestinal cancers such as non-Hodgkin's lymphoma, non-melanoma skin, and urinary tract cancers [6,30,31]. In this regard, it is believed that, while the use of immunosuppressants can guarantee greater protection from tumors in the intestine, acting on chronic inflammation and reducing the risk of neoplastic transformation, the same effect may not be present for extraintestinal tumors, whose pathogenesis could be different from that of chronic inflammation. In contrast, the study by Pedersen et al. suggested a possible bias derived from increased clinical attention in patients undergoing treatment with immunosuppressants and a greater likelihood of being subjected to diagnostic investigations in these patients [4]. Regarding this debated topic, our study seems to deny a possible correlation. There was no significant association between thiopurine treatment and urothelial cancer (OR = 0.57; 95% CI = 0.19–1.69). Our study cannot draw any conclusions regarding a possible association between the use of anti-TNF or anti-integrins and the occurrence of urothelial tumors in patients with IBD due to the insufficient number of patients belonging to these groups.

We want to underline data of particular interest, namely, the age at the diagnosis of IBD in patients in the urothelial cancer group. In these cases, it was found to be 56.0 years (IQR = 40.0–64.8). This was found to be definitely more advanced than the control group: 32.0 years (IQR = 22.0–44.0), much more in line with the epidemiological data regarding IBD [32]. This data is not easy to interpret, but we suggest the particular characteristics of the patients that develop urothelial cancer as a possible explanation: the patients in question are more frequently males, smokers, and workers in industrial activities, patients in whom a late diagnosis is perhaps more frequent for a reduced understanding of risk factors for health and late access to health care for symptom assessment.

From the urological point of view, the results found are in line with the epidemiological characteristics of urothelial tumors in the general population. In our population, patients with bladder cancer were 83.3% and patients with ureteral cancer were 12.5%; in the general population, bladder cancer diagnoses out of total urothelial cancers are 89.9%, while those at ureteral level are 4.4% [33]. Furthermore, the fact that 6 out of 23 patients received a diagnosis of urothelial cancer before the diagnosis of IBD seems to shift the focus more onto the common risk factors of the two diseases, rather than on the action of drugs for IBD treatment.

Our study has some limitations that warrant highlighting. Data loss bias is possible since a retrospective analysis was conducted. The long-time window may have led to non-homogeneous data collection over time. It should be noted, however, that all patients have been followed over the years by the same doctor (A.M.) in the same center, reducing the possibility of having dependent operator data. Another possible bias is linked to the presence of a smaller total population in the study compared to that of multicenter studies; ours, however, is the widest study with data relating to a single center. Finally, data about race, job, and family history (known risk factors of urothelial cancer) could have enriched the study but, due to the retrospective nature, were not available.

5. Conclusions

In conclusion, our study shows that patients with IBD have a similar risk of urothelial cancer compared to the general population. Nonetheless, smoking and being male seem to be risk factors associated with the development of this cancer, despite the fact that it is a single center study it should be taken into consideration. It would therefore be useful to adopt screening methods and prevention strategies for lifestyle changes in this specific population of male smokers with IBD. Finally, our study reassures the use of immunosuppressants in the treatment of IBD since it does not significantly increase the risk of developing urothelial cancer.

Author Contributions: Conceptualization, D.G.R., M.A. and G.M.S.; methodology, D.G.R., G.M. and G.P.C.; software, G.P.C.; validation, A.A. and M.V.; formal analysis, G.M.; investigation, G.M.; resources, G.M.S. and E.B.; data curation, A.A. and C.R.; writing—original draft preparation, G.M.; writing—review and editing, D.G.R., C.R. and M.A.; visualization, E.B.; supervision, G.M.S.; project administration, G.M.S. All authors have read and agreed to the published version of the manuscript.

Funding: This research received no external funding.

Institutional Review Board Statement: The study was conducted according to the guidelines of the Declaration of Helsinki. Patients were included in the "IBD cohort" (Ethics Committee Approval No. 0056924).

Informed Consent Statement: Informed consent was obtained from all subjects involved in the study.

Data Availability Statement: The data was collected anonymously. Anonymous data can be requested in case of need.

Conflicts of Interest: The authors declare no conflict of interest.

References

1. Actis, G.C.; Pellicano, R.; Fagoonee, S.; Ribaldone, D.G. History of Inflammatory Bowel Diseases. *J. Clin. Med.* **2019**, *8*, 1970. [CrossRef] [PubMed]
2. Berkowitz, L.; Schultz, B.M.; Salazar, G.A.; Pardo-Roa, C.; Sebastián, V.P.; Álvarez-Lobos, M.M.; Bueno, S.M. Impact of cigarette smoking on the gastrointestinal tract inflammation: Opposing effects in Crohn's disease and ulcerative colitis. *Front. Immunol.* **2018**, *9*, 74. [CrossRef]
3. Karczewski, J.; Poniedziałek, B.; Rzymski, P.; Rychlewska-Hańczewska, A.; Adamski, Z.; Wiktorowicz, K. The effect of cigarette smoking on the clinical course of inflammatory bowel disease. *Gastroenterol. Rev.* **2014**, *9*, 153–159. [CrossRef]
4. Pedersen, N.; Duricova, D.; Elkjaer, M.; Gamborg, M.; Munkholm, P.; Jess, T. Risk of Extra-Intestinal Cancer in Inflammatory Bowel Disease: Meta-Analysis of Population-Based Cohort Studies. *Am. J. Gastroenterol.* **2010**, *105*, 1480–1487. [CrossRef] [PubMed]
5. Gakis, G. The role of inflammation in bladder cancer. *Adv. Exp. Med. Biol.* **2014**, *816*, 183–196.

6. Bourrier, A.; Carrat, F.; Colombel, J.-F.; Bouvier, A.-M.; Abitbol, V.; Marteau, P.; Cosnes, J.; Simon, T.; Peyrin-Biroulet, L.; Beaugerie, L.; et al. Excess risk of urinary tract cancers in patients receiving thiopurines for inflammatory bowel disease: A prospective observational cohort study. *Aliment. Pharmacol. Ther.* **2016**, *43*, 252–261. [CrossRef] [PubMed]
7. Cumberbatch, M.G.K.; Jubber, I.; Black, P.C.; Esperto, F.; Figueroa, J.D.; Kamat, A.M.; Kiemeney, L.; Lotan, Y.; Pang, K.; Silverman, D.T.; et al. Epidemiology of Bladder Cancer: A Systematic Review and Contemporary Update of Risk Factors in 2018. *Eur. Urol.* **2018**, *74*, 784–795. [CrossRef]
8. Boffetta, P. Tobacco smoking and risk of bladder cancer. *Scand. J. Urol. Nephrol.* **2008**, *42*, 45–54. [CrossRef]
9. Persson, P.-G.; Karlén, P.; Bernell, O.; Leijonmarck, C.-E.; Broström, O.; Ahlbom, A.; Hellers, G. Crohn's disease and cancer: A population-based cohort study. *Gastroenterology* **1994**, *107*, 1675–1679. [CrossRef]
10. Jussila, A.; Virta, L.J.; Pukkala, E.; Färkkilä, M.A. Malignancies in patients with inflammatory bowel disease: A nationwide register study in Finland. *Scand. J. Gastroenterol.* **2013**, *48*, 1405–1413. [CrossRef]
11. Beaugerie, L.; Itzkowitz, S.H. Cancers Complicating Inflammatory Bowel Disease. *N. Engl. J. Med.* **2015**, *372*, 1441–1452. [CrossRef]
12. Biancone, L.; Armuzzi, A.; Scribano, M.L.; Castiglione, F.; D'Incà, R.; Orlando, A.; Papi, C.; Daperno, M.; Vecchi, M.; Riegler, G.; et al. Cancer Risk in Inflammatory Bowel Disease: A 6-Year Prospective Multicenter Nested Case-Control IG-IBD Study. *Inflamm. Bowel Dis.* **2020**, *26*, 450–459. [CrossRef]
13. Maaser, C.; Sturm, A.; Vavricka, S.R.; Kucharzik, T.; Fiorino, G.; Annese, V.; Calabrese, E.; Baumgart, D.C.; Bettenworth, D.; Borralho Nunes, P.; et al. ECCO-ESGAR guideline for diagnostic assessment in IBD part 1: Initial diagnosis, monitoring of known IBD, detection of complications. *J. Crohn's Colitis* **2019**, *13*, 144–164. [CrossRef]
14. Linee Guida Tumore Dell'urotelio. Available online: https://www.aiom.it/wp-content/uploads/2018/11/2018_LG_AIOM_Urotelio.pdf (accessed on 2 July 2021).
15. Kappelman, M.D.; Farkas, D.K.; Long, M.D.; Erichsen, R.; Sandler, R.S.; Sørensen, H.T.; Baron, J.A. Risk of Cancer in Patients With Inflammatory Bowel Diseases: A Nationwide Population-based Cohort Study With 30 Years of Follow-up Evaluation. *Clin. Gastroenterol. Hepatol.* **2014**, *12*, 265–273.e1. [CrossRef] [PubMed]
16. Madanchi, M.; Zeitz, J.; Barthel, C.; Samaras, P.; Scharl, S.; Sulz, M.C.; Biedermann, L.; Frei, P.; Vavricka, S.R.; Rogler, G.; et al. Malignancies in Patients with Inflammatory Bowel Disease: A Single-Centre Experience. *Digestion* **2016**, *94*, 1–8. [CrossRef] [PubMed]
17. Van den Heuvel, T.R.A.; Wintjens, D.S.J.; Jeuring, S.F.G.; Wassink, M.H.H.; Romberg-Camps, M.J.L.; Oostenbrug, L.E.; Sanduleanu, S.; Hameeteman, W.H.; Zeegers, M.P.; Masclee, A.A.; et al. Inflammatory bowel disease, cancer and medication: Cancer risk in the Dutch population-based IBDSL cohort. *Int. J. Cancer* **2016**, *139*, 1270–1280. [CrossRef] [PubMed]
18. Jess, T.; Horváth-Puhó, E.; Fallingborg, J.; Rasmussen, H.H.; Jacobsen, B.A. Cancer Risk in Inflammatory Bowel Disease According to Patient Phenotype and Treatment: A Danish Population-Based Cohort Study. *Am. J. Gastroenterol.* **2013**, *108*, 1869–1876. [CrossRef]
19. Dulai, P.S.; Sandborn, W.J.; Gupta, S. Colorectal Cancer and Dysplasia in Inflammatory Bowel Disease: A Review of Disease Epidemiology, Pathophysiology, and Management. *Cancer Prev. Res.* **2016**, *9*, 887–894. [CrossRef]
20. Carli, E.; Caviglia, G.; Pellicano, R.; Fagoonee, S.; Rizza, S.; Astegiano, M.; Saracco, G.; Ribaldone, D. Incidence of Prostate Cancer in Inflammatory Bowel Disease: A Meta-Analysis. *Medicina* **2020**, *56*, 285. [CrossRef] [PubMed]
21. Algaba, A.; Guerra, I.; Castaño, Á.; de la Poza, G.; Castellano, V.M.; López, M.; Bermejo, F. Risk of cancer, with special reference to extra-intestinal malignancies, in patients with inflammatory bowel disease. *World J. Gastroenterol.* **2013**, *19*, 9359–9365. [CrossRef] [PubMed]
22. Hemminki, K.; Li, X.; Sundquist, J.; Sundquist, K. Cancer risks in ulcerative colitis patients. *Int. J. Cancer* **2008**, *123*, 1417–1421. [CrossRef]
23. Hemminki, K.; Li, X.; Sundquist, J.; Sundquist, K. Cancer risks in Crohn disease patients. *Ann. Oncol.* **2009**, *20*, 574–580. [CrossRef]
24. Jung, Y.S.; Han, M.; Park, S.; Kim, W.H.; Cheon, J.H. Cancer Risk in the Early Stages of Inflammatory Bowel Disease in Korean Patients: A Nationwide Population-based Study. *J. Crohn's Coliti* **2017**, *11*, 954–962. [CrossRef]
25. Ekbom, A.; Helmick, C.; Zack, M.; Adami, H.-O. Extracolonic malignancies in inflammatory bowel disease. *Cancer* **1991**, *67*, 2015–2020. [CrossRef]
26. Mosher, C.A.; Brown, G.R.; Weideman, R.A.; Crook, T.W.; Cipher, D.J.; Spechler, S.J.; Feagins, L.A. Incidence of Colorectal Cancer and Extracolonic Cancers in Veteran Patients With Inflammatory Bowel Disease. *Inflamm. Bowel Dis.* **2018**, *24*, 617–623. [CrossRef]
27. Bernstein, C.N.; Blanchard, J.F.; Kliewer, E.; Wajda, A. Cancer risk in patients with inflammatory bowel disease: A population-based study. *Cancer* **2001**, *91*, 854–862. [CrossRef]
28. Reulen, R.C.; Kellen, E.; Buntinx, F.; Brinkman, M.; Zeegers, M. A meta-analysis on the association between bladder cancer and occupation. *Scand. J. Urol. Nephrol.* **2008**, *42*, 64–78. [CrossRef]
29. Zhang, C.; Liu, S.; Peng, L.; Wu, J.; Zeng, X.; Lu, Y.; Shen, H.; Luo, D. Does inflammatory bowel disease increase the risk of lower urinary tract tumors: A meta-analysis. *Transl. Androl. Urol.* **2021**, *10*, 164–173. [CrossRef]
30. Long, M.D.; Herfarth, H.H.; Pipkin, C.A.; Porter, C.Q.; Sandler, R.S.; Kappelman, M.D. Increased Risk for Non-Melanoma Skin Cancer in Patients With Inflammatory Bowel Disease. *Clin. Gastroenterol. Hepatol.* **2010**, *8*, 268–274. [CrossRef]

31. Lopez, A.; Mounier, M.; Bouvier, A.M.; Carrat, F.; Maynadié, M.; Beaugerie, L.; Peyrin-Biroulet, L. Increased risk of acute myeloid leukemias and myelodysplastic syndromes in patients who received thiopurine treatment for inflammatory bowel disease. *Clin. Gastroenterol. Hepatol.* **2014**, *12*, 1324–1329. [CrossRef]
32. Sands, B.E.; Grabert, S. Epidemiology of inflammatory bowel disease and overview of pathogenesis. *Med. Health R. I.* **2009**, *92*, 73–77.
33. Siegel, R.L.; Miller, K.D.; Jemal, A. Cancer statistics, 2020. *CA Cancer J. Clin.* **2020**, *70*, 7–30. [CrossRef] [PubMed]

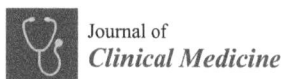

Article

Analysis on Microbial Profiles & Components of Bile in Patients with Recurrent CBD Stones after Endoscopic CBD Stone Removal: A Preliminary Study

Jung Wan Choe [1], Jae Min Lee [2], Jong Jin Hyun [1] and Hong Sik Lee [2,*]

[1] Department of Internal Medicine, Korea University Ansan Hospital, Ansan 15355, Korea; jwchoe@korea.ac.kr (J.W.C.); sean4h@korea.ac.kr (J.J.H.)
[2] Department of Internal Medicine, Korea University Anam Hospital, Seoul 02841, Korea; jmlee1202@gmail.com
* Correspondence: hslee60@korea.ac.kr

Abstract: Background/Aim: Common bile duct (CBD) stone recurrence after endoscopic treatment is a major concern as a late complication. Biliary bacterial factors and biochemical factors determine the path of gallstone formation. The aim of this preliminary study was to investigate the microbial profile and components of bile in patients with and without recurrent CBD stones after endoscopic CBD stone removal. Methods: Among patients who had undergone an initial endoscopic procedure for the removal of CBD stones and were followed up for >2 years, 11 patients who experienced at least two CBD stone recurrences, six months after endoscopic retrograde cholangiopancreatography (ERCP), were categorized into the recurrence group. Nine patients without CBD recurrence events were matched. Results: Polymicrobial infections are generally seen in all patients who have biliary sphincteroplasty. Microbial richness, measured by the numbers of operational taxonomic units (OTUs), was reduced in the recurrence group. The microbial evenness was also significantly lower than in the non-recurrence group. The overall microbial communities in the recurrence group deviated from the non-recurrence group. Infection with bacteria exhibiting β-glucuronidase activity was more frequent in the recurrence group, but there was no statistical significance. In an analysis of the bile components, the bile acid concentration was higher in the non-recurrence group than in the recurrence group. However, the other metabolites were not significantly different. Conclusions: Microbiota dysbiosis and altered bacterial community assembly in bile duct and decreased bile acid in bile juice were associated with recurrence of bile duct stone.

Keywords: gallstones; bile; microbiota; bile acids and salts

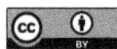

1. Introduction

Endoscopic stone removal by endoscopic retrograde cholangiopancreatography (ERCP) is the standard treatment for patients with cholangitis caused by common bile duct (CBD) stones. However, CBD stone recurrences after endoscopic stone removal is one of the most problematic late complications, with the rate ranging between 3% and 24% [1–3]. The recurred CBD stone could be a burden to both the individual's health and the social healthcare industry.

Many factors have been suggested to be associated with CBD stone recurrence. These factors include abnormal bile duct anatomy (e.g., dilated CBD diameter or sharp angulation of the CBD), retrograde infection from the duodenum with anatomical changes (e.g., periampullary diverticulum (PAD) and manipulated ampulla), altered bile biochemical composition, etc. [3]. Among them, the anatomical risk factors for recurrent CBD stones cannot be changed, whereas biliary bacterial factors and biochemical factors, including bile composition, may be correctable.

Many studies have suggested that different bacterial species and bile composition may augment the formation of recurrent CBD stones [4–6]. Despite the importance of microbial inhabitants of human bile in the pathologic condition, our current knowledge is limited to a few species of culturable bacteria that have been associated with CBD stones. However, as multiple microorganisms coexist in the biliary tract, culture-dependent methods are somewhat insensitive and biased for bacterial identification and are inadequate to study the entire microbial community [7,8]. In this regard, our understanding on the exact contribution of unculturable or difficult to culture bacteria in recurrent CBD stone formation is very limited. Indeed, only a minor fraction (0.1 to 10%) of the bacteria can be cultivated using standard techniques [9]. Recently, the application of next-generation sequencing (NGS) has provided a more comprehensive understanding of the bacterial community and expanded the microbiota detected in humans [10]. Utilizing NGS technology, a total of 3.8 million bacterial species could be discriminated with 16S rRNA sequences discovered from previously collected data and published studies [11]. Unlike conventional methods for identifying microorganisms, NGS provides a comprehensive picture of the unculturable or difficult to culture bacteria by employing bacterial universal primers. The use of this method for the detection and differentiation of bacterial species could increase our understanding on the role of these bacteria and the manner of their pathogenesis in diseases. Nevertheless, there have been few such investigations that have looked into the biliary microbiome. In addition to the importance of microbiome in CBD stone recurrence, the role of bile composition has also not been fully elucidated.

Therefore, this study was carried out to investigate the bacterial communities in bile using NGS and to analyze the metabolic components of bile to elucidate the role of microbiota and bile components in CBD stone recurrence.

2. Materials and Methods

2.1. Patients and Bile Sample Collection

Patients who have been followed-up for at least 2 years after index CBD stone removal and had at least one of the high-risk factors for CBD stone recurrence were included in this study. High-risk factors for CBD stone recurrence were as follows: maximum CBD diameter > 15 mm, CBD angle ≤ 145°, and the presence of periampullary diverticulum (PAD) [12]. Patients included in this study had undergone cholecystectomy at the time of index ERCP since they presented with both GB and CBD stones. These patients were divided up into two groups according to the history of CBD stone recurrence. Patients who belonged to the recurrence group were those who had at least 2 episodes of recurrences during the follow-up period. The non-recurrence group was defined as those who had no recurrence event during the follow-up period. A recurred CBD stone was defined as a particle with a diameter greater than 3 mm which took on the shape of a stone. CBD stones that were found and removed within 6 months after index ERCP were not considered as recurrent stones but as residual stones due to incomplete CBD stone clearance. Only those detected after 6 months following endoscopic CBD stone removal were regarded as recurrent stones [3]. Of the aforementioned patients, 20 who agreed to undergo surveillance endoscopic retrograde cholangiopancreatography (ERCP) procedures to check for CBD stone recurrence were enrolled. All patients were asymptomatic at the time of surveillance ERCP without clinical evidence of biliary tract infection, and had not taken antibiotics nor proton pump inhibitors for at least 3 months prior to bile sample collection.

From these 20 subjects, a total of 20 bile samples (11 from the CBD stone recurrence group and 9 from the non-recurrence group) were collected during scheduled surveillance ERCP from September 2018 to August 2019. After advancing the side-viewing endoscopes (TJF240/JF-260V; Olympus Optical, Tokyo, Japan) into the duodenum 2nd portion and facing the papilla enface, the cannulation catheter was passed through the working channel and inserted into the CBD through the manipulated ampulla. Two to five milliliters of the patients' bile aspirates from bile duct were sucked out via the catheter before the injection of contrast agent for ERCP procedure. A portion of the sample was stored at −80 °C for NGS analysis and the remainder was stored at room temperature for analysis of bile juice components. Afterwards, dye was injected to evaluate for the presence of CBD stones and removed when present. CBD stones were broadly classified as being cholesterol or pigment stones (black or brown) based on their characteristic external appearance by gross inspection [13], and all recurred CBD stones were brown pigment stones.

This study was approved by the Institutional Review Board of Korea University Ansan Hospital (No. 2018AS0208) and the research was conducted in accordance with the Declaration of Helsinki. All patients provided written informed consent upon enrollment.

2.2. Next-Generation Sequencing of Bacterial 16s rRNA Fragments in Bile Samples

To analyze the bacterial community, the V3/V4 regions of the 16S rRNA gene of DNA extracted from the bile samples were amplified, sequenced, and analyzed. The extraction method for bacterial DNA was performed by using a PowerMax Soil DNA Isolation Kit (MO BIO). Each sequenced sample was prepared according to the Illumina 16S Metagenomic Sequencing Library protocols to amplify the V3 and V4 regions (519F-806R). The DNA quality was measured by PicoGreen and NanoDrop. Input genomic DNA (10 ng) was PCR amplified. The barcoded fusion primer sequences used for amplifications were as follows: 341F: 5′ CCTACGGGNGGCWGCAG 3′, and 806R: 5′ GACTACHVGGGTATC-TAATCC 3′ containing forward overhang adapter pair. The final purified product was then quantified using qPCR according to the qPCR Quantification Protocol Guide (KAPA Library Quantification kits for Illumina Sequencing platforms) and qualified using the LabChip GX HT DNA High Sensitivity Kit (PerkinElmer, MA, USA). Then, the paired-end (2×300 bp) sequencing was performed by the Macrogen using the MiSeq™ platform (Illumina, San Diego, CA, USA).

The operational taxonomic units (OTUs) were generated to calculate the number of microbial species in the bile. In order to compare the bacterial community richness of bile between the two groups, observed OTU-based analyses (OTU richness and Chao 1) were performed. OTU richness is the number of bacterial species observed in each individual sample. Chao 1 represents species richness estimators of the expected OTUs present in a group. As Chao 1 measures OTUs expected in samples, given all the bacterial species that were identified in the samples, Chao1 gives more weight to the low abundance species. To determine α-diversity, the Shannon diversity index and the inverse Simpson index were used. The Shannon diversity index is a quantitative measure that shows how evenly the basic individuals are distributed by taking into account and reflecting the number of different species in each sample; a high Shannon diversity index signifies evenness, whereas a low Shannon diversity index denotes unevenness. The Simpson index measures the degree of concentration or dominance of certain species in a sample. Therefore, the inverse Simpson index is an indicator of how evenly the species are distributed; a high inverse Simpson index implies evenness or a lack of dominance, and a low inverse Simpson index suggests unevenness or the presence of dominance. Evaluation of β-diversity, which analyzes community similarity, was performed by calculating pairwise distances using the phylogenetic metric UniFrac.

2.3. Composition of Bile

The bile samples were analyzed for composition of bile, including electrolyte, total bilirubin, total bile acid, cholesterol, phosphorus and Ca^{2+}. Total bilirubin concentration was measured in aliquot on a Cobas 8000 C702 (Roche Diagnostics System, Switzerland). pH, sodium, potassium, chloride, phosphorus, and calcium estimations were carried out on a cobas 8000 ISE (Roche Diagnostics System, Switzerland) using an ion-selective electrode method. For measuring cholesterol and triglycerides, bile was diluted one to five times with methanol and the protein precipitate was removed by centrifugation. The methanol was then evaporated and the residue was taken for analysis. The cholesterol and triglycerides were analyzed by photometric analysis on a Cobas 8000 C702 (Roche Diagnostics System, Switzerland). Total bile acids were also measured with an enzymatic method on a Roche cobas 8000 C702 analyser.

2.4. Statistical Analysis

Statistical analyses were performed using IBM SPSS Statistics version 20.0 (IBM, Armonk, NY, USA). The continuous variables were compared using the Student's t-test. Fisher's exact test was used to analyze the categorical variables. The sequences generated from pyrosequencing were analyzed with variable software for pre-processing (quality-adjustment, barcode split), identification of OTUs, taxonomic assignment, community comparison, and statistical analysis. The FASTP program was used to remove the adapter sequence, and error-correction was performed for areas where the two reads overlap. The paired-end data, separated by each sample, was assembled in one sequence using FLASH (v. 1.2.11). To ensure that any subsequent analysis was highly accurate, sequences shorter than 400 bp were discarded. By using CD-HIT-OTU, after removing the low-quality sequence, ambiguous reads, chimera reads, etc., which are based on errors, the filtered reads were clustered by identity as OTUs at 97% similarity. The representative sequence of each OTU was performed by BALSTN (v. 2.4.0) to the NCBI 16S Microbial DB, performing a taxonomic assignment with the organism information of the most similar subject. The taxonomy is not assigned if the query coverage and identity score matched to the reference are less than 85%. Community diversity was estimated by using the Shannon and inversed Simpson indexes. The weighted UniFrac distance method was used to perform a principal coordinates analysis (PCoA), and trees were built by the unweighted-pair group method with arithmetic mean (UPGMA).

3. Results

3.1. Baseline Characteristics

The mean age of the patients was 62.3 ± 16.6 years (range, 29 to 83 years) and 9 (45.0%) patients were female. The anatomical risk factors for recurrent CBD stones, including CBD diameter, presence of PAD, and angulation of the bile duct $\leq 145°$, were not statistically different between the two groups (Table 1).

Table 1. Baseline characteristics.

	Recurrence Group (N = 11)	Non-Recurrence Group (N = 9)	p-Value
Age, median years (min-max)	62 (32–78)	63 (29–83)	0.12
Gender, male (%)	6 (66.6)	5 (62.5)	0.45
BMI, median kg/m² (min-max)	22.6 (17.6–29.0)	22.5 (16.2–29.4)	0.45
CBD diameter (mm, mean ± SD)	17.7 ± 2.5	17.8 ± 2.2	0.89
Angulation of bile duct ($\leq 145°$) (N, %)	1 (11.1)	0	0.85
PAD (N, %)			0.20
I	2	1	
II	5	4	
III	2	3	

CBD, common bile duct; BMI, body mass index; PAD, periampullary diverticulum.

3.2. Richness of Microbiota in Bile

A total of 303 bacterial species were identified from 20 bile samples. The average OTU, obtained by calculating the mean values after counting the number of observed OTUs in each sample, was reduced in the 11 individuals with CBD stone recurrence compared to the 9 with non-recurrence (29.6 ± 3.6 vs. 60.4 ± 11.6, p = 0.0005, Wilcoxon rank-sum test; Figure 1a). The expected total number of OTUs for each group, as estimated by the Chao1 estimator, was also considerably lower in the recurrence group than in the non-recurrence group (29.8 ± 3.5 vs. 60.5 ± 11.6, p = 0.005, Wilcoxon rank-sum test; Figure 1b).

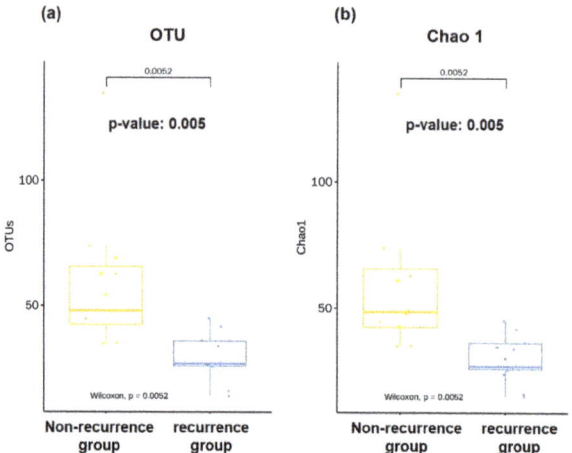

Figure 1. Comparison on richness of microbiota in bile. Microbiota richness, represented as the number of (**a**) observed operational taxonomic units (OTU) and (**b**) Chao 1, was reduced in the recurrent CBD stone group ($n = 11$) compared with the non-recurrence group ($n = 9$).

3.3. Diversities of Microbiota in Bile

The α-diversities of bile samples, as measured by the Shannon diversity index and the inverse Simpson index, were significantly lower in the recurrence group than those of the non-recurrence group samples. The Shannon index, which reflects equal microbial proportional abundance in a species, was lower in the recurrence group compared to the non-recurrence group (0.65 ± 0.36 vs. 3.12 ± 0.45, $p = 0.027$, Figure 2a), signifying that microbial proportional abundance was uneven in the recurrence group. The inverse Simpson index, which is another way of quantifying the evenness of a species, was also lower in the recurrence group compared to the non-recurrence group (0.46 ± 0.10 vs. 0.75 ± 0.06, $p = 0.036$, Figure 2b), meaning that certain species were more dominant than other species in the recurrence group. According to the Shannon index and inverse Simpson index, the diversity index was statistically higher in the bile of the non-recurrence group than that obtained in the patients with recurrent CBD stones.

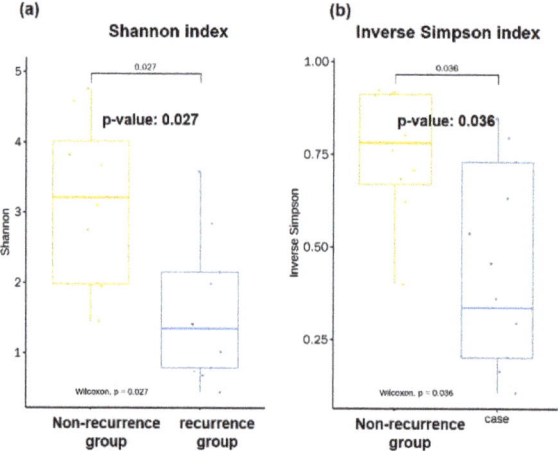

Figure 2. Comparison on evenness and dominance of microbiota in bile. Mean α-diversity, measured by (**a**) Shannon index and (**b**) inverse Simpson index, was reduced in the CBD stone recurrence group compared to the non-recurrence group.

3.4. Microbial Community Similarity

The unweighted UniFrac distance metric, which measures the similarity in the microbial communities of the bile samples (β-diversity), revealed an overall microbial composition difference between the two groups (unweighted UniFrac, PERMANOVAR, pseudo-F: 1.655, $p = 0.05$, Figure 3). This result indicates that the microbiome clustering in the recurrence group was different from that of the non-recurrence group.

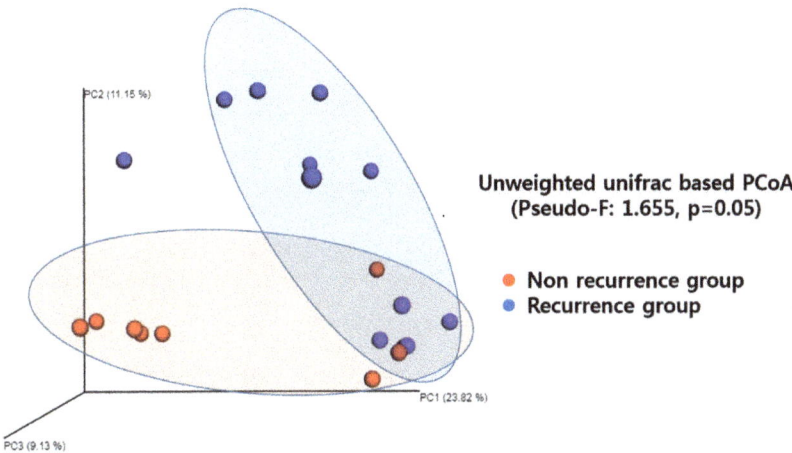

Figure 3. Comparison on community similarity. The unweighted uniFrac distance metric shows difference in microbial communities between the non-recurrence group and recurrence group.

3.5. Microbiome

At the phylum level, Bacteroidetes spp. were significantly decreased in the recurrence group, whereas Actinobacteria and Firmicutes spp. were over-represented in the recurrence group relative to the non-recurrence group (Table 2). At the genus level, three bacterial taxa displayed significantly different abundance between the recurrence group and the non-recurrence group. The three genera, *Neisseria*, *Capnocytophaga*, and *Gemella*, were enriched in the non-recurrence group. Conversely, *E. coli*, *Enterococcus* spp., *Klebsiella* spp., *Acinetobacter* spp., *Streptococcus* spp., and *Staphylococcus*, which exert β-glucuronidase activity, were more frequent in the recurrence group, even though there was no statistical difference (Table 3).

Table 2. List and relative proportion of phylum identified by next-generation sequencing.

Phylum	Recurrence Group		Non-Recurrence Group		*p*-Value
	Mean Proportion	SEM	Mean Proportion	SEM	
Euryarchaeota	<0.001	<0.001	0.001	0.001	0.345
Actinobacteria	0.024	0.005	0.009	0.003	0.048
Bacteroidetes	0.074	0.045	0.188	0.066	0.042
Chloroflexi	<0.001	<0.001	0.002	0.003	0.345
Cyanobacteria	0.001	0.002	<0.001	<0.001	0.084
Deinococcus	<0.001	<0.001	0.001	0.001	0.346
Firmicutes	0.384	0.105	0.178	0.027	0.038
Fusobacteria	0.009	0.006	0.021	0.017	0.311
Gemmatimonadetes	<0.001	<0.001	0.001	0.001	0.345
Proteobacteria	0.504	0.121	0.568	0.094	0.814
Spirochaetes	<0.001	<0.001	0.001	0.001	0.345
Synergistetes	<0.001	<0.001	0.008	0.008	0.409
Tenericutes	<0.001	<0.001	<0.001	<0.001	0.999
Unassigned	0.001	<0.001	0.017	0.013	0.411

SEM, standard error of the mean.

Table 3. List and relative proportion of genus identified by next-generation sequencing.

Genus	Recurrence Group		Non-Recurrence Group		p-Value
	Mean Proportion	SEM	Mean Proportion	SEM	
Neisseria	0.001	0.001	0.162	0.021	0.008
Capnocytophaga	0.001	0.001	0.137	0.004	0.025
Gemella	<0.001	<0.001	0.075	0.003	0.041
Rothia	<0.001	<0.001	0.003	0.001	0.052
Haemophilus	0.041	0.011	0.046	0.033	0.075
Streptococcus	0.132	0.102	0.029	0.009	0.091
Klebsiella	0.134	0.049	0.049	0.026	0.162
Enterococcus	0.033	0.006	0.006	0.003	0.191
Clostridium	0.044	0.029	0.059	0.029	0.201
Pseudomonas	0.081	0.023	0.073	0.048	0.746
Staphylococcus	0.003	0.002	0.002	0.001	0.807
Acinetobacter	0.002	0.001	0.001	0.001	0.957
Lactobacillus	0.034	0.034	0.001	0.001	0.999
Citrobacter	0.163	0.126	0.014	0.009	0.999
Escherichia	0.320	0.123	0.282	0.107	0.999
Aeromonas	0.001	0.001	0.007	0.006	0.473
Fusobacterium	0.009	0.007	0.028	0.018	0.245
Unassigned	0.001	<0.001	0.017	0.013	0.411

SEM, standard error of the mean.

3.6. Bile Composition

Bile acid concentration was higher in the non-recurrence group than in the recurrence group (254.51 ± 82.0 mmol/L vs. 147.1 ± 64.2 mmol/L, $p < 0.01$). Neither the pH values nor Ca^{2+} showed statistical differences between the bile samples of both groups (Table 4).

Table 4. Bile metabolic profile.

	Recurrence Group (N = 11)	Non-Recurrence Group (N = 9)	p-Value
pH	7.8 ± 0.2	7.95 ± 0.4	0.85
Total nucleated cell count	12 ± 5	22 ± 10.4	0.07
Total bilirubin (mg/dL)	37.5 ± 63.5	27.7 ± 80.7	0.85
Cholesterol (mg/dL)	28.1 ± 50.7	34.2 ± 62.1	0.32
Bile acid (mmol/L)	147.1 ± 64.2	254.5 ± 82.0	<0.01
Phospholipid (mg/dL)	324 ± 272	454 ± 350	0.25
Ca^{2+} (mg/dL)	7.7 ± 4.4	5.5 ± 2.2	0.65

CBD, common bile duct.

4. Discussion

In the present study, 16S rRNA gene profiling analysis using NGS allowed us to observe the difference in bile microbiota composition between the CBD stone recurrence group and the non-recurrence group. Although the sample size (N = 20) might not be large enough to generalize the results, the two groups significantly differed in terms of richness and evenness in this preliminary study. The number of species was decreased and the dominance of certain species was present in the bile samples of the recurrence group. On the other hand, all types of species were equally abundant, with no specific species being predominant in the bile samples of the non-recurrence group. In addition, the difference in species composition and clustering between the two groups were also shown.

Recent progress in understanding the symbiosis of human microbiota revealed an important role in immune homeostasis [14,15]. A balance of these commensal microbial species is probably required to prevent infection with pathogens and pathological inflammation. However, this dynamic equilibrium can be altered at any time by environmental factors and external interferences. These microbial alterations and imbalances with decreased richness and diversity in the pathologic condition group is a phenomenon called dysbiosis [16]. There is increasing evidence that the dysbiosis of a microbiome is linked to many gastrointestinal and systemic diseases. An experimental study reported that chemical- and pathogen-induced intestinal inflammation resulted in the loss of microbial density and diversity and led to the proliferation of Gram-negative bacteria which possess β-glucuronidase activity in the intestine [17]. A balance of the microbial species in bile is probably also required to prevent infection with pathogens and pathological inflammation related to the formation of gallstones [10]. Thus, it could be speculated that bacterial dysbiosis with the loss of microbial richness and diversity in bile could lead to inflammation of the bile duct, in favor of biofilm formation with resultant proliferation of bacteria with β-glucuronidase activity. In fact, a notable dysbiosis of the bile microbiome, including decreased richness and diversity in the bile of the recurrence group, was found in the current study. Furthermore, the finding that *E. coli*, *Enterococcus* spp., *Klebsiella* spp., *Pseudomonas* spp., *Acinetobacter* spp., *Streptococcus* spp., and *Staphylococcus*, which exert β-glucuronidase activity, were more frequent in the recurrence group additionally supports the validity of the speculation of this study.

Whereas the abovementioned bacteria were more frequently found in the recurrence group, bacteria in the genera *Neisseria*, *Gemella*, and *Capnocytophaga* were expressed more frequently in the non-recurrence group. All of these three bacteria are part of the normal oral flora associated with periodontitis and dental plaque [18]. There is very little information about the possible clinical significance on the protective role of these bacteria in the formation of biliary stones. Further studies using molecular techniques will be needed and may provide new insights into the pathophysiology of bile duct stone formation and the involvement of microbes or their metabolites in this process.

In addition to differences in the microbiome, the bile component analysis also showed that the two groups had different metabolic profiles with respect to bile acid. Bile acids act as detergents and have an important role in solubilizing dietary lipids and fat-soluble vitamins to facilitate their absorption in the small intestine [19]. Previous studies have shown that decreased concentration of bile salts in the bile diminishes the micellar solubilization of bilirubin, as well as cholesterol, favoring the formation of brown pigment stones [20,21]. In addition to their role in the digestion of lipids, bile acids generally inhibit bacterial growth in the small intestine as a major regulator of the gut microbiota, and prevent retrograde bacterial infections in the CBD [22]. Bile acids themselves can also modulate the composition of the microbiota in the bile duct, directly or indirectly, through the activation of the innate immune system [23,24]. Inflammation in the bile duct could induce oxidative stress in harmful microbiomes, which is related to the formation of gallstones through specific enzymatic activities or the production of biofilm [25,26]. Conversely, other studies have shown that gut microbiota has profound effects on bile acid metabolism and secondary bile acid production [27,28]. The alteration of gut microbiome could change the composition of the bile acid pool with the regulation of secondary bile acid metabolism and inhibition of bile acid synthesis by alleviating FXR inhibition in the ileum [28,29]. Since it seems to be a chicken-and-egg question, to further explore the bile acid functionality, study on the bile acid-bacteria-host interplay at the pathway level would be necessary.

The strength of this study is that microbiological identification of unculturable or difficult to culture bacteria was enhanced using recent advancements in NGS. However, there have been few extensive NGS-based research studies on bile samples. While a recent study focused on the relationships among gut microbiota, bile acids, and cytokines in blood and stool samples of patients with cholangiocarcinoma [30], our study revealed the complexity and specificity of the biliary microecology and metabolites in bile samples of patients with recurrent CBD stones. Therefore, in addition to gaining a better understanding of the disease processes of pathogens, the knowledge gained from this bile research may ultimately lead to the design of new antimicrobial treatments or assist in the development of improved probiotic strains and supplementation of bile acid composition in the future.

Although the abovementioned investigations attempted to provide a comprehensive insight into the potential contribution of the microbiome and metabolic component in bile related to CBD stone recurrence, several limitations need to be addressed. First, aspirated bile samples contain floating bacterial species but cannot detect sessile bacterial populations adhering to the mucosa or those residing in the biofilm. However, since a study demonstrated that bacteria in the bile fluid almost always coincided with the presence of bacteria on the bile duct wall [31], bacteria species floating in bile may sufficiently reflect the total microbial environment of biliary tract. Nevertheless, additional bile duct tissue biopsies can be expected to reveal more accurate microbial communities in the CBD. Second, despite the fact that this study elucidated aspects of the richness and diversity of the biliary microbiota related to recurrent CBD stones by 16S sequencing, a more comprehensive understanding of biliary bacterial function and the microbe–host interaction would require further investigation by methods such as whole-metagenome shotgun sequencing, metatranscriptomic, metametabolomic, and metaproteomic technologies. Third, even though a specific profile of bile salts and their concentrations appear to be key factors in lithogenic potency, exploration on the composition of individual bile salts in the bile was not performed in this study.

In conclusion, polymicrobial infections were seen in all study subjects who underwent ampullary manipulations during ERCP. The patients with recurrent CBD stones showed microbial dysbiosis with a significant reduction in microbial richness and diversity in the bile. The bile composition was also dissimilar between the two groups. A significant difference in the concentration of bile acid was also found between the recurrence group and non-recurrence group. Although the results of this study are preliminary in nature and require confirmation, microbiota dysbiosis and altered bacterial community assembly in bile duct, and decreased bile acid, were associated with recurrence of bile duct stones.

Author Contributions: Each author has been involved in and contributed to this manuscript. Conceptualization, J.W.C. and H.S.L.; Data curation, J.W.C. and J.J.H.; Formal analysis, J.W.C.; Writing—original draft, J.W.C.; Writing—review & editing, J.M.L., J.J.H. and H.S.L. All authors have read and agreed to the published version of the manuscript.

Funding: This research received no external funding.

Institutional Review Board Statement: The study was conducted according to the guidelines of the Declaration of Helsinki, and approved by the Institutional Review Board of Korea University Ansan Hospital (IRB number: 2018AS0208, 8 August 2018).

Informed Consent Statement: Informed consent was obtained from all subjects involved in the study.

Data Availability Statement: The data presented in this study are available on request from the corresponding author.

Acknowledgments: This study was supported by the National Research Foundation of Korea (NRF) grant funded by the Korean government (MSIT) (No. 2019R1C1C1003661).

Conflicts of Interest: The authors declare no conflict of interest.

References

1. Lai, K.H.; Peng, N.J.; Lo, G.H.; Cheng, J.S.; Huang, R.L.; Lin, C.K.; Huang, J.S.; Chiang, H.T.; Ger, L.P. Prediction of recurrent choledocholithiasis by quantitative cholescintigraphy in patients after endoscopic sphincterotomy. *Gut* **1997**, *41*, 399–403. [CrossRef]
2. Ikeda, S.; Tanaka, M.; Matsumoto, S.; Yoshimoto, H.; Itoh, H. Endoscopic sphincterotomy: Long-term results in 408 patients with complete follow-up. *Endoscopy* **1988**, *20*, 13–17. [CrossRef] [PubMed]
3. Cheon, Y.K.; Lehman, G.A. Identification of risk factors for stone recurrence after endoscopic treatment of bile duct stones. *Eur. J. Gastroenterol. Hepatol.* **2006**, *18*, 461–464. [CrossRef] [PubMed]
4. Swidsinski, A.; Lee, S.P. The role of bacteria in gallstone pathogenesis. *Front. Biosci.* **2001**, *6*, E93–E103. [CrossRef] [PubMed]
5. Stewart, L.; Grifiss, J.M.; Jarvis, G.A.; Way, L.W. Biliary bacterial factors determine the path of gallstone formation. *Am. J. Surg.* **2006**, *192*, 598–603. [CrossRef]
6. Maki, T. Pathogenesis of calcium bilirubinate gallstone: Role of *E. coli*, beta-glucuronidase and coagulation by inorganic ions, polyelectrolytes and agitation. *Ann. Surg.* **1966**, *164*, 90–100. [CrossRef]

7. Kaufman, H.S.; Magnuson, T.H.; Lillemoe, K.D.; Frasca, P.; Pitt, H.A. The role of bacteria in gallbladder and common duct stone formation. *Ann. Surg.* **1989**, *209*, 584–591. [CrossRef]
8. Theron, J.; Cloete, T.E. Molecular techniques for determining microbial diversity and community structure in natural environments. *Crit. Rev. Microbiol.* **2000**, *26*, 37–57. [CrossRef]
9. Amann, R.I.; Ludwig, W.; Schleifer, K.H. Phylogenetic Identification and in-Situ Detection of Individual Microbial-Cells without Cultivation. *Microbiol. Rev.* **1995**, *59*, 143–169. [CrossRef]
10. Wu, T.; Zhang, Z.; Liu, B.; Hou, D.; Liang, Y.; Zhang, J.; Shi, P. Gut microbiota dysbiosis and bacterial community assembly associated with cholesterol gallstones in large-scale study. *BMC Genom.* **2013**, *14*, 669. [CrossRef]
11. Lagier, J.C.; Armougom, F.; Million, M.; Hugon, P.; Pagnier, I.; Robert, C.; Bittar, F.; Fournous, G.; Gimenez, G.; Maraninchi, M.J.C.M.; et al. Microbial culturomics: Paradigm shift in the human gut microbiome study. *Clin. Microbiol. Infect.* **2012**, *18*, 1185–1193. [CrossRef]
12. Keizman, D.; Shalom, M.I.; Konikoff, F.M. An angulated common bile duct predisposes to recurrent symptomatic bile duct stones after endoscopic stone extraction. *Surg. Endosc.* **2006**, *20*, 1594–1599. [CrossRef]
13. Trotman, B.W.; Soloway, R.D. Pigment gallstone disease: Summary of the National Institutes of Health–international workshop. *Hepatology* **1982**, *2*, 879–884. [CrossRef]
14. Rooks, M.G.; Garrett, W.S. Gut microbiota, metabolites and host immunity. *Nat. Rev. Immunol.* **2016**, *16*, 341–352. [CrossRef] [PubMed]
15. Marchesi, J.R.; Adams, D.H.; Fava, F.; Hermes, G.D.; Hirschfield, G.M.; Hold, G.; Quraishi, M.N.; Kinross, J.; Smidt, H.; Tuohy, K.M.; et al. The gut microbiota and host health: A new clinical frontier. *Gut* **2016**, *65*, 330–339. [CrossRef] [PubMed]
16. Carding, S.; Verbeke, K.; Vipond, D.T.; Corfe, B.M.; Owen, L.J. Dysbiosis of the gut microbiota in disease. *Microb. Ecol. Health Dis.* **2015**, *26*, 26191. [CrossRef] [PubMed]
17. Lupp, C.; Robertson, M.L.; Wickham, M.E.; Sekirov, I.; Champion, O.L.; Gaynor, E.C.; Finlay, B.B. Host-mediated inflammation disrupts the intestinal microbiota and promotes the overgrowth of Enterobacteriaceae. *Cell Host Microbe* **2007**, *2*, 204. [CrossRef]
18. Lion, C.; Escande, F.; Burdin, J.C. Capnocytophaga canimorsus infections in human: Review of the literature and cases report. *Eur. J. Epidemiol.* **1996**, *12*, 521–533. [CrossRef]
19. Hofmann, A.F. The continuing importance of bile acids in liver and intestinal disease. *Arch. Intern. Med.* **1999**, *159*, 2647–2658. [CrossRef]
20. Akiyoshi, T.; Nakayama, F. Bile acid composition in brown pigment stones. *Dig Dis Sci.* **1990**, *35*, 27–32. [CrossRef]
21. Onochi, S.; Masu, A.; Takahashi, W.; Suzuki, N. Study on bile acid and lipid of gallbladder bile and gallstone in cases with calcium bilirubinate stones. *Nihon Shokakibyo Gakkai Zasshi Jpn. J. Gastro-Enterol.* **1984**, *81*, 2552–2560.
22. Lorenzo-Zuniga, V.; Bartoli, R.; Planas, R.; Hofmann, A.F.; Vinado, B.; Hagey, L.R.; Hernandez, J.M.; Mane, J.; Alvarez, M.A.; Ausina, V.; et al. Oral bile acids reduce bacterial overgrowth, bacterial translocation, and endotoxemia in cirrhotic rats. *Hepatology* **2003**, *37*, 551–557. [CrossRef]
23. Wahlstrom, A.; Sayin, S.I.; Marschall, H.U.; Backhed, F. Intestinal Crosstalk between Bile Acids and Microbiota and Its Impact on Host Metabolism. *Cell Metab.* **2016**, *24*, 41–50. [CrossRef] [PubMed]
24. Ridlon, J.M.; Kang, D.J.; Hylemon, P.B.; Bajaj, J.S. Bile acids and the gut microbiome. *Curr. Opin. Gastroenterol.* **2014**, *30*, 332–338. [CrossRef] [PubMed]
25. Hoogerwerf, W.A.; Soloway, R.D. Gallstones. *Curr. Opin. Gastroenterol.* **1999**, *15*, 442–447. [CrossRef]
26. Vitetta, L.; Best, S.P.; Sali, A. Single and multiple cholesterol gallstones and the influence of bacteria. *Med. Hypotheses* **2000**, *55*, 502–506. [CrossRef] [PubMed]
27. Ramírez-Pérez, O.; Cruz-Ramón, V.; Chinchilla-López, P.; Méndez-Sánchez, N. The Role of the Gut Microbiota in Bile Acid Metabolism. *Ann. Hepatol.* **2017**, *16*, s15–s20. [CrossRef]
28. Sayin, S.I.; Wahlstrom, A.; Felin, J.; Jantti, S.; Marschall, H.U.; Bamberg, K.; Angelin, B.; Hyotylainen, T.; Oresic, M.; Backhed, F. Gut microbiota regulates bile acid metabolism by reducing the levels of tauro-beta-muricholic acid, a naturally occurring FXR antagonist. *Cell Metab.* **2013**, *17*, 225–235. [CrossRef]
29. Islam, K.S.; Fukiya, S.; Hagio, M.; Fujii, N.; Ishizuka, S.; Ooka, T.; Ogura, Y.; Hayashi, T.; Yokota, A.J.G. Bile acid is a host factor that regulates the composition of the cecal microbiota in rats. *Gastroenterology* **2011**, *141*, 1773–1781. [CrossRef]
30. Jia, X.; Lu, S.; Zeng, Z.; Liu, Q.; Dong, Z.; Chen, Y.; Zhu, Z.; Hong, Z.; Zhang, T.; Du, G.; et al. Characterization of Gut Microbiota, Bile Acid Metabolism, and Cytokines in Intrahepatic Cholangiocarcinoma. *Hepatology* **2020**, *71*, 893–906. [CrossRef]
31. Hancke, E.; Nusche, A.; Marklein, G. Bacteria in the gallbladder wall and gallstones–indications for cholecystectomy. *Langenbecks Arch. Chir.* **1986**, *368*, 249–254. [CrossRef] [PubMed]

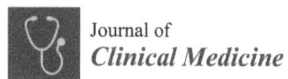

Article

Usefulness of a Hepatitis B Surface Antigen-Based Model for the Prediction of Functional Cure in Patients with Chronic Hepatitis B Virus Infection Treated with Nucleos(t)ide Analogues: A Real-World Study

Gian Paolo Caviglia [1,*], Yulia Troshina [1], Enrico Garro [1], Marcantonio Gesualdo [1], Serena Aneli [1,2], Giovanni Birolo [1], Fabrizia Pittaluga [3], Rossana Cavallo [3], Giorgio Maria Saracco [1,4] and Alessia Ciancio [1,4,*]

1. Department of Medical Sciences, University of Torino, 10123 Turin, Italy; yulia.troshina@unito.it (Y.T.); enrico.garro@edu.unito.it (E.G.); marcantonio.gesualdo@unito.it (M.G.); serena.aneli@unito.it (S.A.); giovanni.birolo@unito.it (G.B.); giorgiomaria.saracco@unito.it (G.M.S.)
2. Department of Biology, University of Padua, 35122 Padova, Italy
3. Microbiology Unit, A.O.U. Città della Salute e della Scienza, 10126 Torino, Italy; fpittaluga@cittadellasalute.to.it (F.P.); rossana.cavallo@unito.it (R.C.)
4. Gastroenterology Unit, A.O.U. Città della Salute e della Scienza, 10126 Torino, Italy
* Correspondence: gianpaolo.caviglia@unito.it (G.P.C.); alessia.ciancio@unito.it (A.C.); Tel.: +39-11-633-3532 (G.P.C.)

Abstract: In patients with chronic hepatitis B (CHB) under long-term treatment with nucleos(t)ide analogues (NAs), the loss of hepatitis B surface antigen (HBsAg) is a rare event. A growing body of evidence supports the use of quantitative HBsAg for the prediction of functional cure, although these results are mainly derived from studies performed on Asian patients with hepatitis B e antigen (HBeAg)-positive CHB. Here, we investigated the clinical role of quantitative HBsAg in a real-life cohort of CHB patients under treatment with NAs in a tertiary care center from North-West Italy. A total of 101 CHB patients (HBeAg-negative, $n = 86$) undergoing NAs treatment were retrospectively enrolled. HBsAg was measured at baseline (T0), 6 months (T1), 12 months (T2) and at the last follow-up (FU). Median FU was 5.5 (3.2–8.3) years; at the end of FU, 11 patients lost the HBsAg (annual incidence rate = 1.8%). Baseline HBsAg levels were significantly different between patients with no HBsAg loss and those achieving a functional cure (3.46, 2.91–3.97 vs. 1.11, 0.45–1.98 Log IU/mL, $p < 0.001$). Similarly, the HBsAg decline (Δ) from T0 to T2 was significantly different between the two groups of patients (0.05, −0.04–0.13, vs. 0.38, 0.11–0.80 Log IU/mL, $p = 0.002$). By stratified cross-validation analysis, the combination of baseline HBsAg and ΔHBsAg T0–T2 showed an excellent accuracy for the prediction of HBsAg loss (C statistic = 0.966). These results corroborate the usefulness of quantitative HBsAg in Caucasian CHB patients treated with antivirals for the prediction of HBsAg seroclearance.

Keywords: antiviral therapy; biomarker; chronic liver disease; HBsAg; HBV

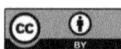

1. Introduction

Hepatitis B virus (HBV) infection is a major health problem [1]. Globally, 257 million people are chronically infected with the virus (estimated prevalence: 3.7%) [2]. However, the epidemiological scenario varies greatly across different geographic regions, mainly due to different socioeconomic conditions and an uneven vaccination coverage [3,4]. In Italy, the prevalence of chronic HBV infection progressively declined in native Italians since the implementation of compulsory vaccination in 1991 [5]. It has then remained stable due to the input of new infections brought by HBV-infected immigrants [6,7]. To date, the clinical presentation of CHB shifted toward older ages and more severe diseases [8].

Therapeutic strategies for CHB include finite treatment with pegylated-interferon (PEG-IFN) and indefinite treatment with nucleos(t)ide analogues (NAs) [9]; the latter allows an effective suppression of viral replication, normalization of alanine aminotransferase (ALT) and thus the prevention of liver disease progression [10]. Despite the low cumulative rate of hepatitis B surface antigen (HBsAg) loss (i.e., functional cure), international guidelines recommend long-term administration of NAs with a high genetic barrier to resistance regardless of liver disease severity [11]. Consistently, previous Italian series showed that NAs therapy was the treatment of choice, not only in IFN-experienced CHB patients but also as first-line approach [12–14].

In the last decade, the measurement of serum HBsAg in patients undergoing NAs treatment gained growing relevance for the prediction of HBsAg clearance [15]. Low pre-treatment HBsAg levels were significantly associated with HBsAg loss, particularly in hepatitis B e antigen (HBeAg)-positive patients [16]. Furthermore, several pieces of evidence suggest that on-treatment HBsAg decline was able to predict HBsAg seroclearance, both in HBeAg–positive and –negative patients [17–19]. However, these results predominantly derive from studies involving Asian patients infected with genotypes B and C. To date, in HBeAg–negative Caucasian patients under long-term treatment with NAs, the predictive value of HBsAg kinetic is less clear [20,21].

The aim of the present study was to investigate the clinical role of quantitative HBsAg in a real-life cohort of CHB patients under treatment with NAs in a tertiary care center from North-West Italy.

2. Materials and Methods

2.1. Patients

This observational study included patients with CHB that underwent treatment with NAs retrospectively recruited at the outpatient clinic of the Unit of Gastroenterology of Città della Salute e della Scienza di Torino–Molinette Hospital, Turin, Italy, between November 2011 and June 2020.

The inclusion criteria included age of ≥18 years, HBsAg–positivity for at least 6 months and having received at least 18 months of consecutive NAs treatment. An additional inclusion criterion was the availability of HBsAg measurement during NAs administration according to the following minimum schedule: baseline (T0), 6th month (T1), 12th month (T2) and last follow-up (FU). No restriction was set concerning previous NAs or IFN-based treatment. Patients were censored in case of death, loss to FU and HBsAg clearance. We excluded patients co-infected with hepatitis C virus or hepatitis D virus (HDV) and those with human immunodeficiency virus infection, patients with a diagnosis of hepatocellular carcinoma, patients receiving NAs as prophylaxis for the risk of HBV reactivation and those with no signed informed consent.

2.2. Study Endpoint

The endpoint of the study was the comparison of baseline HBsAg values and HBsAg kinetics between patients that achieved a functional cure during NAs treatment and those still HBsAg-positive at the last FU.

2.3. Definitions

Functional cure was defined as HBsAg loss, with or without anti-HBs seroconversion. Virologic response was defined as the sustained suppression of HBV DNA to undetectable levels. Biochemical response was defined as the sustained ALT normalization (upper limit of normality, ULN = 40 IU/L) [11].

2.4. Data Collection

A specific database was prepared for the collection of demographic, biochemical, virologic and clinical variables relevant to the study. As per the standard of care, all patients underwent a periodical liver ultrasound examination and esophagogastroduodenoscopy according to their stage of liver disease. The presence of cirrhosis was assessed by liver biopsy, liver elastography (FibroScan®, Echosens™, Paris, France) or by hepatic ultrasound features and endoscopic signs of portal hypertension [11,22].

2.5. Serology and Virology

All the serologic and virologic diagnostics were performed at the centralized reference laboratory of Molinette Hospital. In particular, the ARCHITECT-QT assay (Abbott Diagnostics, Abbott Park, IL, USA) was used for the measurement of HBsAg in serum [23]. Plasma HBV DNA was detected and quantified with the COBAS/AmpliPrepCOBAS TaqMan HBV assay, version 2.0 (Roche Molecular Diagnostics, Branchburg, NJ, USA) [24].

2.6. Statistical Analysis

Data were reported using the median and interquartile range (IQR) or the number and percentage for continuous and categorial variables, respectively. Data normality was checked by the D'Agostino-Pearson test. Comparison between unpaired groups was performed by the Mann-Whitney test for continuous variables and by the Fishers' Exact test or chi-squared test for categorical variables. For paired analysis, we used the Wilcoxon or McNemar test for continuous or categorical data, respectively.

Predictiveness was evaluated by Harrell's concordance index (C-index) and the area under the curve (AUC) of the receiver operating characteristic (ROC) curve. The ROC curve was computed considering events that took place within 10 years and individuals were censored after more than 10 years from the recruitment (10 and 13 individuals, respectively). Cut-off values with maximal Youden *J* statistics were selected from such curve.

Survival analysis was carried out according to the Kaplan-Meier method using the previously selected cut-off values; survival curves were compared using the log-rank test. Multivariate Cox regression analysis was used to evaluate the association between selected variables and the outcome; the strength of the association was reported as a hazard ratio (HR) and a 95% confidence interval (CI). C-index and AUC of the Cox model were estimated using cross-validation (5 splits and shuffling samples 20 times). Confidence intervals at a 95% confidence level have been estimated by bootstrapping 1000 times.

A two-tailed p value < 0.05 was considered statistically significant. All the statistical analyses were performed using MedCalc software, version 18.9.1 (MedCalc bvba, Os-tend, Belgium) and the Python packages scikit-learn (version 0.24.2) and scikit-survival (0.15.0).

3. Results

3.1. Characteristics of the Patients Included in the Study

The clinical records of 171 patients with CHB were screened. A total of 101 (59%) patients were included in the study. Twenty-nine patients were excluded due to chronic HDV infection (anti-HDV-positive/HDV RNA-positive), while 32 patients had a diagnosis of HBeAg–negative chronic infection (i.e., inactive carriers; persistent HBV DNA < 2000 UI/mL and ALT < 40 IU/mL) [11]. Another group of 9 patients had no indication of antiviral treatment due to intermediate HBV DNA levels (2000–20,000 IU/mL), persistently normal ALT and no or mild liver fibrosis (grey zone) [25]. The baseline characteristics of the patients enrolled are reported in Table 1.

The baseline median age was 56 (32–79) years and the male to female ratio was 69/32. Most patients were Caucasian (n = 98; 97%); 79 from Italy and 19 from East Europe. Nine (9%) patients were obese and 7 (7%) patients admitted alcohol abuse. Only 6 (6%) patients had type 2 diabetes requiring therapy while 29 (29%) had a diagnosis of hypertension. The principal risk factor for HBV infection was intrafamily exposure (n = 46; 46%), followed by hospitalization (n = 19; 19%) and sexual exposure (n = 5; 5%).

Only 18 (18%) patients had a diagnosis of cirrhosis. In one patient, the disease was complicated by ascites, while 6 (6%) patients showed esophageal varices at endoscopic examination. Consistently, biochemistry indicated an overall preserved liver function.

Table 1. Baseline characteristics of the overall cohort of patients included in the study and according to HBsAg loss.

Characteristics	Overall	No HBsAg-Loss	Functional Cure	p Value
Patients, n	101	90	11	
Age (years), median (range)	56 (32–79)	57 (32–79)	56 (32–72)	0.624
Male gender, n (%)	69 (68%)	62 (69%)	7 (64%)	0.739
Nationality				
Italian, n (%)	79 (78%)	71 (79%)	8 (73%)	0.643
East Europe, n (%)	19 (19%)	16 (18%)	3 (27%)	
Other, n (%) [A]	3 (3%)	3 (3%)	0	
Risck factors for HBV infection				
Family exposure, n (%)	46 (46%)	42 (47%)	4 (36%)	0.75
Sexual exposure, n (%)	5 (5%)	4 (4%)	1 (9%)	0.445
Hospitalization, n (%)	19 (19%)	15 (17%)	4 (36%)	0.212
Tattoo/Piercing, n (%)	1 (<1%)	1 (1%)	0	1
IVDU, n (%)	1 (<1%)	1 (1%)	0	1
Comorbidities				
Alcohol abuse, n (%) [B]	7 (7%)	6 (7%)	1 (9%)	0.566
Obesity, n (%) [C]	9 (9%)	9 (10%)	0	0.592
T2DM, n (%)	6 (6%)	5 (6%)	1 (9%)	0.09
Hypertension, n (%)	29 (29%)	27 (30%)	2 (18%)	0.505
Cirrhosis, n (%)	18 (18%)	15 (17%)	3 (27%)	0.408
Ascites, n (%)	1 (<1%)	1 (1%)	0	1
Esophageal varices, n (%)	6 (6%)	5 (6%)	1 (9%)	0.509
Serology				
HBsAg (Log IU/mL), median (IQR)	3.25 (2.85–3.88)	3.35 (2.91–3.95)	1.11 (0.45–1.98)	<0.001
HBV DNA (Log IU/mL), median (IQR)	3.45 (1.91–5.63)	3.86 (2.10–6.25)	3.15 (1.57–4.21)	0.13
HBeAg+/anti-HBe+	15/86	14/74	10-1	1
Biochemistry				
ALT (IU/L), median (IQR)	34 (21–68)	32 (21–67)	35 (17–78)	0.87
AST (IU/L), median (IQR)	29 (21–52)	30 (21–53)	24 (17–51)	0.249
γGT (IU/L), median (IQR)	24 (16–39)	24 (16–39)	19 (11–47)	0.33
ALP (IU/L), median (IQR)	65 (57–87)	65 (57–83)	81 (55–158)	0.519
Total bilirubin (mg/dL), median (IQR)	0.7 (0.6–0.9)	0.7 (0.5–0.9)	0.9 (0.7–1.3)	0.077
Albumin (g/L), median (IQR)	4.5 (4.2–4.7)	4.4 (4.1–4.7)	4.5 (4.3–4.7)	0.366
Platelet count (x10^9/L), median (IQR)	181 (133–227)	185 (140–227)	154 (111–225)	0.235
Previous IFN treatment, n (%)	44 (44%)	41 (46%)	4 (36%)	0.75
Previous NAs treatment, n (%)	61 (60%)	53 (59%)	8 (73%)	0.519
Duration of previous NAs (years), median (IQR)	6 (3–10)	6 (3–10)	6 (1–12)	0.602

[A] 2 patients were Asian, 1 was African and 1 was South American. [B] >140 g/week for woman and >210 g/week for men. [C] body mass index $\geq$ 30 kg/m^2. Comparison between continuous variables was performed by the Mann-Whitney test. Comparison between categorical variables was performed by the Fisher's exact test (dichotomous variables) or chi-squared test (non-dichotomous variables). Abbreviations–alkaline phosphatase (ALP), alanine aminotransferase (ALT), aspartate aminotransferase (AST), gamma-glutamyl transpeptidase (γGT), hepatitis B e antigen (HBeAg), hepatitis B surface antigen (HBsAg), hepatitis B virus (HBV), interferon (IFN), interquartile range (IQR), intravenous drug use (IVDU), number (n), nucleos(t)ide analogues (NAs), type 2 diabetes mellitus (T2DM).

The majority of patients were anti-HBe-positive at baseline ($n = 86$; 85%); median HBsAg and HBV DNA levels were 3.25 (2.85–3.88) Log IU/mL and 3.45 (1.91–5.63) Log IU/mL, respectively. Forty-four (44%) patients were IFN-experienced while 61 (60%) patients reported previous NAs therapy. Median FU was 5.5 (3.2–8.3) years; 69 (68%) underwent antiviral treatment with entecavir (ETV), while 32 (32%) with tenofovir disoproxil fumarate (TDF). All the treated patients (100%) achieved virologic response, while 98 (97%) achieved biochemical response. At the end of FU, 11 patients achieved a functional cure (annual incidence rate = 1.8%). The loss of HBsAg was accompanied by seroconversion to anti-HBs in 3/11 (27%) patients (anti-HBs titers: 749 IU/mL, 138 IU/mL, and 124 IU/mL). No differences were observed in treatment duration between patients achieving a functional cure (7.5, 4.3–8.5 years) and those with no HBsAg loss (5.5, 2.9–8.2 years) ($p = 0.433$).

3.2. Comparison between Patients with or without HBsAg-Loss

No significant differences were observed between patients achieving a functional cure and those without HBsAg loss regarding demographic and clinical characteristics (Table 1). At baseline, median HBsAg values were significantly lower in patients that achieved a functional cure compared to those still HBsAg-positive at the last FU (1.11, 0.45–1.98 Log IU/mL vs. 3.353, 2.91–3.95 Log IU/mL, $p < 0.001$). No differences were observed regarding circulating HBV DNA values and ALT levels ($p = 0.130$ and $p = 0.870$, respectively). We further analyzed the kinetics of HBsAg, HBV DNA and ALT from baseline to the last FU. Interestingly, we observed distinct differences according to the achievement of functional cure for HBsAg kinetics, but not for HBV DNA and ALT (Figure 1). HBsAg, HBV DNA and ALT values for each timepoint are reported in Table 2 (HBsAg values and kinetics are reported in absolute numbers in Supplementary Material Table S1).

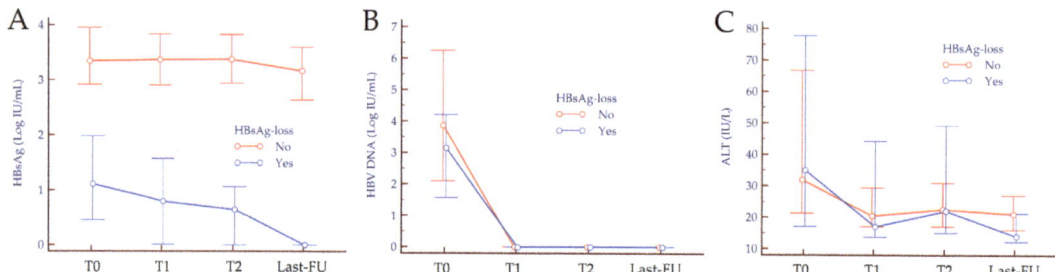

Figure 1. HBsAg (**A**), HBV DNA (**B**) and ALT (**C**) kinetics in patients achieving a functional cure and those with no HBsAg-loss. In both groups, HBsAg, HBV DNA, and ALT levels significantly declined from T0 to the last FU (Friedman test, $p < 0.001$). Data are depicted as the median and interquartile range. Abbreviations–alanine aminotransferase (ALT), follow-up (FU), hepatitis B surface antigen (HBsAg), hepatitis B virus (HBV), timepoint (T).

Table 2. Comparison of HBsAg, HBV DNA and ALT levels according to HBsAg loss.

Biomarker	Timepoint	No HBsAg-Loss	Functional Cure	p Value
HBsAg (Log IU/mL)	T0	3.46 (2.91–3.97)	1.11 (0.45–1.98)	<0.001
	T1	3.39 (2.90–3.92)	0.80 (0.01–1.57)	<0.001
	T2	3.40 (2.95–3.89)	0.65 (0.01–1.06)	<0.001
	Last-FU	3.21 (2.63–3.78)	0 (0–0)	<0.001
HBV DNA (Log IU/mL)	T0	3.86 (2.10–6.25)	3.15 (1.57–4.21)	0.130
	T1	0 (0–0)	0 (0–0)	0.273
	T2	0 (0–0)	0 (0–0)	0.386
	Last-FU	0 (0–0)	0 (0–0)	1.000
ALT (IU/L)	T0	30 (20–67)	35 (17–78)	0.985
	T1	22 (17–31)	17 (14–44)	0.445
	T2	23 (17–31)	22 (15–49)	0.815
	Last-FU	21 (16–28)	14 (12–21)	0.038

p values were calculated by the Mann-Whitney test. Data are reported as the median and interquartile range. Abbreviations–alanine aminotransferase (ALT), follow-up (FU), hepatitis B virus (HBV), hepatitis B surface antigen (HBsAg), timepoint (T).

Focusing on HBsAg, we calculated and compared the magnitude of HBsAg decline (ΔHBsAg) between patients achieving a functional cure and those with no HBsAg loss. We observed no differences between the magnitude of ΔHBsAg from baseline to T1 ($p = 0.082$) and from T1 to T2 ($p = 0.117$) between the two groups of patients, while we observed a significantly higher ΔHBsAg from baseline to T2 in patients achieving a functional cure ($p = 0.002$) (Figure 2). Median ΔHBsAg values in patients with or without HBsAg loss are reported in Table 3.

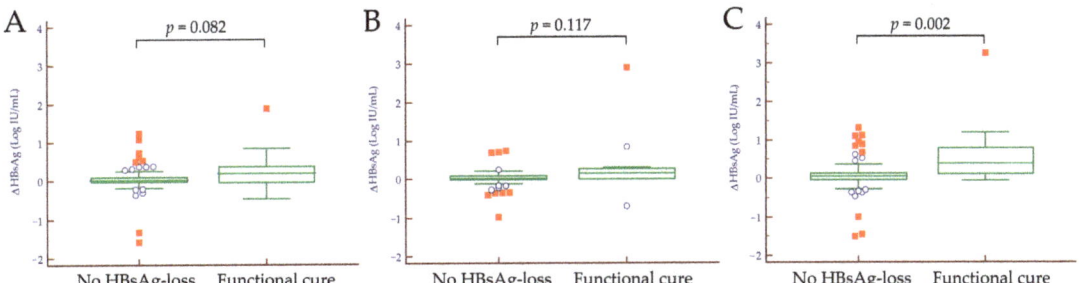

Figure 2. Comparison of HBsAg decline from baseline to T1 (**A**), from T1 to T2 (**B**) and from baseline to T2 (**C**) in patients achieving a functional cure and those with no HBsAg loss. Hollow circles indicate values that are larger than the upper quartile plus 1.5 times the interquartile range while red squares indicate values that are larger than the upper quartile plus 3 times the interquartile range. Abbreviations–HBsAg decline (ΔHBsAg), hepatitis B surface antigen (HBsAg).

Table 3. Comparison of the magnitude of HBsAg decline between patients achieving a functional cure and those with no HBsAg loss.

Biomarker	Time Interval	No HBsAg-Loss	Functional Cure	p Value
ΔHBsAg (Log IU/mL)	T0–T1	0.02 (−0.02–0.10)	0.19 (−0.04–0.37)	0.082
	T1–T2	0.02 (−0.01–0.09)	0.15 (0–0.27)	0.117
	T0–T2	0.05 (−0.04–0.13)	0.38 (0.11–0.80)	0.002

p values were calculated by the Mann-Whitney test. Data are reported as the median and interquartile range. Abbreviations–HBsAg decline (ΔHBsAg), hepatitis B surface antigen (HBsAg), timepoint (T).

3.3. Prediction of HBsAg-Loss

We performed a ROC curve analysis to investigate the performance of baseline HBsAg and ΔHBsAg T0–T2 to identify patients achieving functional cure in ten years. Baseline HBsAg showed a good diagnostic accuracy (AUC = 0.877, 95%CI 0.698–0.992) for the discrimination between patients that lost the HBsAg and those who did not; the optimal cut-off that maximized sensitivity (Se) and specificity (Sp) was ≤2.00 Log IU/mL. ΔHBsAg T0–T2 showed a moderate diagnostic accuracy (AUC = 0.818, 95%CI 0.589–1.000) for the identification of patients that lost the HBsAg; the optimal cut-off that maximized Se and Sp was >0.30 Log IU/mL. Differences between the two survival curves built from such selected cut-offs were significant ($p < 0.001$) (Figure 3). Accordingly, among patients that cleared the HBsAg, 9 out of 11 (82%) and 7 out of 11 (64%) had baseline HBsAg ≤ 2.00 Log IU/mL and ΔHBsAg T0–T2 values >0.30 Log IU/mL, respectively. Among patients still HBsAg-positive at the last FU, only 11 out of 90 (12%) had baseline HBsAg ≤ 2.00 Log IU/mL and 11 out of 90 (12%) had ΔHBsAg T0–T2 values >0.30 Log IU/mL. By multivariate Cox regression analysis, both baseline HBsAg and ΔHBsAg T0–T2 were significantly associated to HBsAg loss (HR = 0.20, 95%CI 0.09–0.44, $p < 0.001$, and HR = 9.40, 95%CI 3.29–26.82, $p < 0.001$, respectively). The prognostic indices obtained from the combination of both parameters were used to assess the discrimination ability of the predictive model; remarkably, we achieved C = 0.965, 95%CI 0.883–0.996.

The score of the multivariate model can be computed by the following formula:

$$-1.62 * (\text{baseline HBsAg Log IU/mL}) + 2.24 * (\Delta\text{HBsAg T0-T2 Log IU/mL})$$

The optimal cut-off was −1.762, which yielded again significant different survival curves ($p < 0.001$) (Figure 4).

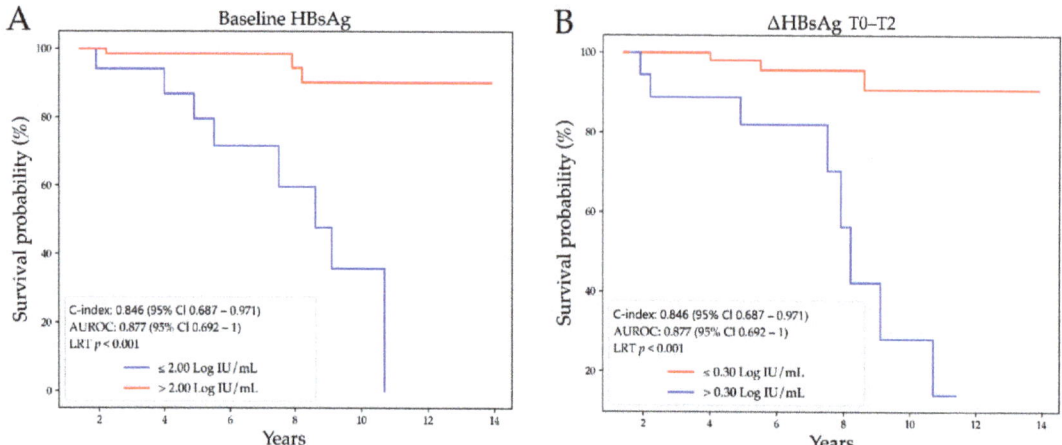

Figure 3. Survival curves for the prediction of HBsAg loss according to baseline HBsAg ≤ 2.00 Log IU/mL (**A**) and ΔHBsAg T0–T2 > 0.30 Log IU/mL (**B**). Survival curve analysis was performed according to the Kaplan–Meier method; the difference between the curves was assessed by a Log rank test. Abbreviations– area under the receiver operating characteristic curve (AUROC), HBsAg decline (ΔHBsAg), hepatitis B surface antigen (HBsAg), log-rank test (LRT), timepoint (T).

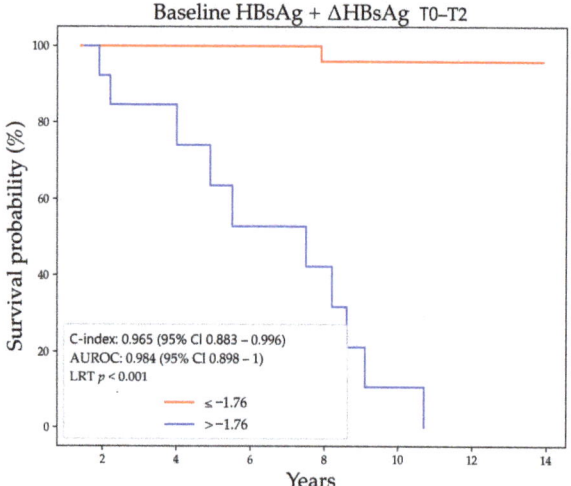

Figure 4. Predictiveness of the model combining baseline HBsAg ≤ 2.00 Log IU/mL and ΔHBsAg T0–T2 > 0.30 Log IU/mL for HBsAg loss. Abbreviations–HBsAg decline (ΔHBsAg), hepatitis B surface antigen (HBsAg), timepoint (T).

4. Discussion

The results of the present study showed that the measurement of baseline serum HBsAg and the magnitude of HBsAg decrease during treatment with third-generation NAs are useful to identify CHB patients with a higher likelihood of achieving functional cure. Our data obtained from a real-world clinical setting confirmed previous results mainly deriving from Asiatic cohorts of HBeAg-positive patients; we were able to confirm the usefulness of the HBsAg measurement in a cohort of CHB patients extremely heterogeneous in term of treatment duration, previous NAs and/or IFN-based treatment. Furthermore, we observed that the combination of both parameters (i.e., baseline HBsAg and HBsAg decline) was able to predict HBsAg seroclearance with high accuracy.

Overall, 11 out of 101 patients cleared the HBsAg during NAs therapy. In our study, the annual incidence rate of HBsAg loss was 1.8%; this result agrees with the estimated annual incidence of 1–2% reported both in Asian and in Western populations [26]. Previous studies showed that baseline HBsAg < 1000 IU/mL was the optimal cut-off for the prediction of HBsAg seroclearance (AUC = 0.860; negative predictive value (NPV) = 98%) in Chinese CHB patients (61.4% HBeAg-positive) undergoing lamivudine (LMV) treatment [27], while lower HBsAg levels after HBeAg seroclearance were associated with HBsAg loss in another Asiatic cohort of CHB patients, irrespectively of antiviral treatment [28]. In 390 Taiwanese HBeAg-positive CHB patients (genotype B and C) who had spontaneously cleared the HBeAg during FU, Tseng and colleagues observed that HBsAg serum levels <100 IU/mL at 1 year after HBeAg seroconversion, were able to predict HBsAg loss (HR = 24.3, 95%CI 8.7–67.5) within 6 years [29]. A recent European study investigated the changes of HBsAg titers in HBeAg-negative CHB patients undergoing low genetic barrier NAs and observed that lower baseline HBsAg levels were associated with on-therapy HBsAg drop <1000 IU/mL [30], while another Chinese study showed that low serum HBsAg level at year 1 of NAs treatment was an independent predictor of subsequent HBsAg <1000 IU/mL at year 8 of FU (HR = 0.24, p = 0.004) [31]. In the present study, we observed that baseline HBsAg values <2.00 Log IU/mL were significantly associated with HBsAg loss in a cohort of CHB patients undergoing ETV or TDF treatment, showing a good performance for seroclearance prediction (C = 0.846); this cut-off allowed us to correctly identify 88 out of 101 patients (accuracy = 87%).

Several studies showed that HBsAg decline is more pronounced in CHB patients treated with PEG-IFN compared to those treated with NAs [16,32]. For most CHB patients under NAs treatment, it has been estimated that a median HBsAg reduction of 0.08 Log IU/mL/year [33] is typical. Nonetheless, a conspicuous body of evidence supports the association between HBsAg decline and favorable therapeutic outcomes in patients under long-term NAs treatment [34]. In 7 out of 70 (10%) patients treated with LMV achieving HBsAg seroclearance, a greater HBsAg reduction (>0.166 Log IU/mL) hs been reported compared to the 63 patients still HBsAg-positive at the end of FU (AUC = 0.794; NPV = 98%) [27]. Another study performed on 266 HBeAg-positive CHB patients treated with TDF showed that an HBsAg decline $\geq$1.00 Log IU/mL at 6 months of therapy was independently associated to HBsAg loss (HR = 14.3, 95%CI 4.7–43.4) [35]. A more recent study including HBeAg-negative CHB patients, showed that an HBsAg decline > 0.3 Log IU/mL at 3 years of NAs treatment had Se = 100%, Sp = 81%, positive predictive value (PPV) = 42% and NPV = 100% for the identification of low HBsAg levels (< 120 IU/mL), and Se = 100%, Sp = 74%, PPV = 17% and NPV = 100% for the identification of HBsAg loss [20]. Finally, in a large cohort of 529 Asian CHB patients (195 HBeAg-positive and 334 HBeAg-negative) receiving ETV, it has been shown that an HBsAg decline $\geq$75% independently predicted HBsAg loss [18]. Furthermore, the authors reported that the combination of baseline HBsAg levels <3000 IU/mL and HBsAg decline $\geq$75% allowed to predict HBsAg seroclearance with PPV = 70% and NPV = 100% [18]. Finally, Jaroszewicz et al. showed that in CHB patients (mostly HBeAg-negative) undergoing treatments with NAs, HBsAg decrease during the first 6 months of NA therapy was not predictive for HBsAg loss, while a strong HBsAg decrease (>0.5 Log IU/mL) 2 years after HBV DNA suppression was associated with HBsAg loss [36]. Although we cannot firmly identify the optimal timing and the exact amount of HBsAg decrease during NAs, all these data highlight the importance of quantitative rather than qualitative HBsAg monitoring during treatment with NAs. Indeed, we observed that HBsAg decline >0.30 Log IU/mL was significantly associated with HBsAg loss (HR = 9.40, p < 0.001). Moreover, the model developed from the combination of baseline HBsAg values and ΔHBsAg T0–T2 used in our study demonstrates an excellent predictiveness for HBsAg loss (C = 0.965). These results further corroborate the usefulness of quantitative HBsAg monitoring in Caucasian CHB patients treated with antivirals; despite the low rate of HBsAg seroclearance during NAs therapy, the quantitative HBsAg qualifies as a reliable predictor of functional cure.

To note, the present research has some limitations including the retrospective design, and the clinical and virologic heterogeneity of the patients enrolled. Nonetheless, our results are in line with previous findings on this topic. Furthermore, the heterogeneity observed in our population resembles the real characteristics of CHB patients currently being referred to most of the tertiary care centers in Italy. Indeed, the majority of these patients have an HBeAg-negative serologic profile and have usually been exposed to previous PEG-IFN and/or NAs therapy. Here, we observed that HBeAg at baseline was not significantly different between patients experiencing HBsAg loss and those still positive at the last FU. However, the number of HBeAg-positive patients at baseline was quite low in our study. Considering that several studies reported that the rate of HBsAg decline is higher in HBeAg-positive vs. HBeAg-negative patients [37–39], we cannot exclude that the rate of HBsAg clearance is similar between HBeAg-negative and -positive CHB patients under NAs therapy. Another limitation may be found in the relatively low number of patients enrolled and the lack of a validation cohort. To overcome this issue, we applied a stratified cross-validation approach to assess the performance of the model; accordingly, the original sample was partitioned into a training set to train the model, and a test set to evaluate its performance, and the procedure was repeated multiple times. As a result, the model showed a high accuracy, with low risk of overfitting, and generalizability to independent datasets. Therefore, we believe that the results of the present study are robust and may be useful for the management of such patients, also in view of the arising concept of NAs cessation in HBsAg-positive patients [40].

5. Conclusions

In the present study, we showed that the measurement of baseline and on-treatment HBsAg decline are useful for the identification of CHB patients achieving a functional cure. Furthermore, the combination of both parameters allowed the prediction of HBsAg-loss with excellent accuracy. Further studies may investigate the applicability of the present findings for the definition of stopping rules for safely discontinuation of NAs therapy.

Supplementary Materials: The following are available online at https://www.mdpi.com/article/10.3390/jcm10153308/s1, Table S1: HBsAg values from baseline to last-FU in the overall population and according to functional cure.

Author Contributions: Conceptualization, A.C.; methodology, G.P.C. and A.C.; software, G.P.C., M.G., S.A. and G.B.; formal analysis, G.P.C., S.A. and G.B.; investigation, G.P.C., Y.T., E.G. and F.P.; resources, A.C.; data curation, Y.T., E.G. and F.P.; writing—original draft preparation, G.P.C.; writing—review and editing, R.C., G.M.S. and A.C.; visualization, G.P.C., S.A. and G.B.; supervision, R.C., G.M.S. and A.C. All authors have read and agreed to the published version of the manuscript.

Funding: This research received no external funding.

Institutional Review Board Statement: The study was conducted according to the guidelines of the Declaration of Helsinki and approved by the Institutional Ethics Committee of A.O.U. Città della Salute e della Scienza di Torino (CEI-135/2019; 03/02/2020).

Informed Consent Statement: Written informed consent was obtained from all subjects involved in the study.

Data Availability Statement: The data presented in this study are available on request from the corresponding author.

Conflicts of Interest: The authors declare no conflict of interest.

References

1. Seto, W.K.; Lo, Y.R.; Pawlotsky, J.M.; Yuen, M.F. Chronic hepatitis B virus infection. *Lancet* **2018**, *392*, 2313–2324. [CrossRef]
2. World Health Organization. *Global Hepatitis Report 2017*; Global Hepatitis Programme: Geneva, Switzerland, April 2017; Available online: http://www.who.int/hepatitis/publications/global-hepatitis-report2017/en/ (accessed on 2 March 2021).
3. Ginzberg, D.; Wong, R.J.; Gish, R. Global HBV burden: Guesstimates and facts. *Hepatol. Int.* **2018**, *12*, 315–329. [CrossRef] [PubMed]

4. Coppola, N.; Corvino, A.R.; De Pascalis, S.; Signoriello, G.; Di Fiore, E.; Nienhaus, A.; Sagnelli, E.; Lamberti, M. The Long-Term Immunogenicity of Recombinant Hepatitis B Virus (HBV) Vaccine: Contribution of Universal HBV Vaccination in Italy. *BMC Infect. Dis.* **2015**, *15*, 149. [CrossRef] [PubMed]
5. Zanetti, A.R.; Tanzi, E.; Romanò, L.; Grappasonni, I. Vaccination against hepatitis B: The Italian strategy. *Vaccine* **1993**, *11*, 521–524. [CrossRef]
6. Zampino, R.; Boemio, A.; Sagnelli, C.; Alessio, L.; Adinolfi, L.E.; Sagnelli, E.; Coppola, N. Hepatitis B virus burden in developing countries. *World J. Gastroenterol.* **2015**, *21*, 11941–11953. [CrossRef]
7. Saracco, G.M.; Evangelista, A.; Fagoonee, S.; Ciccone, G.; Bugianesi, E.; Caviglia, G.P.; Abate, M.L.; Rizzetto, M.; Pellicano, R.; Smedile, A. Etiology of chronic liver diseases in the Northwest of Italy, 1998 through 2014. *World J. Gastroenterol.* **2016**, *22*, 8187–8193. [CrossRef]
8. Sagnelli, E.; Stroffolini, T.; Sagnelli, C.; Morisco, F.; Coppola, N.; Smedile, A.; Pisaturo, M.; Colloredo, G.; Babudieri, S.; Licata, A.; et al. Influence of universal HBV vaccination on chronic HBV infection in Italy: Results of a cross-sectional multicenter study. *J. Med. Virol.* **2017**, *89*, 2138–2143. [CrossRef]
9. Caviglia, G.P.; Abate, M.L.; Pellicano, R.; Smedile, A. Chronic hepatitis B therapy: Available drugs and treatment guidelines. *Minerva Gastroenterol. Dietol.* **2015**, *61*, 61–70.
10. Collo, A.; Belci, P.; Fagoonee, S.; Loreti, L.; Gariglio, V.; Parise, R.; Magistroni, P.; Durazzo, M. Efficacy and safety of long-term entecavir therapy in a European population. *Minerva Gastroenterol. Dietol.* **2018**, *64*, 201–207. [CrossRef]
11. European Association for the Study of the Liver. EASL 2017 Clinical Practice Guidelines on the management of hepatitis B virus infection. *J. Hepatol.* **2017**, *67*, 370–398. [CrossRef]
12. Stroffolini, T.; Spadaro, A.; Di Marco, V.; Scifo, G.; Russello, M.; Montalto, G.; Bertino, G.; Surace, L.; Caroleo, B.; Foti, G.; et al. Current practice of chronic hepatitis B treatment in Southern Italy. *Eur. J. Intern. Med.* **2012**, *23*, e124–e127. [CrossRef]
13. Cuomo, G.; Borghi, V.; Giuberti, T.; Andreone, P.; Massari, M.; Villa, E.; Pietrangelo, A.; Verucchi, G.; Levantesi, F.; Ferrari, C. What to start with in first line treatment of chronic hepatitis B patients: An Italian multicentre observational cohort, HBV-RER study group. *Infez. Med.* **2017**, *25*, 150–157. [PubMed]
14. Caviglia, G.P.; Olivero, A.; Ngatchou, D.; Saracco, G.M.; Smedile, A. Long-term results of chronic hepatitis B antiviral treatment with nucleos(t)ide analogues: A single center experience. *Minerva Gastroenterol. Dietol.* **2019**, *65*, 77–78. [CrossRef] [PubMed]
15. Cornberg, M.; Wong, V.W.; Locarnini, S.; Brunetto, M.; Janssen, H.L.A.; Chan, H.L. The role of quantitative hepatitis B surface antigen revisited. *J. Hepatol.* **2017**, *66*, 398–411. [CrossRef] [PubMed]
16. Martinot-Peignoux, M.; Asselah, T.; Marcellin, P. HBsAg quantification to optimize treatment monitoring in chronic hepatitis B patients. *Liver Int.* **2015**, *35*, S82–S90. [CrossRef]
17. Kim, J.H.; Choi, Y.J.; Moon, H.W.; Ko, S.Y.; Choe, W.H.; Kwon, S.Y. HBsAg level and clinical course in patients with chronic hepatitis B treated with nucleoside analogue: Five years of follow-up data. *Clin. Mol. Hepatol.* **2013**, *19*, 409–416. [CrossRef]
18. Peng, C.Y.; Lai, H.C.; Su, W.P.; Lin, C.H.; Chuang, P.H.; Chen, S.H.; Chen, C.H. Early hepatitis B surface antigen decline predicts treatment response to entecavir in patients with chronic hepatitis B. *Sci. Rep.* **2017**, *7*, 42879. [CrossRef]
19. Lin, T.C.; Chiu, Y.C.; Chiu, H.C.; Liu, W.C.; Cheng, P.N.; Chen, C.Y.; Chang, T.T.; Wu, I.C. Clinical utility of hepatitis B surface antigen kinetics in treatment-naive chronic hepatitis B patients during long-term entecavir therapy. *World J. Gastroenterol.* **2018**, *24*, 725–736. [CrossRef]
20. Broquetas, T.; Garcia-Retortillo, M.; Hernandez, J.J.; Puigvehí, M.; Cañete, N.; Coll, S.; Cabrero, B.; Giménez, M.D.; Solà, R.; Carrión, J.A. Quantification of HBsAg to predict low levels and seroclearance in HBeAg-negative patients receiving nucleos(t)ide analogues. *PLoS ONE* **2017**, *12*, e0188303. [CrossRef]
21. Lee, M.H.; Lee, D.M.; Kim, S.S.; Cheong, J.Y.; Cho, S.W. Correlation of serum hepatitis B surface antigen level with response to entecavir in naive patients with chronic hepatitis B. *J. Med. Virol.* **2011**, *83*, 1178–1186. [CrossRef]
22. Caviglia, G.P.; Touscoz, G.A.; Smedile, A.; Pellicano, R. Noninvasive assessment of liver fibrosis: Key messages for clinicians. *Pol. Arch. Med. Wewn.* **2014**, *124*, 329–335. [CrossRef]
23. Burdino, E.; Ruggiero, T.; Proietti, A.; Milia, M.G.; Olivero, A.; Caviglia, G.P.; Marietti, M.; Rizzetto, M.; Smedile, A.; Ghisetti, V. Quantification of hepatitis B surface antigen with the novel DiaSorin LIAISON XL Murex HBsAg Quant: Correlation with the ARCHITECT quantitative assays. *J. Clin. Virol.* **2014**, *60*, 341–346. [CrossRef]
24. Tandoi, F.; Caviglia, G.P.; Pittaluga, F.; Abate, M.L.; Smedile, A.; Romagnoli, R.; Salizzoni, M. Prediction of occult hepatitis B virus infection in liver transplant donors through hepatitis B virus blood markers. *Dig. Liver. Dis.* **2014**, *46*, 1020–1024. [CrossRef] [PubMed]
25. Carosi, G.; Rizzetto, M.; Alberti, A.; Cariti, G.; Colombo, M.; Craxì, A.; Filice, G.; Levrero, M.; Mazzotta, F.; Pastore, G.; et al. Treatment of chronic hepatitis B: Update of the recommendations from the 2007 Italian Workshop. *Dig. Liver Dis.* **2011**, *43*, 259–265. [CrossRef] [PubMed]
26. Chu, C.M.; Liaw, Y.F. Hepatitis B surface antigen seroclearance during chronic HBV infection. *Antivir. Ther.* **2010**, *15*, 133–143. [CrossRef]
27. Seto, W.K.; Wong, D.K.; Fung, J.; Huang, F.Y.; Lai, C.L.; Yuen, M.F. Reduction of hepatitis B surface antigen levels and hepatitis B surface antigen seroclearance in chronic hepatitis B patients receiving 10 years of nucleoside analogue therapy. *Hepatology* **2013**, *58*, 923–931. [CrossRef]

28. Fung, J.; Wong, D.K.; Seto, W.K.; Kopaniszen, M.; Lai, C.L.; Yuen, M.F. Hepatitis B surface antigen seroclearance: Relationship to hepatitis B e-antigen seroclearance and hepatitis B e-antigen-negative hepatitis. *Am. J. Gastroenterol.* **2014**, *109*, 1764–1770. [CrossRef]
29. Tseng, T.C.; Liu, C.J.; Su, T.H.; Wang, C.C.; Chen, C.L.; Chen, P.J.; Chen, D.S.; Kao, J.H. Serum hepatitis B surface antigen levels predict surface antigen loss in hepatitis B e antigen seroconverters. *Gastroenterology* **2011**, *141*, 517–525. [CrossRef]
30. Striki, A.; Manolakopoulos, S.; Deutsch, M.; Kourikou, A.; Kontos, G.; Kranidioti, H.; Hadziyannis, E.; Papatheodoridis, G. Hepatitis B s antigen kinetics during treatment with nucleos(t)ides analogues in patients with hepatitis B e antigen-negative chronic hepatitis B. *Liver Int.* **2017**, *37*, 1642–1650. [CrossRef]
31. Wang, M.L.; Chen, E.Q.; Tao, C.M.; Zhou, T.Y.; Liao, J.; Zhang, D.M.; Wang, J.; Tang, H. Pronounced decline of serum HBsAg in chronic hepatitis B patients with long-term effective nucleos(t)ide analogs therapy. *Scand. J. Gastroenterol.* **2017**, *52*, 1420–1426. [CrossRef]
32. Reijnders, J.G.; Rijckborst, V.; Sonneveld, M.J.; Scherbeijn, S.M.; Boucher, C.A.; Hansen, B.E.; Janssen, H.L. Kinetics of hepatitis B surface antigen differ between treatment with peginterferon and entecavir. *J. Hepatol.* **2011**, *54*, 449–454. [CrossRef]
33. Chevaliez, S.; Hézode, C.; Bahrami, S.; Grare, M.; Pawlotsky, J.M. Long-term hepatitis B surface antigen (HBsAg) kinetics during nucleoside/nucleotide analogue therapy: Finite treatment duration unlikely. *J. Hepatol.* **2013**, *58*, 676–683. [CrossRef]
34. Chen, C.H.; Chiu, Y.C.; Lu, S.N.; Lee, C.M.; Wang, J.H.; Hu, T.H.; Hung, C.H. Serum hepatitis B surface antigen levels predict treatment response to nucleos(t)ide analogues. *World J. Gastroenterol.* **2014**, *20*, 7686–7695. [CrossRef]
35. Marcellin, P.; Buti, M.; Krastev, Z.; de Man, R.A.; Zeuzem, S.; Lou, L.; Gaggar, A.; Flaherty, J.F.; Massetto, B.; Lin, L.; et al. Kinetics of hepatitis B surface antigen loss in patients with HBeAg-positive chronic hepatitis B treated with tenofovir disoproxil fumarate. *J. Hepatol.* **2014**, *61*, 1228–1237. [CrossRef]
36. Jaroszewicz, J.; Ho, H.; Markova, A.; Deterding, K.; Wursthorn, K.; Schulz, S.; Bock, C.T.; Tillmann, H.L.; Manns, M.P.; Wedemeyer, H.; et al. Hepatitis B surface antigen (HBsAg) decrease and serum interferon-inducible protein-10 levels as predictive markers for HBsAg loss during treatment with nucleoside/nucleotide analogues. *Antivir. Ther.* **2011**, *16*, 915–924. [CrossRef]
37. Zoutendijk, R.; Bettina, E.; Hansen, B.E.; Van Vuuren, A.J.; Charles, A.B.; Boucher, C.A.B.; Janssen, H.L.A. Serum HBsAg decline during long-term potent nucleos(t)ide analogue therapy for chronic hepatitis B and prediction of HBsAg loss. *J. Infect. Dis.* **2011**, *204*, 415–418. [CrossRef]
38. Seto, W.K.; Hui, A.J.; Wong, V.W.; Wong, G.L.; Liu, K.S.; Lai, C.L.; Yuen, M.F.; Chan, H.L. Treatment cessation of entecavir in Asian patients with hepatitis B e antigen negative chronic hepatitis B: A multicentre prospective study. *Gut* **2015**, *64*, 667–672. [CrossRef]
39. Zoulim, F.; Carosi, G.; Greenbloom, S.; Mazur, W.; Nguyen, T.; Jeffers, L.; Brunetto, M.; Yu, S.; Llamoso, C. Quantification of HBsAg in nucleos(t)ide-naïve patients treated for chronic hepatitis B with entecavir with or without tenofovir in the BE-LOW study. *J. Hepatol.* **2015**, *62*, 56–63. [CrossRef]
40. Liu, J.; Li, T.; Zhang, L.; Xu, A. The Role of Hepatitis B Surface Antigen in Nucleos(t)ide Analogues Cessation Among Asian Patients With Chronic Hepatitis B: A Systematic Review. *Hepatology* **2019**, *70*, 1045–1055. [CrossRef]

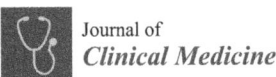

Review

Diagnosis and Management of Achalasia: Updates of the Last Two Years

Amir Mari [1,*], Fadi Abu Baker [2], Rinaldo Pellicano [3] and Tawfik Khoury [4]

1. Department of Gastroenterology, Nazareth Hospital, Faculty of Medicine, Bar-Ilan University, Safed 16100, Israel
2. Hillel Yaffe Medical Center, Department of Gastroenterology and Hepatology, Hadera 38100, Israel; fa_fd@hotmail.com
3. Gastroenterology Unit, Molinette Hospital, 10126 Turin, Italy; rinaldo_pellican@hotmail.com
4. Galilee Medical Center, Department of Gastroenterology, Faculty of Medicine in the Galilee, Bar-Ilan University, Safed 13100, Israel; tawfikkhoury1@hotmail.com
* Correspondence: amir.mari@hotmail.com; Tel.: +972-46028814

Abstract: Achalasia is a rare neurodegenerative disorder causing dysphagia and is characterized by abnormal esophageal motor function as well as the loss of lower esophageal sphincter (LES) relaxation. The assessment and management of achalasia has significantly progressed in recent years due to the advances in high-resolution manometry (HRM) technology along with the improvements and innovations of therapeutic endoscopy procedures. The recent evolution of HRM technology with the inclusion of an adjunctive test, fluoroscopy, and EndoFLIP has enabled more precise diagnoses of achalasia to be made and the subgrouping into therapeutically meaningful subtypes. Current management possibilities include endoscopic treatments such as Botulinum toxin injected to the LES and pneumatic balloon dilation. Surgical treatment includes laparoscopic Heller myotomy and esophagectomy. Furthermore, in recent years, per oral endoscopic myotomy (POEM) has established itself as a principal endoscopic therapeutic alternative to the traditional laparoscopic Heller myotomy. The latest randomized trials report that POEM, pneumatic balloon dilatation, and laparoscopic Heller's myotomy have comparable effectiveness and complications rates. The aim of the current review is to provide a practical clinical approach to dysphagia and to shed light on the most recent improvements in diagnostics and treatment of achalasia over the last two years.

Keywords: dysphagia; achalasia; diagnosis; high resolution manometry (HRM); management; per oral endoscopic myotomy (POEM)

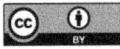

1. Introduction

Achalasia originates from the Greek word a-khalasis, meaning lack of relaxation. It is characterized by a spastic lower esophageal sphincter and a lack of esophageal peristalsis resulting in esophageal outflow obstruction [1,2]. Achalasia is a rare disease, with an estimated incidence of 0.03 to 1.63 per 100,000 persons per year and a prevalence of 10 per 100,000 [1]. Achalasia is generally diagnosed between the third and sixth decades and affects both males and females at equal rates without racial predominance [3,4]. The natural history of achalasia is characterized by a chronic, life-long, but rarely life-threatening disease that seriously affects patients' morbidity and quality of life [5]. When successfully treated, the quality of life almost returns to near normal for a long time; on the other hand, when untreated, the course is usually progressive, leading to esophageal lumen dilatation, which, over time, leads to a burned-out, decompensated sigmoid esophagus with its clinical related consequences, including malnutrition [5,6]. Longstanding achalasia is a significant risk factor for esophageal adenocarcinoma (50 folds) and esophageal squamous cell carcinoma, even when achalasia is adequately managed [7]. Nonetheless, no formal practical guidelines recommend endoscopic surveillance in achalasia patients. However, an endoscopy every three years is considered an acceptable practical surveillance approach for esophageal cancer in longstanding achalasia. In a follow up prospective study that included 32 achalasia patients after surgical treatment for achalasia, Ota and colleagues [8] reported that six patients (18%) developed esophageal cancer in a period of approximately 14.3 years after surgery. Therefore, continuing endoscopic surveillance is required for the detection of malignancy at an early stage. Special clinical awareness is further required in patients with other risk factors for esophageal cancer such as smoking, Barrett's esophagus, alcohol drinking, and family history of esophageal cancer [9].

The main clinical presentations of achalasia are dysphagia, chest pain, vomiting, and weight loss. Despite its chronic course, these profoundly disturb a patient's quality of life [6]. Not uncommonly, the diagnosis of achalasia may not be made for a long time; thus, a high level of clinical suspicion is needed. Esophageal dilation and sigmoid esophagus are considered serious structural consequences of untreated achalasia and eventually may lead to severe nutritional difficulties. Thus far, all treatment options target lower esophageal sphincter (LES) tearing, consequently allowing a bolus to pass through the esophago-gastric junction (EGJ) [6].

2. Medline Search

We performed a MEDLINE/PubMed search for achalasia. Articles discussing and reporting diagnosis, etiology and therapeutic options were extracted and fully accessed. Finally, we generated a comprehensive narrative review by summarizing the most updated data on the diagnosis and management of achalasia focusing on the latest updates from the last two years.

3. Etiology

The etiology of achalasia is still vague, and the precise pathogenesis mechanism of achalasia has been ambiguous up to now. Nevertheless, research findings propose a theory of autoimmune origin, leading to a cascade of a destructive inflammatory processes resulting in destruction of the nitric oxide releasing neurons within the myenteric plexus and the vagus nerve fibers of the lower esophageal sphincter [7]. In end-stage disease, this affects the cholinergic neurons and subsequently progresses to the loss of inhibitory neurons containing nitric oxide synthase and vasoactive intestinal peptide A. This leads to an impaired relaxation of the lower esophageal sphincter [10]. Several patho-mechanisms were proposed as possible triggers of this immuno-destructive process, including underlying viral infection [11], idiopathic autoimmune trigger, and genetic predisposition [12]. Recent data have further addressed the role of autoimmunity and viral infection as the trigger for achalasia development. Innate immune system cells, including eosinophils and mast cells, have been increasingly observed in the esophageal tissue of achalasia patients [13–16]. These cells are already described as important mediators of immune-mediated inflammation and in degenerative neurological diseases [17]. Several studies have reported the involvement of the innate immune system in the pathogenesis of achalasia [13,14,18–20]. Moreover, the adaptive immune (B and T cells) system has recently been shown to play a major role in the development of achalasia. Previous studies using immunohistochemical analysis have shown a strong infiltration of CD3$^+$ T lymphocytes within the esophageal mucosa of achalasia patients, thereby causing myenteric plexitis [21,22]. One recent study showed an increased expression of T lymphocytes (Th22, Th 17, Th 2, Th1 and T regulatory cells) in the lower esophageal sphincter tissue of achalasia patients [23,24]. Additionally, other studies have addressed the emerging role of proinflammatory cytokines (interleukin (IL)-22, IL-17, interferon-gamma, IL-6, and tumor necrosis factor alpha) that were overexpressed in achalasia patients compared with controls [23,25]. However, still more studies are needed to explore the dominant immune cells and cytokines that trigger the development of achalasia and to determine the underlying trigger for the activation of those immune cells and pathways [26]. Still, an underlying viral infection is an acknowledged and reported factor behind achalasia development [27,28]. Based on the existing evidence, the most known viral infections that are associated with achalasia are the herpes virus family (Herpes simplex virus, Epstein–Barr virus, Varicella Zoster virus, and Cytomegalovirus) [29,30], Paramyxoviruses [31], and human immunodeficiency virus (HIV) [32]. In the last few years, evolving new theories have been reported that attempt to address the etiological mechanisms of achalasia, starting from the involvement of the innate immune system. These include mast cells and eosinophils that reach the adaptive immune system and the cytokines that directly induce inhibitory neurons and damage the esophageal muscle layer. Furthermore, studies on the potential role of viral infection in achalasia cannot be ignored. All proofs lead to the conclusion that viruses may lay the foundation for autoimmune responses that attack inhibitory neurons.

4. Diagnostic Approach to Dysphagia and Achalasia

Dysphagia is considered an alarm symptom that mandates the performance of esophago-gastro-duodenoscopy (EGD) as an initial diagnostic modality to exclude structural or mucosal lesions in the esophagus or the stomach cardia. Examples of these include tumors, inflammation, esophageal rings, strictures, and other pathologies that can mimic achalasia, a condition traditionally named pseudochalasia 4. A clinical suspicion of pseudo-achalasia should be sought in patients older than 55 years of age with a prompt onset of solid dysphagia that proceeds to liquid dysphagia and weight loss [33,34]. Classic endoscopic findings of achalasia present in about half of the cases include widening of the esophagus, residue in the esophageal lumen, and obstructed EGJ.

An additional important diagnosis is eosinophilic esophagitis (EoE), an immune-mediated/allergic disorder involving the esophagus causing dysphagia and diagnosed by eosinophils predominant inflammation [35]. Multiple biopsies are mandatory to confirm the diagnosis. Indicative endoscopic findings of EoE include mucosal thickening and edema, ring formation, and white patchy exudates and fibrosis in the late stage [35]. After the exclusion of anatomical, structural, and inflammatory conditions, HRM study is necessary to assess the esophageal motor function and the relaxation of the lower sphincter.

5. High-Resolution Manometry and the Chicago Classification Version 4.0

High-resolution manometry (HRM) is the most accurate investigative system ordinarily utilized in order to study esophageal motility and the LES function when evaluating upper gastrointestinal symptoms including dysphagia when endoscopic and radiologic modalities do not elucidate their cause [36]. The HRM catheter includes 36 pressure sensors disseminated thoroughly over the catheter. The probe is gently entered through the nose and crosses the esophageal body up to the LES. The pressure sensors register pressure changes throughout the swallowing process, and the collected records are processed in a dedicated program that converts these data into a colorful spatiotemporal scheme, where variations in pressure produced by esophageal peristalsis are showed as color distinctions throughout the study duration (Figure 1). The addition of impedance measurement to the HRM studies has enabled impartial valuation of the esophageal clearing capability of fluids to the stomach [33].

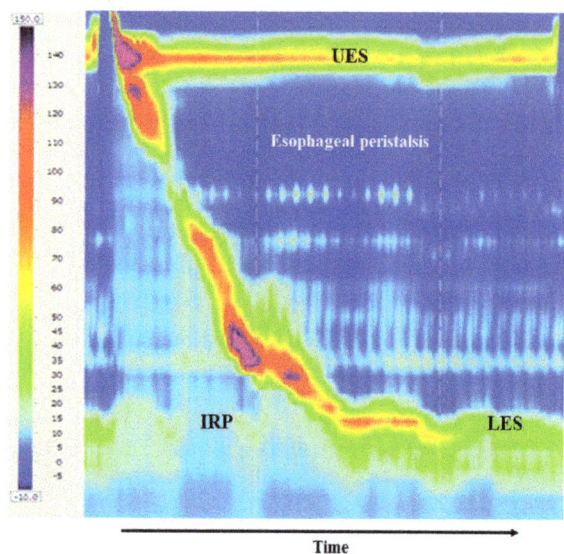

Figure 1. A five milliliter water swallow starts with the opening of the upper esophageal sphincter (UES). One normal esophageal peristalsis and normal lower esophageal sphincter (LES) relaxation is shown. The LES relaxation is measured over a 10 s period, as shown in the box, by measuring the median integrated relaxation pressure (IRP) (supplied from the gastroenterology department at EMMS Nazareth hospital).

The Chicago classification, currently in its fourth version (CCv4.0), is a conceptualized and standardized approach to interpreting HRM findings [10]. One major improvement of the CCv 4.0 is providing rigorous definition and diagnosis for various manometric findings and highlighting their clinical significance and relevance. Conveyed by the expanding knowledge and experience with HRM, the CCv4.0 aimed to provide an updated classification scheme as well as to apply a more rigorous standardized HRM protocol, with the inclusion of provocative tests aiming to reproduce the natural behavior of drinking and eating. These tests include water swallows in various positions, setting and supine; the multiple rapid swallow test (MRS), a repetitive and rapid swallow of water that assesses the deglutitive inhibition function of the LES; and the rapid drink challenge of 200 mL water (RDC), which assesses the deglutitive inhibition function of the LES in addition to depicting the 'recovery capability' of the esophagus by the production of a powerful clearing swallow. Additionally, the addition of bread swallows or a test meal is optional when there is high suspicion of EGJ outflow obstruction (EGJOO). The inclusion of provocation or 'adjunctive tests' in the HRM protocol is based on the fact that the standard 5 mL water swallow is unrepresentative of the normal esophageal physiology and performance, infrequently induces esophageal symptoms, and might under-diagnose motility disorders of clinical significance. The previous Chicago classification version 3 (CCv3.0) included only 10 mL water swallows in the supine position [37]. However, many studies suggested that adjunctive tests could improve the diagnostic yield of HRM for the detection of motility disorders and for better defining the clinical relevance of these findings [38–42]. Furthermore, to ease the implementation of solid swallows in routine clinical practice, Hollenstein et al. performed a development and validation study that aimed to define normal values of esophageal metrics for solid swallows. The authors developed a classification of motility disorders (named the Chicago classification) and this was adapted for solids. The developed classification was applied in the assessment of patients (750) with esophageal symptoms, and the authors confirmed that the inclusion of a solid swallow test improved the diagnosis of clinically pertinent esophageal motility disorders in a cohort with dysphagia and reflux symptoms [43].

Since the introduction of the Chicago classification, three subtypes of achalasia could be identified, depending on the esophageal peristalsis failure type. According to the last Chicago classification (CCv4.0), achalasia type I is defined as an increased intergrade relaxation pressure (IRP—an indicator of the relaxation capability of the LES) and the complete absence of esophageal contractility (totally failed peristalsis with loss of LES relaxation). Type II achalasia is characterized by the production of 'pressure columns' due to pan-esophageal pressure through the hollow esophagus. According to the CCv4.0, type II achalasia is defined as an elevated IRP associated with defective esophageal peristalsis (pan-esophageal pressure in at least 20% of swallows). Achalasia type III is characterized by the presence of premature and/or spastic contractions and a conclusive diagnosis is obtained through the detection of an elevated IRP and the presence of at least 20% premature contractions (Figure 2). This subtyping has improved our understanding of achalasia and, furthermore, has influenced the management plan, enabling a more personalized therapeutic approach. Functional or idiopathic EGJOO—previously called "variant achalasia"—is a disorder more commonly encountered than achalasia and specified by normal esophageal contractility alongside distal obstruction at the level of the LES. Possible etiologies for functional EGJOO include a true idiopathic failure of the LES to relax (a condition that could be treated as achalasia) or the result of technical issues such as the patient's position or the angulation of the catheter [39,44–46]. Secondary causes of outflow obstructions include mucosal or submucosal lesions, EOE, external compression, strictures, post-surgical complications, as well as medications such as opioids [47–49] (Table 1). Treatment should target the source of the outflow obstruction, such as surgical corrections of anatomical abnormalities, endoscopic dilation of strictures, EOE management, and opioid cessation [36].

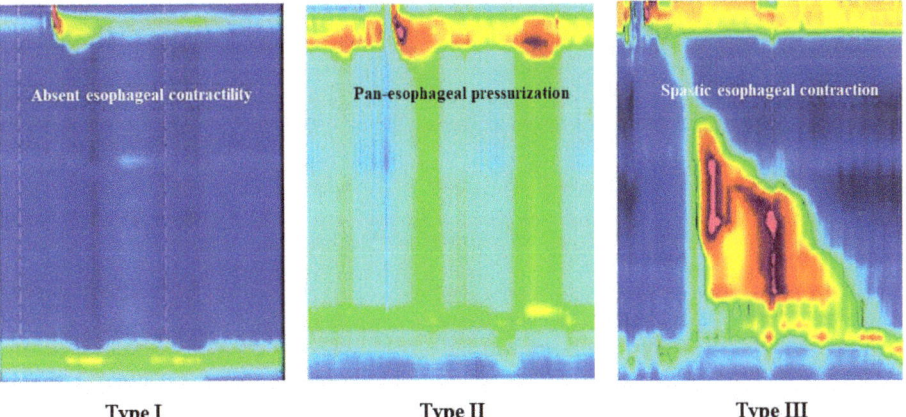

Figure 2. The three achalasia subtypes determined by the Chicago classification (supplied from the gastroenterology department at EMMS Nazareth hospital).

Table 1. Achalasia subtypes.

	Achalasia	
	Manometric Findings	Treatment *
Type I (classic)	Non-relaxing LES and absent peristalsis	LHM, PD, POEM
Type II (pan-esophageal pressurizations)	Non relaxing LES and pressurization	LHM, PD, POEM
Type III (spastic)	Non-relaxing LES and spastic contractions	POEM

* Botox injection use is limited to elderly, frail patients and could be offered to all achalasia subtypes. LES: Lower esophageal Sphincter; LHM: Laparoscopic Hiller Myotomy; PD: Pneumatic Dilation; POEM: Per-Oral Endoscopic Myotomy (POEM).

6. Barium Swallows

Barium esophagography has commonly been used to evaluate esophageal morphology prior to surgery. Recently, the timed barium swallow (TBS) has been used to assess treatment success by evaluating esophageal emptying. Measurement of the retained barium column at several time points after the swallow has been accepted as a reliable tool to objectively assess the level of obstruction at the esophagogastric junction. Moreover, barium emptying studies have gained special popularity in the post treatment period, and they correlate well with treatment response [50]. TBS has several advantages: it is simple, practical, reproducible, economic, non-invasive and well-tolerated by patients. A latest work by Sanagapali et al. that aimed to study the role of barium surface area compared with the traditional barium column as an indicator of treatment response revealed that barium surface area decrease predicted a more precise treatment response [51].

7. EndoFLIP

Endoflip is a novel diagnostic device that permits measurement of the level of distensibility at the esophagogastric junction as well as is capable of detecting the various achalasia subtypes with a high level of confidence and accuracy, particularly with the advent of combining distensibility sensors to manometry sensors [52]. The test is performed while the patient is sedated, eliminating the inconvenience related to HRM and potentially replacing it in select patients.

8. Treatment of Achalasia

The most fundamental goals of treating achalasia are to attain symptomatic relief and to improve patients' quality of life and work capability. Since the repair and the rehabilitation of the defective contractility are impractical and unrealistic, the eventual target of treating achalasia is to release the resistance at the esophagogastric junction. This treatment choice is not straightforward, and a personalized approach should be adopted that takes into account factors including the demographics and medical background of the patient, the achalasia subtype, and the patient's predilection (Table 1) [53]. Importantly, when describing treatment outcomes in achalasia, most previous trials relied on subjective symptom relief as reported by patients, generally by applying the EKARDT score. The EKARDT score includes the four main achalasia symptoms of dysphagia, regurgitation, weight loss, and chest pain. The score points relied on the frequency of each symptom reported by patients and ranges from 3 to 12 (worst symptoms) [54,55]. Nonetheless, despite the widespread implementation of the EKARDT score in clinical practice, it has not been validated yet for this purpose (I). Moreover, most trials considered an Eckardt score of >3 or a reduction in symptoms of <50% as treatment failure. However, several limitations exist with this instrument of assessing treatment outcomes, including using subjective symptoms that could be perceived differently between patients. It can be also be misleading, frequency and time intervals of applying the EKARDT core have yet to be defined, and the cardinal achalasia symptoms could be provoked by pathologies other than achalasia.

Botulinum toxin (Botox) is a well-known therapeutic option for achalasia that has been used for decades [56]. When injected into the distal esophagus and to the LES, the toxin inhibits the release of acetylcholine, which eventually leads to a transitory inhibition of the contractility of LES smooth muscle fibers. Despite the excellent safety profile of Botox injection, the key drawback of this therapeutic option is its short-term durability given a substantial decline in symptoms relief after 6 and 12 months [56]. Therefore, Botox use is restricted to special cases such as comorbid elderly patients or as a temporarily relief before surgery, POEM, or balloon dilation.

Pneumatic balloon dilation is a therapeutic option where a pneumatic balloon is placed in the LES under the guidance of fluoroscopy. The gradual inflation of the balloon leads to mechanical disruption of the LES and relieves the obstruction at the esophagogastric junction. Currently, the preferred protocol for dilation is using a graded attitude, where dilation starts with the 30 mm balloon but the balloon diameter increases in subsequent sessions to 35 mm and up to 40 mm. The gradual dilation approach has been shown to have greater efficacy and a higher safety profile [57]. Pneumatic balloon dilation is long-lasting, with a symptomatic relief over 80% after 2 and 5 years [58]. The long-standing clinical success of pneumatic balloon dilation after 2 and 5 years is satisfactory and similar to surgical outcomes [59]. Complications related to balloon dilation are rare and may include the development of esophageal reflux symptoms in 15–35% of patients. Esophageal perforation is rare and occurs in about 2% of cases and very rarely leads to bleeding [60].

Heller myotomy is an well-established procedure for achalasia treatment that has been performed for more than a century and involves the dissection of the LES smooth muscle fibers. The incidence of esophageal reflux symptoms and the development of erosive esophagitis after the myotomy have been significant; therefore, surgeons also complete a partial fundoplication wrap of the posterior (Toupet) or the anterior (Dor) to prevent reflux symptoms and complications. LHM is a safe and effective therapeutic modality with durable symptomatic relief, estimated to be over 85% after 5 years [59].

Recently, POEM has been acknowledged as an efficient novel treatment modality with an excellent safety profile [61]. This procedure is performed by an invasive gastroenterologist or a surgeon and normally in an operating room while the patient is under sedation and intubated. The procedure involves the creation of a tunnel located at the submucosa using an endoscopic knife. The tunnel generally originates at the middle or lower esophagus and ends up at the stomach cardia, commonly 2–3 cm beyond the LES. Endoscopic myotomy is completed by either anterior or posterior dissection of the circular muscle's fibers. Ujiki et al. performed a pooled data analysis of three comparative studies that aimed to assess various clinical outcomes of POEM and LHM. The analysis revealed comparable results of therapeutic options including success rate, complications, perforation rate, as well as procedure time [62]. Kumbhari et al. performed a comparative study over 75 patients and showed that POEM seems to be a better therapeutic option for achalasia type III when compared with LHM [63]. Even though it is suggested that there is an increased trend towards the development of GERD after POEM, when looking carefully at the reported results, most reflux esophagitis cases were mild and responded well to conservative treatment with proton pump inhibitor drugs. However, the main difficulty of the POEM technique is the operator learning curve; a recent study reported that mastering POEM in Latin America requires approximately 61 procedures both for POEM efficiency and to accomplish the procedure within 97 min [64]. Another previous study reported that 40 POEMs are needed to achieve efficiency and that 60 POEMS are needed to attain mastery [65].

Lastly, surgical esophagectomy is a radical procedure that is considered a last resort therapeutic option for longstanding advanced achalasia cases, which are rarely encountered and estimated to occur in 2–5% of cases. End-stage achalasia generally involves pathological dilation of the esophageal tubular structure and that even could be associated with alterations of the esophageal morphology (creating a sigmoid shape or mega-esophagus). Even though LHM could still be considered and performed successfully in end-stage achalasia with morphologic distortion of the esophagus, the radical esophagectomy might be the final possibility to improve patients' nutritional status, to ease their symptoms, and to improve their general performance and quality of life. Notably, esophagectomy is a major chest surgery and is associated with high adverse events including hospital-acquired pneumonia in 10% of cases, leaks at the surgical site causing chest infections in about 7% of cases, and finally, a mortality risk of 2% [6].

9. Treatment Decision-Making and Predictors of Outcomes

Recent published data from retrospective, prospective, and randomized studies indicate that there is no superiority between the three options of pneumatic dilation, LHM, and POEM. Considerations regarding the choice of therapy are largely determined by the achalasia subtype; clinical presentation; patient's age and fitness; the available expertise; and importantly, the patient's preferences. Significantly, the emerging data from the last decade points toward an association between the achalasia type and post-therapy clinical outcomes [43]. A post-hoc analysis by Rohof et al. of the European achalasia registry study found an association between achalasia subtype and treatment outcomes; the efficacy of pneumatic dilation was outstandingly excellent in type II achalasia but significantly decreased to 40% in type III achalasia [66]. Conversely, Kumbhari et al. conducted a multi-center comparative study that aimed to evaluate the treatment outcomes of 75 patients with type III achalasia and showed an excellent treatment success (98%) following POEM in comparison to 80% after LHM during both short-term (8.6 months) and long-term (21.5 months) ($p < 0.01$) follow-up [63]. This added value of POEM over LHM is logically explained by the capability of the endoscopic approach to achieve a tailored proximal extension of the myotomy. Oude and colleagues conducted a systematic review and meta-analysis that aimed to study various factors that might be associated with achalasia treatment outcomes. The analysis included 75 published studies and revealed that only the manometric pattern of achalasia and patient age were recognized as the most applicable predictors of clinical response [67].

10. Conclusions

Achalasia is an long-standing disease that has attracted much interest in the last two decades due to the revolutionary progress in its understanding and management. The introduction of the HRM with impedance along with the construction of the Chicago classification and their implementation in clinical practice has profoundly enriched our understanding of the esophageal and LES functions and has eventually led to classifying achalasia into three different types based on diverse manometric patterns. Moreover, EndoFLIP and the improved methodology in barium studies added to our knowledge, and these modalities complement HRM in specific clinical scenarios. The introduction of the POEM to the therapeutic arsenal has drastically reformed the attitude to achalasia therapy. The POEM procedure seems to be promising, with outcomes comparable to conventional procedures such as LHM and pneumatic balloon dilation. Nonetheless, more prospective studies are required to properly determine the long-term efficacy and safety of POEM. The treatment choice of achalasia should be tailored, taking into account several clinical and manometric factors.

Author Contributions: A.M. and T.K. contributed to the design and conception of the manuscript. A.M., R.P. and F.A.B. contributed to data collection, analysis, and interpretation. T.K. and A.M. wrote the first draft of the manuscript. R.P. and F.A.B. performed scientific criticism and language editing. All authors approved the final version to be published. All authors have read and agreed to the published version of the manuscript.

Funding: This research did not receive any funding.

Institutional Review Board Statement: Not applicable for a review article.

Informed Consent Statement: Not applicable for a review article.

Conflicts of Interest: The authors declare no conflict of interest regarding this manuscript.

Abbreviations

LES	Lower esophageal sphincter
EGJ	Esophago-gastric junction
EGJOO	Esophago-gastric outflow obstruction
HRM	High-Resolution Manometry
POEM	Per oral endoscopic myotomy
EOE	Eosinophilic Esophagitis
EGD	Esophago-Gastro-Duodenoscopy
LHM	Laparoscopic Heller myotomy
RDC	Rapid drinking challenge
MRS	Multiple rapid swallows
TBS	Timed barium swallow

References

1. Pandolfino, J.E.; Gawron, A.J. Achalasia: A systematic review. *JAMA* **2015**, *313*, 1841–1852. [CrossRef] [PubMed]
2. Williams, V.A.; Peters, J.H. Achalasia of the esophagus: A surgical disease. *J. Am. Coll. Surg.* **2009**, *208*, 151–162. [CrossRef]
3. Khashab, M.A.; Vela, M.F.; Thosani, N.; Agrawal, D.; Buxbaum, J.L.; Abbas Fehmi, S.M.; Fishman, D.S.; Gurudu, S.R.; Jamil, L.H.; Jue, T.L.; et al. ASGE guideline on the management of achalasia. *Gastrointest. Endosc.* **2020**, *91*, 213–227. [CrossRef] [PubMed]
4. Vaezi, M.F.; Pandolfino, J.E.; Yadlapati, R.H.; Greer, K.B.; Kavitt, R.T. ACG Clinical Guidelines: Diagnosis and Management of Achalasia. *Am. J. Gastroenterol.* **2020**, *115*, 1393–1411. [CrossRef]
5. Eckardt, V.F.; Hoischen, T.; Bernhard, G. Life expectancy, complications, and causes of death in patients with achalasia: Results of a 33-year follow-up investigation. *Eur. J. Gastroenterol. Hepatol.* **2008**, *20*, 956–960. [CrossRef] [PubMed]
6. Zaninotto, G.; Bennett, C.; Boeckxstaens, G.; Costantini, M.; Ferguson, M.K.; Pandolfino, J.E.; Patti, M.G.; Ribeiro, U., Jr.; Richter, J.; Swanstrom, L.; et al. The 2018 ISDE achalasia guidelines. *Dis. Esophagus* **2018**, *31*. [CrossRef]
7. Cassella, R.R.; Ellis, F.H., Jr.; Brown, A.L., Jr. Fine-Structure Changes in Achalasia of Esophagus. Ii. Esophageal Smooth Muscle. *Am. J. Pathol.* **1965**, *46*, 467–475. [PubMed]
8. Ota, M.; Narumiya, K.; Kudo, K.; Yagawa, Y.; Maeda, S.; Osugi, H.; Yamamoto, M. Incidence of Esophageal Carcinomas After Surgery for Achalasia: Usefulness of Long-Term and Periodic Follow-up. *Am. J. Case Rep.* **2016**, *17*, 845–849. [CrossRef] [PubMed]
9. Torres-Aguilera, M.; Remes Troche, J.M. Achalasia and esophageal cancer: Risks and links. *Clin. Exp. Gastroenterol.* **2018**, *11*, 309–316. [CrossRef]
10. Francis, D.L.; Katzka, D.A. Achalasia: Update on the disease and its treatment. *Gastroenterology* **2010**, *139*, 369–374. [CrossRef]
11. Gockel, I.; Becker, J.; Wouters, M.M.; Niebisch, S.; Gockel, H.R.; Hess, T.; Ramonet, D.; Zimmermann, J.; Vigo, A.G.; Trynka, G.; et al. Common variants in the HLA-DQ region confer susceptibility to idiopathic achalasia. *Nat. Genet.* **2014**, *46*, 901–904. [CrossRef]
12. Raymond, L.; Lach, B.; Shamji, F.M. Inflammatory aetiology of primary oesophageal achalasia: An immunohistochemical and ultrastructural study of Auerbach's plexus. *Histopathology* **1999**, *35*, 445–453. [CrossRef]
13. Jin, H.; Wang, B.; Zhang, L.L.; Zhao, W. Activated Eosinophils are Present in Esophageal Muscle in Patients with Achalasia of the Esophagus. *Med. Sci. Monit.* **2018**, *24*, 2377–2383. [CrossRef]
14. Liu, Z.Q.; Chen, W.F.; Wang, Y.; Xu, X.Y.; Zeng, Y.G.; Lee Dillon, D.; Cheng, J.; Xu, M.D.; Zhong, Y.S.; Zhang, Y.Q.; et al. Mast cell infiltration associated with loss of interstitial cells of Cajal and neuronal degeneration in achalasia. *Neurogastroenterol. Motil.* **2019**, *31*, e13565. [CrossRef]
15. Clayton, S.; Cauble, E.; Kumar, A.; Patil, N.; Ledford, D.; Kolliputi, N.; Lopes-Virella, M.F.; Castell, D.; Richter, J. Plasma levels of TNF-alpha, IL-6, IFN-gamma, IL-12, IL-17, IL-22, and IL-23 in achalasia, eosinophilic esophagitis (EoE), and gastroesophageal reflux disease (GERD). *BMC Gastroenterol.* **2019**, *19*, 28. [CrossRef] [PubMed]
16. Spechler, S.J.; Konda, V.; Souza, R. Can Eosinophilic Esophagitis Cause Achalasia and Other Esophageal Motility Disorders? *Am. J. Gastroenterol.* **2018**, *113*, 1594–1599. [CrossRef]
17. Skaper, S.D.; Facci, L.; Zusso, M.; Giusti, P. Neuroinflammation, Mast Cells, and Glia: Dangerous Liaisons. *Neuroscientist* **2017**, *23*, 478–498. [CrossRef] [PubMed]
18. Nakajima, N.; Sato, H.; Takahashi, K.; Hasegawa, G.; Mizuno, K.; Hashimoto, S.; Sato, Y.; Terai, S. Muscle layer histopathology and manometry pattern of primary esophageal motility disorders including achalasia. *Neurogastroenterol. Motil.* **2017**, *29*. [CrossRef] [PubMed]
19. Goldblum, J.R.; Rice, T.W.; Richter, J.E. Histopathologic features in esophagomyotomy specimens from patients with achalasia. *Gastroenterology* **1996**, *111*, 648–654. [CrossRef] [PubMed]
20. Zarate, N.; Wang, X.Y.; Tougas, G.; Anvari, M.; Birch, D.; Mearin, F.; Malagelada, J.R.; Huizinga, J.D. Intramuscular interstitial cells of Cajal associated with mast cells survive nitrergic nerves in achalasia. *Neurogastroenterol. Motil.* **2006**, *18*, 556–568. [CrossRef] [PubMed]
21. Villanacci, V.; Annese, V.; Cuttitta, A.; Fisogni, S.; Scaramuzzi, G.; De Santo, E.; Corazzi, N.; Bassotti, G. An immunohistochemical study of the myenteric plexus in idiopathic achalasia. *J. Clin. Gastroenterol.* **2010**, *44*, 407–410. [CrossRef]

22. Clark, S.B.; Rice, T.W.; Tubbs, R.R.; Richter, J.E.; Goldblum, J.R. The nature of the myenteric infiltrate in achalasia: An immunohistochemical analysis. *Am. J. Surg. Pathol.* **2000**, *24*, 1153–1158. [CrossRef] [PubMed]
23. Furuzawa-Carballeda, J.; Aguilar-Leon, D.; Gamboa-Dominguez, A.; Valdovinos, M.A.; Nunez-Alvarez, C.; Martin-del-Campo, L.A.; Enriquez, A.B.; Coss-Adame, E.; Svarch, A.E.; Flores-Najera, A.; et al. Achalasia–An Autoimmune Inflammatory Disease: A Cross-Sectional Study. *J. Immunol. Res.* **2015**, *2015*, 729217. [CrossRef]
24. Torres-Landa, S.; Furuzawa-Carballeda, J.; Coss-Adame, E.; Valdovinos, M.A.; Alejandro-Medrano, E.; Ramos-Avalos, B.; Martinez-Benitez, B.; Torres-Villalobos, G. Barrett's Oesophagus in an Achalasia Patient: Immunological Analysis and Comparison with a Group of Achalasia Patients. *Case Rep. Gastrointest. Med.* **2016**, *2016*, 5681590. [CrossRef] [PubMed]
25. Kilic, A.; Owens, S.R.; Pennathur, A.; Luketich, J.D.; Landreneau, R.J.; Schuchert, M.J. An increased proportion of inflammatory cells express tumor necrosis factor alpha in idiopathic achalasia of the esophagus. *Dis. Esophagus* **2009**, *22*, 382–385. [CrossRef] [PubMed]
26. Wu, X.Y.; Liu, Z.Q.; Wang, Y.; Chen, W.F.; Gao, P.T.; Li, Q.L.; Zhou, P.H. The etiology of achalasia: An immune-dominant disease. *J. Dig. Dis.* **2021**, *22*, 126–135. [CrossRef]
27. Ganem, D.; Kistler, A.; DeRisi, J. Achalasia and viral infection: New insights from veterinary medicine. *Sci. Transl. Med.* **2010**, *2*, 33ps24. [CrossRef] [PubMed]
28. Pressman, A.; Behar, J. Etiology and Pathogenesis of Idiopathic Achalasia. *J. Clin. Gastroenterol.* **2017**, *51*, 195–202. [CrossRef]
29. Facco, M.; Brun, P.; Baesso, I.; Costantini, M.; Rizzetto, C.; Berto, A.; Baldan, N.; Palu, G.; Semenzato, G.; Castagliuolo, I.; et al. T cells in the myenteric plexus of achalasia patients show a skewed TCR repertoire and react to HSV-1 antigens. *Am. J. Gastroenterol.* **2008**, *103*, 1598–1609. [CrossRef]
30. Kahrilas, P.J.; Boeckxstaens, G. The spectrum of achalasia: Lessons from studies of pathophysiology and high-resolution manometry. *Gastroenterology* **2013**, *145*, 954–965. [CrossRef]
31. Jones, D.B.; Mayberry, J.F.; Rhodes, J.; Munro, J. Preliminary report of an association between measles virus and achalasia. *J. Clin. Pathol.* **1983**, *36*, 655–657. [CrossRef]
32. Wang, A.J.; Tu, L.X.; Yu, C.; Zheng, X.L.; Hong, J.B.; Lu, N.H. Achalasia secondary to cardial tuberculosis caused by AIDS. *J. Dig. Dis.* **2015**, *16*, 752–753. [CrossRef]
33. Mari, A.; Patel, K.; Mahamid, M.; Khoury, T.; Pesce, M. Achalasia: Insights into Diagnostic and Therapeutic Advances for an Ancient Disease. *Rambam Maimonides Med. J.* **2019**, *10*. [CrossRef]
34. Woodfield, C.A.; Levine, M.S.; Rubesin, S.E.; Langlotz, C.P.; Laufer, I. Diagnosis of primary versus secondary achalasia: Reassessment of clinical and radiographic criteria. *AJR Am. J. Roentgenol.* **2000**, *175*, 727–731. [CrossRef] [PubMed]
35. Mari, A.; Abu Baker, F.; Mahamid, M.; Khoury, T.; Sbeit, W.; Pellicano, R. Eosinophilic esophagitis: Pitfalls and controversies in diagnosis and management. *Minerva Med.* **2020**, *111*, 9–17. [CrossRef] [PubMed]
36. Mari, A.; Sweis, R. Assessment and management of dysphagia and achalasia. *Clin. Med.* **2021**, *21*, 119–123. [CrossRef]
37. Yadlapati, R.; Kahrilas, P.J.; Fox, M.R.; Bredenoord, A.J.; Prakash Gyawali, C.; Roman, S.; Babaei, A.; Mittal, R.K.; Rommel, N.; Savarino, E.; et al. Esophageal motility disorders on high-resolution manometry: Chicago classification version 4.0((c)). *Neurogastroenterol. Motil.* **2021**, *33*, e14058. [CrossRef] [PubMed]
38. Kahrilas, P.J.; Bredenoord, A.J.; Fox, M.; Gyawali, C.P.; Roman, S.; Smout, A.J.; Pandolfino, J.E.; International High Resolution Manometry Working, G. The Chicago Classification of esophageal motility disorders, v3.0. *Neurogastroenterol. Motil.* **2015**, *27*, 160–174. [CrossRef]
39. Sanagapalli, S.; McGuire, J.; Leong, R.W.; Patel, K.; Raeburn, A.; Abdul-Razakq, H.; Plumb, A.; Banks, M.; Haidry, R.; Lovat, L.; et al. The Clinical Relevance of Manometric Esophagogastric Junction Outflow Obstruction Can Be Determined Using Rapid Drink Challenge and Solid Swallows. *Am. J. Gastroenterol.* **2021**, *116*, 280–288. [CrossRef]
40. Ang, D.; Misselwitz, B.; Hollenstein, M.; Knowles, K.; Wright, J.; Tucker, E.; Sweis, R.; Fox, M. Diagnostic yield of high-resolution manometry with a solid test meal for clinically relevant, symptomatic oesophageal motility disorders: Serial diagnostic study. *Lancet Gastroenterol. Hepatol.* **2017**, *2*, 654–661. [CrossRef]
41. Wang, Y.T.; Tai, L.F.; Yazaki, E.; Jafari, J.; Sweis, R.; Tucker, E.; Knowles, K.; Wright, J.; Ahmad, S.; Kasi, M.; et al. Investigation of Dysphagia After Antireflux Surgery by High-resolution Manometry: Impact of Multiple Water Swallows and a Solid Test Meal on Diagnosis, Management, and Clinical Outcome. *Clin. Gastroenterol. Hepatol.* **2015**, *13*, 1575–1583. [CrossRef]
42. Araujo, I.K.; Roman, S.; Napoleon, M.; Mion, F. Diagnostic yield of adding solid food swallows during high-resolution manometry in esophageal motility disorders. *Neurogastroenterol. Motil.* **2021**, *33*, e14060. [CrossRef]
43. Hollenstein, M.; Thwaites, P.; Butikofer, S.; Heinrich, H.; Sauter, M.; Ulmer, I.; Pohl, D.; Ang, D.; Eberli, D.; Schwizer, W.; et al. Pharyngeal swallowing and oesophageal motility during a solid meal test: A prospective study in healthy volunteers and patients with major motility disorders. *Lancet Gastroenterol. Hepatol.* **2017**, *2*, 644–653. [CrossRef]
44. Ang, D.; Hollenstein, M.; Misselwitz, B.; Knowles, K.; Wright, J.; Tucker, E.; Sweis, R.; Fox, M. Rapid Drink Challenge in high-resolution manometry: An adjunctive test for detection of esophageal motility disorders. *Neurogastroenterol. Motil.* **2017**, *29*. [CrossRef]
45. Babaei, A.; Szabo, A.; Yorio, S.D.; Massey, B.T. Pressure exposure and catheter impingement affect the recorded pressure in the Manoscan 360 system. *Neurogastroenterol. Motil.* **2018**. [CrossRef]
46. Lynch, K.L.; Yang, Y.X.; Metz, D.C.; Falk, G.W. Clinical presentation and disease course of patients with esophagogastric junction outflow obstruction. *Dis. Esophagus* **2017**, *30*, 1–6. [CrossRef]

47. DeLay, K.; Austin, G.L.; Menard-Katcher, P. Anatomic abnormalities are common potential explanations of manometric esophagogastric junction outflow obstruction. *Neurogastroenterol. Motil.* **2016**, *28*, 1166–1171. [CrossRef]
48. Biasutto, D.; Mion, F.; Garros, A.; Roman, S. Rapid drink challenge test during esophageal high resolution manometry in patients with esophago-gastric junction outflow obstruction. *Neurogastroenterol. Motil.* **2018**, *30*, e13293. [CrossRef] [PubMed]
49. Triggs, J.R.; Carlson, D.A.; Beveridge, C.; Jain, A.; Tye, M.Y.; Kahrilas, P.J.; Pandolfino, J.E. Upright Integrated Relaxation Pressure Facilitates Characterization of Esophagogastric Junction Outflow Obstruction. *Clin. Gastroenterol. Hepatol.* **2019**, *17*, 2218–2226.e2212. [CrossRef] [PubMed]
50. Rohof, W.O.; Lei, A.; Boeckxstaens, G.E. Esophageal stasis on a timed barium esophagogram predicts recurrent symptoms in patients with long-standing achalasia. *Am. J. Gastroenterol.* **2013**, *108*, 49–55. [CrossRef]
51. Sanagapalli, S.; Plumb, A.; Maynard, J.; Leong, R.W.; Sweis, R. The timed barium swallow and its relationship to symptoms in achalasia: Analysis of surface area and emptying rate. *Neurogastroenterol. Motil.* **2020**, *32*, e13928. [CrossRef]
52. Carlson, D.A.; Kahrilas, P.J.; Lin, Z.; Hirano, I.; Gonsalves, N.; Listernick, Z.; Ritter, K.; Tye, M.; Ponds, F.A.; Wong, I.; et al. Evaluation of Esophageal Motility Utilizing the Functional Lumen Imaging Probe. *Am. J. Gastroenterol.* **2016**, *111*, 1726–1735. [CrossRef]
53. O'Neill, O.M.; Johnston, B.T.; Coleman, H.G. Achalasia: A review of clinical diagnosis, epidemiology, treatment and outcomes. *World J. Gastroenterol.* **2013**, *19*, 5806–5812. [CrossRef] [PubMed]
54. Eckardt, V.F.; Gockel, I.; Bernhard, G. Pneumatic dilation for achalasia: Late results of a prospective follow up investigation. *Gut* **2004**, *53*, 629–633. [CrossRef] [PubMed]
55. Patel, D.A.; Sharda, R.; Hovis, K.L.; Nichols, E.E.; Sathe, N.; Penson, D.F.; Feurer, I.D.; McPheeters, M.L.; Vaezi, M.F.; Francis, D.O. Patient-reported outcome measures in dysphagia: A systematic review of instrument development and validation. *Dis. Esophagus* **2017**, *30*, 1–23. [CrossRef]
56. Pasricha, P.J.; Ravich, W.J.; Hendrix, T.R.; Sostre, S.; Jones, B.; Kalloo, A.N. Intrasphincteric botulinum toxin for the treatment of achalasia. *N. Engl. J. Med.* **1995**, *332*, 774–778. [CrossRef] [PubMed]
57. Boeckxstaens, G.E.; Annese, V.; des Varannes, S.B.; Chaussade, S.; Costantini, M.; Cuttitta, A.; Elizalde, J.I.; Fumagalli, U.; Gaudric, M.; Rohof, W.O.; et al. Pneumatic dilation versus laparoscopic Heller's myotomy for idiopathic achalasia. *N. Engl. J. Med.* **2011**, *364*, 1807–1816. [CrossRef] [PubMed]
58. Vaezi, M.F.; Pandolfino, J.E.; Vela, M.F. ACG clinical guideline: Diagnosis and management of achalasia. *Am. J. Gastroenterol.* **2013**, *108*, 1238–1249, quiz 1250. [CrossRef]
59. Kilic, A.; Schuchert, M.J.; Pennathur, A.; Gilbert, S.; Landreneau, R.J.; Luketich, J.D. Long-term outcomes of laparoscopic Heller myotomy for achalasia. *Surgery* **2009**, *146*, 826–831. [CrossRef] [PubMed]
60. Lynch, K.L.; Pandolfino, J.E.; Howden, C.W.; Kahrilas, P.J. Major complications of pneumatic dilation and Heller myotomy for achalasia: Single-center experience and systematic review of the literature. *Am. J. Gastroenterol.* **2012**, *107*, 1817–1825. [CrossRef]
61. Campos, G.M.; Vittinghoff, E.; Rabl, C.; Takata, M.; Gadenstatter, M.; Lin, F.; Ciovica, R. Endoscopic and surgical treatments for achalasia: A systematic review and meta-analysis. *Ann. Surg.* **2009**, *249*, 45–57. [CrossRef]
62. Ujiki, M.B.; Yetasook, A.K.; Zapf, M.; Linn, J.G.; Carbray, J.M.; Denham, W. Peroral endoscopic myotomy: A short-term comparison with the standard laparoscopic approach. *Surgery* **2013**, *154*, 893–897. [CrossRef]
63. Kumbhari, V.; Tieu, A.H.; Onimaru, M.; El Zein, M.H.; Teitelbaum, E.N.; Ujiki, M.B.; Gitelis, M.E.; Modayil, R.J.; Hungness, E.S.; Stavropoulos, S.N.; et al. Peroral endoscopic myotomy (POEM) vs laparoscopic Heller myotomy (LHM) for the treatment of Type III achalasia in 75 patients: A multicenter comparative study. *Endosc. Int. Open* **2015**, *3*, E195–E201. [CrossRef]
64. Kahaleh, M.; Tyberg, A.; Suresh, S.; Lambroza, A.; Casas, F.R.; Rey, M.; Nieto, J.; Martinez, G.M.; Zamarripa, F.; Arantes, V.; et al. The Learning Curve for Peroral Endoscopic Myotomy in Latin America: A Slide to the Right? *Clin. Endosc.* **2021**. [CrossRef]
65. Patel, K.S.; Calixte, R.; Modayil, R.J.; Friedel, D.; Brathwaite, C.E.; Stavropoulos, S.N. The light at the end of the tunnel: A single-operator learning curve analysis for per oral endoscopic myotomy. *Gastrointest. Endosc.* **2015**, *81*, 1181–1187. [CrossRef]
66. Rohof, W.O.; Salvador, R.; Annese, V.; Bruley des Varannes, S.; Chaussade, S.; Costantini, M.; Elizalde, J.I.; Gaudric, M.; Smout, A.J.; Tack, J.; et al. Outcomes of treatment for achalasia depend on manometric subtype. *Gastroenterology* **2013**, *144*, 718–725. [CrossRef]
67. Oude Nijhuis, R.A.B.; Prins, L.I.; Mostafavi, N.; van Etten-Jamaludin, F.S.; Smout, A.; Bredenoord, A.J. Factors Associated With Achalasia Treatment Outcomes: Systematic Review and Meta-Analysis. *Clin. Gastroenterol. Hepatol.* **2020**, *18*, 1442–1453, quiz e713–714. [CrossRef]

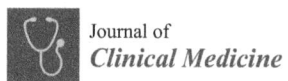

Article

Prothrombotic and Inflammatory Markers in Elderly Patients with Non-Alcoholic Hepatic Liver Disease before and after Weight Loss: A Pilot Study

Antonio Gidaro [1], Roberto Manetti [2], Alessandro Palmerio Delitala [2], Emanuele Salvi [1], Luigi Bergamaschini [1], Gianpaolo Vidili [2] and Roberto Castelli [2,*]

[1] Department of Biomedical and Clinical Sciences Luigi Sacco, Luigi Sacco Hospital, University of Milan, Via G.B. Grassi N° 74, 20157 Milan, Italy; gidaro.antonio@asst-fbf-sacco.it (A.G.); emalele29@gmail.com (E.S.); luigi.bergamaschini@unimi.it (L.B.)

[2] University of Sassari Department of Medical, Surgical and Experimental Science University Hospital of Sas-sari, Piazza Università N° 21, 07100 Sassari, Italy; rmanetti@uniss.it (R.M.); aledelitala@tiscali.it (A.P.D.); gianpaolovidili@uniss.it (G.V.)

* Correspondence: rcastelli@uniss.it; Tel.: +39-079-228446

Citation: Gidaro, A.; Manetti, R.; Delitala, A.P.; Salvi, E.; Bergamaschini, L.; Vidili, G.; Castelli, R. Prothrombotic and Inflammatory Markers in Elderly Patients with Non-Alcoholic Hepatic Liver Disease before and after Weight Loss: A Pilot Study. *J. Clin. Med.* **2021**, *10*, 4906. https://doi.org/10.3390/jcm10214906

Academic Editors: Davide Giuseppe Ribaldone and Gian Paolo Caviglia

Received: 13 September 2021
Accepted: 21 October 2021
Published: 25 October 2021

Publisher's Note: MDPI stays neutral with regard to jurisdictional claims in published maps and institutional affiliations.

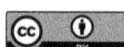

Copyright: © 2021 by the authors. Licensee MDPI, Basel, Switzerland. This article is an open access article distributed under the terms and conditions of the Creative Commons Attribution (CC BY) license (https://creativecommons.org/licenses/by/4.0/).

Abstract: Background: Non-alcoholic fatty liver disease (NAFLD) is a pathological condition, ranging from fatty liver to chronic steatohepatitis (NASH), liver cirrhosis, and eventually to hepatocellular carcinoma. Recent findings suggest that patients with NAFLD have an increased risk of cardiovascular events and thromboembolism, which is independent of metabolic diseases that are frequently associated with NAFLD, such as diabetes, hyperlipidemia, and obesity. Methods: We evaluated 30 NAFLD patients, before and after weight loss. Plasma levels of C-reactive protein (CRP), fibrinogen, plasminogen activator inhibitor-1 (PAI-1), von Willebrand factor (VWF), homocysteine, coagulation protein S, Thrombin activable fibrinolysis inhibitor (TAFI), and factor VII (FVII) were assessed to evaluate whether they should be responsible of the prothrombotic state of NAFLD after weight loss. Results: At baseline, patients affected by NAFLD had a significantly higher levels of CRP, fibrinogen, PAI-1, VWF antigen, and FVII levels. After weight reduction, we observed a significant drop of inflammatory and prothrombotic markers, as well as glucometabolic, lipid profile. Conclusion: These findings provide evidence for a link between NAFLD/NASH and thromboembolism. The association seems to be linked with primitive thrombotic state and hypercoagulation due to increased levels of coagulation factors and reduced levels of PAI-1. This hypercoagulation state might explain increased levels of thrombosis and splanchnic thrombosis observed in NASH correlated cirrhosis.

Keywords: non-alcoholic fatty liver disease (NAFLD); insulin resistance; plasminogen activator inhibitor-1 (PAI-1); von Willebrand factor (VWF); factor VII (FVII); slimming; weight loss; TAFI; protein S

1. Introduction

Non-alcoholic fatty liver disease (NAFLD) is a pathological condition, ranging from fatty liver (FL) to chronic steatohepatitis (NASH), liver cirrhosis, and eventually to hepatocellular carcinoma (HCC) [1].

Nonalcoholic fatty liver disease (NAFLD), on its whole spectrum of conditions ranging from steatosis to steatohepatitis (nonalcoholic steatohepatitis; NASH) and cirrhosis, is the most frequent liver disease in developed countries, now regarded as the liver manifestation of the metabolic syndrome [2]. Several studies indicate that NAFLD, especially in its necro-inflammatory form (NASH), is associated with a systemic proinflammatory/prothrombotic state, leading to atherothrombosis such as cardiovascular disease. The pathogenesis seems to be mediated through systemic release of proinflammatory and procoagulant factors from the steatosis liver (C-reactive protein, plasminogen activator inhibitor-1, interleukin-6, fibrinogen, and other proinflammatory cytokines) and is responsible for immunomodulated thrombosis [3–7]. Strong epidemiological, biochemical, and therapeutic evidences support the hypothesis that the primary pathophysiological derangement in most patients with NAFLD is insulin resistance. Insulin resistance leads to increased lipolysis, triglyceride synthesis, increased hepatic uptake of free fatty acids (FFA), and accumulation of hepatic triglycerides [8].

Fat-derived hormones, such as adiponectin, leptin, and resistin, are important co-regulators of hepatic insulin sensitivity. Insulin resistance may lead to activation of the coagulation cascade via increased levels of plasminogen activator inhibitor 1 (PAI-1) and factor VIII, whereas anticoagulant levels of protein Care decreased [9]. The topic, however, remains matter of debate and there are no consistent epidemiological or clinical data to support increased rates of venous thrombosis in NASH [10–13]. Aggressive lifestyle modifications focused on weight reduction and increased physical activities may reduce the inflammatory state of NAFLD, the insulin resistance, and the prothrombotic state which characterize NAFLD [14–18]. The vascular involvement of NAFLD might be considered its systemic burden, conditioning higher mortality in patients affected by the disease. High physical activity (PA) levels or exercise training (ET) should be a pivotal role of any treatment plan for obese individuals regardless of weight loss goals, and is associated with numerous CV benefits [14–18]. On the other hand, physical inactivity, obesity and disability correlate with institutionalization and loss of independence [19].

The aims of this study are to evaluate the parameters of the coagulation, fibrinolysis and inflammation in a group of NAFLD patients and to verify whether dietary modification or lifestyle change such as increased physical activity affects these parameters

2. Materials and Methods

2.1. Study Population

From 2 February to 5 May 2020, we prospectively enrolled patients with: (1) Age over 60 years, (2) certain diagnosis of NAFLD defined by: (i) Demonstration of hepatic steatosis by abdominal ultra-sonography or liver biopsy. Abdominal ultra-sonography was preferred to CT scanning due to its capability to detect mild to moderate steatosis. According to the general guidelines [19], we performed liver biopsy with the following indications: to confirm or exclude the diagnosis of NAFLD when ultra-sonography was not conclusive, to diagnose other liver diseases, and to determine amounts of damage to the liver when necessary for treatment and prognosis. The last includes necro inflammatory activity, which is potentially reversible, and collagen deposition with varying degrees of remodeling, which is potentially less reversible. (ii) Exclusion of significant alcohol consumption (<140 g/week. For men and <70 g/week for women). (iii) Exclusion of other causes of hepatic steatosis including drug-induced steatosis. (iv) Absence of coexisting chronic liver disease.

The exclusion criteria were: (1) Ongoing therapy with at least one between: anti-inflammatory, anti-fibrinolytic, anti-coagulant, anti-platelet, anti-diabetic drugs, or anti-hypertensive agents. (2) History of smoking (active or previous), chronic obstructive pulmonary disease, renal failure, chronic inflammatory diseases, or neoplasms. (3) Non responders to diet and change of lifestyle, defined as a weight loss of less than 10% of the basal body weight after one year of follow-up.

The study participants gave a written informed consent and local ethical committee approved the study (Ospedale Maggiore Policlinico di Milano; N 206 date 29 June 2013).

2.2. Sample Collection and Storage

Blood samples were collected after 12 h of fasting. Using sodium citrate 3.8% as an anti-coagulant, antecubital venous blood samples were drawn from patients affected by NAFLD, at baseline. Additional blood samples were collected when patients obtained 10% in decreased of basal body weight. Plasma was obtained by centrifuging the samples at

2000× g for 20 min at room temperature, frozen in small aliquots and stored at −80 °C until testing.

2.3. Measurements

Measurements included BMI, waist girth, and blood pressure. C reactive protein was measured by ELISA (Zymutest CRP, Hyphen BioMed, Andresy, France) with intra- and inter-assay coefficients of variation (CVs) of 7–11%. Fibrinogen was measured by a commercial coagulometric method (Diagnostica Stago, Asnières, France) with intra- and inter-assay CVs of 4% and 7%. Serum lipids were measured with the standardized methods of the Centers for Disease Control and Prevention, including total cholesterol, HDL cholesterol, and triglycerides. LDL cholesterol was estimated by the Friedewald equation [20]. When triglycerides were >400 mg/dL, LDL cholesterol was measured directly using an automated spectrophotometric assay. Glucose tolerance, insulin sensitivity, insulin secretion and insulin clearance were assessed by frequently sampled 75 g oGTT. Fasting serum glucose was determined using the hexokinase-glucose 6 phosphate dehydrogenase enzymatic assay, and insulin was determined using radioimmunoassay (Linc Research, St. Charles, MO, USA). Plasminogen activator inhibitor 1 (PAI-1) activity was measured using a commercial bio-immunoassay (Chromolize PAI-1, Bio pool, Umea, Sweden) with intra- and inter- assay CVs of 2.4% and 4.5%. Von Willebrand factor (VWF) antigen was measured in citrated plasma by an "in-house" sandwich ELISA using two monoclonal antibodies directed against different VWF epitopes (11B6.18 and 7G10.8). The intra- and inter-assay CVs were both 8%. Factor VII (FVII) activity was measured using a commercially available one-stage prothrombin time-based assay (Instrumentation Laboratory Company, Lexington, MA, USA) in accordance with the manufacturer's instructions. The intra- and inter-assay CVs were 10%. Total homocysteine values were determined by high performance liquid chromatography (HPLC) with fluorometric detection and isocratic elution. Free protein S antigen was measured using the Asserachrom Free Protein S assay (Stago), a one-step ELISA assay that uses 2 monoclonal antibodies specific for distinct epitopes of the free form of protein S to directly measure free protein S in plasma. Thrombin-activatable fibrinolysis inhibitor (TAFI) was purified from fresh-frozen plasma by immunoaffinity chromatography followed by further purification on protein G-Sepharose and Q-Sepharose (Amersham Pharmacia Biotech, Uppsala, Sweden). TAFI antigen levels were determined by a sandwich-type enzyme linked immunosorbent assay using a monoclonal capturing antibody and a polyclonal detection antibody.

2.4. Physical Activity Quantification

The self-estimation of physical activity levels was assessed while using the German Physical Activity Questionnaire 50+ (GPAQ 50+) [21], a self-administered questionnaire assessing older adults' PA level per week.

2.5. Statistical Analysis

Kolmogorov–Smirnov test was performed to evaluate the normality of distribution of data. Quantitative data were expressed as mean, standard deviation, median and range. Student T-test and Mann–Whitney test (for non-parametric data) were used for comparison between groups. p-value less than 0.05 was considered statistically significant. Data are shown as median values and interquartile ranges (25th and 75th percentiles). The between-group differences were analyzed using Mann–Whitney non-parametric tests for independent samples, and the effects of weight loss were assessed using multivariate analysis of variance, Friedman's test and Wilcoxon's test for paired samples. Data were analyzed using the SPSS PC statistical package, version 17.00 (SPSS Inc., Chicago, IL, USA). Univariate analysis of coagulation, metabolic parameter was performed to assess relationship between obesity, NAFLD, physical activity and prothrombotic state.

3. Results

During the observational period, sixty-five patients with certain diagnosis of NAFLD were evaluated, but only 30 met the inclusion criteria. In particular, 30 patients were excluded because ongoing therapy or history, five were non responders to diet and change of lifestyle, reducing the eligible number to 30 patients, (nine females and 21 males).

Median age of the examined population was 72 years (IQR 70–73) (Table 1). Thirteen patients had NASH, two patients had liver cirrhosis (all those 15 patients performed liver biopsy before the study beginning), and 11 patients had hepatic steatosis. In our case series, liver biopsy was performed during observational time in four cases, showing NASH in two cases and liver cirrhosis in two cases.

Table 1. Reports coagulation, fibrinolysis and inflammatory parameters, basal and after 10% of weight loss secondary to increase of PA. Data are reported as "median (IQR)".

	Before Weight Loss	After Weight Loss	p Value
age (years)	72 (70–73)		
Waist circumference (cm)	112.0 (91.5–116.0)	94.0 (86.0–105.0)	<0.0001
BMI (Kg/m^2)	37.0 (34.0–38.0)	31.5 (30.0–34.0)	<0.0001
Blood glucose (mg/dL)	126.00 (124.00–130.00)	96.00 (90.00–115.75)	<0.0001
OGTT (mg/dL)	180.00 (180.00–185.00)	160.00 (145.75–174.00)	<0.0001
CRP (mg/dL)	13.0 (12.0–16.5)	8.0 (6.0–10.0)	<0.0001
Fibrinogen (mg/dL)	450 (400–450)	300 (280–340)	<0.0001
PAI (UI/mL)	46.0 (44.0–50.0)	26.0 (21.5–31.5)	<0.0001
vWF (%)	160 (160–180)	115 (110–120)	<0.0001
F VII (%)	160 (150–160)	110 (110–110)	<0.0001
TAFI (%)	65.00 (60.00–70.00)	79.00 (78–82.25)	<0.0001
Homocysteine (μmol/L)	16 (14–18)	20 (17–22)	0.006
Protein S (%)	45.0 (42.0–46.5)	48.0 (44.0–48.0)	0.021
HDL (mg/dL)	25.00 (21.00–28.00)	36.00 (32.75–38.00)	<0.0001
Triglycerides (mg/dL)	156.00 (153.75–158.00)	127.00 (125.00–129.00)	<0.0001
PAS (mmHg)	140 (130–140)	120 (110–120)	<0.0001
PAD (mmHg)	90.00 (85.00–91.25)	75.00 (75.00–80.00)	<0.0001

Among NAFLD patients, two were normal-weight, (BMI among 18.5 to < 25.0), five patients were over-weight (BMI among 25 to < 30), and 23 patients were obese having BMI > 30.

BMI positively correlated with CRP (r = 0.57, p = < 0.0001), fibrinogen (r = 0.31, p = 0.0001), and PAI-1 levels (r = 0.75, p = 0.0001), vWF (r = 0.56, p = 0.001), F VII (r = 0.68, p = 0.001); basal glucose (r = 0.35, p = 0.0001), OGGT (r = 0.79, p = 0.0001), and TAFI (r = 0.49, p = 0.02). Waist circumference significantly correlated with basal glucose (r = 0.51, p = 0.0001), and OGTT (r = 0.45, p = 0.0001), systolic blood pressure (r = 0.49, p = 0.0001), and diastolic blood pressure (r = 0.51, p = 0.0001) as well as with coagulation parameters: PAI-1 (r = 0.52, p = 0.0001), vWF (r = 0.42, p = 0.0001), FVII (r = 0.53, p = 0.0001), TAFI (r = 0.29, p = 0.0001).

Protein S was correlated to BMI (r = 0.46, p = < 0.0001), but not to waist circumference (r = 0.17, p = 0.19).

Both BMI and waist circumference were not correlated to homocysteine (respectively, r = 0.07, p = 0.58; r = 0.06, p = 0.67).

After lifestyle modification was reached after one year of follow up, which was focused on a weight reduction to at least 10% of the basal and increased physical activity, we observed a significant reduction of BMI (p = 0.0001), waist circumference (p = 0.0001), as well as glucometabolic (p = 0.0001), lipid (p = 0.0001), and inflammatory (p = 0.0001), and prothrombotic markers (p = 0.0001), Figures 1–3.

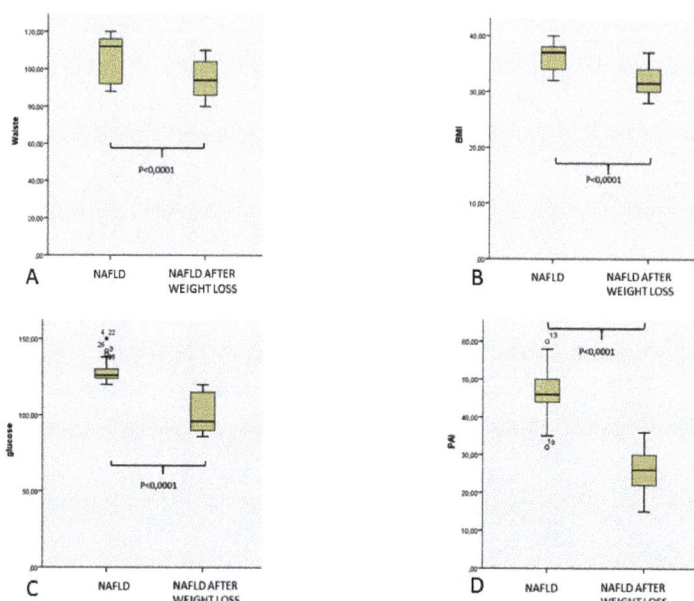

Figure 1. (**A**) Waist circumference. (**B**) body mass index. (**C**) glucose. (**D**) PAI 1 in 30 patients affected by NAFLD in basal control and after weight loss.

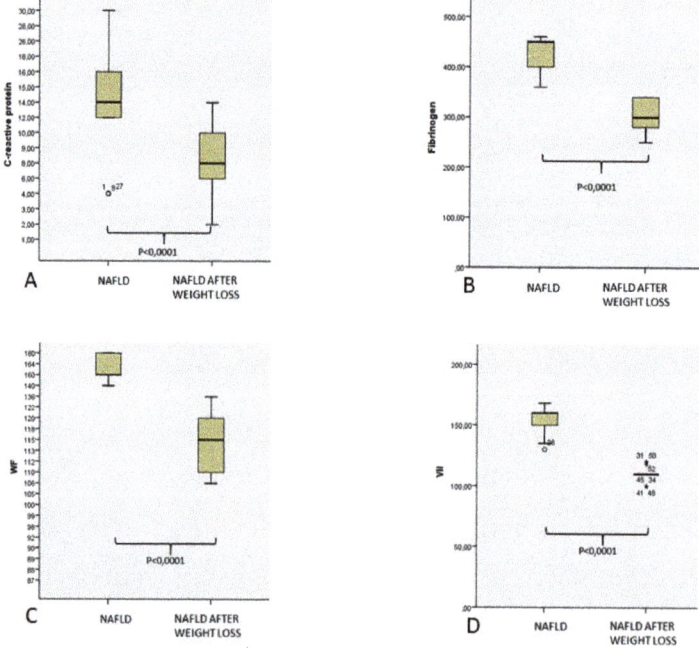

Figure 2. Plasma C-reactive protein levels (**A**), fibrinogen (**B**), von Willebrand factor (**C**), and factor VII levels (**D**) in 30 patients affected by NAFLD in basal control and after weight loss.

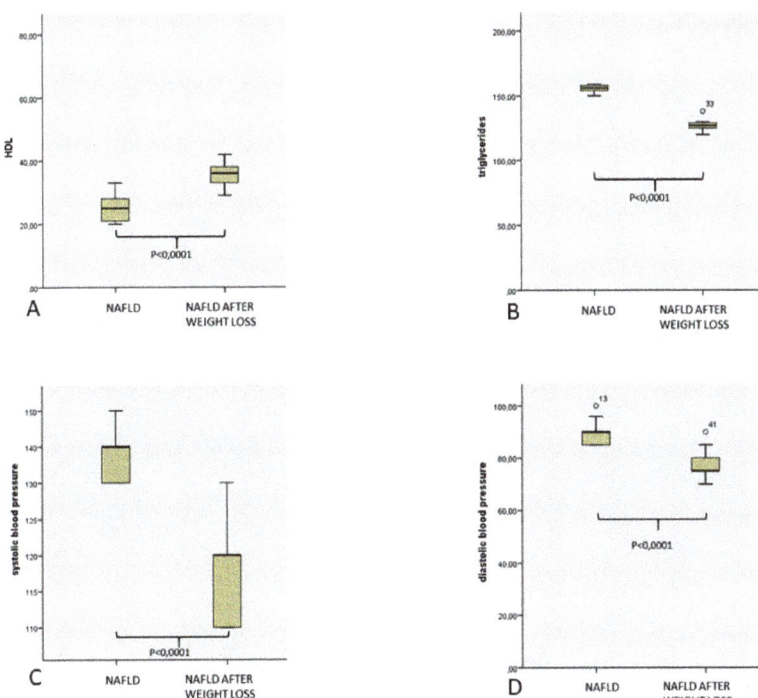

Figure 3. HDL cholesterol (**A**), triglycerides (**B**), systolic blood pressure (**C**), and diastolic blood pressure (**D**) of 30 patients affected by NAFLD in basal control and after weight loss.

In this time frame, BMI had decreased from 36.4 Kg/m^2 (34.2–38.6) to 32 Kg/m^2 (29.4–34.6) (p = 0.0001), waist abdominal circumference from 106.3 cm (94.6–118.1) to 95.3 cm (85.7–104.9) (p = 0.0001). Similarly, inflammatory markers, as well as coagulation parameters, significantly decreased after weight loss: CRP from 14.7 mg/dL (8.3–21.1) to 8.1 mg/dL (4.7–11.5) (p = 0.0001), fibrinogen from 429.9 mg/dL (400.4–459.5 mg/dL) to 301.5 (272.8–330.9) mg/dL (p = 0.0001), PAI 1 from 46.9 UI/mL (40.3–53.5) to 26.7 U/l (20.4–33), von Willebrand factor 163.7% (149.8%–177.2) to 115.5% (109.1–121.9) (p = 0.0001), factor VII from 155.6% (146.6–164.5) to 109.9% (103.6–116.3) (p = 0.0001).

TAFI value increased after slimming, from 65.6% (52-80) to 79.7% (74–88) (p = 0.0001).

Statistical regression analysis showed that at 12 months, the changes in BMI positively correlated with those of CRP (r = 0.46, p = 0.025), fibrinogen (r = 0.44, p = 0.026), PAI-1 levels (r = 0.47, p = 0.019), VWF (r = 0.47, p = 0.045). Statistical analysis revealed significant gender and BMI interaction effects.

4. Discussion

The relationship between NAFLD and venous thrombosis, particularly portal vein thrombosis (PVT), is described in a limited number of patients. [22]. Nevertheless, splanchnic venous thromboembolism greatly contributes to the outcome and clinical course of liver cirrhosis.

The clinical observation by Dentali et al. [23], that metabolic syndrome was diagnosed in 50.5% of patients with idiopathic vein thrombosis, underlies the pathogenetic role of the metabolic syndrome in venous thromboembolism, but the real incidence of thrombotic events among NAFLD remains relatively unexplored.

It has long been known that diabetes, obesity, and hypertension increase the prothrombotic risk [11], but, to the best of our knowledge, this is the first study aimed at correlating coagulation assessment in the NAFLD and offering an overview of the interactions between coagulation factors and fibrinolysis with inflammatory system in these setting.

The present study indicates that patients affected by NAFLD have elevated levels of CRP, fibrinogen, PAI-1, von Willebrand factors, and F VII, which are known to be associated with an increased risk of thrombosis. This further supports the in vivo data for a hypercoagulable state existing in NAFLD [7]. On the other side, this study suggests that systemic inflammation predisposes patients to endothelial dysfunction and thrombosis. Recent data [9] examining plasma for levels of procoagulants and anticoagulants in patients across the spectrum of NAFLD, including those with cirrhosis, support this. Although the exact clinical implications of this finding remain unclear, we postulate that the imbalance may be due to increased factor VIII and reduced protein C levels, which may lead to the downstream hallmark effects of adverse cardiovascular events. The relationship between coagulation and liver fibrosis in NASH patients remains to be explained.

Weight loss (at least 10% of basal body weight) induced by physical exercise is linked with reduction in inflammatory and coagulation parameters thus reducing the thrombotic risk. Similar findings were observed by a previous paper in obese patients undergoing gastric banding after weight loss [24].

Data from the present studies show a highly significant and direct correlation between fibrinogen, PAI-I, von Willebrand factor, and Factor VII, with morphometric parameters such as BMI and waist circumference. On the other side, we observed a significant reduction of coagulation factors and a decreased level of PAI-1 after weight loss induced by diet and physical exercise. Conflicting results have also been observed regarding fibrinogen levels in obese patients after dietary treatment [25].

The reduction of PAI-1 and von Willebrand factors (both markers of vascular/endothelial damage) after weight loss strongly suggests an improvement of the endothelial dysfunction, as already reported in a similar paper on metabolic syndrome and inflammation [26].

The reversibility of the damage remains to be explained. We cannot exclude that increasing coagulation factors may be due to the fact that they are acute phase proteins, in response to a chronic inflammatory state linked with metabolic syndrome. Similarly, NAFLD is regarded as an inflammatory condition capable of activating coagulation and impairing fibrinolysis. As a consequence, we observed significant increased levels of PCR with a statistically significant correlation with BMI and waist circumference.

Nevertheless, the high prevalence of NAFLD among idiopathic vein thrombosis, as observed by Dentali et al., corroborates the pathogenetic link between metabolic syndrome and thrombogenesis [23].

Our patients with NAFLD have higher levels of PAI-1. The link between PAI-1 and the metabolic syndrome with obesity was established many years ago [27], and increased PAI-1 level can be now considered a true component of the syndrome. The production of PAI-1 by adipose tissue, in particular by tissue from omentum, has been demonstrated and could be an important contributor to the elevated plasma PAI-1 levels observed in insulin resistant patients supporting the notion that PAI-1 can be a link between NAFLD, insulin resistance and cardiovascular disease [28,29].

The increase of TAFI values after slimming in our cohort confirm that data of Lisman et al. [30], which reported a deficiency of this inhibitor in cirrhosis patients.

Other gastroenterological autoimmune conditions (such as Celiac disease [31] and inflammatory bowel disease [32]) are at an increased risk of venous thromboembolism; the genetic link between those disease is well established. If the hypercoagulability is confirmed in a future study, the genetic landscape of NAFLD patients has to be investigated to discover a possible link.

Gut microbiota dysregulation plays a key role in the pathogenesis of nonalcoholic fatty liver disease (NAFLD) [33] and in hypercoagulability [34] through its metabolites. Therefore, the restoration of the gut microbiota and supplementation with commensal bacterial metabolites, due to diet and change of lifestyle during our study, can be of therapeutic benefit against the disease.

Another consideration on our series regards the age. There are few reports on NAFLD in the elderly population [35], although immobilization and comorbidities, well known hypercoagulability risk factors, greatly impact on the course of these patients [19].

The main limitation of this study is the small number of patients. This is the result of the highly selective criteria designed to ensure the absence of comorbidities and of the classification of NAFLD in different subtypes according to histologic findings.

5. Conclusions

The originality of the paper lies in the observation that NAFLD is correlated with increased prothrombotic and inflammatory factors, directly correlated with BMI and waist circumference, which decrease after weight loss induced by physical exercise.

The second key message is that weight loss is linked to amelioration blood pressure, metabolic control, and reduction of the prothrombotic state also in NAFLD. However, larger studies are needed to confirm the observation and establish differences in subgroups of NAFLD (steatosis; steatohepatitis (nonalcoholic steatohepatitis; NASH) and cirrhosis.

Author Contributions: R.C. defined the design of the study, studied and analyzed the results and wrote the paper. A.G., R.M., A.P.D., E.S. and G.V. managed the data collection process and analyzed data. L.B., A.P.D. and R.M. and reviewed the manuscript. All authors have read and agreed to the published version of the manuscript.

Funding: This research received no external funding.

Institutional Review Board Statement: The study was conducted according to the guidelines of the Declaration of Helsinki, and approved by the Institutional Ethics Committee of Ospedale Maggiore Policlinico di Milano (N 206 date 29 June 2013).

Informed Consent Statement: Informed consent was obtained from all subjects involved in the study.

Data Availability Statement: The study data will be made available upon request to the corresponding author.

Conflicts of Interest: The authors have no competing interests.

References

1. Ekstedt, M.; Franzén, L.E.; Mathiesen, U.L.; Thorelius, L.; Holmqvist, M.; Bodemar, G.; Kechagias, S. Long-term follow-up of patients with NAFLD and elevated liver enzymes. *Hepatology* **2006**, *44*, 865–873. [CrossRef]
2. Caldwell, S.H.; Lee, V.D.; Kleiner, D.; Al-Osaimi, A.M.; Argo, C.K.; Northup, P.G.; Berg, C.L. NASH and cryptogenic cirrhosis: A histological analysis. *Ann. Hepatol.* **2009**, *8*, 346–352. [CrossRef]
3. Wang, B.; Zhao, Z.; Liu, S.; Wang, S.; Chen, Y.; Xu, Y.; Xu, M.; Wang, W.; Ning, G.; Li, M.; et al. Impact of diabetes on subclinical atherosclerosis and major cardiovascular events in individuals with and without non-alcoholic fatty liver disease. *Diabetes Res. Clin. Pract.* **2021**, *177*, 108873. [CrossRef] [PubMed]
4. Hsiao, C.-C.; Teng, P.-H.; Wu, Y.-J.; Shen, Y.-W.; Mar, G.-Y.; Wu, F.-Z. Severe, but not mild to moderate, non-alcoholic fatty liver disease associated with increased risk of subclinical coronary atherosclerosis. *BMC Cardiovasc. Disord.* **2021**, *21*, 1–9. [CrossRef] [PubMed]
5. Targher, G.; Tilg, H.; Byrne, C.D. Non-alcoholic fatty liver disease: A multisystem disease requiring a multidisciplinary and holistic approach. *Lancet Gastroenterol. Hepatol.* **2021**, *6*, 578–588. [CrossRef]
6. Tomeno, W.; Imajo, K.; Takayanagi, T.; Ebisawa, Y.; Seita, K.; Takimoto, T.; Honda, K.; Kobayashi, T.; Nogami, A.; Kato, T.; et al. Complications of Non-Alcoholic Fatty Liver Disease in Extrahepatic Organs. *Diagnostics* **2020**, *10*, 912. [CrossRef] [PubMed]
7. Han, A.L. Association of Cardiovascular Risk Factors and Metabolic Syndrome with non-alcoholic and alcoholic fatty liver disease: A retrospective analysis. *BMC Endocr. Disord.* **2021**, *21*, 1–8. [CrossRef] [PubMed]
8. Gilbert, M. Role of skeletal muscle lipids in the pathogenesis of insulin resistance of obesity and type 2 diabetes. *J. Diabetes Investig.* **2021**, *9*, 15. [CrossRef]
9. Hörber, S.; Lehmann, R.; Stefan, N.; Machann, J.; Birkenfeld, A.L.; Wagner, R.; Heni, M.; Häring, H.-U.; Fritsche, A.; Peter, A. Hemostatic alterations linked to body fat distribution, fatty liver, and insulin resistance. *Mol. Metab.* **2021**, *53*, 101262. [CrossRef] [PubMed]
10. Tripodi, A.; Primignani, M.; Mannucci, P.M.; Caldwell, S.H. Changing Concepts of Cirrhotic Coagulopathy. *Am. J. Gastroenterol.* **2017**, *112*, 274–281. [CrossRef] [PubMed]

11. Targher, G.; Zoppini, G.; Moghetti, P.; Day, C.P. Disorders of Coagulation and Hemostasis in Abdominal Obesity: Emerging Role of Fatty Liver. *Semin. Thromb. Hemost.* **2010**, *36*, 041–048. [CrossRef] [PubMed]
12. Tripodi, A.; Fracanzani, A.L.; Primignani, M.; Chantarangkul, V.; Clerici, M.; Mannucci, P.M.; Peyvandi, F.; Bertelli, C.; Valenti, L.; Fargion, S. Procoagulant imbalance in patients with non-alcoholic fatty liver disease. *J. Hepatol.* **2014**, *61*, 148–154. [CrossRef] [PubMed]
13. Targher, G.; Chonchol, M.; Miele, L.; Zoppini, G.; Pichiri, I.; Muggeo, M. Nonalcoholic Fatty Liver Disease as a Contributor to Hypercoagulation and Thrombophilia in the Metabolic Syndrome. *Semin. Thromb. Hemost.* **2009**, *35*, 277–287. [CrossRef] [PubMed]
14. Swift, D.L.; Lavie, C.J.; Johannsen, N.M.; Arena, R.; Earnest, C.; O'Keefe, J.H.; Milani, R.V.; Blair, S.N.; Church, T.S. Physical Activity, Cardiorespiratory Fitness, and Exercise Training in Primary and Secondary Coronary Prevention. *Circ. J.* **2013**, *77*, 281–292. [CrossRef]
15. Blair, S.N.; Brodney, S. Effects of physical inactivity and obesity on morbidity and mortality: Current evidence and research issues. *Med. Sci. Sports Exerc.* **1999**, *31*, S646. [CrossRef]
16. Wei, M.; Kampert, J.B.; Barlow, C.E. Relationship between low cardio respiratory fitness and mortality in normal-weight, over-weight, and obese men. *JAMA* **1999**, *282*, 1547–1553. [CrossRef]
17. Ainsworth, B.E.; Haskell, W.L.; Herrmann, S.D.; Meckes, N.; Bassett, D.R.; Tudor-Locke, C.; Greer, J.L.; Vezina, J.; Whitt-Glover, M.C.; Leon, A.S. 2011 Compendium of Physical Activities. *Med. Sci. Sports Exerc.* **2011**, *43*, 1575–1581. [CrossRef] [PubMed]
18. Li, X.; Weber, N.; Cohn, D.; Hollmann, M.; DeVries, J.; Hermanides, J.; Preckel, B. Effects of Hyperglycemia and Diabetes Mellitus on Coagulation and Hemostasis. *J. Clin. Med.* **2021**, *10*, 2419. [CrossRef] [PubMed]
19. Chalasani, N.; Younossi, Z.; Lavine, J.E.; Diehl, A.M.; Brunt, E.M.; Cusi, K.; Charlton, M.; Sanyal, A.J. The Diagnosis and Management of Non-alcoholic Fatty Liver Disease: Practice Guideline by the American Gastroenterological Association, American Association for the Study of Liver Diseases, and American College of Gastroenterology. *Gastroenterology* **2012**, *142*, 1592–1609. [CrossRef]
20. Friedewald, W.T.; Levy, R.I.; Fredrickson, D.S. Estimation of the concentration of low-density lipoprotein cholesterol in plasma, without use of the preparative ultracentrifuge. *Clin. Chem.* **1972**, *18*, 499–502. [CrossRef]
21. Huy, C.; Schneider, S. Instrument Für Die Erfassung Der Physischen Aktivität Bei Personen Im Mittleren Und Höheren Erwachsenenalter: Entwicklung, Prüfung Und Anwendung Des "German-PAQ-50+". *Z. Gerontol. Geriatr.* **2008**, *41*, 208–216. [CrossRef] [PubMed]
22. Zocco, M.A.; Di Stasio, E.; De Cristofaro, R.; Novi, M.; Ainora, M.E.; Ponziani, F.R.; Riccardi, L.; Lancellotti, S.; Santoliquido, A.; Flore, R.A.; et al. Thrombotic risk factors in patients with liver cirrhosis: Correlation with MELD scoring system and portal vein thrombosis development. *J. Hepatol.* **2009**, *51*, 682–689. [CrossRef]
23. Dentali, F.; Romualdi, E.; Ageno, W. The metabolic syndrome and the risk of thrombosis. *Haematologica* **2007**, *92*, 297–299. [CrossRef] [PubMed]
24. Cugno, M.; Castelli, R.; Mari, D.; Mozzi, E.; Zappa, M.A.; Boscolo-Anzoletti, M.; Roviaro, G.; Mannucci, P.M. Inflammatory and prothrombotic parameters in normotensive non-diabetic obese women: Effect of weight loss obtained by gastric banding. *Intern. Emerg. Med.* **2011**, *7*, 237–242. [CrossRef]
25. Svendsen, O.L.; Hassager, C.; Christiansen, C.; Nielsen, J.D.; Winther, K. Plasminogen activator inhibitor-1, tissue-type plasminogen activator, and fibrinogen. Effect of dieting with or without exercise in overweight postmenopausal women. *Arterioscerl. Thromb. Vasc. Biol.* **1996**, *16*, 381–385. [CrossRef]
26. Zhang, X.; Gao, B.; Xu, B. Association between plasminogen activator inhibitor-1 (PAI-1) 4G/5G polymorphism and risk of Alzheimer's disease, metabolic syndrome, and female infertility. *Medicine* **2020**, *99*, e23660. [CrossRef]
27. Juhan-Vague, I.; Alessi, M.-C. PAI-1, Obesity, Insulin Resistance and Risk of Cardiovascular Events. *Thromb. Haemost.* **1997**, *78*, 656–660. [CrossRef]
28. Ciavarella, A.; Gnocchi, D.; Custodero, C.; Lenato, G.M.; Fiore, G.; Sabbà, C.; Mazzocca, A. Translational insight into prothrombotic state and hypercoagulation in nonalcoholic fatty liver disease. *Thromb. Res.* **2020**, *198*, 139–150. [CrossRef] [PubMed]
29. Campbell, P.T.; VanWagner, L.B.; Colangelo, L.A.; Lewis, C.E.; Henkel, A.; Ajmera, V.H.; Lloyd-Jones, D.M.; Vaughan, D.E.; Khan, S.S. Association between plasminogen activator inhibitor-1 in young adulthood and nonalcoholic fatty liver disease in midlife: CARDIA. *Liver Int.* **2020**, *40*, 1111–1120. [CrossRef]
30. Lisman, T.; Leebeek, F.W.G.; Mosnier, L.O.; Bouma, B.N.; Meijers, J.C.M.; Janssen, H.L.A.; Nieuwenhuis, H.K.; De Groot, P.G. Thrombin-Activatable Fibrinolysis Inhibitor Deficiency in Cirrhosis Is Not Associated with Increased Plasma Fibrinolysis. *Gastroenterology* **2001**, *121*, 131–139. [CrossRef]
31. Dumic, I.; Martin, S.; Salfiti, N.; Watson, R.; Alempijevic, T. Deep Venous Thrombosis and Bilateral Pulmonary Embolism Revealing Silent Celiac Disease: Case Report and Review of the Literature. *Case Rep. Gastrointest. Med.* **2017**, *2017*, 1–8. [CrossRef] [PubMed]
32. Cheng, K.; Faye, A.S. Venous thromboembolism in inflammatory bowel disease. *World J. Gastroenterol.* **2020**, *26*, 1231–1241. [CrossRef] [PubMed]
33. Chen, J.; Vitetta, L. Gut Microbiota Metabolites in NAFLD Pathogenesis and Therapeutic Implications. *Int. J. Mol. Sci.* **2020**, *21*, 5214. [CrossRef] [PubMed]

34. Hasan, R.A.; Koh, A.Y.; Zia, A. The gut microbiome and thromboembolism. *Thromb. Res.* **2020**, *189*, 77–87. [CrossRef]
35. Golabi, P.; Paik, J.; Reddy, R.; Bugianesi, E.; Trimble, G.; Younossi, Z.M. Prevalence and long-term outcomes of non-alcoholic fatty liver disease among elderly individuals from the United States. *BMC Gastroenterol.* **2019**, *19*, 56. [CrossRef]

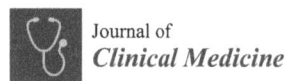

Review

Risk and Prevention of Hepatitis B Virus Reactivation during Immunosuppression for Non-Oncological Diseases

Lorenzo Onorato [1,2], Mariantonietta Pisaturo [1], Clarissa Camaioni [1], Pierantonio Grimaldi [1], Alessio Vinicio Codella [2], Federica Calò [2] and Nicola Coppola [1,2,*]

[1] Department of Mental Health and Public Medicine, Faculty of Medicine, University of Campania Luigi Vanvitelli, Via L. Armanni 5, 80138 Naples, Italy; lorenzoonorato@libero.it (L.O.); mariantonietta.pisaturo@unicampania.it (M.P.); clarissacamaioni91@gmail.com (C.C.); peogrimaldi@me.com (P.G.)
[2] Infectious Diseases Unit, Azienda Ospedaliera Universitaria Luigi Vanvitelli, Via Pansini 5, 80138 Naples, Italy; alessiovinicio.codella@studenti.unicampania.it (A.V.C.); fede.calo85@gmail.com (F.C.)
* Correspondence: nicola.coppola@unicampania.it

Abstract: Reactivation of overt or occult HBV infection (HBVr) is a well-known, potentially life-threatening event which can occur during the course of immunosuppressive treatments. Although it has been described mainly in subjects receiving therapy for oncological or hematological diseases, the increasing use of immunosuppressant agents in non-oncological patients observed in recent years has raised concerns about the risk of reactivation in several other settings. However, few data can be found in the literature on the occurrence of HBVr in these populations, and few clear recommendations on its management have been defined. The present paper was written to provide an overview of the risk of HBV reactivation in non-neoplastic patients treated with immunosuppressive drugs, particularly for rheumatological, gastrointestinal, dermatological and neurological diseases, and for COVID-19 patients receiving immunomodulating agents; and to discuss the potential strategies for prevention and treatment of HBVr in these settings.

Keywords: HBV infection; HBV reactivation; rheumatological diseases; gastrointestinal diseases; neurological diseases; dermatological diseases

Citation: Onorato, L.; Pisaturo, M.; Camaioni, C.; Grimaldi, P.; Codella, A.V.; Calò, F.; Coppola, N. Risk and Prevention of Hepatitis B Virus Reactivation during Immunosuppression for Non-Oncological Diseases. *J. Clin. Med.* **2021**, *10*, 5201. https://doi.org/10.3390/jcm10215201

Academic Editors: Davide Giuseppe Ribaldone and Gian Paolo Caviglia

Received: 3 September 2021
Accepted: 3 November 2021
Published: 8 November 2021

Publisher's Note: MDPI stays neutral with regard to jurisdictional claims in published maps and institutional affiliations.

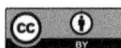

Copyright: © 2021 by the authors. Licensee MDPI, Basel, Switzerland. This article is an open access article distributed under the terms and conditions of the Creative Commons Attribution (CC BY) license (https://creativecommons.org/licenses/by/4.0/).

1. Introduction

Hepatitis B virus (HBV) represents one of the most important threats for public health. According to the WHO estimates, approximately 3.5% of the global population was living with a chronic HBV infection in 2015, and about 900,000 people died during the same year from HBV-related cirrhosis or hepatocellular carcinoma [1]. Furthermore, after HBsAg loss, the viral genome may persist in the hepatocytes, leading to a condition known as "occult HBV infection" (OBI), which is defined as the presence of replication of competent HBV DNA in the liver and/or blood of subjects testing negative for HBsAg [2].

In recent years, the increasing use of immunosuppressive treatments has led to a growing incidence of HBV reactivation (HBVr) in patients with overt or occult infection [3]. As a systematic review recently published by our group estimated a prevalence of OBI in Western countries ranging from 19% to 51% [4], and considering the incidence of immunosuppressive diseases and/or the use of immunosuppressive treatments, the risk of HBVr has become high. Life-threatening reactivation episodes have frequently been described in subjects undergoing immune suppression for oncological or hematological diseases [5,6]; however, little is known about the risk of HBVr in patients treated with immunosuppressants in other settings, such as rheumatological, gastroenterological, neurological, or dermatological diseases, and most recently for SARS-CoV-2 pneumonia.

The present paper was written to provide an overview of the risk of reactivation of HBV infection in non-oncological and non-hematological settings, and to discuss the strategies for preventing and treating these life-threatening events.

2. Epidemiology of HBV Infection

HBV belongs to the Hepadnaviridae family, which includes viruses with double-stranded DNA and lipoprotein envelopes. It mainly infects hepatocytes and is one of the most widespread viruses in the world. Despite the incisive vaccination programs that have been carried out, HBV still remains a global health problem due to its enormous burden in terms of morbidity and mortality. In fact, this virus can cause various clinical manifestations: acute hepatitis B, inactive carrier state, and chronic hepatitis B, which can lead to liver cirrhosis and hepatocellular carcinoma [7].

The WHO estimated that in 2015, chronic HBV infections affected about 257 million people in the world, 68% of whom lived in Africa and the Western Pacific [8]. We should point out that the prevalence of infection varies considerably by geographical area: in the African regions, it is 4.6–8.5%; in the Western Pacific region, 6.2–7.6%; in the East Mediterranean regions, the prevalence fluctuates between 2.6% and 4.3%; in South East Asia between 1.5% and 4%; in Europe between 1.2% and 2.6%; and finally, in North America, between 0.7% and 1.6% of the population is estimated to be HBsAg-positive [8].

In the regions with the highest prevalence, infection is mainly transmitted through the vertical route or as a result of intrafamily contacts, and therefore, it is acquired at birth or at an early age. These transmission routes contribute to maintaining high endemicity in these areas, especially given the high rate of chronicization reported when the infection is contracted during the first years of life. In regions with low prevalence, on the other hand, HBV is acquired mainly in adulthood by sexual or parenteral contact; but in these regions high HBsAg prevalence can be found in specific groups, such as among immigrants from areas with high endemicity [9], people who inject drugs (PWID), men who have sex with men (MSM), and people living with HIV (PLWHIV) [10].

Thanks to the extensive vaccination programs carried out, the prevalence of chronic hepatitis B among children under the age of 5 fell to below 1% in 2019 (compared to 5% in the pre-vaccination period or up to 2000), but the goal planned by the WHO—to eliminate HBV infection as a major health problem—is still far from being achieved [11].

3. Natural History of HBV Infection

The natural history of chronic HBV infection has been divided into five phases, according to the HBeAg serostatus, the viral load, the transaminase levels, and the grading and staging of liver disease [12]. A HBeAg-positive chronic infection, previously called "immunotolerant phase", is characterized by a limited or absent immune response against the virus, which leads to intense viral replication, with HBeAg positivity, ALT persistently in the normal range, and no or minimal liver necroinflammation or fibrosis. During the second phase, currently named "HBeAg-positive chronic hepatitis", the host produces an active immune response against viral antigens, causing a consequent reduction in viral load, and elevation of transaminase levels and liver inflammation. The immune response can eventually lead to control of the infection, with HBeAg seroclearance, low level replication (HBV DNA < 2000 UI/mL), absence of ALT elevation, and mild or no necroinflammation in the liver: these features define the phase of "HBeAg-negative chronic infection". The acquisition of mutations in the pre-core or basal core promoter regions, however, may allow high-level viral replication despite the presence of antibodies against HBeAg, and lead to elevation of the viral load and liver enzymes, concurrent moderate to severe liver inflammation, and rapid progression of disease. Finally, as previously described, after the HBsAg clearance, the viral genome can still remain detectable in the liver or plasma, defining the "HBsAg-negative phase" or "occult B infection"; several data suggest that the persistence of low-level replication in patients with occult infections can contribute to the advancement of liver fibrosis and the development of hepatocellular cancer in patients with other etiologies of liver disease, particularly hepatitis C virus (HCV) infections [13,14].

In patients with chronic hepatitis, the cumulative 5-year incidence of progression to cirrhosis is estimated to be 8–20%. The wide variability can be determined by the viral load, the HBeAg serostatus, and the presence of concomitant alcohol abuse or coinfection with

HCV, hepatitis Delta virus (HDV), or human immunodeficiency virus (HIV) [15]. Once cirrhosis occurs, the risk of decompensation is estimated to be around 20–25% per year, and the 5-year survival is 20–30% [16]. Moreover, about 5–15% of cirrhotic patients develop hepatocellular cancer during their lives [17].

4. HBV Reactivation following Immunosuppressive Treatments

Although many definitions have been proposed, HBV reactivation commonly refers to either the de novo detection of HBV DNA or a ≥10-fold increase in HBV DNA level compared with the baseline value in HBsAg-positive patients, and seroconversion to HBsAg-positive status in previously negative subjects [18]. The biological basis of HBVr is the persistence of the viral genome as ccc-DNA in liver cells.

Several risks factors for the occurrence of reactivation after immune suppression have been identified [19].

As regards the host characteristics, the most important factor is the HBV immune control preceding the treatment. Obviously, patients with chronic HBV infections are significantly more at risk of reactivation compared to subjects with OBI, as demonstrated by several studies in both oncological [20] and non-oncological settings [21,22]. Furthermore, among HBsAg-negative subjects, the presence of anti-HBs has been related to a lower risk of reactivation, as demonstrated by Seto et al. [23] among 63 patients receiving rituximab for hematological malignancies. Other host factors that have been related to increased risk of reactivation include male gender [24], older age [25], and underlying lymphoproliferative diseases [5].

According to the agent used and the serostatus of the patient, the risk of HBVr can be roughly classified into high risk (frequency of reactivation > 10% in the absence of prophylaxis), medium risk (1–10%), or low risk (<1%) [18,26,27]. It is well known that the use of specific drugs, such as B-cell depleting agents, is associated with a high risk of reactivation in patients with both overt and occult infections [28]. Other drug classes that can cause reactivation in more than 10% of cases among HBsAg-positive subjects include anthracycline derivatives [20] and high dose corticosteroids (20 mg daily of prednisone or equivalent) administered for more than 4 weeks of treatment [18]. In particular, glucocorticoids have been demonstrated to directly stimulate HBV replication in hepatoma cells through the activation of regulatory elements [29]. Additional drug classes that have been related to reactivation in patients with overt and/or occult HBV infections include inhibitors of TNF-alfa [22] or other cytokine or integrin inhibitors [30], and tyrosine kinases [31] and JAK inhibitors [21]. Many of these agents have been used increasingly in recent years in non-oncological settings, such as rheumatological diseases or inflammatory bowel diseases, but less clear data on their impacts on HBV infection are available so far among non-oncological populations.

5. Strategies for the Prevention and Treatment of HBV Reactivation

Since the likelihood of HBV reactivation depends on the type, duration, and intensity of the immunosuppression, therapeutic strategies aimed at avoiding HBV reactivation are modulated according to the risk profile of reactivation. The algorithm of HBVr prevention according to HBsAg serostatus and risk of reactivation is shown in Figure 1.

Considering the phases of HBV infection, the patients with chronic hepatitis are at high risk for HBVr and progression of liver damage, so and they should be evaluated for treatment. Those with HBeAg-positive or HBeAg–negative chronic infections and those with previous infections show various risks of reactivation, and should be evaluated for HBV prophylaxis or pre-emptive therapy according to the immunosuppressive regimens they will undergo [12].

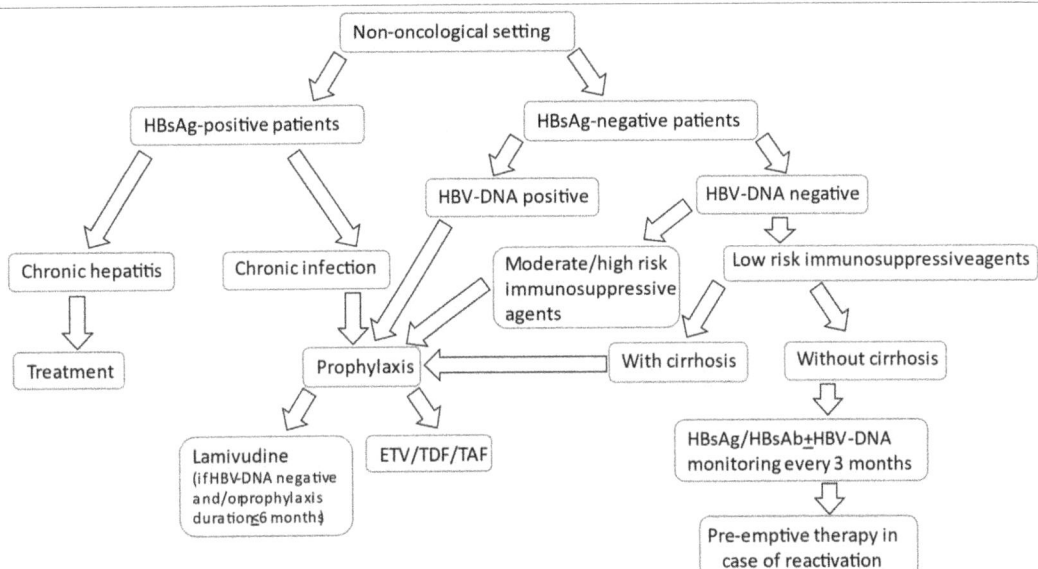

Figure 1. Algorithm of HBVr management in patients undergoing immunosuppression for non-oncological diseases.

In the patients with HBV-related hepatitis, a therapy with high genetic barrier nucleos(t)ide analogues (entecavir (ETV), tenofovir (TDF), or tenofovir alafenamide (TAF)) should be started as soon as possible, as for non-immunocompromised subjects, so this is considered therapy and not prophylaxis [12,32–35].

Instead, in patients with HBV infections undergoing treatments that involve moderate–high risks of reactivation, some form of prophylaxis should be prescribed, preferably an antiviral drug with a high genetic barrier, i.e., ETV, TDF, or TAF, as recommended by international guidelines [12,32]. Lamivudine was the first nucleoside analogue used as antiviral prophylaxis to reduce HBVr complications; however, the development of resistance in patients requiring prolonged duration of therapy may lead to a re-emergence of HBV DNA and a risk of HBVr, so newer nucleoside agents with high barriers to resistance may provide additional options for antiviral prophylaxis [36]. According to the guidelines of the American Gastroenterological Association (AGA), the use of lamivudine should be limited to the prophylaxis of patients with undetectable viral loads at baseline or with expected durations of prophylaxis of less than 6 months [32].

The prophylaxis should be started before the prescription of the immunosuppressive regimen and continued until 12–18 months after the discontinuation of the treatment [32,37–39].

HBsAg-negative, anti-HBc-positive patients should be considered for antiviral prophylaxis or pre-emptive therapy according to the HBV DNA at baseline.

Patients with positive HBV DNA at baseline should receive prophylaxis similarly to patients with overt infections. Conversely, the management depends on the risk of HBV reactivation: when the risk of reactivation is high (e.g., the use of B-cell depleting agents), a prophylactic agent should be prescribed. In the case of a moderate risk of reactivation, the correct strategy is still a matter of debate. The guidelines of the European Association for Study of Liver (EASL) recommend a pre-empitve therapy strategy [12], although a prophylaxis can be considered, according to the AGA guidelines [32]. Instead, with a low risk of reactivation, a strategy based on pre-emptive therapy is generally recommended. Patients should undergo close monitoring during and after the immunosuppression. If HBsAg seroreversion occurs, antiviral therapy with a nucleos(t)ide analogue should be initiated.

However, in select patients with previous infection and low risk of reactivation, but with advanced liver disease due to a different etiology, lamivudine prophylaxis may be considered, to avoid the risk of a life-threatening hepatic failure following the reactivation [12,32,40,41].

As regards the monitoring of the patients for whom prophylaxis is envisaged, liver function tests and HBV DNA for patients with HBV infections and HBV DNA/HBsAg tests for patients with resolved HBV infection should be performed every 3–6 months during prophylaxis and up to 12–18 months after stopping the antiviral treatment, as an episode of reactivation can still occur after the interruption of the antiviral therapy. Instead, in patients with HBV related diseases for whom therapy is envisaged, virological and biochemical monitoring is lifelong [12,32].

In the following sections we discuss the risk of reactivation related to the use of immunosuppressant agents in non-oncological settings and provide an overview of the possible management strategies.

5.1. Risk of HBV Reactivation in Gastroenterological Diseases

Autoimmune and inflammatory disorders, such as Crohn's disease and ulcerative colitis, are common gastroenterological conditions that often require the use of immunosuppressive therapies. Disease severity and the relapsing and remitting course affect the selection of the right drug. Agents commonly used include corticosteroids, immunomodulator agents (e.g., azathioprine/mercaptopurine and methotrexate), biological therapies (i.e., tumor necrosis factor (TNF) inhibitors), anti-adhesion therapy, anti-IL12/23 p40 antibody, and Janus kinase (JAK) inhibitor in the ultra-refractory cases.

A list of studies evaluating the risk of HBV reactivation in patients with gastroenteric diseases treated with immunosuppressive agents is reported in Table 1. In a retrospective study of 8887 patients treated with TNF inhibitors for autoimmune disorders, HBVr was observed in 9 of the 23 HBsAg-positive patients and 2 of 4267 patients in the unknown HBV status group [22]. Concomitant immunosuppressives, including steroids and non-biological immunosuppressants, were also associated with HBVr.

In a Spanish multicenter analysis of 162 patients with inflammatory bowel disease (IBD) treated with different immunosuppressant drugs, the authors described HBVr in 9 (36%) out of the 25 HBsAg-positive patients; however, none of the HBsAg-negative but anti-HBc positive subjects patients reported HBVr [42]. In addition, the authors found that treatment with ≥ 2 immunosuppressive agents was an independent predictor of HBVr (OR 8.75; 95% CI 1.16–65.66).

Morisco et al. [43], in a retrospective study, evaluated 5096 patients with IBD and found a lower rate of HBVr; indeed, HBVr was detected in only one of six (16%) HBsAg-positive patients treated with a therapeutic regimen that included infliximab and azathioprine.

In a systematic review evaluating 257 subjects with positive hepatitis B markers (89 were HBsAg-positive and 168 were HBsAg-negative/anti-HBc-positive carriers) treated with anti-TNF inhibitors for IBD and other autoimmune disorders, Perez-Alvarez et al. [44] found a lower rate of reactivation in patients who had antiviral prophylaxis (23% vs. 62%, $p = 0.003$) but a higher rate in those already treated with immunosuppressive drugs (96% vs. 70%, $p = 0.033$).

In a national cohort of 3357 patients with IBD in the USA, Shah et al. did not identify a single case of confirmed clinically relevant HBVr after anti-TNF starting [45].

As regards HBsAg-negative/anti-HBc-positive subjects with IBD, only a few cases of HBVr have been described. Clarke et al. [46] investigated the prevalence of HBVr in a single-center retrospective cohort analysis of 120 HBsAg-negative/anti-HBc-positive subjects (anti-TNF treatment in 19% of the cases), and found a low rate of HBV reactivation (0.8%). Solay et al. [47] assessed 29 cases of patients with resolved HBV infection who received biological treatment: HBVr was observed in five patients (17.2). Pauly et al. reported that not one of the 178 HBsAg-negative/anti-HBc-positive subjects treated with TNF antagonists had documented HBVr [22]. Additionally, Papa et al. [48] reported no cases of HBV reactivation in 22 HBsAg-negative/anti-HBc-positive IBD patients treated with anti-TNF. Additionally, no HBVr and/or associated biochemical breakthrough was detected in a retrospective study that evaluated 90 patients (of whom 13 with IBD) with past HBV infection who received anti-TNF treatment [49]. In the above-mentioned systematic review [44], the authors reported an HBVr rate of 39% in HBsAg-positive patients and 5% in HBsAg-negative/anti-HBc-positive patients.

In conclusion, complete serology for HBV is required in IBD patients to determine the virological status (active carrier, inactive carrier or anti-HBc positivity), since the HBV profile affects the choice of HBV therapy, prophylaxis, or monitoring. In fact, in consideration of the higher risk of reactivation, IBD patients who are HBsAg-positive carriers should receive prophylactic antiviral treatment with nucleotide or nucleoside analogues before the introduction steroids at moderate to high doses (>20 mg/die of prednisone or equivalent) for more than 4 weeks, azathioprine, anti-TNF therapy, or ustekinumab. Treatment may be lifelong in patients with chronic HBV and for at least one year after discontinuing immunosuppressive therapy in HBsAg asymptomatic carriers.

The approach to IBD patients who are HBsAg-negative and anti-HBc-positive is not standardized across the various guidelines. The American Gastroenterological Association recommends antiviral prophylaxis for HBsAg-negative/anti-HBc-positive patients treated with anti-TNF or with corticosteroids (10–20 mg or >20 mg prednisone daily for 4 weeks); there is a moderate risk of reactivation in this population [32]. The European Association for the Study of the Liver [12] and the European Crohn and Colitis Organization guidelines [50] suggest the strategy of active monitoring of viremia and recommend that antiviral agents be initiated once HBV DNA or seroconversion to positive HBsAg is detected. Therefore, considering the indications of the published guidelines and the scant data available in the literature in support of antiviral prophylaxis, HBsAg monitoring every 2–3 months may be recommended for such patients.

5.2. Risk of HBV Reactivation in Dermatological Diseases

Immunosuppressive drugs, both conventional and biological, are used in many different dermatological diseases, among which psoriasis is the most common and affects approximately 125 million people worldwide [51]. Conventional disease modifying drugs (cDMARDs) include acitretine, cyclosporin A, and methotrexate; and biological DMARDs (bDMARDs) include etanercept, adalimumab, infliximab, ustekinumab, golimumab, certolizumab, and secukinumab. Trials investigating new drugs do not usually involve HBV patients, so data on their safety regarding HBV reactivation in patients with psoriasis are based mostly on case reports and small retrospective cohort studies.

Table 2 summarizes the studies evaluating reactivation of current and past HBV infections in the setting of dermatological disease.

Chiu et al. [52] evaluated the risk of reactivation of HBV in 14 psoriatic patients undergoing therapy with ustekinumab. Two out of the seven (29%) HBsAg-positive patients not receiving prophylaxis showed HBVr during ustekinumab treatment, whereas no reactivation was observed among the 3 HBsAg-negative/HBcAb-positive patients.

In a retrospective cohort study, Ting et al. [53] included 54 subjects with active or previous infections. Only three patients experienced virological reactivation. The calculated incidence rate of annual HBV reactivation with ustekinumab was 17.4% among inactive HBV carriers without prophylaxis and 1.5% in the occult hepatitis B infection group.

A retrospective study by Snast et al. [54] reported no reactivation among 25 psoriatic patients with past infections and one with a current HBV infection treated with biological therapies. Similar results were observed in an Italian study among patients with psoriasis and chronic HBV infection treated with adalimumab [55].

In a cohort study published in 2018 [56], the authors followed-up 32 patients with psoriasis and concurrent positive HBV markers (chronic inactive and occult cases) treated with biological agents (adalimumab, etanercept, ustekinumab) for at least 24 weeks and found no evidence of viral reactivation 3 months after stopping treatment.

Finally, a meta-analysis performed by Cantini et al. [57] estimated a pooled prevalence of HBVr of 3% among subjects with previous HBV infections, and of 15.4% in patients with overt infections during treatment with anti TNF for dermatological and rheumatological diseases.

Although the reliability of many of these studies is limited by small numbers of subjects and short periods of follow-up, the available evidence suggests that in HBsAg-positive patients who receive treatment with immunosuppressive drugs associated with moderate risk of HBV reactivation (anti-TNFα, including etanercept, adalimumab, and golimumab; and cytokine or integrin inhibitors, such as ustekinumab or secukinumab), antiviral prophylaxis would be preferable; for HBsAg-negative/anti-HBc–positive patients, both antiviral prophylaxis and close monitoring with pre-emptive therapy are feasible options.

5.3. Risk of Reactivation in Rheumatological Diseases

Rheumatological drugs include corticosteroids, non-steroidal anti-inflammatory drugs (NSAIDs), analgesic drugs, and disease-modifying antirheumatic drugs (DMARDs). The latter are divided into conventional synthetics (cs) and biological (b) drugs.

The csDMARDs include sulfasalazine; methotrexate; hydroxychloroquine; leflunomide; and less frequently, azathioprine, gold salts, and minocycline [58]. The bDMARDs can instead be distinguished on the basis of mechanism of action into TNF inhibitors (etanercept, infliximab, adalimumab, certolizumab, and golimumab), IL-1 inhibitors (anakinra, and canakinumab), IL-6 and IL-6R inhibitors (tocilizumab and sarilumab, respectively), inhibitors of IL-17 (secukinumab and ixekizumab), IL-23 inhibitors (ustekinumab and guselkumab), and JAK kinase inhibitors (tofacitinib, baricitinib, upadacitinib, filgotinib, and peficitinib [59,60].

Studies that provided data on HBVr in patients with rheumatological diseases are shown in Table 3. HBVr has been found in rheumatological patients receiving both csDMARD and bDMARD treatment. Among the csDMARDs, methotrexate has been widely used, but its impact on HBVr has not yet been clarified. A Thai study did not report episodes of reactivation among 65 HBcAb-positive, HbsAg-negative rheumatological patients treated for nine years with methotrexate [61], whereas seven cases of reactivation, five of which were severe, were described in the literature among patients with overt HBV infections treated with the same drug [62–66].

A study by Chen et al. [67] enrolling 123 HbsAg-positive subjects with rheumatoid arthritis from 2006 to 2012 demonstrated a higher risk of HBVr (occurring in 30 patients) when csDMARDS were combined with other immunosuppressants: in particular, low-dose glucocorticoids with csDMARDs and bDMARDs (excluding rituximab) caused an HBV reactivation in 54.5% of cases, bDMARDs (excluding rituximab) associated with csDMARDs coincided with reactivation in 5.9% of patients, and the risk of HBVr for csDMARDs associated with glucocorticoids was 12.5%. Regarding outcomes, despite antiviral treatment being initiated at the time of HBVr appearance, 13 (43.3%) patients developed severe hepatitis and 5 (16.7%) hepatic decompensation, with death in three cases.

As regards anti-TNF bDMARDs, a study by Ryu et al. [68] recorded two (6.9%) cases of HBVr within one year of anti-TNF treatment among 29 patients not receiving a primary prophylaxis. Only one reactivation (9%) was recorded in the prophylaxis group (20 patients) at the 64th week of therapy with bDMARDs.

Regarding HbsAg-negative patients, a prospective multicenter study by Fukuda et al. [69] described an HBVr rate of 1.93/100 people/year among 1042 patients undergoing immunosuppressive treatment for rheumatological diseases. The incidence of reactivation among patients testing negative for HBsAb was significantly higher than that of HBsAb-positive subjects (4.32 vs. 1.42/100 persons/year). No liver dysfunction occurred during HBVr. In a subsequent paper on the same group, 57 cases of HBVr (0.43/100 persons/year) occurred over the course of 4 years; age >70 years [70]. The presence of isolated anti-HBc antibodies and immunosuppressive therapy other than monotherapy with methotrexate were found to be independent risk factors for HBVr. The authors proposed a scoring system to distinguish between patients at higher and lower risks of reactivation. Finally, in a meta-analysis published in 2013, Lee et al. [71] reported eight (1.7%) cases of HBV reactivation among 468 patients with previous HBV infections who underwent anti-TNF treatment for rheumatic disease.

In a study by Varisco et al. [72], HBVr was evaluated in patients with previous HBV infections treated with methotrexate plus rituximab (with or without steroids) for rheumatoid arthritis. None of the subjects received antiviral prophylaxis for HBV. No case of seroreversion to HbsAg positivity was observed, but 6 out of 28 (21%) HBsAb-positive patients presented a decrease (>50%) in the antibody titer. Only one patient was positive for HBV DNA after 6 months of treatment with rituximab; the subject was promptly treated with lamivudine, avoiding an exacerbation of hepatitis.

In a study by Urata et al. [73], 135 HBsAg-negative and anti-HBc-positive patients undergoing immunosuppressive treatment for rheumatoid arthritis were prospectively evaluated. HBV DNA was positive during follow-up in seven cases (5.1%). The patients who received bDMARDs had a significantly higher rate of HBV reactivation compared with those who were treated with other immunosuppressants ($p = 0.008$), with a hazard ratio of 10.9 (1.4–87.7).

Nakamura et al. [74] evaluated 57 patients with rheumatoid arthritis treated with bDMARDs and a previous HBV infection, with a median observation of 18 months. No antiviral prophylaxis was prescribed. HBV DNA became positive in 5.3% of the population, specifically in two patients treated with tocilizumab and in one patient treated with etanercept. However, there were no significant changes in markers of liver function, and no patient required antiviral therapy.

Regarding the JAK kinase inhibitors, a study by Harigai et al. [75] included 215 patients with previous or current HBV infections, treated with baricitinib (with or without csDMARDs) for rheumatoid arthritis, in four clinical trials. All patients tested negative for HBV DNA at baseline. During the follow-up, 32 (14.9%) patients tested positive for HBV DNA, but only four of them met the HBV reactivation criteria (HBV DNA $\geq$ 100 IU/mL). The use of baricitinib was discontinued temporarily in two patients and permanently in four. In no case was there clinical evidence of hepatitis.

In conclusion, the risk of HBVr depends on the subject's immunosuppressive status and the baseline condition of HBV infection. For both HBsAg-positive and HBsAg-negative patients, the risk of HBVr is low with csDMARDs, including methotrexate, leflunomide, and azathioprine; and short (<4 weeks), low-dose (<10 mg/day of prednisone or equivalent) cortisone-based therapies. However, it is moderate with anti-TNFs (etanercept, infliximab, and adalimumab) or tyrosine kinase inhibitors (such as baricitinib), and is even higher with combination therapies; thus, an antiviral prophylaxis should be recommended in these cases [18,76].

5.4. Risk of HBV Reactivation in Neurological Diseases

Multiple sclerosis (MS) is a chronic inflammatory disease of the central nervous system (CNS) causing demyelination, that causes progressive neurodegeneration and disability. Glucocorticoids have been widely used to manage the acute phases of the disease, although their effectiveness tends to decrease over time. However, disease modifying drugs acquired a central role in the treatment of MS outpatients. So far, a series of biological therapies have been approved which are distributed in the first, second, and third lines of treatment. All have some degree of immunosuppressive potential: they mainly include anti-CD20 monoclonal antibodies (ocrelizumab, ofatumumab), anti-CD52 antibodies (alemtuzumab), a4b1 integrin inhibitor (Natalizumab), DNA intercalator (Mitoxantrone), and sphingosine-1 phosphate inhibitor (fingolimod) and its modulators (siponimod, ozanimod) [77].

Table 1. Studies on HBV reactivation in patients with gastroenteric diseases.

First Author, Year [Reference]	Study Design	N. Patients	Gastroenteric Disease (n, %)	Immunosuppressive Treatment	HBV Status (n, %)	HBVr Definition	HBVr (n, %)	HBVr among Pts Receiving Prophylaxis (n, %)	HBVr among Pts Not Receiving Prophylaxis (n, %)
Pauly MP, 2018 [22]	Retrospective	8887	1186 (13.4)	Anti-TNF α agents ± steroids and non-biological immunosuppressants	HBsAg+: 23 (0.3) HBsAg−/HBcAb+: 178 (2)	>1 log increase in serum HBV DNA from baseline OR serum HBV DNA detectable when previously undetectable OR HBV DNA >2000 IU/mL if no baseline OR reverse seroconversion from HBsAg negative to HBsAg+.	HBsAg+: 9 (39.1) HBsAg−/HBcAb+: 0 (0)	HBsAg+: 1 (11.1) HBsAg−/HBcAb+: 0 (0)	HBsAg+: 8 (88.9) HBsAg−/HBcAb+: 0 (0)
Loras C, 2010 [42]	Retrospective	162	162 (100)	Steroids ± anti-TNF α agents ± non-biological immunosuppressants	HBsAg+: 25 (15.4) HBsAg−/HBcAb+: 65 (40.1)	1.5–2 fold the baseline value of alanine transaminase (ALT) plus an increase of >2000 IU/ml HBV DNA levels or DNA reappearance in a negative patient.	HBsAg+: 9 (36) HBsAg−/HBcAb+: 0 (0)	HBsAg+: 1 (11.1) HBsAg−/HBcAb+: 0 (0)	HBsAg+: 8 (88.9) HBsAg−/HBcAb+: 0 (0)
Morisco F, 2013 [43]	Retrospective	5096	5096 (100)	Anti-TNF α agents ± non-biological immunosuppressants	HBsAg+: 6 (0.1) HBsAg−/HBcAb+: 4 (0.07)	In HBsAg−positive patients >1 log10 increase HBV DNA with or without the concomitant increase in transaminases; in isolated anti-HBc-positive, the re-emergence of HBsAg or appearance or at least >1 log10 increase HBV DNA	HBsAg+: 1 (16.6) HBsAg−/HBcAb+: 1 (25)	HBsAg+: 0 (0) HBsAg−/HBcAb+: 0 (0)	HBsAg+: 1 (100) HBsAg−/HBcAb+: 0 (0)
Perez-Alvarez, 2011 [44]	Retrospective	257	20 *	Anti-TNF α agents	HBsAg+: 89 (34.6) HBsAg−/HBcAb+: 168 (65.3)	The reappearance of serum HBV-DNA in a patient with previously inactive or resolved HBV infection, and either as an increase of >1 log10 of viral load or >400 IU/mL (2000 copies/mL) with respect to the baseline HBV-DNA load before anti-TNF therapy, or as the appearance of serum HBV DNA above standard cutoff values (>60 IU/L, equivalent to >300 copies/mL).	HBsAg+: 35 (39.3) HBsAg−/HBcAb+: 9 (5.3)	HBsAg+: 7 (20) HBsAg−/HBcAb+: 0 (0)	HBsAg+: 28 (80) ** HBsAg−/HBcAb+: 0 (0)
Shah R, 2018 [45]	Retrospective	3357	3357 (100)	Anti-TNF α agents	HBsAg+: NA HBsAg−/HBcAb+: NA	Using ICD-9 codes for HBV (070.2×, 070.3×), acute liver failure (670.×), or filled prescriptions for medications used in the treatment of HBV. Potential cases of HBV reactivation were verified using manual EMR through CAPRI.	HBsAg+: 0 (0) HBsAg−/HBcAb+: 0 (0)	HBsAg+: 0 (0) HBsAg−/HBcAb+: 0 (0)	HBsAg+: 0 (0) HBsAg−/HBcAb+: 0 (0)
Clarke WT, 2018 [46]	Retrospective	3171	23 ***	Anti-TNF α agents ± immunomodulators	HBsAg+: NA HBsAg−/HBcAb+: 120 (3.8)	Demonstration of reverse seroconversion to positive HBsAg status OR development of detectable HBV DNA	HBsAg+: NA HBsAg−/HBcAb+: 1 (0.8)	HBsAg+: NA HBsAg−/HBcAb+: NA	HBsAg+: NA HBsAg−/HBcAb+: NA

Table 1. Cont.

First Author, Year [Reference]	Study Design	N. Patients	Gastroenteric Disease (n, %)	Immunosuppressive Treatment	HBV Status (n, %)	HBVr Definition	HBVr (n, %)	HBVr among Pts Receiving Prophylaxis (n, %)	HBVr among Pts Not Receiving Prophylaxis (n, %)
Solay AH, 2018 [47]	Retrospective	278	1 ****	Anti-TNF α agents	HBsAg+: NA HBsAg−/HBcAb+: 29	Detection of HBV DNA and/or HBsAg conversion in blood analysis during the follow-up.	HBsAg+: NA HBsAg−/HBcAb+: 5 (17.2)	HBsAg+: NA HBsAg−/HBcAb+: 0 (0)	HBsAg+: NA HBsAg−/HBcAb+: 0 (0)
Papa A, 2013 [48]	Prospective	301	301 (100)	Anti-TNF α agents	HBsAg+: 1 (0.3) HBsAg−/HBcAb+: 22 (7.3)	HBsAg or HBV-DNA detection in patients previously negative for HBsAg or with undetectable levels of HBV DNA	HBsAg+: 0 (0) HBsAg−/HBcAb+: 0 (0)	HBsAg+: 0 (0) HBsAg−/HBcAb+: NA	HBsAg+: 0 (0) HBsAg−/HBcAb+: NA
Sayar S, 2020 [49]	Retrospective	653	13 *****	Anti-TNF α agents ± corticosteroid and/or immunomodulator.	HBsAg+: 5 (0.8) HBsAg−/HBcAb+: 90 (13.8)	An increase of >1 log10 IU/mL in the HBV DNA level compared with the past value OR positivity in those who were HBV DNA negative OR detection of any positive HBV DNA level in patients whose baseline HBV DNA level was not studied	HBsAg+: NA HBsAg−/HBcAb+: 0 (0)	HBsAg+: NA HBsAg−/HBcAb+: 0 (0)	HBsAg+: NA HBsAg−/HBcAb+: 0 (0)

NA: not available; * number of IBD patients out of 44 patients with HBVr; ** in two patients, whether antiviral prophylaxis was done was not specified; *** number of IBD patients out of the 120 HBsAg−/HBcAb+ patients; **** number of IBD patients out of the 29 HBsAg−/HBcAb+ patients; ***** number of IBD patients out of the 90 HBsAg−/HBcAb+ patients.

Table 2. Studies on HBV reactivation in patients with dermatological diseases.

First Author, Year [Reference]	Study Design	N. Patients	Dermatological Disease	Immunosuppressive Treatment	HBV Status (n, %)	HBVr Definition	HBVr (n, %)	HBVr among Pts Receiving Prophylaxis (n, %)	HBVr among Pts Not Receiving Prophylaxis (n, %)
Chiu, 2013 [52]	Retrospective cohort	14	Psoriasis	Ustekinumab	HBsAg+: 11 HBsAg−/HBcAb+: 3	One of the following: 1. ALT elevation with increase in serum HBV DNA level to >1 log10 copies/mL higher than before therapy; 2. Absolute increase in HBV DNA level exceeding 6 log10 copies /mL; 3. Conversion of serum HBV-DNA test results from negative to positive.	HBsAg+: 2 (14.3) HBsAg−/HBcAb+: 0 (0)	HBsAg+: 0 (0) HBsAg−/HBcAb+:0 (0)	HBsAg+: 2 (28.6) HBsAg−/HBcAb+:0 (0)
Ting, 2018 [53]	Prospective cohort	54	Psoriasis	Ustekinumab	HBsAg+: 10 HBsAg−/HBcAb+: 44	One of the following: 1. >2 log increase in HBV replication from baseline levels, 2. New appearance of HBV DNA at a level of >100 IU/mL in a person with previously stable or undetectable levels 3. Detection of HBV DNA at a level >20,000 IU/mL in a person with no baseline HBV DNA	HBsAg+: 2 (20) HBsAg−/HBcAb+: 1 (2.3)	HBsAg+: 0 (0) HBsAg−/HBcAb+:0 (0)	HBsAg+: 2 (25) HBsAg−/HBcAb+:1 (2.3)

Table 2. Cont.

First Author, Year [Reference]	Study Design	N. Patients	Dermatological Disease	Immunosuppressive Treatment	HBV Status (n, %)	HBVr Definition	HBVr (n, %)	HBVr among Pts Receiving Prophylaxis (n, %)	HBVr among Pts Not Receiving Prophylaxis (n, %)
Snast, 2017 [54]	Retrospective cohort	26	Psoriasis	Adalimumab, Etanercept, Golimumab, Infliximab, Secukinumab, Ustekinumab	HBsAg+: 1 HBsAg−/HBcAb+: 26	One of the following: 1. Increase in HBV replication of at least 1 log10 copies/mL 2. Conversion of serum HBV DNA results from negative to positive	HBsAg+: 0 (0) HBsAg−/HBcAb+: 0 (0)	HBsAg+: 0 (0) HBsAg−/HBcAb+: 0 (0)	HBsAg+: 0 (0) HBsAg−/HBcAb+: 0 (0)
Piaserico, 2017 [55]	Retrospective cohort	17	Psoriasis	Adalimumab	HBsAg+: 10 HBsAg−/HBcAb+: 7	One of the following: 1. ALT elevation with increase in serum HBV DNA level to >1 log10 copies/mL higher than before therapy; 2. Absolute increase in HBV DNA level exceeding 6 log10 copies/mL; 3. Conversion of serum HBV-DNA test results from negative to positive.	HBsAg+: 0 (0) HBsAg−/HBcAb+: 0 (0)	HBsAg+: 0 (0)	HBsAg+: 0 (0) HBsAg−/HBcAb+: 0 (0)
AlMutairi, 2018 [56]	Prospective cohort	32	Psoriasis	Adalimumab, Etanercept, Ustekinumab	HBsAg+: 4 HBsAg−/HBcAb+: 28	One of the following: 1. Increase in serum HBV DNA level to >1 log10 copies/mL higher than before therapy; 2. Absolute increase in HBV DNA level exceeding 6 log10 copies/mL; 3. Conversion of serum HBV-DNA test results from negative to positive.	HBsAg+: 0 (0) HBsAg−/HBcAb+: 0 (0)	HBsAg−/HBcAb+: 0 (0)	HBsAg+: 0 (0)

Table 3. Studies on HBV reactivation in patients with rheumatological diseases.

First Author, Year [Reference]	Study Design	N. Patients	Rheumatological Disease	Immunosuppressive Treatment	HBV Status (n, %)	HBVr Definition	HBVr (n, %)	HBVr among Pts Receiving Prophylaxis (n, %)	HBVr among Pts Not Receiving Prophylaxis (n, %)
Laohapand, 2015 [61]	Cross-sectional	173	RA, spondyloarthropathies, systemic lupus erythematosus, others	Methotrexate	HBsAg+: 1 (0.6) HBsAg−/HBcAb+: 65 (37.6)	Not reported	HBsAg+: 0 (0) HBsAg−/HBcAb+: 0 (0)	HBsAg+: 0 (0) HBsAg−/HBcAb+: 0 (0)	HBsAg+: 0 (0) HBsAg−/HBcAb+: 0 (0)
Chen, 2017 [67]	Retrospective cohort	123	RA	Glucocorticoids: 51 (41.5) bDMARDs: 36 (29.3) csDMARDs: 123 (100)	HBsAg+: 123 (100)	One of the following: 1. Increase in HBV DNA >1 Log10 IU/mL, compared with baseline 2. 3-fold increase in serum alanine aminotransferase (ALT) level accompanied by HBV DNA >20,000 copies/mL	HBsAg+: 30 (24.4)		HBsAg+: 30 (24.4)

Table 3. Cont.

First Author, Year [Reference]	Study Design	N. Patients	Rheumatological Disease	Immunosuppressive Treatment	HBV Status (n, %)	HBVr Definition	HBVr (n, %)	HBVr among Pts Receiving Prophylaxis (n, %)	HBVr among Pts Not Receiving Prophylaxis (n, %)
Ryu, 2012 [68]	Retrospective cohort	49	RA, ankylosing spondylitis	Etanercept, Infliximab, adalimumab	HBsAg+: 49 (100)	Both the following: 1. 10-fold rise in HBV DNA compared with baseline resulting in HBV DNA greater than 20,000 IU/mL (HBeAg-positive patients) or 2000 IU/mL (HBeAg-negative patients). 2. Increase in AST or ALT to above twice the upper normal limit (40 IU/l)	HBsAg+: 3 (6.1)	HBsAg+: 1 (5.0)	HBsAg+: 2 (6.9)
Fukuda, 2019 [70]	Prospective cohort	1127	RA, others	Glucocorticoids: 373 (38.9) bDMARDS: 274 (28.8) csDMARDS: 751 (79.1)	HBsAg−/HBcAb+: 1127 (100)	Positive conversion of HBV-DNA	HBsAg−/HBcAb+: 57 (5.1)		HBsAg−/HBcAb+: 57 (5.1)
Varisco, 2016 [72]	Retrospective cohort	33	RA	Rituximab ± DMSARDs	HBsAg−/HBcAb+: 33 (100)	HBsAg seroreversion or serum HBV-DNA positivity	HBsAg−/HBcAb+: 0 (0)		HBsAg−/HBcAb+: 0 (0)
Urata, 2011 [73]	Prospective cohort	123	RA	Glucocorticoids, bDMARDS, csDMARDs	HBsAg−/HBcAb+: 123 (100)	Not reported	HBsAg−/HBcAb+: 7 (5.2)		HBsAg−/HBcAb+: 7 (5.2)
Nakamura, 2016 [74]	Retrospective cohort	57	RA	bDMARDs	HBsAg−/HBcAb+: 57 (100)	Serum HBV-DNA positivity	HBsAg−/HBcAb+: 3 (5.3)		HBsAg−/HBcAb+: 3 (5.3)
Harigai 2020 [75]	Prospective cohort	290	RA	Baricitinib, Methotrexate	HBsAg−/HBcAb+: 215 (74.1) HBsAg−/HBcAb−: 75 (25.9)	≥2 log increase from baseline levels or new appearance of HBV DNA to a level of ≥100 IU/mL	HBsAg−/HBcAb+: 32 (14.8) HBsAg−/HBcAb−: 4 (5.3)		HBsAg−/HBcAb+: 32 (14.8) HBsAg−/HBcAb−: 4 (5.3)

Footnotes: RA: rheumatoid arthritis.

Although all these drugs seem to be related to HBVr, limited data are available in the literature concerning the risk of HBVr when used in a neurological setting. Ciardi et al. [78] reported a case of HBVr in a patient with a previous HBV infection treated with ocrelizumab for multiple sclerosis who did not receive prophylaxis. Although many authors agree on the need for antiviral prophylaxis in patients treated with ocrelizumab, similarly to what is recommended for other anti-CD20 antibodies, no clear and definitive consensus exists on the best prevention strategies in subjects receiving other immunosuppressive drugs in this setting [79]. Further studies are needed to clarify this point.

5.5. Risk of HBV Reactivation in COVID-19 Patients

The SARS-CoV-2 pandemic has been responsible for more than 150 million cases and over 3 million deaths as of April 2021, according to the data reported on the online dashboard implemented by the Johns Hopkins University [80]. Several immunosuppressive and immunomodulating agents have been adopted for the treatment of COVID-19, such as corticosteroids, which are currently recommended by the WHO guidelines for severe or critical diseases [81], and interleukin-6 (IL-6) inhibitors, which have been tested in several clinical trials compared to the standard of care [82].

As already stated, high dose glucocorticoids significantly increase the risk of reactivation in both overt and occult B infections [18]. However, limited data are available in the literature on the HBVr rate of COVID-19 patients treated with corticosteroids. A retrospective study reported three cases of HBVr, two of whom had received methylprednisolone treatment, among 20 Chinese HBsAg-positive, treatment-naïve patients hospitalized for SARS-CoV-2 pneumonia between January and March 2020 [83].

Regarding the IL-6 inhibitors, several studies have reported an increased risk of HBVr in patients receiving tocilizumab for rheumatological diseases [84]. However, a retrospective cohort study [85] including 29 HBsAg-negative/anti-HBc-positive patients receiving immunosuppressive treatment for COVID-19 (mostly tocilizumab or siltuximab) reported no case of HBVr requiring antiviral treatment. Only two patients showed detectable HBV DNA during the follow-up, in both cases below the limit of quantification (<15 UI/mL). Most probably, the short duration of treatment limits the risk of reactivation in this setting. No data are available on the risks related to other immunosuppressive agents that have been used in COVID-19 patients, such as baricitinib, ruxolitinib, and tofacitinib; however, these drugs have been associated with significant risks of HBVr reactivation in other settings [75]. Therefore, all patients expected to be treated with corticosteroids for more than 7–10 days or with other immunosuppressive drugs for COVID-19 pneumonia should be screened for current and previous HBV infections, in order to evaluate the risk of reactivation and implement preventive strategies when needed.

6. Conclusions

The growing use of immunosuppressive treatments in patients with a large variety of non-oncological diseases has drawn attention to the risk of reactivation of HBV infection in many settings. However, the available data on the risk of HBVr related to the different drugs are limited and fragmentary. Further prospective studies are needed to assess the best preventive strategies to reduce the occurrence of these potentially life-threatening events.

Author Contributions: L.O., M.P., and N.C. were involved in conceptualization and design, and drafting of the manuscript; C.C., P.G., A.V.C., and F.C. were involved in acquisition of data, analysis and interpretation of data, and critical revision of the manuscript. All authors have read and agreed to the published version of the manuscript.

Funding: This research received no external funding.

Institutional Review Board Statement: Not applicable.

Informed Consent Statement: Not applicable.

Conflicts of Interest: The authors declare no conflict of interest.

References

1. Stone, G.M.; Mullin, S.A.; Teran, A.A.; Hallinan, D.T., Jr.; Minor, A.M.; Hexemer, A.; Balsara, N.P. Resolution of the Modulus versus Adhesion Dilemma in Solid Polymer Electrolytes for Rechargeable Lithium Metal Batteries. *J. Electrochem. Soc.* **2012**, *159*, A222–A227. [CrossRef]
2. Raimondo, G.; Locarnini, S.; Pollicino, T.; Levrero, M.; Zoulim, F.; Lok, A.S.; Allain, J.-P.; Berg, T.; Bertoletti, A.; Brunetto, M.R.; et al. Update of the Statements on Biology and Clinical Impact of Occult Hepatitis B Virus Infection. *J. Hepatol.* **2019**, *71*, 397–408. [CrossRef]
3. Pisaturo, M.; Onorato, L.; Russo, A.; Chiodini, P.; Coppola, N. An Estimation of the Prevalence of Occult HBV Infection in Western Europe and in Northern America: A Meta-Analysis. *J. Viral Hepat.* **2020**, *27*, 415–427. [CrossRef] [PubMed]
4. Loomba, R.; Liang, T.J. Hepatitis B Reactivation Associated with Immune Suppressive and Biological Modifier Therapies: Current Concepts, Management Strategies, and Future Directions. *Gastroenterology* **2017**, *152*, 1297–1309. [CrossRef] [PubMed]
5. Wang, B.; Mufti, G.; Agarwal, K. Reactivation of Hepatitis B Virus Infection in Patients with Hematologic Disorders. *Haematologica* **2019**, *104*, 435–443. [CrossRef]
6. Sagnelli, C.; Pisaturo, M.; Calò, F.; Martini, S.; Sagnelli, E.; Coppola, N. Reactivation of Hepatitis B Virus Infection in Patients with Hemo-Lymphoproliferative Diseases, and its Prevention. *World J. Gastroenterol.* **2019**, *25*, 3299–3312. [CrossRef] [PubMed]
7. Fattovich, G. Natural History and Prognosis of Hepatitis B. *Semin. Liver Dis.* **2003**, *23*, 47–58. [CrossRef] [PubMed]
8. World Health Organization. Hepatitis C. Available online: https://www.who.int/en/news-room/fact-sheets/detail/hepatitis-c (accessed on 4 March 2019).
9. Coppola, N.; Monari, C.; Alessio, L.; Onorato, L.; Gualdieri, L.; Sagnelli, C.; Minichini, C.; Sagnelli, E.; Di Caprio, G.; Surace, L.; et al. Blood-borne Chronic Viral Infections in a Large Cohort of Immigrants in Southern Italy: A Seven-Centre, Prospective, Screening Study. *Travel Med. Infect. Dis.* **2020**, *35*, 101551. [CrossRef] [PubMed]
10. van Houdt, R.; Bruisten, S.M.; Speksnijder, A.G.; Prins, M. Unexpectedly High Proportion of Drug Users and Men Having Sex with Men who Develop Chronic Hepatitis B Infection. *J. Hepatol.* **2012**, *57*, 529–533. [CrossRef] [PubMed]
11. WHO. Global Health Sector Strategy on Viral Hepatitis 2016–2021 Towards Ending Viral Hepatitis. 2017. Available online: https://apps.who.int/iris/bitstream/handle/10665/246177/WHO-HIV-2016.06-eng.pdf?sequence=1&isAllowed=y (accessed on 28 October 2021).
12. Lampertico, P.; Agarwal, K.; Berg, T.; Buti, M.; Janssen, H.L.; Papatheodoridis, G.; Zoulim, F.; Tacke, F. EASL 2017 Clinical Practice Guidelines on the Management of Hepatitis B Virus Infection. *J. Hepatol.* **2017**, *67*, 370–398. [CrossRef] [PubMed]
13. Coppola, N.; Onorato, L.; Pisaturo, M.; Macera, M.; Sagnelli, C.; Martini, S.; Sagnelli, E. Role of Occult Hepatitis B Virus Infection in Chronic Hepatitis C. *World J. Gastroenterol.* **2015**, *21*, 11931–11940. [CrossRef]
14. Coppola, N.; Onorato, L.; Sagnelli, C.; Sagnelli, E.; Angelillo, I.F. Association Between Anti-HBc Positivity and Hepatocellular Carcinoma in HBsAg-negative Subjects with Chronic Liver Disease: A Meta-Analysis. *Medicine* **2016**, *95*, e4311. [CrossRef] [PubMed]
15. Di Marco, V.; Iacono, O.L.; Camma, C.; Vaccaro, A.; Giunta, M.; Martorana, G.; Fuschi, P.; Almasio, P.L.; Craxi, A. The Long-Term Course of Chronic Hepatitis B. *Hepatology* **1999**, *30*, 257–264. [CrossRef]
16. Fattovich, G.; Brollo, L.; Giustina, G.; Noventa, F.; Pontisso, P.; Alberti, A.; Realdi, G.; Ruol, A. Natural History and Prognostic Factors for Chronic Hepatitis Type B. *Gut* **1991**, *32*, 294–298. [CrossRef] [PubMed]
17. Fattovich, G.; Bortolotti, F.; Donato, F. Natural History of Chronic Hepatitis B: Special Emphasis on Disease Progression and Prognostic Factors. *J. Hepatol.* **2008**, *48*, 335–352. [CrossRef] [PubMed]
18. Perrillo, R.P.; Gish, R.; Falck-Ytter, Y.T. American Gastroenterological Association Institute Technical Review on Prevention and Treatment of Hepatitis B Virus Reactivation During Immunosuppressive Drug Therapy. *Gastroenterology* **2015**, *148*, 221–244.e3. [CrossRef] [PubMed]
19. Shi, Y.; Zheng, M. Hepatitis B Virus Persistence and Reactivation. *BMJ* **2020**, *370*. [CrossRef] [PubMed]
20. Paul, S.; Saxena, A.P.; Terrin, N.; Viveiros, K.; Balk, E.M.; Wong, J.B. Hepatitis B Virus Reactivation and Prophylaxis during Solid Tumor Chemotherapy. *Ann. Intern. Med.* **2016**, *164*, 30–40. [CrossRef] [PubMed]
21. Chen, Y.-H.; Huang, W.-N.; Wu, Y.-D.; Lin, C.-T.; Chen, D.-Y.; Hsieh, T.-Y. Reactivation of Hepatitis B Virus Infection in Patients with Rheumatoid Arthritis Receiving Tofacitinib: A Real-World Study. *Ann. Rheum. Dis.* **2018**, *77*, 780–782. [CrossRef] [PubMed]
22. Pauly, M.P.; Tucker, L.-Y.; Szpakowski, J.-L.; Ready, J.B.; Baer, D.; Hwang, J.; Lok, A.S.-F. Incidence of Hepatitis B Virus Reactivation and Hepatotoxicity in Patients Receiving Long-term Treatment with Tumor Necrosis Factor Antagonists. *Clin. Gastroenterol. Hepatol.* **2018**, *16*, 1964–1973.e1. [CrossRef] [PubMed]
23. Seto, W.-K.; Chan, T.S.; Hwang, Y.-Y.; Wong, D.K.-H.; Fung, J.; Liu, K.S.-H.; Gill, H.; Lam, Y.-F.; Lie, A.K.; Lai, C.-L.; et al. Hepatitis B Reactivation in Patients with Previous Hepatitis B Virus Exposure Undergoing Rituximab-Containing Chemotherapy for Lymphoma: A Prospective Study. *J. Clin. Oncol.* **2014**, *32*, 3736–3743. [CrossRef] [PubMed]
24. Yeo, W.; Chan, P.K.; Zhong, S.; Ho, W.M.; Steinberg, J.L.; Tam, J.S.; Hui, P.; Leung, N.W.; Zee, B.; Johnson, P.J. Frequency of Hepatitis B Virus Reactivation in Cancer Patients Undergoing Cytotoxic Chemotherapy: A Prospective Study of 626 Patients with Identification of Risk Factors. *J. Med. Virol.* **2000**, *62*, 299–307. [CrossRef]

25. Yeo, W.; Zee, B.C.-Y.; Zhong, S.; Chan, P.; Wong, W.-L.; Ho, W.M.; Lam, K.C.; Johnson, P.J. Comprehensive Analysis of Risk Factors Associating with Hepatitis B Virus (HBV) Reactivation in Cancer Patients Undergoing Cytotoxic Chemotherapy. *Br. J. Cancer* **2004**, *90*, 1306–1311. [CrossRef]
26. Pisaturo, M.; Di Caprio, G.; Calò, F.; Portunato, F.; Martini, S.; Coppola, N. Management of HBV Reactivation in Non-Oncological Patients. *Expert Rev. Anti-Infect. Ther.* **2018**, *16*, 611–624. [CrossRef]
27. Smalls, D.J.; Kiger, R.E.; Norris, L.B.; Bennett, C.L.; Love, B.L. Hepatitis B Virus Reactivation: Risk Factors and Current Management Strategies. *Pharmacother. J. Hum. Pharmacol. Drug Ther.* **2019**, *39*, 1190–1203. [CrossRef]
28. Mozessohn, L.; Chan, K.K.W.; Feld, J.J.; Hicks, L.K. Hepatitis B Reactivation in HBsAg-Negative/HBcAb-Positive Patients Receiving Rituximab for Lymphoma: A Meta-Analysis. *J. Viral Hepat.* **2015**, *22*, 842–849. [CrossRef]
29. Tur-Kaspa, R.; Burk, R.D.; Shaul, Y.; Shafritz, D.A. Hepatitis B Virus DNA Contains a Glucocorticoid-Responsive Element. *Proc. Natl. Acad. Sci. USA* **1986**, *83*, 1627–1631. [CrossRef] [PubMed]
30. Navarro, R.; Vilarrasa, E.; Herranz, P.; Puig, L.; Bordas, X.; Carrascosa, J.; Taberner, R.; Ferrán, M.; García-Bustinduy, M.; Romero-Maté, A.; et al. Safety and Effectiveness of Ustekinumab and Antitumour Necrosis Factor Therapy in Patients with Psoriasis and Chronic Viral Hepatitis B or C: A Retrospective, Multicentre Study in a Clinical Setting. *Br. J. Dermatol.* **2013**, *168*, 609–616. [CrossRef] [PubMed]
31. Orlandi, E.M.; Elena, C.; Bono, E. Risk of Hepatitis B Reactivation under Treatment with Tyrosine-Kinase Inhibitors for Chronic Myeloid Leukemia. *Leuk. Lymphoma* **2017**, *58*, 1764–1766. [CrossRef] [PubMed]
32. Reddy, K.R.; Beavers, K.L.; Hammond, S.; Lim, J.K.; Falck-Ytter, Y.T. American Gastroenterological Association Institute Guideline on the Prevention and Treatment of Hepatitis B Virus Reactivation during Immunosuppressive Drug Therapy. *Gastroenterology* **2015**, *148*, 215–219. [CrossRef]
33. Brost, S.; Schnitzler, P.; Stremmel, W.; Eisenbach, C. Entecavir as Treatment for Reactivation of Hepatitis B in Immunosuppressed Patients. *World J. Gastroenterol.* **2010**, *16*, 5447–5451. [CrossRef] [PubMed]
34. Chen, F.W.; Coyle, L.; Jones, B.E.; Pattullo, V. Entecavir Versus Lamivudine for Hepatitis B Prophylaxis in Patients with Haematological Disease. *Liver Int.* **2013**, *33*, 1203–1210. [CrossRef] [PubMed]
35. Koskinas, J.; Deutsch, M.; Adamidi, S.; Skondra, M.; Tampaki, M.; Alexopoulou, A.; Manolakopoulos, S.; Pectasides, D. The Role of Tenofovir in Preventing and Treating Hepatitis B Virus (HBV) Reactivation in Immunosuppressed Patients. A Real Life Experience from a Tertiary Center. *Eur. J. Intern. Med.* **2014**, *25*, 768–771. [CrossRef] [PubMed]
36. Tseng, C.; Chen, T.; Hsu, Y.; Chang, C.; Lin, J.; Mo, L. Comparative Effectiveness of Nucleos(t)ide Analogues in Chronic Hepatitis B Patients Undergoing Cytotoxic Chemotherapy. *Asia-Pac. J. Clin. Oncol.* **2016**, *12*, 421–429. [CrossRef] [PubMed]
37. Marrone, A.; Capoluongo, N.; D'Amore, C.; Pisaturo, M.; Esposito, M.; Guastafierro, S.; Siniscalchi, I.; Macera, M.; Boemio, A.; Onorato, L.; et al. Eighteen-Month Lamivudine Prophylaxis on Preventing Occult Hepatitis B Virus Infection Reactivation in Patients with Haematological Malignancies Receiving Immunosuppression Therapy. *J. Viral Hepat.* **2018**, *25*, 198–204. [CrossRef]
38. Chew, E.; Thursky, K.; Seymour, J.F. Very Late Onset Hepatitis-B Virus Reactivation Following Rituximab despite Lamivudine Prophylaxis: The Need for Continued Vigilance. *Leuk. Lymphoma* **2014**, *55*, 938–939. [CrossRef] [PubMed]
39. Dai, M.-S.; Chao, T.-Y.; Kao, W.-Y.; Shyu, R.-Y.; Liu, T.-M. Delayed Hepatitis B Virus Reactivation after Cessation of Preemptive Lamivudine in Lymphoma Patients Treated with Rituximab Plus CHOP. *Ann. Hematol.* **2004**, *83*, 769–774. [CrossRef]
40. Sarmati, L.; Andreoni, M.; Antonelli, G.; Arcese, W.; Bruno, R.; Coppola, N.; Gaeta, G.; Galli, M.; Girmenia, C.; Mikulska, M.; et al. Recommendations for Screening, Monitoring, Prevention, Prophylaxis and Therapy of Hepatitis B Virus Reactivation in Patients with Haematologic Malignancies and Patients who Underwent Haematologic Stem Cell Transplantation—A Position Paper. *Clin. Microbiol. Infect.* **2017**, *23*, 935–940. [CrossRef]
41. Pawłowska, M.; Flisiak, R.; Gil, L.; Horban, A.; Hus, I.; Jaroszewicz, J.; Lech-Maranda, E.; Styczyński, J. Prophylaxis of Hepatitis B Virus (HBV) Infection Reactivation—Recommendations of the Working Group for Prevention of HBV Reactivation. *Clin. Exp. Hepatol.* **2019**, *5*, 195–202. [CrossRef] [PubMed]
42. Loras, C.; Gisbert, J.P.; Minguez, M.; Merino, O.; Bujanda, L.; Saro, C.; Domenech, E.; Barrio, J.; Andreu, M.; Ordas, I.; et al. Liver Dysfunction Related to Hepatitis B and C in Patients with Inflammatory Bowel Disease Treated with Immunosuppressive Therapy. *Gut* **2010**, *59*, 1340–1346. [CrossRef]
43. Morisco, F.; Castiglione, F.; Rispo, A.; Stroffolini, T.; Sansone, S.; Vitale, R.; Guarino, M.; Biancone, L.; Caruso, A.; D'Inca, R.; et al. Effect of Immunosuppressive Therapy on Patients with Inflammatory Bowel Diseases and Hepatitis B or C Virus Infection. *J. Viral Hepat.* **2013**, *20*, 200–208. [CrossRef] [PubMed]
44. Pérez-Alvarez, R.; Díaz-Lagares, C.; Garcia-Hernandez, F.J.; Lopez-Roses, L.; Zeron, P.B.; Pérez-De-Lis, M.; Retamozo, S.; Bové, A.; Bosch, X.; Sanchez-Tapias, J.-M.; et al. Hepatitis B Virus (HBV) Reactivation in Patients Receiving Tumor Necrosis Factor (TNF)-Targeted Therapy. *Medicine* **2011**, *90*, 359–371. [CrossRef] [PubMed]
45. Shah, R.; Ho, E.Y.; Kramer, J.R.; Richardson, P.; Sansgiry, S.; El-Serag, H.B.; Hou, J.K. Hepatitis B Virus Screening and Reactivation in a National VA Cohort of Patients with Inflammatory Bowel Disease Treated with Tumor Necrosis Factor Antagonists. *Dig. Dis. Sci.* **2018**, *63*, 1551–1557. [CrossRef] [PubMed]
46. Clarke, W.T.; Amin, S.S.; Papamichael, K.; Feuerstein, J.D.; Cheifetz, A.S. Patients with Core Antibody Positive and Surface Antigen Negative Hepatitis B (anti-HBc+, HBsAg−) on Anti-TNF Therapy have a Low Rate of Reactivation. *Clin. Immunol.* **2018**, *191*, 59–62. [CrossRef] [PubMed]

47. Solay, A.H.; Acar, A.; Eser, F.; Kuscu, F.; Tutuncu, E.E.; Kul, G.; Senturk, G.C.; Gurbuz, Y.; Solay, A.H. Reactivation Rates in Patients Using Biological Agents, with Resolved HBV Infection or Isolated Anti-HBc IgG Positivity. *Turk. J. Gastroenterol.* **2018**, *29*, 561–565. [CrossRef]
48. Papa, A.; Felice, C.; Marzo, M.; Andrisani, G.; Armuzzi, A.; Covino, M.; Mocci, G.; Pugliese, D.; De Vitis, I.; Gasbarrini, A.; et al. Prevalence and Natural History of Hepatitis B and C Infections in a Large Population of IBD Patients Treated with Anti-Tumor Necrosis Factor-α Agents. *J. Crohns Coliti* **2013**, *7*, 113–119. [CrossRef] [PubMed]
49. Sayar, S.; Kurbuz, K.; Kahraman, R.; Ozturk, O.; Caliskan, Z.; Doganay, H.L.; Ozdil, K. Risk of Hepatitis B Reactivation during Anti-TNF Therapy; Evaluation of Patients with Past Hepatitis B Infection. *Turk. J. Gastroenterol.* **2020**, *31*, 522–528. [CrossRef] [PubMed]
50. Rahier, J.; Magro, F.; Abreu, C.; Armuzzi, A.; Ben-Horin, S.; Chowers, Y.; Cottone, M.; De Ridder, L.G.D.; De Ehehalt, R. Second European Evidence-Based Consensus on the Prevention, Diagnosis and Management of Opportunistic Infections in Inflammatory Bowel Disease. *J. Crohns Coliti* **2014**, *8*, 443–468. [CrossRef] [PubMed]
51. Armstrong, A.W.; Read, C. Pathophysiology, Clinical Presentation, and Treatment of Psoriasis. *JAMA* **2020**, *323*, 1945–1960. [CrossRef] [PubMed]
52. Chiu, H.-Y.; Chen, C.-H.; Wu, M.-S.; Cheng, Y.-P.; Tsai, T.-F. The Safety Profile of Ustekinumab in the Treatment of Patients with Psoriasis and Concurrent Hepatitis B or C. *Br. J. Dermatol.* **2013**, *169*, 1295–1303. [CrossRef] [PubMed]
53. Ting, S.-W.; Chen, Y.-C.; Huang, Y.-H. Risk of Hepatitis B Reactivation in Patients with Psoriasis on Ustekinumab. *Clin. Drug Investig.* **2018**, *38*, 873–880. [CrossRef] [PubMed]
54. Snast, I.; Atzmony, L.; Braun, M.; Hodak, E.; Pavlovsky, L. Risk for Hepatitis B and C Virus Reactivation in Patients with Psoriasis on Biologic Therapies: A Retrospective Cohort Study and Systematic Review of the Literature. *J. Am. Acad. Dermatol.* **2017**, *77*, 88–97.e5. [CrossRef] [PubMed]
55. Piaserico, S.; Dapavo, P.; Conti, A.; Gisondi, P.; Russo, F.P. Adalimumab is a Safe Option for Psoriasis Patients with Concomitant Hepatitis B or C Infection: A Multicentre Cohort Study of 37 Patients and Review of the Literature. *J. Eur. Acad. Dermatol. Venereol.* **2017**, *31*, 1853–1859. [CrossRef] [PubMed]
56. Almutairi, N.; Abouzaid, H.A. Safety of Biologic Agents for Psoriasis in Patients with Viral Hepatitis. *J. Dermatol. Treat.* **2018**, *29*, 553–556. [CrossRef]
57. Cantini, F.; Boccia, S.; Goletti, D.; Iannone, F.; Leoncini, E.; Panic, N.; Prignano, F.; Gaeta, G.B. HBV Reactivation in Patients Treated with Antitumor Necrosis Factor-Alpha (TNF-α) Agents for Rheumatic and Dermatologic Conditions: A Systematic Review and Meta-Analysis. *Int. J. Rheumatol.* **2014**, *2014*, 926836. [CrossRef] [PubMed]
58. Singh, J.A.; Saag, K.G.S.L.B., Jr.; Akl, E.A.; Bannuru, R.; Sullivan, E.; Vaysbrot, E.; McNaughton, C.; Osani, M.; Shmerling, R.H. 2015 American College of Rheumatology Guideline for the Treatment of Rheumatoid Arthritis. *Arthritis Rheum.* **2016**, *68*, 1–25. [CrossRef]
59. Ramiro, S.; Smolen, J.S.; Landewé, R.; Van Der Heijde, D.; Dougados, M.; Emery, P.; De Wit, M.; Cutolo, M.; Oliver, S.; Gossec, L. Pharmacological Treatment of Psoriatic Arthritis: A Systematic Literature Review for the 2015 Update of the EULAR Recommendations for the Management of Psoriatic Arthritis. *Ann. Rheum. Dis.* **2016**, *75*, 490–498. [CrossRef] [PubMed]
60. Lee, Y.H.; Song, G.G. Comparative Efficacy and Safety of Tofacitinib, Baricitinib, Upadacitinib, Filgotinib and Peficitinib as Monotherapy for Active Rheumatoid Arthritis. *J. Clin. Pharm. Ther.* **2020**, *45*, 674–681. [CrossRef] [PubMed]
61. Laohapand, C.; Arromdee, E.; Tanwandee, T. Long-Term Use of Methotrexate does not Result in Hepatitis B Reactivation in Rheumatologic Patients. *Hepatol. Int.* **2015**, *9*, 202–208. [CrossRef] [PubMed]
62. Flowers, M.A.; Heathcote, J.; Wanless, I.R.; Sherman, M.; Reynolds, W.J.; Cameron, R.G.; Levy, G.A.; Inman, R.D. Fulminant Hepatitis as a Consequence of Reactivation of Hepatitis B Virus Infection after Discontinuation of Low-Dose Methotrexate Therapy. *Ann. Intern. Med.* **1990**, *112*, 381. [CrossRef] [PubMed]
63. Hagiyama, H.; Kubota, T.; Komano, Y.; Kurosaki, M.; Watanabe, M.; Miyasaka, N. Fulminant Hepatitis in an Asymptomatic Chronic Carrier of Hepatitis B Virus Mutant after Withdrawal of Low-Dose Methotrexate Therapy for Rheumatoid Arthritis. *Clin. Exp. Rheumatol.* **2004**, *22*, 375–376.
64. Ito, S.; Nakazono, K.; Murasawa, A.; Mita, Y.; Hata, K.; Saito, N.; Kikuchi, M.; Yoshida, K.; Nakano, M.; Gejyo, F. Development of Fulminant Hepatitis B (Precore Variant Mutant Type) after the Discontinuation of Low-Dose Methotrexate Therapy in a Rheumatoid Arthritis Patient. *Arthritis Rheum.* **2001**, *44*, 339–342. [CrossRef]
65. Narvaez, J.; Rodriguez-Moreno, J.; Martinez-Aguilá, M.D.; Clavaguera, M.T. Severe Hepatitis Linked to B Virus Infection after Withdrawal of Low Dose Methotrexate Therapy. *J. Rheumatol.* **1998**, *25*, 2037–2038. [PubMed]
66. Gwak, G.-Y.; Koh, K.C.; Kim, H.-Y. Fatal Hepatic Failure Associated with Hepatitis B Virus Reactivation in a Hepatitis B Surface Antigen-Negative Patient with Rheumatoid Arthritis receiving Low Dose Methotrexate. *Clin. Exp. Rheumatol.* **2007**, *25*, 888–889. [PubMed]
67. Chen, M.-H.; Chen, M.-H.; Liu, C.-Y.; Tsai, C.-Y.; Huang, D.-F.; Lin, H.-Y.; Lee, M.-H.; Huang, Y.-H. Hepatitis B Virus Reactivation in Rheumatoid Arthritis Patients undergoing Biologics Treatment. *J. Infect. Dis.* **2017**, *215*, 566–573. [CrossRef] [PubMed]
68. Ryu, H.H.; Lee, E.Y.; Shin, K.; Choi, I.A.; Lee, Y.J.; Yoo, B.; Park, M.-C.; Park, Y.-B.; Bae, S.-C.; Yoo, W.H.; et al. Hepatitis B Virus Reactivation in Rheumatoid Arthritis and Ankylosing Spondylitis Patients treated with Anti-TNFα Agents: A Retrospective Analysis of 49 Cases. *Clin. Rheumatol.* **2012**, *31*, 931–936. [CrossRef] [PubMed]

69. Fukuda, W.; Hanyu, T.; Katayama, M.; Mizuki, S.; Okada, A.; Miyata, M.; Handa, Y.; Hayashi, M.; Koyama, Y.; Arii, K.; et al. Incidence of Hepatitis B Virus Reactivation in Patients with Resolved Infection on Immunosuppressive Therapy for Rheumatic Disease: A Multicentre, Prospective, Observational Study in Japan. *Ann. Rheum. Dis.* **2017**, *76*, 1051–1056. [CrossRef] [PubMed]
70. Fukuda, W.; Hanyu, T.; Katayama, M.; Mizuki, S.; Okada, A.; Miyata, M.; Handa, Y.; Hayashi, M.; Koyama, Y.; Arii, K.; et al. Risk Stratification and Clinical Course of Hepatitis B Virus Reactivation in Rheumatoid Arthritis Patients with Resolved Infection: Final Report of a Multicenter Prospective Observational Study at Japanese Red Cross Hospital. *Arthritis Res.* **2019**, *21*, 255. [CrossRef] [PubMed]
71. Lee, Y.H.; Bae, S.-C.; Song, G.G. Hepatitis B Virus Reactivation in HBsAg-Positive Patients with Rheumatic Diseases Undergoing Anti-Tumor Necrosis Factor Therapy or DMARDs. *Int. J. Rheum. Dis.* **2013**, *16*, 527–531. [CrossRef]
72. Varisco, V.; Viganò, M.; Batticciotto, A.; Lampertico, P.; Marchesoni, A.; Gibertini, P.; Pellerito, R.; Rovera, G.; Caporali, R.; Todoerti, M.; et al. Low Risk of Hepatitis B Virus Reactivation in HBsAg-negative/Anti-HBc–Positive Carriers Receiving Rituximab for Rheumatoid Arthritis: A Retrospective Multicenter Italian Study. *J. Rheumatol.* **2016**, *43*, 869–874. [CrossRef] [PubMed]
73. Urata, Y.; Uesato, R.; Tanaka, D.; Kowatari, K.; Nitobe, T.; Nakamura, Y.; Motomura, S. Prevalence of Reactivation of Hepatitis B Virus Replication in Rheumatoid Arthritis Patients. *Mod. Rheumatol.* **2011**, *21*, 16–23. [CrossRef] [PubMed]
74. Nakamura, J.; Nagashima, T.; Nagatani, K.; Yoshio, T.; Iwamoto, M.; Minota, S. Reactivation of Hepatitis B Virus in Rheumatoid Arthritis Patients Treated with Biological Disease-Modifying Antirheumatic Drugs. *Int. J. Rheum. Dis.* **2016**, *19*, 470–475. [CrossRef] [PubMed]
75. Harigai, M.; Winthrop, K.; Takeuchi, T.; Hsieh, T.-Y.; Chen, Y.-M.; Smolen, J.S.; Burmester, G.; Walls, C.; Wu, W.-S.; Dickson, C.; et al. Evaluation of Hepatitis B Virus in Clinical Trials of Baricitinib in Rheumatoid Arthritis. *RMD Open* **2020**, *6*, e001095. [CrossRef]
76. Chen, Y.-M.; Yang, S.-S.; Chen, D.-Y. Risk-Stratified Management Strategies for HBV Reactivation in RA Patients receiving Biological and Targeted Therapy: A Narrative Review. *J. Microbiol. Immunol. Infect.* **2019**, *52*, 1–8. [CrossRef] [PubMed]
77. McGinley, M.P.; Goldschmidt, C.H.; Rae-Grant, A.D. Diagnosis and Treatment of Multiple Sclerosis: A Review. *JAMA* **2021**, *325*, 765–779. [CrossRef]
78. Ciardi, M.R.; Iannetta, M.; Zingaropoli, M.A.; Salpini, R.; Aragri, M.; Annecca, R.; Pontecorvo, S.; Altieri, M.; Russo, G.; Svicher, V.; et al. Reactivation of Hepatitis B Virus with Immune-Escape Mutations After Ocrelizumab Treatment for Multiple Sclerosis. *Open Forum Infect Dis.* **2018**, *6*, 365. [CrossRef] [PubMed]
79. Epstein, D.J.; Dunn, J.; Deresinski, S. Infectious Complications of Multiple Sclerosis Therapies: Implications for Screening, Prophylaxis, and Management. *Open Forum Infect. Dis.* **2018**, *5*, ofy174. [CrossRef]
80. Dong, E.; Du, H.; Gardner, L. An Interactive Web-Based Dashboard to Track COVID-19 in Real Time. *Lancet Infect. Dis.* **2020**, *20*, 533–534. [CrossRef]
81. World Health Organization. *COVID-19 Clinical Management: Living Guidance*; WHO: Geneve, Switzerland, 2021.
82. Ghosn, L.; Chaimani, A.; Evrenoglou, T.; Davidson, M.; Graña, C.; Schmucker, C.; Bollig, C.; Henschke, N.; Sguassero, Y.; Nejstgaard, C.H.; et al. Interleukin-6 Blocking Agents for Treating COVID-19: A Living Systematic Review. *Cochrane Database Syst. Rev.* **2021**, *2021*, CD013881. [CrossRef]
83. Liu, J.; Wang, T.; Cai, Q.; Sun, L.; Huang, D.; Zhou, G.; He, Q.; Wang, F.; Liu, L.; Chen, J. Longitudinal Changes of Liver Function and Hepatitis B Reactivation in COVID-19 Patients with Pre-Existing Chronic Hepatitis B Virus Infection. *Hepatol. Res.* **2020**, *50*, 1211–1221. [CrossRef] [PubMed]
84. Mori, S. Hepatitis B Virus Reactivation Associated with Antirheumatic Therapy: Risk and Prophylaxis Recommendations. *World J. Gastroenterol.* **2015**, *21*, 10274–10289. [CrossRef] [PubMed]
85. Rodríguez-Tajes, S.; Miralpeix, A.; Costa, J.; López-Suñé, E.; Laguno, M.; Pocurull, A.; Lens, S.; Mariño, Z.; Forns, X. Low Risk of Hepatitis B Reactivation in Patients with Severe COVID-19 who Receive Immunosuppressive Therapy. *J. Viral Hepat.* **2021**, *28*, 89–94. [CrossRef] [PubMed]

Article

Gastric Xanthoma Is Related to the Rapid Growth of Gastric Cancer

Ko Miura, Tadayuki Oshima *, Akio Tamura, Ken Hara, Takuya Okugawa, Masashi Fukushima, Toshihiko Tomita, Hirokazu Fukui and Hiroto Miwa

Division of Gastroenterology and Hepatology, Department of Internal Medicine, Hyogo College of Medicine, Nishinomiya 663-8501, Japan; i.move.mountain@gmail.com (K.M.); akio@hyo-med.ac.jp (A.T.); k-hara@hyo-med.ac.jp (K.H.); okugawat@hyo-med.ac.jp (T.O.); ma-fukushima@hyo-med.ac.jp (M.F.); tomita@hyo-med.ac.jp (T.T.); hfukui@hyo-med.ac.jp (H.F.); miwahgi@hyo-med.ac.jp (H.M.)
* Correspondence: t-oshima@hyo-med.ac.jp; Tel.: +81-798-45-6662

Abstract: Early detection of gastric cancer is important. However, rapid growth of gastric cancers that cannot be resected endoscopically occurs even with periodic check-ups. Accordingly, we assessed factors associated with the speed of gastric cancer growth by examining historical endoscopic images. A total of 1996 gastric cancer cases were screened, and characteristics of lesions with slow and rapid growth were assessed. A total of 114 lesions from 114 patients were included in the assessment. Sixty slow-growing and fifty-four rapidly growing gastric cancers were compared. Female sex and incidence of lesions in the lower part of the stomach were significantly less frequent in the rapid-growth group than in the slow-growth group. History of endoscopic treatment tended to be more frequent in the rapid-growth group. Age, body mass index, histology, *Helicobacter pylori* status, and medications did not differ significantly between groups. Xanthoma was significantly related to rapid growth of gastric cancer, and map-like redness tended to be more frequent in the rapid-growth group in univariate analysis. Xanthoma was significantly related to rapid growth of gastric cancer on multivariate analysis. Further studies are warranted to clarify the pathophysiological mechanisms involved in the speed of gastric cancer growth.

Keywords: gastric cancer; growth; xanthomatosis

1. Introduction

Gastric cancer remains an important cancer worldwide, responsible for over 1,000,000 new cases and an estimated 783,000 deaths in 2018 (equivalent to 1 in every 12 deaths globally), making it the fifth most frequently diagnosed cancer and the third leading cause of cancer death [1]. On a global scale, the incidence of gastric cancer is higher in Asia than in Europe or Northern America. In a previous report, cases of *Helicobacter pylori* gastritis from seven countries were evaluated and the highest scores for antral atrophy were found in Japan [2]. Chronic atrophic gastritis is strongly associated with gastric cancer, and the incidence of gastric cancer is high in East Asia [3].

Early detection of gastric cancer has therefore recently been the focus of screening examinations. Subjects in Korea who underwent upper gastrointestinal endoscopy were less likely to die from gastric cancer [4]. Upper gastrointestinal endoscopy screening achieved a 30% reduction in gastric cancer mortality within 36 months before the date of gastric cancer diagnosis [5]. Based on such data, health check-ups by upper gastrointestinal endoscopy are currently recommended every other year in Japan and Korea [6]. When cancers are detected at an early stage and can be treated endoscopically, quality of life is significantly better after endoscopic submucosal resection compared to surgery [7].

However, rapid growth of gastric cancers that could not be resected endoscopically has been reported even in patients receiving periodic check-ups [8]. Previous reports have shown the natural history of gastric cancers in specific subjects who were not treated for various reasons [9]. A report showed that the median time to progression from tumor-node-metastasis stage I to stage II was 34 months, and no risk factors for cancer progression were found [10]. Cases of gastric cancer remained as mucosal cancer for 3–9 years [11,12]. As cancers that remain untreated necessarily show specific conditions and the patients are often not in a good state of health, outcomes from these patients cannot be generalized as representing the natural history of gastric cancer. Furthermore, no studies have assessed the speed of gastric cancer growth and prospective follow-up of cases is ethically unacceptable.

Studies assessing patients and endoscopic factors (e.g., sex, gastric xanthoma, atrophy, and intestinal metaplasia) associated with the speed of gastric cancer growth are therefore needed to reveal those high-risk gastric cancer patients who should be followed closely. Accordingly, the present study was conducted to identify factors associated with the speed of gastric cancer growth by examining historical images from endoscopy.

2. Materials and Methods

2.1. Study Design, Setting and Participants

Patients who underwent esophagogastroduodenoscopy (EGD) at Hyogo College of Medicine (Nishinomiya, Japan) from March 2012 to December 2019 were assessed. During the study period, 49,587 EGDs were performed, and 1996 cases of gastric cancer were diagnosed. After excluding cases with no history of EGD 1 year or more before detection, cases and lesions with a history of EGD were counted.

Patients were excluded if they satisfied any of the following exclusion criteria: remnant stomach, familial adenomatous polyposis (FAP), or lack of data years before detection (including cases without identified lesion location in the initial EGD). Included cases were classified as a slow-growth group, comprising patients whose findings showed cancer in previous endoscopic images (Figure 1), or a rapid-growth group, comprising cases whose findings showed no cancer in previous endoscopic images (Figure 1) [6,13,14]. The study protocol was approved by the ethics committee/institutional review board at Hyogo College of Medicine, Japan (approval no. 201909-047) on 24 June 2019.

2.2. Definition of Lesion

The date of EGD examination that led to the diagnosis of gastric cancer was used as the index data for endoscopy. The slow-growth group comprised cases in which the lesion was detectable with careful retrospective inspection at least 2 years before the index EGD examination as initial data [8]. We used a period of 2 years because the current recommended interval for screening upper gastrointestinal endoscopy for health check-ups is every other year [6]. The color and surface structure observed during the initial EGD examination were compared between the expected location and surrounding mucosa using saved images, and lesions were defined as present when findings were different from those of the surrounding mucosa. The rapid-growth group comprised cases in which no lesions were detected 1–2 years before the index EGD.

The definition of no lesion at two years before the index EGD was dependent on the review of the two experts. To make the decision more objective, differences in color on images, as one of the factors used to distinguish lesions, were assessed using image-analysis software (ImageJ; National Institutes of Health, Bethesda, MD, USA). The method for evaluating objectivity was based on a previously reported technique [15]. Briefly, endoscopic images were converted into JPEG images. Using the default method, i.e., the "Measure" tool in the "Analyze" menu, mean gray values (MGVs) of the lesion and perilesional normal mucosa were calculated. MGV of the lesion was measured at one location, and the perilesional mucosa was calculated as the average of MGVs from four locations. Color index was defined using the following equation: color index = |(lesion MGV/mean perilesional MGV) − 1|. With this method, an absence of any color difference between the lesion and perilesional mucosa would provide a value of 0 (Figure 2).

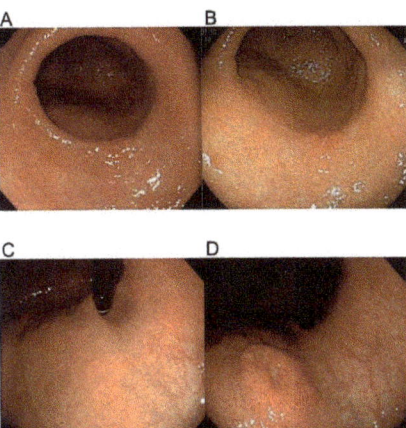

Figure 1. Representative lesions showing slow and rapid gastric cancer growth. A slow-growing lesion at two years before diagnosis (**A**) and at the time of diagnosis (**B**). The site of a rapidly growing lesion at two years before diagnosis (**C**) and at the time of diagnosis (**D**).

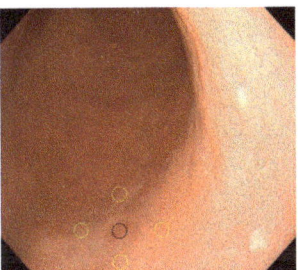

Figure 2. Assessment of color index. One central lesion and 4 surrounding points were evaluated to determine the color index. Black circle, lesion area. Yellow circles, surrounding areas.

2.3. Definition of Related Factors

Factors were identified by comparing the slow- and rapid-growth groups. Factors used in the present study were the characteristics of the patient and lesion, including age, sex, body mass index (BMI), family history of gastric cancer, history of endoscopic treatment, location, size, macroscopic type [16], histology, *H. pylori* infection, use of proton pump inhibitors (PPIs), use of statins, use of steroids, use of aspirin, and use of non-steroidal anti-inflammatory drugs (NSAIDs). The characteristics of endoscopic findings were defined using the Kyoto classification of gastritis [17] and confirmed by index endoscopies. Cancer location was classified into two types: lower part (angle and antrum) and other parts. *H. pylori* infection was detected based on endoscopic features, rapid urease test, urea breath test, or serum antibody. The use of PPIs, statins, steroids, aspirin, or NSAIDs was defined when these factors were present for more than 6 months before the detection of gastric cancer.

2.4. Statistical Analysis

To determine factors related to the rapid growth of gastric cancer, we estimated odds ratios and 95% confidence intervals (CI). Age and BMI were compared using Student's *t*-test, and macroscopic type was compared using Fisher's exact test. Sex, family history of gastric cancer, history of endoscopic treatment, location, histology, *H. pylori* infection, PPI, statin, steroid, aspirin, NSAID, atrophy, xanthoma, map-like redness, intestinal metaplasia, diffuse redness, enlarged fold and nodularity were compared using the chi-square test for univariate analyses and unconditional logistic regression for multivariate analysis. Factors showing values of $p < 0.1$ on univariate analysis were used in the multivariate analysis. All reported p-values were two-sided, and values less than 0.05 were considered statistically significant. JMP® was used for all statistical analyses (version 14; SAS Institute Inc., Cary, NC, USA).

3. Results

3.1. Characteristics of Patients and Lesions

During the study period, 49,587 EGDs were performed, and 1996 cases were diagnosed with gastric cancer. Patients were excluded if they satisfied any of the following exclusion criteria: no history of EGD $\geq$ 1 year before detection (n = 1747), remnant stomach (n = 25), FAP (n = 2), or no data 2 years before detection (n = 108). A total of 114 lesions from 114 patients were finally included in the present study (Figure 3). The mean age of patients was 72.1 years, and 42 patients were female. Three cases were not infected with *H. pylori*, 19 showed present infection, and 92 were post-eradication. The pathological diagnoses of the slow-growth group obtained from index data were pap, 1; tub1, 47; tub2, 4; por1, 2; por2, 2; sig, 2; and gastric adenocarcinoma of fundic gland type (GA-FG), 2. The pathological diagnoses of the rapid-growth group were pap, 2; tub1, 38; tub2, 5; por1, 1; por2, 4; sig, 2; and GA-FG, 2. Gastric xanthoma was detected in 53 (46.5%) of the 114 patients included in the present study. Reasons for undergoing EGD were periodic check-up due to *H. pylori* infection and eradication history in 97.4%.

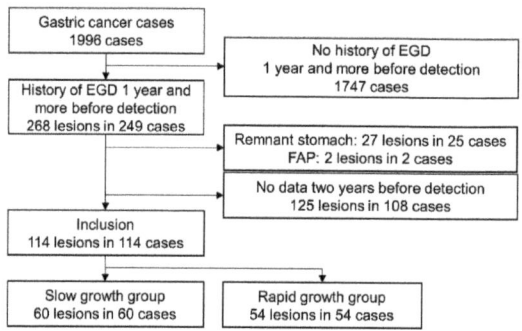

Figure 3. Patient flowchart. EGD, esophagogastroduodenoscopy; FAP, familial adenomatous polyposis.

3.2. Factors Related to Speed of Gastric Cancer Progression

Data for the initial endoscopy were extracted at 41 months (interquartile range (IQR), 29–64 months) before the index endoscopy for the slow-growth group and at 16 months (IQR, 13–24 months) for the rapid-growth group. To make identifying the presence of the initial lesion more objective, differences in color were assessed by color index in the areas of lesions. Color index was significantly higher in the slow-growth group than in the rapid-growth group (0.16, 95% CI 0.11–0.21 vs. 0.04, 95% CI 0.03–0.06, respectively; $p < 0.01$).

The demographics and characteristics of the slow-growth group (n = 60) and rapid-growth group (n = 54) are summarized in Table 1. Female sex and presence of the lesion in the lower stomach were significantly less frequent in the rapid-growth group than in the slow-growth group (Table 1). History of endoscopic treatment tended to be more frequent in the rapid-growth group, although the difference was not significant. Age, BMI, histology of the lesion, *H. pylori* infectious status, and use of medications likewise did not differ between groups. In cases after *H. pylori* eradication, the duration until the detection of gastric cancer after eradication did not differ between groups. Lesion depth did not differ between slow- and rapid-growth groups (slow growth: m, 51; sm1, 5; sm2, 2; and ss, 2 vs. rapid growth: m, 43; sm1, 1; sm2, 5; mp, 1; and ss, 4).

Table 1. Characteristics of patients and lesions.

	Slow Growth (n = 60)	Rapid Growth (n = 54)	Univariate OR (95% CI)	p-Value
Age, mean (SD), years	72.4 (10.1)	71.9 (7.8)	0.99 (0.95–1.04)	0.785
Sex (female), n (%)	28 (46.7)	14 (25.9)	0.40 (0.18–0.88)	0.023
BMI, mean (SD)	22.9 (3.6)	23.4 (3.6)	1.04 (0.94–1.16)	0.439
Endoscopy interval, months, median (IQR)	41 (29–64)	16 (13–24)	0.65 (0.52–0.81)	<0.001
Family history of GC, n (%)	1 (1.7)	1 (1.9)	1.11 (0.07–18.2)	0.940
History of endoscopic treatment, n (%)	12 (20.0)	20 (37.0)	2.04 (0.89–4.66)	0.092
Location (lower part), n (%)	38 (63.3)	22 (40.7)	0.40 (0.19–0.85)	0.017
Size, median (IQR), mm	12 (5.3–15.8)	10 (6.0–16.0)	0.98 (0.95–1.02)	0.274
Macroscopic type, n (%)				
0–I	3 (5.0)	0		0.246 [†]
0–IIa	19 (31.7)	14 (25.9)		0.540 [†]
0–IIc	32 (43.3)	34 (57.4)		0.345 [†]
0–IIa + IIc	4 (6.7)	1 (1.9)		0.367 [†]
Type 1	1 (1.7)	0		1.000 [†]
Type 2	0	4 (7.4)		0.253 [†]
Type 3	1 (1.7)	0		1.000 [†]
Type 4	0	0		-
Type 5	0	1 (1.9)		0.473 [†]
Histology (diffuse), n (%)	6 (10.0)	7 (13.0)	1.34 (0.42–4.27)	0.620
H. pylori infection, n (%)				
Negative	3 (5.0)	0 (0.0)	-	-
Eradication	44 (73.3)	48 (88.9)	1.00	-
Positive	13 (21.7)	6 (11.1)	0.42 (0.15–1.21)	0.108
PPI, n (%)	29 (48.3)	18 (33.3)	0.53 (0.25–1.14)	0.106
Statin, n (%)	23 (38.3)	14 (25.9)	0.56 (0.25–1.25)	0.160
Steroid, n (%)	7 (11.7)	10 (18.5)	1.72 (0.60–4.89)	0.309
Aspirin, n (%)	8 (13.3)	5 (9.3)	0.66 (0.20–2.17)	0.497
NSAID, n (%)	7 (11.7)	2 (3.7)	0.29 (0.06–1.47)	0.135

[†] Fisher's exact test. OR, odds ration; SD, standard deviation; BMI, body mass index; GC, gastric cancer; IQR, interquartile range; PPI, proton pump inhibitor; NSAID, non-steroidal anti-inflammatory drug.

Univariate analyses of characteristics from endoscopic images showed that xanthoma correlated significantly with rapid growth of gastric cancer (Table 2). The incidence of map-like redness tended to be greater in the rapid-growth group, although the difference was not significant. Atrophy, intestinal metaplasia, and diffuse redness did not differ between groups. Multivariate analysis showed that xanthoma was significantly related to rapid growth of gastric cancer (Table 3).

Table 2. Characteristics of endoscopic image.

	Slow Growth (n = 60)	Rapid Growth (n = 54)	Univariate OR (95% CI)	p-Value
Atrophy (open), n (%)	48 (80.0)	46 (85.2)	0.70 (0.26–1.86)	0.469
Xanthoma, n (%)	22 (36.7)	31 (57.4)	2.33 (1.10–4.94)	0.028
Map-like redness, n (%)	8 (13.3)	15 (27.8)	2.50 (0.96–6.49)	0.060
Intestinal metaplasia, n (%)	51 (85.0)	40 (74.1)	0.50 (0.20–1.28)	0.151
Diffuse redness, n (%)	11 (18.3)	8 (14.8)	0.77 (0.29–2.10)	0.615
Enlarged fold, n (%)	2 (3.3)	0 (0.0)	-	-
Nodularity, n (%)	0 (0.0)	0 (0.0)	-	-

OR, odds ratio; CI, confidence interval.

Table 3. Multivariate analysis.

	Multivariate OR (95% CI)	p-Value
Sex (female)	0.49 (0.21–1.16)	0.103
Location (lower part)	0.53 (0.24–1.20)	0.129
History of endoscopic treatment	1.26 (0.50–3.14)	0.627
Xanthoma	2.39 (1.06–5.39)	0.037
Map-like redness	1.96 (0.69–5.54)	0.207

OR, odds ratio.

4. Discussion

The present study assessed the speed of gastric cancer growth by assessing previous upper gastrointestinal endoscopic images to reveal characteristics of rapidly progressing cancers that were found by surveillance approaches. Xanthoma was found to be associated with rapid growth of gastric cancer. Although the natural history of gastric cancer was first assessed 65 years ago [18], no reports appear to have described factors related to the speed of gastric cancer growth. The present study is the first to reveal factors affecting the speed of gastric cancer progression.

4.1. H. pylori Infection

H. pylori infection could be one factor related to the speed of gastric cancer growth, as *H. pylori* itself causes chronic inflammation and acts to promote stomach carcinogenesis [19], while eradication of *H. pylori* infection reduces the incidence of gastric cancer [20]. However, this infection was not associated with the speed of gastric cancer growth in the present study. Therefore, speed of gastric cancer growth may be unrelated to active *H. pylori* infection. Recent studies have shown that map-like redness represents a risk factor for the development of gastric cancer after successful eradication of *H. pylori* [21,22]. However, besides xanthoma, these endoscopic characteristics were not associated with the speed of gastric cancer growth in the present study.

4.2. Gastric Xanthoma

Gastric xanthoma, also known as xanthelasma or lipid island, is a small, yellowish-white plaque or nodule characterized by accumulation of lipid, including oxidized low-density lipoprotein, in histiocytic foam cells [23,24]. The incidence of gastric xanthomas varies from 0.23% to 7% [25,26]. Previous reports have indicated that the presence of gastric xanthoma and the incidence of gastric cancer are significantly associated [27,28], and gastric xanthoma offers a predictive marker for metachronous and synchronous gastric cancer [29]. However, no reports have clarified the relationship to the speed of gastric cancer progression. Kaiserling et al. reported that increased release of oxygen free radicals may be involved in the formation of gastric xanthoma [24]. Oxygen free radicals are well known to cause DNA damage and to play roles in the pathogenesis of various malignancies [30]. Such mechanisms of xanthoma might also be related to the speed of gastric cancer progression. The present data showed that xanthoma was independently related to the speed of gastric cancer growth after adjustment by sex. Although some reports have described a male predominance in gastric xanthoma [31,32], the data remain conflicting [25–27]. Further studies are warranted to clarify the relationship between xanthoma and the speed of gastric cancer progression.

4.3. Histological Type

Interestingly, histological types were not associated with speed of lesion growth in the present study, although diffuse-type gastric cancer was speculated to be more common in the rapid-growth group. Multivariate analysis indicated that among pathological variables of the tumor, a histological type of poorly differentiated gastric cancer was one independent prognostic factor [33]. As all new lesions that were not apparent in the index examination were defined as rapidly growing lesions in the present study, newly identified slow-progressing cancers might have also been included in the rapid-growth group. Furthermore, signet-ring cells confer favorable prognosis in the early stage [34,35]. These factors might have contributed to the lack of significant differences in histological types between the two groups.

4.4. Screening Examination

Recently, although screening examinations have been performed to identify various cancers in the early stages, reports have indicated that small cancers found by screening examinations do not affect the overall survival of patients [36–38]. Therefore, to prevent overdiagnosis and overtreatment, there is a movement to avoid categorizing lesions that do not affect survival as cancers [37]. Conversely, gastric cancers that progress rapidly exist, and a background mucosa with xanthoma is one factor related to rapid growth. As surgical resection can negatively affect the quality of life of patients, early detection of lesions that have potential to grow rapidly is of great significance. Strict follow-up and detailed observation are needed to detect lesions in the early stage among such high-risk patients.

4.5. Limitations

Several limitations to the present study must be considered. First, the study was retrospective, although a prospective study to follow cancer progression would be ethically unworkable. Second, data were extracted from one tertiary care center, so various selection biases would be present, and some patients have a history of endoscopic treatment or other concomitant diseases. The initial EGD may have been for reasons other than screening for cancers in some cases. These factors were therefore also assessed in this analysis, revealing no correlations. Third, the rapid-growth group might have also included some newly identified slow-growing lesions, because the rapid growth in the present study only meant no lesion for at least 1 year before detection. Some factors not identified as significant in the multivariate analysis of the present study might still be candidates for affecting the speed of gastric cancer growth. Fourth, xanthoma would not be the only factor affecting the speed of gastric cancer growth. Examination of genetic, genomic alteration, or DNA methylation in the background gastric mucosa might reveal biomarkers related to rapid cancer growth.

5. Conclusions

Xanthoma was identified as a factor related to the rapid growth of gastric cancer. As prospective studies evaluating the natural history of gastric cancer cannot be performed due to ethical problems, the present study revealed a potentially important clinical factor that affects the speed of gastric cancer growth. Further studies are warranted to reveal the pathophysiological mechanisms involved in the speed of gastric cancer growth.

Author Contributions: K.M. performed experiments, analyzed data, prepared figures, and drafted the manuscript. T.O. (Tadayuki Oshima) designed the research, interpreted results, and edited the manuscript. A.T., K.H., T.O. (Takuya Okugawa), M.F., T.T. and H.F. interpreted the data and revised the manuscript; H.M. designed the research and edited the manuscript. All authors have read and agreed to the published version of the manuscript.

Funding: This research received no external funding.

Institutional Review Board Statement: The study was conducted according to the guidelines of the Declaration of Helsinki and approved by the Ethics Committee/Institutional Review Board of Hyogo College of Medicine, Japan (No. 201909-047) on 24 June 2019.

Informed Consent Statement: Informed consent was obtained from all subjects involved in the study.

Data Availability Statement: The data presented in this study are available on request from the corresponding author. The data are not publicly available due to ethical restrictions.

Conflicts of Interest: The authors declare no conflict of interest.

References

1. Bray, F.; Ferlay, J.; Soerjomataram, I.; Siegel, R.L.; Torre, L.A.; Jemal, A. Global cancer statistics 2018: GLOBOCAN estimates of incidence and mortality worldwide for 36 cancers in 185 countries. *CA Cancer J. Clin.* **2018**, *68*, 394–424. [CrossRef]
2. Liu, Y.; Ponsioen, C.I.J.; Xiao, S.-D.; Tytgat, G.N.; Ten Kate, F.J. Geographic Pathology of Helicobacter pylori Gastritis. *Helicobacter* **2005**, *10*, 107–113. [CrossRef]
3. Suzuki, H.; Mori, H. Different Pathophysiology of Gastritis between East and West? An Asian Perspective. *Inflamm. Intest. Dis.* **2016**, *1*, 123–128. [CrossRef]
4. Jun, J.K.; Choi, K.S.; Lee, H.-Y.; Suh, M.; Park, B.; Song, S.H.; Jung, K.W.; Lee, C.W.; Choi, I.J.; Park, E.-C.; et al. Effectiveness of the Korean National Cancer Screening Program in Reducing Gastric Cancer Mortality. *Gastroenterology* **2017**, *152*, 1319–1328.e7. [CrossRef]
5. Hamashima, C.; Shabana, M.; Okada, K.; Okamoto, M.; Osaki, Y. Mortality reduction from gastric cancer by endoscopic and radiographic screening. *Cancer Sci.* **2015**, *106*, 1744–1749. [CrossRef] [PubMed]
6. Park, C.H.; Kim, E.H.; Chung, H.; Lee, H.; Park, J.C.; Shin, S.K.; Lee, Y.C.; An, J.Y.; Kim, H.-I.; Cheong, J.-H.; et al. The optimal endoscopic screening interval for detecting early gastric neoplasms. *Gastrointest. Endosc.* **2014**, *80*, 253–259. [CrossRef]
7. Tae, C.H.; Shim, K.-N.; Kim, B.-W.; Kim, J.-H.; Hong, S.J.; Baik, G.H.; Song, H.J.; Kim, Y.S.; Jang, S.-H.; Jung, H.-K. Comparison of subjective quality of life after endoscopic submucosal resection or surgery for early gastric cancer. *Sci. Rep.* **2020**, *10*, 6680. [CrossRef] [PubMed]
8. Iida, T.; Yamashita, K.; Ohwada, S.; Ohkubo, Y.; Hirano, T.; Miyake, T.; Onodera, K.; Kubo, T.; Yamano, H.; Nakase, H. Natural history of gastric cancer from a retrospective review of endoscopic images of older patients with interval gastric cancer. *Geriatr. Gerontol. Int.* **2018**, *18*, 997–1002. [CrossRef]
9. Tsukuma, H.; Oshima, A.; Narahara, H.; Morii, T. Natural history of early gastric cancer: A non-concurrent, long term, follow up study. *Gut* **2000**, *47*, 618–621. [CrossRef]
10. Oh, S.-Y.; Lee, J.-H.; Lee, H.-J.; Kim, T.H.; Huh, Y.-J.; Ahn, H.-S.; Suh, Y.-S.; Kong, S.-H.; Kim, G.H.; Ahn, S.J.; et al. Natural History of Gastric Cancer: Observational Study of Gastric Cancer Patients Not Treated During Follow-Up. *Ann. Surg. Oncol.* **2019**, *26*, 2905–2911. [CrossRef] [PubMed]
11. Fujisaki, J.; Nakajima, T.; Hirasawa, T.; Yamamoto, Y.; Ishiyama, A.; Tsuchida, T.; Hoshino, E.; Igarashi, M.; Yamaguchi, T. Natural history of gastric cancer—a case followed up for eight years: Early to advanced gastric cancer. *Clin. J. Gastroenterol.* **2012**, *5*, 351–354. [CrossRef] [PubMed]
12. Iwagami, H.; Ishihara, R.; Nakagawa, K.; Ohmori, M.; Matsuno, K.; Inoue, S.; Arao, M.; Iwatsubo, T.; Nakahira, H.; Matsuura, N.; et al. Natural history of early gastric cancer: Series of 21 cases. *Endosc. Int. Open* **2019**, *7*, E43–E48. [CrossRef] [PubMed]
13. Hamashima, C.; Narisawa, R.; Ogoshi, K.; Kato, T.; Fujita, K. Optimal interval of endoscopic screening based on stage distributions of detected gastric cancers. *BMC Cancer* **2017**, *17*, 740. [CrossRef]
14. Kim, J.; Kim, S.M.; Ha, M.H.; Seo, J.E.; Choi, M.-G.; Lee, J.H.; Sohn, T.S.; Kim, S.; Jung, S.-H.; Bae, J.M. Does the interval of screening endoscopy affect survival in gastric cancer patients?: A cross-sectional study. *Medicine* **2016**, *95*, e5490. [CrossRef] [PubMed]
15. Watari, J.; Kobayashi, M.; Nakai, K.; Ito, C.; Tamura, A.; Ogawa, T.; Yamasaki, T.; Okugawa, T.; Kondo, T.; Kono, T.; et al. Objective image analysis of non-magnifying image-enhanced endoscopy for diagnosis of small depressed early gastric cancers. *Endosc. Int. Open* **2018**, *06*, E1445–E1453. [CrossRef] [PubMed]
16. Japanese Gastric Cancer Association Japanese classification of gastric carcinoma: 3rd English edition. *Gastric Cancer* **2011**, *14*, 101–112. [CrossRef] [PubMed]
17. Haruma, K.; Kato, M.; Inoue, K.; Murakami, K.; Shibata, T. *Kyoto Classification of Gastritis*, 2nd ed.; Nihon Medical Center: Tokyo, Japan, 2018.
18. Meiselas, L.E. Observations on the natural history of gastric cancer. *Am. J. Med. Sci.* **1953**, *226*, 383–386. [CrossRef]
19. Tsukamoto, T.; Mizoshita, T.; Tatematsu, M. Animal Models of Stomach Carcinogenesis. *Toxicol. Pathol.* **2007**, *35*, 636–648. [CrossRef] [PubMed]
20. Lee, Y.-C.; Chiang, T.-H.; Chou, C.-K.; Tu, Y.-K.; Liao, W.-C.; Wu, M.-S.; Graham, D.Y. Association Between Helicobacter pylori Eradication and Gastric Cancer Incidence: A Systematic Review and Meta-analysis. *Gastroenterology* **2016**, *150*, 1113–1124.e5. [CrossRef]
21. Yan, X.; Hu, X.; Duan, B.; Zhang, X.; Pan, J.; Fu, J.; Xu, M.; Xu, Q. Exploration of endoscopic findings and risk factors of early gastric cancer after eradication of Helicobacter pylori. *Scand. J. Gastroenterol.* **2021**, *56*, 356–362. [CrossRef]
22. Majima, A.; Dohi, O.; Takayama, S.; Hirose, R.; Inoue, K.; Yoshida, N.; Kamada, K.; Uchiyama, K.; Ishikawa, T.; Takagi, T.; et al. Linked color imaging identifies important risk factors associated with gastric cancer after successful eradication of Helicobacter pylori. *Gastrointest. Endosc.* **2019**, *90*, 763–769. [CrossRef] [PubMed]

23. Yamashita, K.; Suzuki, R.; Kubo, T.; Onodera, K.; Iida, T.; Saito, M.; Arimura, Y.; Endo, T.; Nojima, M.; Nakase, H. Gastric Xanthomas and Fundic Gland Polyps as Endoscopic Risk Indicators of Gastric Cancer. *Gut Liver* **2019**, *13*, 409–414. [CrossRef] [PubMed]
24. Kaiserling, E.; Heinle, H.; Itabe, H.; Takano, T.; Remmele, W. Lipid islands in human gastric mucosa: Morphological and immunohistochemical findings. *Gastroenterology* **1996**, *110*, 369–374. [CrossRef]
25. Gencosmanoglu, R.; Sen-Oran, E.; Kurtkaya-Yapicier, O.; Tözün, N. Xanthelasmas of the upper gastrointestinal tract. *J. Gastroenterol.* **2004**, *39*, 215–219. [CrossRef]
26. Yi, S.Y. Dyslipidemia andH pyloriin gastric xanthomatosis. *World J. Gastroenterol.* **2007**, *13*, 4598–4601. [CrossRef]
27. Sekikawa, A.; Fukui, H.; Maruo, T.; Tsumura, T.; Kanesaka, T.; Okabe, Y.; Osaki, Y. Gastric xanthelasma may be a warning sign for the presence of early gastric cancer. *J. Gastroenterol. Hepatol.* **2014**, *29*, 951–956. [CrossRef] [PubMed]
28. Sekikawa, A.; Fukui, H.; Sada, R.; Fukuhara, M.; Marui, S.; Tanke, G.; Endo, M.; Ohara, Y.; Matsuda, F.; Nakajima, J.; et al. Gastric atrophy and xanthelasma are markers for predicting the development of early gastric cancer. *J. Gastroenterol.* **2015**, *51*, 35–42. [CrossRef] [PubMed]
29. Shibukawa, N.; Ouchi, S.; Wakamatsu, S.; Wakahara, Y.; Kaneko, A. Gastric xanthoma is a predictive marker for metachronous and synchronous gastric cancer. *World J. Gastrointest. Oncol.* **2017**, *9*, 327–332. [CrossRef]
30. Farinati, F.; Cardin, R.; Degan, P.; Rugge, M.; Di Mario, F.; Bonvicini, P.; Naccarato, R. Oxidative DNA damage accumulation in gastric carcinogenesis. *Gut* **1998**, *42*, 351–356. [CrossRef]
31. Oviedo, J.; Swan, N.; Farraye, F.A. Gastric xanthomas. *Am. J. Gastroenterol.* **2001**, *96*, 3216–3218. [CrossRef]
32. Chen, Y.S.; Lin, J.B.; Dai, K.S.; Deng, B.X.; Xu, L.Z.; Lin, C.D.; Jiang, Z.G. Gastric xanthelasma. *Chin. Med. J.* **1989**, *102*, 639–643.
33. Adachi, Y.; Yasuda, K.; Inomata, M.; Sato, K.; Shiraishi, N.; Kitano, S. Pathology and prognosis of gastric carcinoma: Well versus poorly differentiated type. *Cancer* **2000**, *89*, 1418–1424. [CrossRef]
34. Chon, H.J.; Hyung, W.J.; Kim, C.; Park, S.; Kim, J.-H.; Park, C.H.; Ahn, J.B.; Kim, H.; Chung, H.; Rha, S.Y.; et al. Differential Prognostic Implications of Gastric Signet Ring Cell Carcinoma: Stage adjusted analysis from a single high-volume center in Asia. *Ann. Surg.* **2017**, *265*, 946–953. [CrossRef]
35. Kunisaki, C.; Shimada, H.; Nomura, M.; Matsuda, G.; Otsuka, Y.; Akiyama, H. Therapeutic strategy for signet ring cell carcinoma of the stomach. *BJS* **2004**, *91*, 1319–1324. [CrossRef] [PubMed]
36. Srivastava, S.; Reid, B.J.; Ghosh, S.; Kramer, B.S. Research Needs for Understanding the Biology of Overdiagnosis in Cancer Screening. *J. Cell. Physiol.* **2015**, *231*, 1870–1875. [CrossRef] [PubMed]
37. Esserman, L.J.; Thompson, I.M.; Reid, B.; Nelson, P.; Ransohoff, D.F.; Welch, H.G.; Hwang, S.; A Berry, D.; Kinzler, K.W.; Black, W.C.; et al. Addressing overdiagnosis and overtreatment in cancer: A prescription for change. *Lancet Oncol.* **2014**, *15*, e234–e242. [CrossRef]
38. Welch, H.G.; Black, W.C. Overdiagnosis in Cancer. *J. Natl. Cancer Inst.* **2010**, *102*, 605–613. [CrossRef] [PubMed]

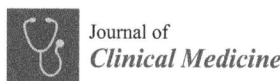

Article

Risk Factors Associated with the Development of Metastases in Patients with Gastroenteropancreatic Neuroendocrine Tumors: A Retrospective Analysis

Shuzo Kohno [1,*], Masahiro Ikegami [2], Toru Ikegami [3], Hiroaki Aoki [1], Masaichi Ogawa [1], Fumiaki Yano [3] and Ken Eto [3]

1. Department of Surgery, The Jikei University Katsushika Medical Center, Tokyo 125-8061, Japan; halm@jikei.ac.jp (H.A.); 0gamasa@jikei.ac.jp (M.O.)
2. Department of Pathology, The Jikei University Katsushika Medical Center, Tokyo 125-8061, Japan; ikegami@jikei.ac.jp
3. Department of Surgery, The Jikei University School of Medicine, Tokyo 105-8461, Japan; tikesurg@icloud.com (T.I.); f-yano@live.jp (F.Y.); etoken@jikei.ac.jp (K.E.)
* Correspondence: s-kohno@jikei.ac.jp; Tel.: +81-3-3603-2111; Fax: +81-03-3838-9945

Abstract: Neuroendocrine tumors develop from systemic endocrine and nerve cells, and their occurrence has increased recently. Since these tumors are heterogeneous, pathological classification has been based on the affected organ. In 2019, the World Health Organization introduced a change expected to influence neuroendocrine tumor research, as gastroenteropancreatic neuroendocrine tumors are now included within a unified classification. This retrospective study aimed to investigate the characteristics (e.g., lymph node metastases and all other metastases) of gastroenteropancreatic neuroendocrine tumors using this new classification in 50 cases. Tumor size, depth, MIB-1 index, lymphatic invasion, venous invasion, and neuroendocrine tumor grade were significantly correlated with lymph node metastasis and other metastases. The venous invasion was more strongly correlated with lymph node metastasis and all other types of metastases than with lymphatic invasion. Identification rates for lymphatic invasion were considered lower because of structural problems such as lymphatic vessels being much thinner than veins. However, venous invasion was considered effective in compensating for the low identification rate in cases of lymphatic invasion. In future research, a unified classification and standardized framework for assessment will be important when analyzing the characteristics of neuroendocrine tumors, and large-scale studies are required.

Keywords: neuroendocrine tumor; metastasis; lymphatic invasion; venous invasion

1. Introduction

Neuroendocrine tumors (NETs) are heterogeneous malignancies with various pathological and clinical features [1–3] that arise from systemic endocrine and nerve cells, and their prevalence has been increasing of late [4]. Previously, NET classification was based on the organ in which the tumor developed. However, according to the 2019 World Health Organization (WHO) classification, NETs occurring in all gastroenteropancreatic (GEP) organs have been grouped and reclassified [5]. Basic and clinical studies have promoted advancements in the diagnosis and treatment of NETs [6,7], and the reclassification of NETs is expected to further advance this research [6].

Treatment guidelines have been created for NETs in each organ, mainly in Europe and the United States [8–11]. Tumor resection is an effective and important treatment option, with radical treatment involving complete removal of the tumor [8]. Localized NETs are an indication for endoscopic and surgical resection. Indications for endoscopic treatment are determined by the grade, depth, and size of the tumor. For localized tumors that are not indicated for endoscopic resection, the indication for surgical resection is determined based on whether the metastatic lesion can be completely resected [8,12,13]. Thus, the diagnosis and prediction of metastasis, especially lymph node metastasis, is important when selecting the treatment option for a particular NET. Lymph node metastases may be surgically removed, which can improve prognosis; however, it is difficult to surgically remove other metastases, often not indicated for surgery, thus highlighting the need for preoperative evaluation.

Therefore, in the present study, we aimed to examine the factors related to lymph node metastases and all other types of metastases in the new GEP-NET classification and determine problems that can arise when identifying these factors.

2. Materials and Methods

2.1. Patients

The medical histories of 48 patients with 50 consecutive cases of GEP-NET treated via endoscopic or surgical resection at our institution between January 2010 and March 2021 were retrospectively collected and compared. Patients who refused treatment and cases in which the tumor size was unknown were excluded. Data related to age, sex, body mass index, and pathological tumor findings (site, size, depth of invasion, lymphatic invasion, venous invasion, and MIB-1 index) were obtained from electronic medical records for all patients.

2.2. Pathological Classification and Staging

The diagnosis and treatment of patients were evaluated based on contemporary standards. The NET classification was based on the 2019 World Health Organization classification [14]. All GEP-NETs were classified into well-differentiated NETs, poorly differentiated neuroendocrine carcinomas, and mixed endocrine/non-endocrine neoplasms. Well-differentiated NETs were classified into grades 1, 2, and 3 (G1, G2, and G3) based on the mitotic rate and Ki-67 index (G1, mitotic rate of <2 per 10 high-power fields and/or Ki67 index of <3%; G2, mitotic rate of 2 to 20 per 10 high-power fields and/or Ki67 index of 3 to 20%; and G3, mitotic rate of >20 per 10 high-power fields and/or Ki67 index of >20%). Neuroendocrine carcinomas were classified as small- or large-cell types. Mixed endocrine/non-endocrine neoplasms consisted of either neuroendocrine or non-neuroendocrine components, such as adenocarcinoma. For endoscopically resected specimens, a cut surface was created at the center of the lesion. In addition to hematoxylin and eosin staining, synaptophysin, chromogranin, CD56, and Ki67 staining were performed for all resected lesions. The lymphatic invasion was diagnosed via D2-40 staining [15], and venous invasion was diagnosed via Elastica van Gieson staining [16].

2.3. Statistical Analysis

Univariate and multivariate analyses for age, sex, body mass index, tumor size, site of origin, depth, MIB-1 index, lymphatic invasion, venous invasion, and NET grade for lymph node metastases and all metastases were performed using logistic regression analysis. The effects of lymphatic invasion and venous invasion on lymph node metastases and all metastases were analyzed using Fisher's exact test. Statistical significance was set at $p < 0.05$. Statistical analyses were performed using SPSS Statistics version 22.0 (IBM Japan, Ltd., Tokyo, Japan).

3. Results

3.1. Background Data

The background data of all patients with GEP-NET who underwent endoscopic or surgical resection at our institution during the study period are shown in Table 1. Fifty resections were performed in 48 patients with NETs. One case had multiple NET occurrences in the duodenum, ileum and rectum, and the other 49 cases had a NET from a single site.

Table 1. Background characteristics of neuroendocrine tumors (n = 50).

Characteristic		Value
Age (years)	Mean ± SD	60.3 ± 14.1
Sex, n (%)	Male (%)	35 (70)
	Female (%)	15 (30)
Body mass index	Mean ± SD	23.67 ± 4.11
Size (mm)	Mean ± SD	9.06 ± 9.22
Excision method	Endoscopic resection	36 (72%)
	Surgical resection	14 (28%)
Location	Esophagus	2 (3.8%)
	Stomach	6 (11.5%)
	Duodenum	7 (13.5%)
	Small intestine	2 (3.8%)
	Pancreas	3 (5.8%)
	Colon	1 (1.9%)
	Rectum	31 (59.6%)
Depth	T1a	7 (14%)
	T1b(+c)	34 (68%)
	T2	6 (12%)
	T3	2 (4%)
	T4	1 (2%)
MIB-1 index	<3%	36 (72%)
	>3%	14 (28%)
Grade	Grade 1	39 (78%)
	Grade 2	7 (14%)
	Grade 3	0
	NEC	4 (8%)
Characteristic	Yes	No
Lymphatic invasion (n)	10 (20%)	40 (80%)
Venous invasion (n)	13 (26%)	37 (74%)

SD, standard deviation; NEC, neuroendocrine carcinoma. T1a, intramucosal; T1b, submucosal; T2, muscularis propria; T3, subserosal; T4, extraserosal infiltration. In the pancreas, T1: localized to the pancreas (maximum diameter ≤2 cm), T2 (localized to the pancreas, 2 cm < maximum diameter ≤ 4 cm), T3: (localized to the pancreas, 4 cm < maximum diameter/duodenum/bile duct infiltration).

Three deaths were noted in our study. The first patient died due to brain metastasis of esophageal neuroendocrine carcinoma three years and ten months after a subtotal esophagectomy; the second patient died of sepsis due to a perianal abscess with rectal, duodenal, and intraperitoneal recurrence seven years and five months after endoscopic resection for rectal NET G2; and the third patient died two months after sigmoid resection for a perforated intraperitoneal abscess of a sigmoid colon NET with liver and multiple lymph node metastases.

The average observation period was 925.3 (36~3000) days. There were 35 (70%) men and 15 (30%) women, and the patient age ranged from 33–88 years (average, 60.4 years). The mean body mass index was 23.67 ± 4.11. The resection method was endoscopic resection in 36 cases and surgical resection in 14 cases. Surgical resection was considered in cases performed after endoscopic resection and those performed after examination without endoscopic resection. The esophagus was resected in two cases, the stomach in six, the duodenum in seven, the small intestine in two, the pancreas in three, the colon in two, and rectum in 31. The invasion depth was intramucosal in seven cases, submucosal (in the pancreas, the tumor remained in the organ and did not infiltrate adjacent organs) in 34 cases, up to the muscularis propria in six cases, up to the serosa in two cases, and extraserosal in one case. Metastasis was observed in eight cases (16.7%). The metastatic sites were observed in the lymph nodes, liver, lung, and brain in six, three, one, and one case, respectively, and there was one case of dissemination.

3.2. Venous and Lymphatic Invasion

Lymphatic invasion of resected specimens was reported in eight cases before this study, but two small metastatic lesions (Figure 1) were diagnosed again by a different pathologist, indicating a total of 10 cases (20%). The lesions identified via repeat microscopy with D2-40 staining exhibited very small amounts of NET cells in vertically or diagonally cut lymphatic vessels. Intravenous invasion was observed in 13 cases (26%). Venous invasion was identified in all six cases of lymph node metastasis, while lymphatic invasion was identified in four cases.

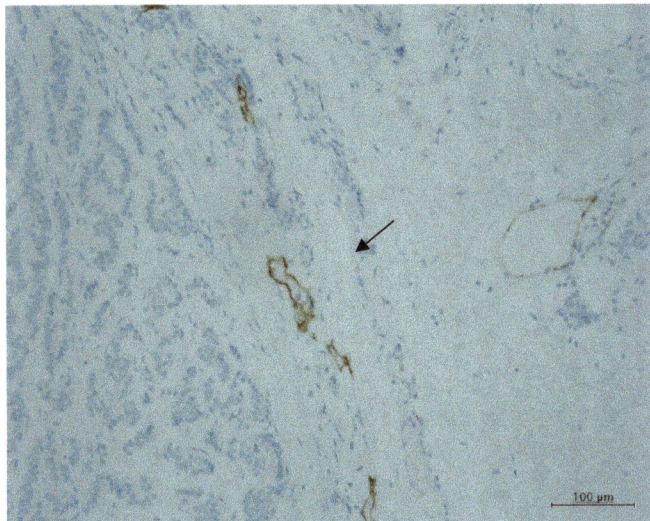

Figure 1. Rectal G1 NET 6 mm. D2-40 immunohistochemical stain showing lymphatic invasion (arrow) in the lymphatic vessels that had been cut diagonally. (×100).

The univariate analysis revealed significant differences in tumor size (Odds ratio [OR] = 1.033, 95% confidence interval [CI]: 1.001–1.066, p = 0.044), depth (OR = 3.957, 95% CI: 1.306–11.992, p = 0.015), MIB-1 index (OR =6.800, 95% CI: 1.082–42.731, p = 0.041), lymphatic invasion (OR = 12.677, 95% CI: 1.888–84.965, p = 0.009), and NET grade (OR = 1.724, 95% CI: 1.874–24.131, p = 0.003) in cases of lymph node metastases, although statistical values could not be obtained for venous invasion (Table 2). Similarly, for all other metastases, the univariate analysis identified significant differences in tumor size (OR = 1.097, 95% CI: 1.020–1.180, p = 0.013), depth (OR = 9.253, 95% CI: 2.038–42.013, p = 0.004), MIB-1 index (OR = 6.111, 95% CI: 1.222–30.572, p = 0.028), lymphatic invasion (OR = 6.000, 95% CI: 1.172–30.725, p = 0.032), venous invasion (OR = 35.000, 95% CI: 3.700–331.059, p = 0.002), and NET grade (OD = 14.900, 95% CI: 2.979–74.529, p = 0.001) (Table 3). However, only NET grade exhibited a significant difference in the multivariate analysis. In the multivariate analysis, we used the variable increase method, and each variable was included in the multivariate model based on the likelihood ratio. Therefore, the OR was only calculated for the NET grade.

Table 2. Logistic regression analysis for lymph node metastases.

	Univariate Analysis				Multivariate Analysis			
	OR	95% CI		p-Value	OR	95% CI		p-Value
Age (per 1 year)	1.074	0.988	1.166	0.092	–			
Sex, Male (vs. Female)	0.375	0.066	2.120	0.267	–			
Body mass index (per 1 kg/m^2)	0.866	0.682	1.100	0.239	–			
Size (per 1 mm)	1.033	1.001	1.066	0.044	n.e.			
Location					–			
Rectum	1.000		ref					
Stomach	n.c.							
Duodenum	6.000	0.321	112.258	0.231				
Esophagus	n.c.							
Intestine	n.c.							
Large intestine	n.c.							
Pancreas	n.c.							
Depth (per 1)	3.957	1.306	11.992	0.015	n.e.			
MIB-1 index, >3% (vs. <3%)	6.800	1.082	42.731	0.041	n.e.			
Lymphatic invasion, Yes (vs. No)	12.667	1.888	84.965	0.009	n.e.			
Venous invasion, Yes (vs. No)	n.c.				–			
Lymphatic invasion/Venous invasion					–			
Neither	1.000		ref					
Either one/Both	n.c.							
Grade (per 1)	6.724	1.874	24.131	0.003	6.724	1.874	24.131	0.003

OR, odds ratio; 95% CI, 95% confidence interval; ref, reference; n.c., not calculable; n.e., not entered. Variables that were significant in the univariate analysis were used in the multivariate analysis (variable increase method: likelihood ratio). Values in bold indicate significant factors.

Table 3. Logistic regression analysis for all metastases.

	Univariate Analysis				Multivariate Analysis			
	OR	95% CI		p-Value	OR	95% CI		p-Value
Age (per 1 year)	1.066	0.993	1.145	0.077	–			
Sex, Male (vs. Female)	0.355	0.076	1.667	0.189	–			
Body mass index (per 1 kg/m^2)	0.901	0.737	1.102	0.309	–			
Size (per 1 mm)	1.097	1.020	1.180	0.013	n.e.			
Tumor location					–			
Rectum	1.000		ref					
Stomach	n.c.							
Duodenum	2.900	0.219	38.320	0.419				
Esophagus	n.c.							
Intestine	n.c.							
Large intestine	n.c.							
Pancreas	7.250	0.443	118.700	0.165				
Depth (per 1)	9.253	2.038	42.013	0.004	n.e.			
MIB-1 index, >3% (vs. <3%)	6.111	1.222	30.572	0.028	n.e.			
Lymphatic invasion, Yes (vs. No)	6.000	1.172	30.725	0.032	n.e.			
Venous invasion, Yes (vs. No)	35.000	3.700	331.059	0.002	n.e.			
Lymphatic invasion/Venous invasion					n.e.			
Neither	1.000		ref					
Either one/both	17.500	1.940	157.881	0.011				
Grade (per 1)	14.900	2.979	74.529	0.001	14.900	2.979	74.529	0.001

OR, odds ratio; 95% CI, 95% confidence interval; ref, reference; n.c., not calculable; n.e., not entered. Variables that were significant in the univariate analysis were used in the multivariate analysis (variable increase method: likelihood ratio). Values in bold indicate significant factors.

3.3. Correlations with Lymph Node Metastasis and All Other Types of Metastases

We investigated the relationship between lymph node invasion and venous invasion in cases of lymph node metastasis (Table 4) and all other types of metastases (Table 5). For lymph node metastases, the *p*-value for lymphatic invasion was 0.011, whereas that for venous invasion was 0.000, indicating a stronger correlation with venous invasion. Furthermore, for all metastases, the *p*-value for lymphatic invasion was 0.041, whereas that for venous invasion was 0.000, indicating a stronger correlation with venous invasion.

Table 4. Comparison of cases with and without lymph node metastases.

	Without Lymph Node Metastases ($n = 44$)		With Lymph Node Metastases ($n = 6$)		*p*-Value
Lymphatic invasion					**0.011**
No	38	86.4	2	33.3	
Yes	6	13.6	4	66.7	
Venous invasion					**0.000**
No	36	81.8	0	0.0	
Yes	8	18.2	6	100.0	
Lymphatic invasion/Venous invasion					**0.000**
Neither	31	70.5	0	0.0	
Either one	12	27.3	2	33.3	
Both	1	2.3	4	66.7	
Lymphatic invasion/Venous invasion					**0.002**
Neither	31	70.5	0	0.0	
Either one/both	13	29.5	6	100.0	

Data are presented as *n* %; *p*-value: Fisher's exact test. Values in bold are significant.

Table 5. Comparison of cases with and without all metastases.

	Without All Metastases ($n = 42$)		With All Metastases ($n = 8$)		*p*-Value
Lymphatic invasion					**0.041**
No	36	85.7	4	50.0	
Yes	6	14.3	4	50.0	
Venous invasion					**0.000**
No	35	83.3	1	12.5	
Yes	7	16.7	7	87.5	
Lymphatic invasion /Venous invasion					**0.000**
Neither	30	71.4	1	12.5	
Either one	11	26.2	3	37.5	
Both	1	2.4	4	50.0	
Lymphatic invasion /Venous invasion					**0.003**
Neither	30	71.4	1	12.5	
Either one/both	12	28.6	7	87.5	

Data are presented as *n* %; *p*-value: Fisher's exact test. Values in bold are significant.

4. Discussion

The curative treatment for GEP-NET is complete resection. However, given the heterogeneous nature of the lesions, indications for resection have been examined based on the organ affected. We believe that it is necessary to examine the entire NET to define its characteristics. In this study, we investigated the factors that influence lymph node metastasis and other types of metastases in patients with GEP-NET. Our analysis revealed that both categories of metastasis were significantly associated with tumor size, depth,

MIB-1 index, lymphatic invasion, venous invasion, and NET grade. This result is consistent with currently reported organ-specific results [10].

The prognosis of lymph node metastasis is important for treating NETs [13,17]. A localized NET indicates endoscopic or surgical resection; however, surgical resection requires complete resection of lymph node metastases; therefore, optimal methods for lymph node dissection are being investigated [9,11,18]. NETs in the stomach, duodenum, pancreas, colon, and rectum that are <1 cm in size and intramucosal ly0 and v0 tumors are indicated for endoscopic treatment [19–24]. There is no treatment algorithm for esophageal NETs due to the scarcity of cases [25]. Endoscopic resection is not indicated for NETs in the small intestine—even if the tumor's major axis is 1 cm or less—due to the high rate of lymph node metastasis [26], a large number of multiple lesions [27], and technical difficulty. The amount of tumor remaining in the small intestine after resection may be larger than the piece resected; therefore, it may be necessary to consider the depth and size of the whole tumor when analyzing the data. In pancreatic NET staging, the criteria for invasion depth differ from the diagnostic criteria in other areas of the gastrointestinal tract, making them difficult to evaluate using the same criteria. For these reasons, when considering treatment options for a GEP-NET as a whole, it is necessary to consider the organ in which the tumor is situated.

Our findings indicated that venous invasion was more strongly correlated with lymph node metastases and all other metastases than lymphatic invasion. Previous studies have demonstrated that immunostaining increases the detection rate of vascular invasion [16,28]. However, other studies have reported contradictory data regarding the pathological identification of vascular invasion with and without immunostaining, and this discrepancy must be fully considered when comparing the data reported. Overexpression of a large number of angiogenesis-promoting molecules has been reported in NET cells, suggesting a link to metastasis [29]. A study on early-stage colorectal cancer noted that venous invasion was more useful than lymphatic invasion as a predictor of lymph node metastasis [30]. For small rectal NETs of 1.5 cm or less, those with vascular infiltration have been reported to have a high potential for lymph node metastasis, as high as 48.8% [31], but the authors did not compare lymphatic infiltration and venous invasion. Most studies have examined the possibility of metastasis in cases of vascular invasion, which is a combination of lymphatic invasion and venous invasion, and few have compared lymphatic invasion with venous invasion. In venous invasion, a large number of tumor cells are identified in the lumen, and the number is greater than that observed in lymphatic vessels. In lymphatic invasion, a few tumor cells are often found in the smaller lymphatic lumen. The difficulty in identifying lymphatic invasion, especially when the lymphatic vessels are cut vertically, may be related to the low rate at which lymphatic invasion is identified. These factors may explain the higher identification rate for venous invasion than for lymphatic invasion. Improving the rate at which lymphatic invasion is identified requires careful tumor identification using D2-40 immunostaining for all diagnoses. Combined evaluation with synaptophysin and other immunostaining methods can also be effective. In this study, venous invasion was observed in all cases of lymph node metastasis, and venous invasion correlates well with lymph node metastasis at present; therefore, simultaneous evaluation of vascular invasion is considered a sufficient index.

A previous study reported that lymphatic invasion and lymph node metastasis rates increase significantly in cases of multiple lesions in patients with rectal NETs [32]. Furthermore, lymph node metastasis of rectal NETs has been associated with tumor size, depth of invasion, vascular invasion, and WHO grade, which is consistent with our findings for GEP-NET [33]. In addition, lymph node metastasis has been reported to affect prognosis. In patients with gastric NETs undergoing gastrectomy and lymph node dissection, the prognosis is related to type I and type III of the Rindi classification, tumor size, and grade [34]. For gastric NETs, the Rindi classification is based on the presence or absence of atrophic gastritis and gastrin secretion. A treatment algorithm has been created based on this classification [23]. Comparing findings for tumors based on this classification and those based on the entire NET may provide insight into methods for improving NET classification. Previous research has indicated that venous invasion is a poor prognostic indicator in patients with pancreatic NETs [35]. In the current study, results for GEP-NET metastasis were similar to those for individual organs. In particular, the results were quite similar to those for the rectum, although most of our data were from rectal cases. Although differences in organ specificity may influence GEP-NET research, we believe that these findings are important for the study of tumor specificity and reflect the GEP-NET group.

The present study had some limitations, including its retrospective design and the low number of cases for certain organs. Further, lymph node dissection was not performed in all cases, suggesting that the rate of metastasis was not accurate in the lymph node metastasis group and that standardized and appropriate diagnostic imaging methods for lymph node metastasis remain unclear. Additionally, follow-up for recurrence may have been insufficient, and the overall assessment may have included unsuitable organs. Randomized controlled studies are difficult, given that the guidelines indicate appropriate treatments. Further studies are warranted to obtain necessary and sufficient data based on very accurate common diagnostic criteria. These studies should employ appropriate follow-up periods and a thorough, unified method for investigating recurrence.

5. Conclusions

This study investigated factors related to the metastasis of GEP-NETs based on 2019 WHO classification. The most important factors were found to be tumor grade and vascular invasion. Of the types of vascular invasion, venous invasion was more highly correlated with metastasis than lymphatic invasion, and the analysis indicated that pathological examination of lymphatic invasion might be problematic. At present, it may be better to evaluate vascular invasion to assess NET metastasis, as it combines lymphatic and venous invasion. The development of a unified classification system for NETs and a standardized method for evaluating them is important for the future of NET research.

Author Contributions: Conceptualization, S.K.; investigation, methodology, writing and analysis, S.K.; validation and pathological analysis, M.I.; investigation and validation; H.A., M.O.; supervision; T.I., F.Y. and K.E. All authors have read and agreed to the published version of the manuscript.

Funding: This research received no external funding.

Institutional Review Board Statement: The study was conducted according to the guidelines of the Declaration of Helsinki and approved by the Institutional Review Board of Jikei University School of Medicine (protocol code 33-039 [10649], approval date 10 May 2021).

Informed Consent Statement: The requirement for patient consent was waived by Jikei University School of Medicine (IRB No. 33-039 [10649]) due to the retrospective nature of the study and the use of anonymized data.

Data Availability Statement: The data presented in this study are available in this article.

Acknowledgments: We would like to thank Koji Nomura for his pathological assessment.

Conflicts of Interest: The authors declare no conflict of interest. The funders had no role in the design of the study; in the collection, analyses, or interpretation of data; in the writing of the manuscript, or in the decision to publish the results.

References

1. Basuroy, R.; Srirajaskanthan, R.; Ramage, J.K. Neuroendocrine Tumors. *Gastroenterol. Clin. N. Am.* **2016**, *45*, 487–507. [CrossRef] [PubMed]
2. Gonzalez, R.S. Diagnosis and Management of Gastrointestinal Neuroendocrine Neoplasms. *Surg. Pathol. Clin.* **2020**, *13*, 377–397. [CrossRef] [PubMed]
3. Cives, M.; Strosberg, J.R. Gastroenteropancreatic Neuroendocrine Tumors. *CA Cancer J. Clin.* **2018**, *68*, 471–487. [CrossRef]
4. Das, S.; Dasari, A. Epidemiology, Incidence, and Prevalence of Neuroendocrine Neoplasms: Are There Global Differences? *Curr. Oncol. Rep.* **2021**, *23*, 43. [CrossRef]

5. Nagtegaal, I.D.; Odze, R.D.; Klimstra, D.; Paradis, V.; Rugge, M.; Schirmacher, P.; Washington, K.M.; Carneiro, F.; Cree, I.A.; WHO Classification of Tumours Editorial Board. The 2019 WHO Classification of Tumours of the Digestive System. *Histopatholog.* **2020**, *76*, 182–188. [CrossRef] [PubMed]
6. Rindi, G.; Inzani, F. Neuroendocrine Neoplasm Update: Toward Universal Nomenclature. *Endocr. Relat. Cancer* **2020**, *27*, R211–R218. [CrossRef] [PubMed]
7. Walter, M.A.; Spanjol, M.; Kollár, A.; Bütikofer, L.; Gloy, V.L.; Dumont, R.A.; Seiler, C.A.; Christ, E.R.; Radojewski, P.; Briel, M.; et al. Treatment for Gastrointestinal and Pancreatic Neuroendocrine Tumours:a Network Meta-Analysis. *Cochrane Database Syst. Rev.* **2020**. [CrossRef]
8. Shah, M.H.; Goldner, W.S.; Benson, A.B.; Bergsland, E.; Blaszkowsky, L.S.; Brock, P.; Chan, J.; Das, S.; Dickson, P.V.; Fanta, P.; et al. Neuroendocrine and Adrenal Tumors, Version 2.2021, NCCN Clinical Practice Guidelines in Oncology. *J. Natl. Compr. Cancer Netw.* **2021**, *19*, 839–868. [CrossRef]
9. Zandee, W.T.; de Herder, W.W. The Evolution of Neuroendocrine Tumor Treatment Reflected by Enets Guidelines. *Neuroendocrinology* **2018**, *106*, 357–365. [CrossRef]
10. Garcia-Carbonero, R.; Sorbye, H.; Baudin, E.; Raymond, E.; Wiedenmann, B.; Niederle, B.; Sedlackova, E.; Toumpanakis, C.; Anlauf, M.; Cwikla, J.M.; et al. Vienna Consensus Conference participants. ENETS Consensus Guidelines for High-Grade Gastroenteropancreatic Neuroendocrine Tumors and Neuroendocrine Carcinomas. *Neuroendocrinology* **2016**, *103*, 186–194. [CrossRef]
11. Shah, M.H.; Goldner, W.S.; Halfdanarson, T.R.; Bergsland, E.; Berlin, J.D.; Halperin, D.; Chan, J.; Kulke, M.H.; Benson, A.B.; Blaszkowsky, L.S.; et al. NCCN Guidelines Insights: Neuroendocrine and Adrenal Tumors, Version 2.2018. *J. Natl. Compr. Cancer Netw.* **2018**, *16*, 693–702. [CrossRef] [PubMed]
12. Eto, K.; Yoshida, N.; Ikegami, S.; Iwatsuki, M.; Baba, H. Surgical Treatment for Gastrointestinal Neuroendocrine Tumors. *Ann. Gastroenterol. Surg.* **2020**, *4*, 652–659. [CrossRef]
13. Martin, J.A.; Warner, R.R.P.; Aronson, A.; Wisnivesky, J.P.; Kim, M.K. Lymph Node Metastasis in the Prognosis of Gastroenteropancreatic Neuroendocrine Tumors. *Pancreas* **2017**, *46*, 1214–1218. [CrossRef]
14. WHO Classification of Tumors Editorial Board. *WHO Classification of Tumors. Digestive System Tumors*, 5th ed.; International Agency for Research on Cancer (LARC): Lyon, France, 2019.
15. Raica, M.; Cimpean, A.M.; Ribatti, D. The Role of Podoplanin in Tumor Progression and Metastasis. *Anticancer Res.* **2008**, *28*, 2997–3006.
16. Kitagawa, Y.; Ikebe, D.; Hara, T.; Kato, K.; Komatsu, T.; Kondo, F.; Azemoto, R.; Komoda, F.; Tanaka, T.; Saito, H.; et al. Enhanced Detection of Lymphovascular Invasion in Small Rectal Neuroendocrine Tumors Using D2-40 and Elastica Van Gieson Immunohistochemical Analysis. *Cancer Med.* **2016**, *5*, 3121–3127. [CrossRef]
17. Sohn, B.; Kwon, Y.; Ryoo, S.B.; Song, I.; Kwon, Y.H.; Lee, D.W.; Moon, S.H.; Park, J.W.; Jeong, S.Y.; Park, K.J.; et al. Predictive Factors for Lymph Node Metastasis and Prognostic Factors for Survival in Rectal Neuroendocrine Tumors. *J. Gastrointest. Surg.* **2017**, *21*, 2066–2074. [CrossRef]
18. Dasari, A.; Shen, C.; Halperin, D.; Zhao, B.; Zhou, S.; Xu, Y.; Shih, T.; Yao, J.C. Trends in the Incidence, Prevalence, and Survival Outcomes in Patients with Neuroendocrine Tumors in the United States. *JAMA Oncol.* **2017**, *3*, 1335–1342. [CrossRef]
19. Zhou, X.; Xie, H.; Xie, L.; Li, J.; Fu, W. Factors Associated with Lymph Node Metastasis in Radically Resected Rectal Carcinoids: A Systematic Review and Meta-Analysis. *J. Gastrointest. Surg.* **2013**, *17*, 1689–1697. [CrossRef]
20. Konishi, T.; Watanabe, T.; Kishimoto, J.; Kotake, K.; Muto, T.; Nagawa, H.; Japanese Society for Cancer of the Colon and Rectum. Prognosis and Risk Factors of Metastasis in Colorectal Carcinoids: Results of a Nationwide Registry Over 15 Years. *Gut* **2007**, *56*, 863–868. [CrossRef] [PubMed]
21. Soga, J. Carcinoids of the Rectum: An Evaluation of 1271 Reported Cases. *Surg. Today* **1997**, *27*, 112–119. [CrossRef] [PubMed]
22. Shields, C.J.; Tiret, E.; Winter, D.C.; International Rectal Carcinoid Study Group. Carcinoid Tumors of the Rectum: A Multi-Institutional International Collaboration. *Ann. Surg.* **2010**, *252*, 750–755. [CrossRef] [PubMed]
23. Sato, Y.; Hashimoto, S.; Mizuno, K.; Takeuchi, M.; Terai, S. Management of Gastric and Duodenal Neuroendocrine Tumors. *World J. Gastroenterol.* **2016**, *22*, 6817–6828. [CrossRef]
24. Falconi, M.; Eriksson, B.; Kaltsas, G.; Bartsch, D.K.; Capdevila, J.; Caplin, M.; Kos-Kudla, B.; Kwekkeboom, D.; Rindi, G.; Klöppel, G.; et al. Enets Consensus Guidelines Update for the Management of Patients with Functional Pancreatic Neuroendocrine Tumors and Non-Functional Pancreatic Neuroendocrine Tumors. *Neuroendocrinology* **2016**, *103*, 153–171. [CrossRef] [PubMed]
25. Giannetta, E.; Guarnotta, V.; Rota, F.; de Cicco, F.; Grillo, F.; Colao, A.; Faggiano, A.; NIKE. A Rare Rarity: Neuroendocrine Tumor of the Esophagus. *Crit. Rev. Oncol. Hematol.* **2019**, *137*, 92–107. [CrossRef]
26. Walsh, J.C.; Schaeffer, D.F.; Kirsch, R.; Pollett, A.; Manzoni, M.; Riddell, R.H.; Albarello, L. Ileal "Carcinoid" Tumors-Small Size Belies Deadly Intent: High Rate of Nodal Metastasis in Tumors ≤1 Cm in Size. *Hum. Pathol.* **2016**, *56*, 123–127. [CrossRef] [PubMed]
27. Pasquer, A.; Walter, T.; Rousset, P.; Hervieu, V.; Forestier, J.; Lombard-Bohas, C.; Poncet, G. Lymphadenectomy during Small Bowel Neuroendocrine Tumor Surgery: The Concept of Skip Metastases. *Ann. Surg. Oncol.* **2016**, *23*, 804–808. [CrossRef]
28. Kang, H.S.; Kwon, M.J.; Kim, T.H.; Han, J.; Ju, Y.S. Lymphovascular Invasion as a Prognostic Value in Small Rectal Neuroendocrine Tumor Treated by Local Excision: A Systematic Review and Meta-Analysis. *Pathol. Res. Pract.* **2019**, *215*, 152642. [CrossRef] [PubMed]

29. Cives, M.; Pelle', E.; Quaresmini, D.; Rizzo, F.M.; Tucci, M.; Silvestris, F. The Tumor Microenvironment in Neuroendocrine Tumors: Biology and Therapeutic Implications. *Neuroendocrinology* **2019**, *109*, 83–99. [CrossRef]
30. Gleeson, F.C.; Levy, M.J.; Dozois, E.J.; Lason, D.W.; Michel, L.; Song, W.K.; Boardman, L.A. Endoscopically identified well-differentiated rectal carcinoid tumors: Impact of tumor size on the natural history and outcomes. *Gastrointest Endosc.* **2014**, *80*, 144–151. [CrossRef]
31. Nam, S.J.; Kim, C.K.; Chang, H.J.; Jeon, H.H.; Kim, J.; Kim, S.Y. Risk Factors for Lymph Node Metastasis and Oncologic Outcomes in Small Rectal Neuroendocrine Tumors with Lymphovascular Invasion. *Gut Liver* **2021**. [CrossRef]
32. Nishikawa, Y.; Chino, A.; Ide, D.; Saito, S.; Igarashi, M.; Takamatsu, M.; Fujisaki, J.; Igarashi, Y. Clinicopathological Characteristics and Frequency of Multiple Rectal Neuroendocrine Tumors: A Single-Center Retrospective Study. *Int. J. Colorectal Dis.* **2019**, *34*, 1887–1894. [CrossRef] [PubMed]
33. Wang, Y.; Zhang, Y.; Lin, H.; Xu, M.; Zhou, X.; Zhuang, J.; Yang, Y.; Chen, B.; Liu, X.; Guan, G. Risk factors for lymph node metastasis in rectal neuroendocrine tumors: A recursive partitioning analysis based on multicenter data. *J. Surg. Oncol.* **2021**, *124*, 1098–1105. [CrossRef] [PubMed]
34. Hanna, A.; Kim-Kiselak, C.; Tang, R.; Metz, D.C.; Yang, Z.; DeMatteo, R.; Fraker, D.L.; Roses, R.E. Gastric Neuroendocrine Tumors: Reappraisal of Type in Predicting Outcome. *Ann. Surg. Oncol.* **2021**, *13*. [CrossRef] [PubMed]
35. Nanno, Y.; Toyama, H.; Otani, K.; Asari, S.; Goto, T.; Terai, S.; Ajiki, T.; Zen, Y.; Fukumoto, T.; Ku, Y. Microscopic Venous Invasion in Patients with Pancreatic Neuroendocrine Tumor as a Potential Predictor of Postoperative Recurrence. *Pancreatology* **2016**, *16*, 882–887. [CrossRef]

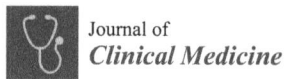

Article

Crosstalk between Irisin Levels, Liver Fibrogenesis and Liver Damage in Non-Obese, Non-Diabetic Individuals with Non-Alcoholic Fatty Liver Disease

Angelo Armandi [1,2,*], Chiara Rosso [1,*], Aurora Nicolosi [1], Gian Paolo Caviglia [1], Maria Lorena Abate [1], Antonella Olivero [1], Daphne D'Amato [1,3], Marta Vernero [1,3], Melania Gaggini [4], Giorgio Maria Saracco [1,3], Davide Giuseppe Ribaldone [1,3], Diana Julie Leeming [5], Amalia Gastaldelli [4] and Elisabetta Bugianesi [1,3]

[1] Department of Medical Sciences, University of Turin, 10126 Turin, Italy; aurora.nicolosi@unito.it (A.N.); gianpaolo.caviglia@unito.it (G.P.C.); marialorena.abate@unito.it (M.L.A.); antonella.olivero@unito.it (A.O.); daphne.damato@unito.it (D.D.); marta.vernero@gmail.com (M.V.); giorgiomaria.saracco@unito.it (G.M.S.); davrib_1998@yahoo.com (D.G.R.); elisabetta.bugianesi@unito.it (E.B.)
[2] Metabolic Liver Research Program, University Medical Center, Department of Internal Medicine I, Johannes Gutenberg University, 55131 Mainz, Germany
[3] Division of Gastroenterology, Città della Salute e della Scienza University-Hospital, 10100 Turin, Italy
[4] Cardiometabolic Risk Unit, Institute of Clinical Physiology, CNR, 56121 Pisa, Italy; mgaggini@ifc.cnr.it (M.G.); amalia@ifc.cnr.it (A.G.)
[5] Nordic Bioscience, 2730 Herlev, Denmark; djl@nordicbio.com
* Correspondence: angelo.armandi@unito.it (A.A.); chiara.rosso@unito.it (C.R.); Tel.: +39-011-633-3572 (ext. 10100) (A.A. & C.R.)

Abstract: Background: Insulin resistance plays a relevant role in the onset of non-alcoholic fatty liver disease (NAFLD) and its progression to non-alcoholic steatohepatitis (NASH) and fibrosis. Irisin is an exercise-induced myokine involved in the regulation of energy homeostasis and glucose metabolism. Additionally, pre-clinical models have shown a potential role of irisin in the pathogenesis of NAFLD. The aim of this study is to explore the association between irisin, histological features and biomarkers of liver fibrogenesis in non-diabetic, non-obese, biopsy-proven NAFLD individuals. Methods: Forty-one patients with histological evidence of NAFLD were included. Circulating irisin and direct markers of fibrogenesis N-terminal type III collagen propeptide (PRO-C3) and type VI collagen cleavage product (PRO-C6) were measured by ELISA. Results: Median age of the cohort was 45 years (41–51) and 80.4% were male. Significant fibrosis (stage $\geq$ 2) was present in 36.6% of cases. Circulating irisin, PRO-C3 and PRO-C6 levels were significantly higher in subjects with fibrosis stage $\geq$ 2 when compared to those with fibrosis stage < 2 (5.96 ng/mL (95% CI = 4.42–9.19) vs. 2.42 ng/mL (95% CI = 1.73–5.95), p = 0.033; 9.5 ng/mL (95% CI = 7.7–13.6) vs. 6.2 ng/mL (95% CI = 4.9–8.9), p = 0.016; 6.6 ng/mL (95% CI = 5.6–7.9) vs. 5.1 ng/mL (95% CI = 4.2–5.4), p = 0.013, respectively). Irisin levels were similarly distributed between the features of NASH. Circulating irisin positively correlated with both PRO-C3 and PRO-C6 levels (r = 0.47, p = 0.008 and r = 0.46, p = 0.002). Conclusions: Increased circulating irisin levels may identify a more aggressive phenotype of liver disease with increased fibrogenesis and more severe liver damage.

Keywords: irisin; insulin resistance; non-invasive biomarkers; liver fibrosis; liver fibrogenesis; PRO-C3; PRO-C6; NAFLD

Citation: Armandi, A.; Rosso, C.; Nicolosi, A.; Caviglia, G.P.; Abate, M.L.; Olivero, A.; D'Amato, D.; Vernero, M.; Gaggini, M.; Saracco, G.M.; et al. Crosstalk between Irisin Levels, Liver Fibrogenesis and Liver Damage in Non-Obese, Non-Diabetic Individuals with Non-Alcoholic Fatty Liver Disease. *J. Clin. Med.* **2022**, *10*, 635. https://doi.org/10.3390/jcm11030635

Academic Editor: Jiangao Fan

Received: 31 December 2021
Accepted: 26 January 2022
Published: 27 January 2022

Publisher's Note: MDPI stays neutral with regard to jurisdictional claims in published maps and institutional affiliations.

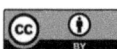

Copyright: © 2022 by the authors. Licensee MDPI, Basel, Switzerland. This article is an open access article distributed under the terms and conditions of the Creative Commons Attribution (CC BY) license (https://creativecommons.org/licenses/by/4.0/).

1. Introduction

Non-Alcoholic Fatty Liver Disease (NAFLD) is currently the most common chronic liver disease, tightly associated with type 2 diabetes mellitus (T2DM) and the metabolic syndrome (MetS). Liver necro-inflammatory changes superimposed to fat accumulation (Non-Alcoholic Steatohepatitis, NASH) leads to scar tissue deposition in the parenchyma (fibrosis) and to the progression towards end-stage liver disease and its complications.

Liver fibrosis is the most relevant prognostic factor and its early recognition is a mainstay of management in NAFLD patients [1].

Insulin resistance (IR) in the adipose tissue, liver and skeletal muscle (SM) is a well-recognized pathophysiological mechanism underlying both the onset and progression of NAFLD [2]. The study of the metabolic cross-talks between insulin-sensitive tissues can unveil potential targets for biomarkers or therapy. Irisin is a recently discovered cytokine mainly synthesized in the SM in response to physical exercise and it is involved in energy metabolism, favoring thermogenesis and browning of adipose tissue [3]. Irisin is also produced in the adipose tissue, where it regulates lipid metabolism and glucose uptake [4] and may be involved in the regulation of pancreatic beta-cell activity [5].

In animal studies, irisin reduced gluconeogenesis and stimulated glycogen synthesis [6], reduced cholesterol content from hepatocytes of both lean and obese mice [7] and modulated oxidative stress [8]. These findings are remarkable, as oxidative stress is the main source of lipid-driven hepatocyte damage, leading to chronic inflammation and ultimately to fibrogenesis. However, studies conducted on NAFLD individuals have yielded conflicting results. Zhang et al. found that serum irisin levels are inversely associated with intrahepatic fat content detected by magnetic resonance spectroscopy (MRS) [9], also confirmed by Metwally et al., in patients with liver biopsy [10]. On the contrary, another study found a positive association between irisin levels and steatosis, NASH and liver fibrosis [11]. Finally, a recent meta-analysis reported that irisin levels are increased in mild NAFLD with respect to moderate–severe NAFLD, but specifically in the Asian population [12].

In this study, we assessed the association between circulating irisin levels and metabolic parameters of IR, markers of fibrogenesis and histological fibrosis in a well-characterized cohort of biopsy-proven NAFLD individuals in the absence of major metabolic confounders (obesity and T2DM).

2. Materials and Methods

2.1. Study Population

This is a retrospective, cross-sectional study of biopsy-proven NAFLD individuals. These patients had been prospectively and consecutively enrolled from 2010 to 2015 at the Division of Gastroenterology and Hepatology of the University of Turin as part of the EU-funded FLIP/EPOS cohort. The present study includes 41 patients selected from the whole cohort (n = 135) according to the absence of T2DM and obesity, and with metabolomic data and fibrogenesis markers available for analysis. A flow chart of the study is provided in Supplementary Figure S1.

Other causes of liver disease, including viral (hepatitis B and C virus infection), autoimmune, cholestatic, genetic and drug-induced diseases, were excluded, and only features of NAFLD were detected at histology. Significant alcohol consumption was excluded according to established thresholds (less than 210 g/week for males and 140 g/week for females) through direct questioning of patients and close relatives. At the time of biopsy, no clinical, biochemical or imaging-supported evidence of cirrhosis was present. A diagnosis of cirrhosis was made solely based on the histology findings. Physical examination and blood samples were collected at the time of biopsy. Obesity was defined by body mass index (BMI) equal or above 30 kg/m^2. IR was assessed by homeostatic model assessment (HOMA)-IR according to the following formula: ((fasting plasma insulin in mU/L) × (fasting plasma glucose in mmol/L)/22.5) [13]; a HOMA-IR value higher or equal to 2.5 indicates IR.

The study was carried out according to the principles of the Declaration of Helsinki, and it was approved by the ethics committee of the University Hospital "Città della Salute e della Scienza" of Torino (CEI/522, 23 December 2009). All patients gave signed consent for the collection of personal data in the database and for the use of blood samples for research purposes and for participation in the tracer study.

2.2. Analytical Determinations

Plasma samples for laboratory investigations were collected at the time of liver biopsy and stored at −80 °C for the investigations. Irisin was measured by the commercially available competitive human enzyme linked immunosorbent assay (ELISA) kit (Phoenix Pharmaceuticals, Inc., Burlingame, CA, USA) according to manufacturer's instructions. Irisin concentration was determined with an ELISA reader at 450 nm and the final concentration was derived by the 4 parameter logistics method analysis. The intra- and inter-assay coefficients of variation were below 10% and 15%, respectively.

The concentration of free fatty acids (FFAs), was determined by enzymatic colorimetric assays (WAKO diagnostic, Richmond, VA, USA).

Liver fibrogenesis was evaluated by interstitial matrix turnover biomarkers: N-terminal type III collagen propeptide (PRO-C3) and type VI collagen cleavage product (PRO-C6) (Nordic Bioscience competitive ELISA assays, Nordic Bioscience Laboratory, Herlev, Denmark) [14,15].

2.3. Histology

All liver biopsies were analyzed by a local pathologist with experience in liver disease and blinded to patients' clinical information. The average length of liver tissue was 25 mm (range 14–45 mm) with at least 11 portal tracts. Histological features of NAFLD, including steatosis, ballooning, lobular inflammation and fibrosis, were assessed and scored according to the Clinical Research Network scoring system (NAFLD Activity Score (NAS)) [16]. The diagnosis of NASH was made according to the joint presence of steatosis, hepatocyte ballooning, and lobular inflammation. Significant fibrosis was defined as fibrosis stage equal or above 2.

2.4. Statistical Analysis

Data are reported as mean ± standard deviation (SD) for continuous normally distributed variables, as median and 95% confidence interval (CI) for the median for continuous not-normally distributed variables or as frequency and percentage (%) for categorical variables. Comparisons between two groups were performed by Mann–Whitney test for non-normally distributed variables and by t test for normally distributed variables. The Fisher's exact test or the Chi-square test were used for categorical data. Spearman or Pearson correlations were performed as appropriate to evaluate the correlation between all the metabolic parameters. A multivariate regression analysis, adjusted for age and gender, was performed to assess the association between irisin levels and liver fibrogenesis.

Values of $p < 0.05$ were considered statistically significant. All the analyses were performed with MedCalc Software bvba version 18.9.1 (Mariakerke, Belgium).

3. Results

A total of 41 non-diabetic, non-obese NAFLD patients were included in this study. Significant fibrosis, defined as $F \geq 2$, was present in 36.6% of subjects. The clinical and biochemical characteristics of the cohort are reported in Table 1.

Table 1. Clinical, biochemical and histological characteristics of the study cohort according to degree of liver fibrosis ($n = 41$).

Variables	All ($n = 41$)	F0/F1 ($n = 26$)	$F \geq 2$ ($n = 15$)	p Value
Age (years), median (95% CI)	45 (41–51)	44 (38–48)	51 (38–64)	0.068
BMI (kg/m^2), median (95% CI)	25.7 (24.6–26.6)	25.6 (23.6–27.6)	25.7 (20.1–26.4)	0.705
Male/Female gender, n (%)	33/8 (80.4/19.6)	24/4 (85.7/14.3)	9/4 (69.2/30.8)	0.221
AST (IU/L), median (95% CI)	31 (28–36)	31 (26–35)	31 (25–58)	0.424
ALT (IU/L), median (95% CI)	48 (41–67)	47 (41–70)	53 (27–99)	0.801
Platelets ($\times 10^9$/L), median (95% CI)	230 (216–261)	230 (206–270)	218 (201–283)	0.889

Table 1. Cont.

Variables	All (n = 41)	F0/F1 (n = 26)	F ≥ 2 (n = 15)	p Value
Insulin (mU/L), median (95% CI)	10.2 (9–11.8)	9.7 (8.1–10.5)	12.2 (10.1–17)	0.004
Glucose (mg/dL), median (95% CI)	94 (90–98)	92 (90–97)	97 (89–121)	0.165
HOMA-IR	2.5 (2.08–2.73)	2.15 (1.71–2.4)	2.92 (2.26–3.6)	0.012
HOMA-IR ≥ 2.5, n (%)	16 (39)	7 (25)	9 (69)	0.008
Total-Chol (mg/dL), median (95% CI)	184 (177–200)	184 (175–201)	190 (178–213)	0.268
HDL-Chol (mg/dL), median (95% CI)	46 (42–49)	47 (41–50)	44 (39–51)	0.492
Triglycerides (mg/dL), median (95% CI)	100 (86–117)	93 (79–118)	116 (90–178)	0.179
FFAs (mmol/L), mean (sd)	0.627 ± 0.225	0.61 ± 0.24	0.66 ± 0.2	0.449
Irisin (ng/mL), median (95% CI)	5.8 (2.87–5.96)	2.42 (1.73–5.95)	5.96 (4.42–9.19)	0.033
PRO-C3 (ng/mL), median (95% CI)	8.65 (6.32–9.64)	6.2 (4.9–8.9)	9.5 (7.7–13.6)	0.016
PRO-C6 (ng/mL), median (95% CI)	5.6 (5.1–6.74)	5.1 (4.2–5.4)	6.6 (5.6–7.9)	0.013

Note. Data are reported as mean and standard deviation, as median and 95% confidence interval of the median or as number and percentage. Abbreviations. ALT, alanine aminotransferase; AST, aspartate aminotransferase; BMI, body mass index; Chol, cholesterol; CI, confidence interval; FFAs, free fatty acids; HDL-Chol, high density lipoprotein cholesterol; HOMA-IR, homeostasis model of assessment of insulin resistance; PRO-C3, N-terminal type III collagen propeptide; PRO-C6, type VI collagen cleavage product.

The median age of the whole cohort was 45 years (95% CI of the median, 41–51), 80.4% of cases male gender. Patients with F ≥ 2 had significantly higher levels of insulin and HOMA-IR. The overall prevalence of IR (by HOMA-IR ≥2.5) was higher in patients with significant fibrosis compared to those with F0/F1 fibrosis ($p = 0.008$).

3.1. Histological Features Versus Circulating Irisin and Biomarkers of Fibrogenesis

Irisin levels were higher in the population with F ≥ 2 (5.96 ng/mL (4.42–9.19) versus 2.42 ng/mL (1.73–5.95) in patients with F0/F1 fibrosis ($p = 0.033$)). Similarly, the levels of the two biomarkers of fibrogenesis, PRO-C3 and PRO-C6, were increased in NAFLD with significant fibrosis (Table 1).

Overall, NASH was found in 76% of cases, without differences between the two groups. Hepatic steatosis and ballooning degeneration were similar in the individuals with significant fibrosis vs F0/F1 fibrosis, while lobular inflammation was higher in patients with F ≥ 2 (Table 2). Circulating irisin as well as the biomarkers of fibrogenesis PRO-C3 and PRO-C6 had no correlation with hepatic steatosis, ballooning and lobular inflammation, Supplementary Table S1.

Table 2. Histological characteristics of NAFLD patients according to liver fibrosis (n = 41).

Histological Features	All (n = 41)	F0/F1 (n = 26)	F ≥ 2 (n = 15)	p Value
Hepatic steatosis (%), median (95% CI)	25 (10–40)	22 (10–40)	32 (15–45)	0.583
Lobular Inflammation (0/1/2), n (%)	8/31/2 (19/76/5)	6/20/- (23/77/-)	2/11/2 (13/74/13)	0.005
Ballooning (0/1/2), n (%)	4/21/16 (10/51/39)	3/14/9 (11/54/35)	1/7/7 (6/47/47)	0.091
NASH, n (%)	31 (76)	19 (73)	12 (80)	0.623

Note. Data are reported as median and 95% confidence interval of the median or as number and percentage. NASH, non-alcoholic steatohepatitis.

3.2. Circulating Irisin Versus Metabolic Profile and Biomarkers of Fibrogenesis

Correlations between circulating irisin and metabolic parameters are reported in Figure 1.

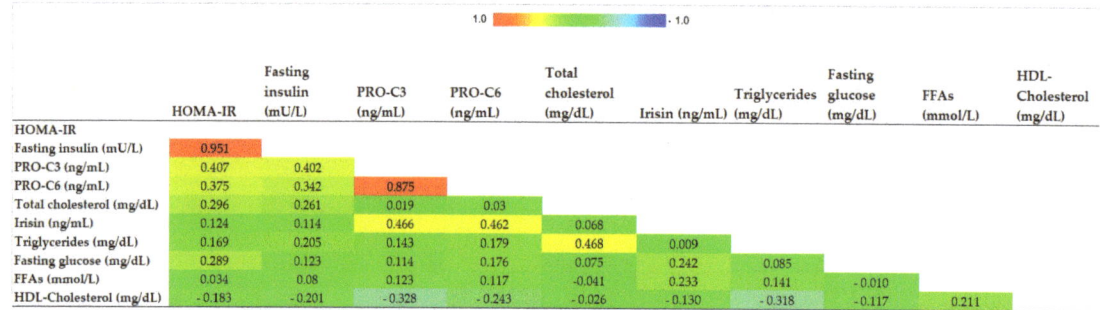

Figure 1. Correlogram representing the correlations between irisin levels and metabolic parameters. Abbreviations. HDL, high density lipoprotein cholesterol; FFAs, free fatty acids; HOMA-IR, homeostasis model of assessment of insulin resistance; PRO-C3, N-terminal type III collagen propeptide; PRO-C6, type VI collagen cleavage product.

No significant correlation was found between irisin levels and both glucose and lipid profile. On the other hand, circulating irisin directly correlated with both PRO-C3 and PRO-C6 levels ($r_S = 0.47$, $p = 0.008$ and $r_S = 0.46$, $p = 0.002$, respectively) (Figure 2a,b).

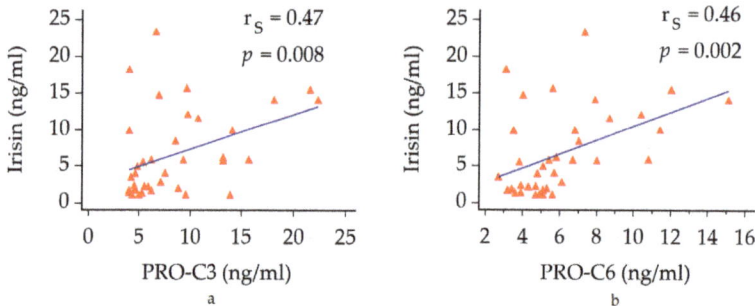

Figure 2. Correlations between circulating irisin with biomarkers of fibrogenesis. (**a**) correlation between irisin and PRO-C3. (**b**) correlation between irisin and PRO-C6. Abbreviations: PRO-C3, N-terminal type III collagen propeptide; PRO-C6, type VI collagen cleavage product.

4. Discussion

We have conducted a retrospective, cross-sectional study with the aim to explore the mechanistic role of the myokine irisin in a population of biopsy-established NAFLD, in the absence of major metabolic burdens (obesity and T2DM). We found that irisin levels were significantly higher in individuals with significant fibrosis. Similarly, we found a positive correlation between circulating irisin and novel markers of collagen remodeling PRO-C3 and PRO-C6. Current evidence from the literature assesses the role of these two peptides for the quantification of liver fibrogenesis [14,15]. Our results suggest a harmonic relationship between irisin and liver fibrogenesis, which is the hepatic response to the inflammatory injury. This remarks the hypothesis that irisin is potentially a hallmark of a more severe phenotype of liver disease, which is suggested by the increased irisin levels in individuals with advanced fibrosis.

Given the tight link between IR, liver injury and fibrogenesis, the increased irisin synthesis may represent a continuum in the damage-response role that is exerted at a mechanistic level. The increase of irisin in significant fibrosis is consistent with the results described by Petta et al. [11], where irisin was overexpressed in hepatic stellate cells of individuals with significant fibrosis. With regard to other histological features, we did not find any association between irisin and liver steatosis, differently from other studies reporting an inverse association between irisin levels and intrahepatic fat [9,10].

In mice, about 70% of total circulating irisin derives from SM and the remaining part mainly secreted by adipose tissue [3]. In humans, adipose tissue seems to be a relevant source of irisin synthesis only in obese individuals, due to the expansion of visceral adipose tissue [17]. In addition, a liver production of irisin has also been described [18]. In particular, in individuals with advanced liver disease, where sarcopenia is a common clinical finding, irisin levels seem to lack correlation with SM mass and with the diverse stages of liver disease severity [19]. However, similar studies remark a positive association between irisin levels and sarcopenia [20]. The heterogeneity of the study population due to either different clinical features or the severity of liver disease, in association with extraepatic co-morbidities, may significantly affect the circulating pool of irisin. In this study, it is plausible that the main source of irisin is represented by SM, potentially with a liver contribution in its synthesis, in relation to the disease activity.

The strength of this work is the well-characterized cohort of biopsy-proven NAFLD patients who were selected for the absence of the major metabolic confounders, that could have affected the interpretations of the results. In fact, irisin seems to be involved in the regulation of IR, with conflicting results [21,22]. It seems to promote lipolysis and glucose uptake in both adipocytes and SM through GLUT4 upregulation and translocation [4]. As a result, irisin levels have been found to be associated with the risk of MetS and major cardiovascular events [23,24], but a plausible interpretation of the results is limited by the heterogeneity in MetS population, which features can significantly impact the circulating irisin pool. Male gender and age higher than 50 years are two hallmarks of higher risk for MetS development, but we did not find any difference in the distribution of irisin levels in these subgroups, when compared to the counterparts (data not shown). Our study has some limitations. The small number of patients limits the strength of the results. In addition, we did not investigate the concomitant role of SM, which is affected by IR in the setting of NAFLD. In fact, SM is a major source of peripheral IR, and the rise of sarcopenia is the hallmark of the suffering SM protein synthesis along with the metabolic disturbances. Sarcopenia may cause reduction in irisin synthesis, as described in literature, even if without strong evidence [25,26]. However, the retrospective nature of this study did not allow for further investigations at the time of liver biopsy. In conclusion, in a well-characterized cohort of non-obese, non-diabetic, biopsy-proven NAFLD individuals, increased irisin levels are found in individuals with significant fibrosis and are correlated with increased liver fibrogenesis, potentially identifying a more aggressive phenotype of liver disease. Larger studies are needed to confirm the results. The role of major metabolic confounders, such as obesity and T2DM, demands a careful selection of study populations and needs further investigations. The involvement of irisin in multiple cross talks makes it difficult to underline a target population where it would be evaluated without confounders. In addition, obesity and T2DM are the commonest features linked to NAFLD onset and progression. However, given the association with liver fibrosis in this cohort of lean individuals, is it plausible that higher levels of irisin in the absence of sarcopenia may be a potential biomarker for liver disease severity, both among regular phenotypes and for non-obese, non-diabetic patients.

Supplementary Materials: The following are available online at https://www.mdpi.com/article/10.3390/jcm11030635/s1. Supplementary Figure S1: Flow chart of the study. Supplementary Table S1: Correlations between irisin, PRO-C3 and PRO-C6 with the histological features of NASH.

Author Contributions: Conceptualization, A.A.; methodology, A.A., C.R.; software, C.R., G.P.C.; data collection, A.N., M.V., D.D.; formal analysis, C.R.; investigation, A.A., C.R., G.P.C.; resources, C.R., M.L.A., A.O., D.J.L.; data curation, A.A., C.R., M.V.; writing—original draft preparation, A.A., C.R.; writing—review and editing, A.G., E.B.; visualization, M.G., D.G.R., G.M.S., A.G., D.J.L.; supervision, E.B.; funding acquisition, E.B. All authors have read and agreed to the published version of the manuscript.

Funding: This research has been supported by the Italian Ministry for Education, University and Research (Ministero dell'Istruzione, dell'Università e della Ricerca—MIUR) under the programme "Dipartimenti di Eccellenza 2018–2022", project code D15D18000410001 and by the Elucidating Pathways of Steatohepatitis (EPoS) project. The EPoS project was funded by Horizon 2020-EU.3.1.1 under grant agreement n. 634413.

Institutional Review Board Statement: The study was conducted according to the guidelines of the Declaration of Helsinki, and approved by the Institutional Ethics Committee of the University Hospital "Città della Salute e della Scienza" of Torino (CEI/522, 23 December 2009).

Informed Consent Statement: Informed consent was obtained from all subjects involved in the study.

Conflicts of Interest: The authors declare no conflict of interest.

References

1. Hagström, H.; Nasr, P.; Ekstedt, M.; Hammar, U.; Stål, P.; Hultcrantz, R.; Kechagias, S. Fibrosis stage but not NASH predicts mortality and time to development of severe liver disease in biopsy-proven NAFLD. *J. Hepatol.* **2017**, *67*, 1265–1273. [CrossRef]
2. Armandi, A.; Rosso, C.; Caviglia, G.P.; Bugianesi, E. Insulin Resistance across the Spectrum of Nonalcoholic Fatty Liver Disease. *Metabolites* **2021**, *11*, 155. [CrossRef] [PubMed]
3. Boström, P.; Wu, J.; Jedrychowski, M.P.; Korde, A.; Ye, L.; Lo, J.C.; Rasbach, K.A.; Boström, E.A.; Choi, J.H.; Long, J.Z.; et al. A PGC1-α-dependent myokine that drives brown-fat-like development of white fat and thermogenesis. *Nature* **2012**, *11*, 463–468. [CrossRef] [PubMed]
4. Huh, J.Y.; Dincer, F.; Mesfum, E.; Mantzoros, C.S. Irisin stimulates muscle growth-related genes and regulates adipocyte differentiation and metabolism in humans. *Int. J. Obes.* **2014**, *38*, 1538–1544. [CrossRef] [PubMed]
5. Yang, M.; Chen, P.; Jin, H.; Xie, X.; Gao, T.; Yang, L.; Yu, X. Circulating levels of irisin in middle-aged first-degree relatives of type 2 diabetes mellitus—Correlation with pancreatic β-cell function. *Diabetol. Metab. Syndr.* **2014**, *5*, 133. [CrossRef] [PubMed]
6. Liu, T.; Shi, C.; Gao, R.; Sun, H.; Xiong, X.; Ding, L.; Chen, Q.; Li, Y.H.; Wang, J.J.; Kang, Y.M.; et al. Irisin inhibits hepatic gluconeogenesis and increases glycogen synthesis via the PI3K/Akt pathway in type 2 diabetic mice and hepatocytes. *Clin. Sci.* **2015**, *129*, 839–850. [CrossRef] [PubMed]
7. Tang, H.; Yu, R.; Liu, S.; Huwatibieke, B.; Li, Z.; Zhang, W. Irisin Inhibits Hepatic Cholesterol Synthesis via AMPK-SREBP2 Signaling. *EBioMedicine* **2016**, *6*, 139–148. [CrossRef]
8. Batirel, S.; Bozaykut, P.; Altundag, E.M.; Ozer, N.K.; Mantzoros, C.S. The effect of Irisin on antioxidant system in liver. *Free Radic. Biol. Med.* **2014**, *75*, S16. [CrossRef]
9. Zhang, H.-J.; Zhang, X.-F.; Ma, Z.-M.; Pan, L.-L.; Chen, Z.; Han, H.-W.; Han, C.-K.; Zhuang, X.-J.; Lu, Y.; Li, X.-J.; et al. Irisin is inversely associated with intrahepatic triglyceride contents in obese adults. *J. Hepatol.* **2013**, *59*, 557–562. [CrossRef]
10. Metwally, M.; Bayoumi, A.; Romero-Gomez, M.; Thabet, K.; John, M.; Adams, L.A.; Huo, X.; Aller, R.; García-Monzón, C.; Arias-Loste, M.T.; et al. A polymorphism in the Irisin-encoding gene (FNDC5) associates with hepatic steatosis by differential miRNA binding to the 3′UTR. *J. Hepatol.* **2019**, *70*, 494–500. [CrossRef]
11. Petta, S.; Valenti, L.; Svegliati-Baroni, G.; Ruscica, M.; Pipitone, M.R.; Dongiovanni, P.; Rychlicki, C.; Ferri, N.; Cammà, C.; Fracanzani, A.L.; et al. Fibronectin Type III Domain-Containing Protein 5 rs3480 A > G Polymorphism, Irisin, and Liver Fibrosis in Patients with Nonalcoholic Fatty Liver Disease. *J. Clin. Endocrinol. Metab.* **2017**, *102*, 2660–2669. [CrossRef] [PubMed]
12. Hu, J.; Ke, Y.; Wu, F.; Liu, S.; Ji, C.; Zhu, X.; Zhang, Y. Circulating Irisin Levels in Patients with Nonalcoholic Fatty Liver Disease: A Systematic Review and Meta-Analysis. *Gastroenterol. Res. Pract.* **2020**, *2020*, 8818191. [CrossRef] [PubMed]
13. Matthews, D.R.; Hosker, J.P.; Rudenski, A.S.; Naylor, B.A.; Treacher, D.F.; Turner, R.C. Homeostasis model assessment: Insulin resistance and β-cell function from fasting plasma glucose and insulin concentrations in man. *Diabetologia* **1985**, *28*, 412–419. [CrossRef] [PubMed]
14. Bril, F.; Leeming, D.J.; Karsdal, M.A.; Kalavalapalli, S.; Barb, D.; Lai, J.; Rabe, M.; Cusi, K. Use of Plasma Fragments of Propeptides of Type III, V, and VI Procollagen for the Detection of Liver Fibrosis in Type 2 Diabetes. *Diabetes Care* **2019**, *42*, 1348–1351. [CrossRef]
15. Caussy, C.; Bhargava, M.; Villesen, I.F.; Gudmann, N.S.; Leeming, D.J.; Karsdal, M.A.; Faulkner, C.; Bao, D.; Liu, A.; Lo, M.; et al. Collagen Formation Assessed by N-Terminal Propeptide of Type 3 Procollagen Is a Heritable Trait and Is Associated with Liver Fibrosis Assessed by Magnetic Resonance Elastography. *Hepatology* **2019**, *70*, 127–141. [CrossRef]
16. Kleiner, D.E.; Brunt, E.M.; Van Natta, M.; Behling, C.; Contos, M.J.; Cummings, O.W.; Ferrell, L.D.; Liu, Y.-C.; Torbenson, M.S.; Unalp-Arida, A.; et al. Design and validation of a histological scoring system for nonalcoholic fatty liver disease. *Hepatology* **2005**, *41*, 1313–1321. [CrossRef]
17. Kurdiova, T.; Balaz, M.; Vician, M.; Maderova, D.; Vlcek, M.; Valkovič, L.; Srbecky, M.; Imrich, R.; Kyselovicova, O.; Belan, V.; et al. Effects of obesity, diabetes and exercise on *Fndc5* gene expression and irisin release in human skeletal muscle and adipose tissue: In vivo and in vitro studies. *J. Physiol.* **2014**, *592*, 1091–1107. [CrossRef]
18. Mo, L.; Shen, J.; Liu, Q.; Zhang, Y.; Kuang, J.; Pu, S.; Cheng, S.; Zou, M.; Jiang, W.; Jiang, C.; et al. Irisin Is Regulated by CAR in Liver and Is a Mediator of Hepatic Glucose and Lipid Metabolism. *Mol. Endocrinol.* **2016**, *30*, 533–542. [CrossRef]

19. Kukla, M.; Skladany, L.; Menżyk, T.; Derra, A.; Stygar, D.; Skonieczna, M.; Hudy, D.; Nabrdalik, K.; Gumprecht, J.; Marlicz, W.; et al. Irisin in Liver Cirrhosis. *J. Clin. Med.* **2020**, *9*, 3158. [CrossRef]
20. Zhao, M.; Zhou, X.; Yuan, C.; Li, R.; Ma, Y.; Tang, X. Association between serum irisin concentrations and sarcopenia in patients with liver cirrhosis: A cross-sectional study. *Sci. Rep.* **2020**, *10*, 16093. [CrossRef]
21. Moreno-Navarrete, J.M.; Ortega, F.; Serrano, M.; Guerra, E.; Pardo, G.; Tinahones, F. Irisin is expressed and produced by human muscle and adipose tissue in association with obesity and insulin resistance. *J. Clin. Endocrinol. Metab.* **2013**, *98*, E769–E778. [CrossRef] [PubMed]
22. Qiu, S.; Cai, X.; Yin, H.; Zügel, M.; Sun, Z.; Steinacker, J.M.; Schumann, U. Association between circulating irisin and insulin resistance in non-diabetic adults: A meta-analysis. *Metabolism* **2016**, *65*, 825–834. [CrossRef] [PubMed]
23. Moreno, M.; Moreno-Navarrete, J.M.; Serrano, M.; Ortega, F.; Delgado, E.; Sanchez-Ragnarsson, C.; Valdés, S.; Botas, P.; Ricart, W.; Fernández-Real, J.M. Circulating irisin levels are positively associated with metabolic risk factors in sedentary subjects. *PLoS ONE* **2015**, *10*, e0124100. [CrossRef] [PubMed]
24. Aronis, K.N.; Moreno, M.; Polyzos, S.A.; Moreno-Navarrete, J.M.; Ricart, W.; Delgado, E.; de La Hera, J.; Sahin-Efe, A.; Chamberland, J.P.; Berman, R.; et al. Circulating irisin levels and coronary heart disease: Association with future acute coronary syndrome and major adverse cardiovascular events. *Int. J. Obes.* **2015**, *39*, 156–161. [CrossRef]
25. Chang, J.S.; Kim, T.H.; Nguyen, T.T.; Park, K.-S.; Kim, N.; Kong, I.D. Circulating irisin levels as a predictive biomarker for sarcopenia: A cross-sectional community-based study. *Geriatr. Gerontol. Int.* **2017**, *17*, 2266–2273. [CrossRef]
26. Choi, H.Y.; Kim, S.; Park, J.W.; Lee, N.S.; Hwang, S.Y.; Huh, J.Y.; Hong, H.C.; Yoo, H.J.; Baik, S.H.; Youn, B.S.; et al. Implication of Circulating Irisin Levels with Brown Adipose Tissue and Sarcopenia in Humans. *J. Clin. Endocrinol. Metab.* **2014**, *99*, 2778–2785. [CrossRef]

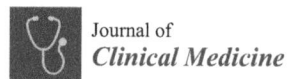 Journal of
Clinical Medicine

Review

Celiac Disease in Juvenile Idiopathic Arthritis and Other Pediatric Rheumatic Disorders

Dimitri Poddighe [1,2,*], Micol Romano [3], Kuanysh Dossybayeva [1], Diyora Abdukhakimova [1], Dinara Galiyeva [1] and Erkan Demirkaya [3,4]

1. Department of Medicine, Nazarbayev University School of Medicine (NUSOM), Nur-Sultan 010000, Kazakhstan; kuanysh.dossybayeva@nu.edu.kz (K.D.); dabdukhakimova@nu.edu.kz (D.A.); d.galiyeva@nu.edu.kz (D.G.)
2. Clinical Academic Department of Pediatrics, National Research Center for Maternal and Child Health (NRCMCH), University Medical Center (UMC), Nur-Sultan 010000, Kazakhstan
3. Division of Pediatric Rheumatology, Schulich School of Medicine & Dentistry, University of Western Ontario, London, ON N6A 5W9, Canada; micol.romano@lhsc.on.ca (M.R.); erkan.demirkaya@lhsc.on.ca (E.D.)
4. Department of Epidemiology and Biostatistics, Schulich School of Medicine & Dentistry, University of Western Ontario, London, ON N6A 5W9, Canada
* Correspondence: dimitri.poddighe@nu.edu.kz or d.poddighe@umc.kz.org; Tel.: +7-7172-6946-37

Abstract: Celiac Disease (CD) is an immune-mediated and gluten-related disorder whose prevalence is higher in children affected with other autoimmune disorders, including diabetes mellitus type 1, autoimmune thyroiditis, and others. As regards Juvenile Idiopathic Arthritis (JIA) and other pediatric rheumatic disorders, there is no clear recommendation for CD serological screening. In this review, we analyze all the available clinical studies investigating CD among children with JIA (and other rheumatic diseases), in order to provide objective data to better understand the necessity of CD serological screening during the follow-up. Based on the present literature review and analysis, >2.5% patients with JIA were diagnosed with CD; however, the CD prevalence in JIA patients may be even higher (>3–3.5%) due to several study limitations that could have underestimated CD diagnosis to a variable extent. Therefore, serological screening for CD in children affected with JIA could be recommended due to the increased CD prevalence in these patients (compared to the general pediatric population), and because these JIA patients diagnosed with CD were mostly asymptomatic. However, further research is needed to establish a cost-effective approach in terms of CD screening frequency and modalities during the follow-up for JIA patients. Conversely, at the moment, there is no evidence supporting a periodical CD screening in children affected with other rheumatic diseases (including pediatric systemic lupus erythematosus, juvenile dermatomyositis, and systemic sclerosis).

Keywords: celiac disease; juvenile idiopathic arthritis; pediatric systemic lupus erythematosus; juvenile dermatomyositis; systemic scleroderma; screening; prevalence

Citation: Poddighe, D.; Romano, M.; Dossybayeva, K.; Abdukhakimova, D.; Galiyeva, D.; Demirkaya, E. Celiac Disease in Juvenile Idiopathic Arthritis and Other Pediatric Rheumatic Disorders. *J. Clin. Med.* **2022**, *11*, 1089. https://doi.org/10.3390/jcm11041089

Academic Editors: Gian Paolo Caviglia, Davide Giuseppe Ribaldone and Matteo Neri

Received: 21 January 2022
Accepted: 16 February 2022
Published: 18 February 2022

Publisher's Note: MDPI stays neutral with regard to jurisdictional claims in published maps and institutional affiliations.

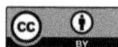

Copyright: © 2022 by the authors. Licensee MDPI, Basel, Switzerland. This article is an open access article distributed under the terms and conditions of the Creative Commons Attribution (CC BY) license (https:// creativecommons.org/licenses/by/ 4.0/).

1. Introduction

Celiac Disease (CD) is an immune-mediated and gluten-related disorder occurring in around 3% of patients who are carriers of specific HLA-DQ alleles (DQA1*0501-DQB1*02 and/or DQA1*0301-DQB1*0302) [1,2]. The hallmark of CD is the development of consistent histopathological alterations of the small bowel mucosa, including increased intraepithelial lymphocytes (IELs), crypts hyperplasia, and shortened/atrophic intestinal villi, as reflected by the Marsh–Oberhuber classification [3]. However, CD is not only a gastrointestinal disorder but also a systemic disease: indeed, the gastrointestinal manifestations are only one component of the clinical picture in these patients (including children), who often display extra-gastrointestinal involvement, including musculoskeletal complaints [4–6]. Conversely, there are several reports describing patients affected with rheumatic disorders who resulted to be concomitantly affected with CD and, thus, are claimed to deserve periodical screening for it by some authors [7].

Several autoimmune disorders were included in the European Society for Pediatric Gastroenterology, Hepatology, and Nutrition (ESPGHAN) guidelines for the Diagnosis of Coeliac Disease (published in 2012), as "conditions associated with CD". Notably, Juvenile Idiopathic Arthritis (JIA) was listed among those in this position paper, where 1.5–2.5% CD prevalence was reported among these patients; however, this information was supported by only two studies dated back to 1996 and 1997, respectively [8–10]. Unlike other autoimmune disorders (such as type 1 diabetes mellitus, autoimmune thyroiditis, and autoimmune liver disease), no recommendation was given about CD screening in JIA patients in this position paper; moreover, JIA is not cited at all in the recently updated ESPGHAN guidelines for CD screening and management [8–11]. However, the growing availability of serological tests for CD promoted and increased its screening in a larger number of children, including those with rheumatic disorders, even though no clear recommendations or guidelines have been published in this regard. This gap of knowledge can cause both CD under-diagnosis (with potentially negative long-term consequences for rheumatic children in whom CD is overlooked) and/or inappropriate use of CD serological tests (with consequent waste of resources and/or diagnostic concerns).

In this review, we analyzed all the available clinical studies investigating CD among children with JIA, in order to provide objective data to better understand the necessity of CD serological screening during the follow-up of this rheumatic disorder. Moreover, in order to make our analysis more complete, we also assessed whether there is any evidence regarding the potential association between CD and other rheumatic diseases in children.

2. Juvenile Idiopathic Arthritis and Celiac Disease

Juvenile idiopathic arthritis (JIA) is the most common chronic rheumatic disorder in children. It is diagnosed in patients aged up to 16 years with chronic arthritis (lasting 6 weeks or more), which is not associated to any specific and recognizable etiology (e.g., infectious, neoplastic, metabolic). According to the International League of Associations for Rheumatology (ILAR), five main subtypes can be defined inside the JIA classification: systemic (sJIA); oligoarticular (oJIA), which may be persistent or extended; polyarticular (pJIA), which is usually rheumatoid factor (RF) negative and, much less frequently, positive; psoriatic (PsJIA); and enthesitis-related (ERA). Additionally, JIA may be categorized as undifferentiated, if arthritis does not fulfill the diagnostic criteria for any of the aforementioned subtypes [12]. Like CD, HLA system plays a role in JIA etiopathogenesis; however, the HLA genetic predisposition to JIA is mainly due to other HLA class II molecules (HLA-DRB1, HLA-DPB1), which are differentially involved according to the JIA subtype [13,14].

In order to investigate the epidemiological burden of CD in JIA patients, the literature search was performed using PubMed with the keywords (["children"] AND "Celiac Disease" AND "arthritis" OR "Juvenile Idiopathic Arthritis") restricted between 2000 and 2021 (31 December). Only the clinical studies describing cohorts (not case reports or series) of JIA patients screened for CD were included for data extraction, as summarized in Table 1 [15–28].

The study by Stagi et al. reported a relatively high prevalence (6.7%) of CD in their cohort of JIA patients [15]. A comparable result emerged from the research by Skrabl-Baumgartne et al., who found a 4.2% prevalence of CD in their JIA patients [20]. Notably, both studies included a control group, where no CD cases were identified: moreover, these were among the largest studies (JIA: $n = 151$ and $n = 95$, respectively; controls: $n = 158$ and $n = 100$, respectively) of the present selection [15,22]. Actually, in terms of JIA cohort, the second largest research was the prospective study published by Alpegiani et al. ($n = 108$), who reported a CD prevalence of 2.8%; however, no control group was available in this research [16]. A third study (by Stoll et al.) included a control group, but patients' number (JIA: $n = 32$; controls: $n = 10$) was among the smallest ones; here, no CD diagnoses were made in either group [18].

Table 1. Clinical studies assessing CD in children affected with JIA.

Author-1st-(Year) [Country]	Study Design	CD Tests	JIA Pts.	JIA M/F & Age *	JIA Duration	CD Pts.	CD Symptoms	Comments
Stagi [15] (2005) [Italy]	CROSS	AGA EmA tTG	151	21/120 8.3 (2.4–16.9)	n/a	10 (6.7%)	n/a	CD: M/F = 1/9; oJIA: n = 5, pJIA: n = 5; Marsh: n/a.
Alpigiani [16] (2008) [Italy]	PRO	EmA tTG	108	37/71 5.7 (1–15)	-	3 (2.8%)	No (n = 2) Yes (n = 1)^	Annual serological screening Study follow-up: 5.3 yrs. (0.15–12.3) No further information on CD pts.
Koehne [17] (2012) [Brazil]	CROSS	AGA (IgA/IgG) EmA [tTG (IgA)]	32	n/a	n/a	0	-	Only EmA+ patients underwent tTG IgA test.
Stoll [18] (2012) [USA]	CROSS	tTG IgA	42 (n = 11) [E]	11/30 8.8 (4.6–21) [E] 2.8 (1.5–5.9) [NE]	2.1 ± 2.2 [E] 2.2 ± 2.7 [NE]	0	-	-
Robazzi [19] (2013) [Brazil]	CROSS	tTG	53	28/25 10.4 (2.3–17.9)	3.4 ± 3.1	1 (1.9%)	No	CD: M; 10 yrs; sJIA; Marsh: 3c.
Moghtaderi [20] (2016) [Iran]	CROSS	tTG IgA	53	27/26 10.6 (1.5–16)	3.5 ± 3.0	0	-	One patient was anti-tTG IgA+, but endoscopy was normal
Nisihara [21] (2017) [Brazil]	CROSS	EmA tTG IgG	45	16/29 12 (3–16)	0.5–10	0	-	Four patients were serologically positive (EmA, n = 2; tTG IgG, n = 2), but all declined endoscopy.
Skrabl-Baumgartner [22] (2017) [Austria]	CROSS	tTG IgA	95	29/66 12.3 (2.3–17.9)	n/a	4 (4.2%)	No (n = 3) Yes (n = 1)^	Only tTG IgA+ pts. were tested for EmA (all+) CD: M/F = 2/2; oJIA: n = 2, pJIA: n = 1, PsJIA: n = 1; Marsh 3c: n = 2, 3b: n = 1, 2b: n = 1.
Tronconi [23] (2017) [Italy]	RETRO	tTG IgA	79	28/51 10.7 (2.8–21)	-	3 (2.4%)	n/a	annual serological screening CD: M/F = 0:3; oJIA, n = 2; PsJIA, n = 1.
Sahin [24] (2019) [Turkey]	CROSS	tTG IgA	96	40/56 11.6 (n/a)	n/a	0	-	-
Oman [25] (2019) [Sweden]	CROSS	tTG IgA/IgG	216	81/135 8.4 (3.1–13.3)	n/a	6 (2.8%)	No (n = 3) Yes (n = 3)^	CD: oJIA: n = 4, PsJIA: n = 1; ERA, n = 1; M/F = 0/6; Marsh III: n = 6.
AlEnzi [25] (2020) [Saudi Arabia]	CROSS	AGA IgA/IgG EmA tTG	73	28/45 10.0 ± 2.6	n/a	1 (1.4%)	n/a	8 pts. had one or more positive CD markers. All underwent endoscopy, but all resulted Marsh neg.
Pagnini [27] (2021) [Italy]	RETRO	tTG/Ema/AGA	53 (ERA)	33/20 10.9 (3–16)	-	1 (1.8%)	n/a	Unclear if all patients received serological screening
Sadeghi [28] (2021) [Iran]	CROSS	tTG IgA	78	[1:2] 7.9 (1.6–16)	2.8 ± 2.8	1 (1.3%)	No	3 pts. resulted tTG IgA+, but only one accepted endoscopy CD: M; oJIA.

* Age is expressed as mean age (age range), except in two articles (Oman et al.: inter-quartile range between brackets; AlEnzi study: mean and standard deviation). ^ Patients already diagnosed with CD before JIA onset; [E] JIA patients diagnosed as ERA in the study by Stoll ([NE] JIA patients diagnosed as non-ERA). Abbreviations: M, male; F, female; pts, patients; AGA, anti-gliadin antibody; EmA, anti-endomysium antibody; tTG, anti-tissue transglutaminase antibody; SpA, Spondylo-arthritis; n/a: information not available; PsJIA: psoriatic arthritis; oJIA: oligoarticular arthritis; pJIA: polyarticular arthritis; sJIA: systemic arthritis; ERA: entesitis-related arthritis; CROSS, cross-sectional study; RETRO, retrospective study; PRO, prospective study.

Among the remaining studies included in our selection, no one included a control group, and CD cases were identified in six studies, showing a CD prevalence ranging between 1.3% and 2.8% [19,23,25–27]. All the other studies did not identify any CD patient; however, these were basically the least numerous studies [17,18,20,21], except the one published by Sahin et al. (n = 96) [24]. Notably, these studies adopted an incomplete CD screening strategy: indeed, Khoene et al. and Nisihara et al., respectively, performed the serological screening by using anti-gliadin antibody(AGA)/anti-endomysia antibody (EmA) and EmA/anti-tissue transglutaminase IgG (tTG IgG), which are not the most sensitive serological markers for CD [17,21]. Currently, anti-tissue transglutaminase IgA (tTG IgA) is considered the most accurate serological marker (in terms of both sensitivity and specificity) for CD in children [11,29,30]. Sahin et al., Stoll et al., and Moghdateri et al. actually used tTG IgA to screen their JIA patients [18,20,24]; however, some patients may be positive for EmA only (and tTG-IgA negative, at least in the initial stage of disease) [5,31,32] and, therefore, a cross-sectional study where EmA or tTG IgA are not used together may have lost these CD patients, even if they are very few.

Considering the sum of all articles included our literature research, there were 1174 JIA patients, and 30 of them were concomitantly diagnosed with CD, suggesting a CD prevalence as high as 2.6% in JIA patients. This prevalence may be an estimation by defect: in addition to the aforementioned concerns about the serological screening in several studies, some tTG IgA and/or EmA serologically positive patients did not undergo or declined the upper gastrointestinal endoscopy (overall, around 10 serologically positive patients declined this procedure in these studies, whereas this information is not available in at least four studies). Finally, it is worth reporting that the total IgA measurement is clearly confirmed in only half of the studies (7 out of 14), whereas in the remaining ones, such an important aspect is not specified. Indeed, as emphasized by several authors and guidelines, the concomitant measurement of total serum IgA is an essential step for a complete CD serological screening, since IgA deficiency impairs the reliability of the most sensitive markers, namely EmA and tTG IgA [11,33,34]. In this regard, JIA patients could also be characterized by an increased prevalence of IgA deficiency, as it occurs in several autoimmune disorders [33,35]. Unfortunately, recent data investigating IgA levels in JIA are missing, but a dated report by Pelkonen et al. reported >7% frequency of persistent or transient IgA deficiency in their study population (including 350 patients with JIA) [36]. If this finding could be confirmed, that may represent an additional reason for under-estimating CD prevalence in JIA.

In summary, based on the present literature review and analysis, >2.5% patients with JIA were diagnosed with CD; however, considering the suboptimal strategy for CD serological screening and the incomplete diagnostic work-up (without upper GI endoscopy and, thus, duodenal biopsy), as discussed above, the CD prevalence in JIA patients may be even higher (>3–3.5%). Anyway, even the actual CD prevalence of 2.6% emerging from our analysis in JIA patients is higher than CD prevalence in the general pediatric population, which is estimated to be around 1% [37]. Therefore, JIA patients seem to be at greater risk of developing CD during the pediatric age. Even though this increased risk is not as high as in other conditions reported in the aforementioned ESPGHAN CD guidelines (such as type 1 diabetes mellitus, autoimmune thyroiditis, and autoimmune liver disorders) [8], JIA patients could be eligible for periodic CD screening, although the frequency of these serological tests may be debated. Methodologically standardized and controlled prospective studies with larger sample sizes are needed to confirm this number and assess the most cost-effective approach to monitor JIA patients as regards the potential occurrence of CD.

Notably, in the present analysis, all JIA patients concomitantly diagnosed with CD were reported to be asymptomatic for the latter condition (see Table 1), which would further support the indication to screen JIA patients for CD during their rheumatological follow-up. Although this clinical practice has been already implemented in some rheumatological centers, this approach is neither systematic nor standardized since it is not supported by clear evidence. Indeed, as mentioned above, additional research may lead to specific algorithms to screen JIA patients for CD, which could also consider some demographic, clinical, and laboratory parameters to implement a cost-effective approach for this purpose.

As regards the JIA subtypes, among those 30 ascertained CD diagnoses in JIA patients, the JIA subtype is declared for 25 of them (oJIA: $n = 14$, pJIA: $n = 6$; PsJIA: $n = 3$; ERA: $n = 1$; sJIA: $n = 1$). Accordingly, oJIA represents >55% of CD/JIA patients, whereas this subtype is considered to account for around 40% of JIA patients, regardless of the ethnicity; conversely, sJIA is diagnosed in around 13% of JIA patients [38], whereas only 1 JIA patient (4%) was diagnosed with CD. Again, >75% (19 out of these 25) JIA patients diagnosed with CD were female, which corresponds to a female-to-male ratio greater than 3:1, which is higher than the gender ratios previously reported for JIA patients in both European (7:3) and non-European (3:2) populations [38]. Finally, information about additional autoimmune disorders (e.g., thyroiditis) and/or family history and/or some laboratory parameters commonly assessed during JIA follow-up (e.g., liver enzymes, specific autoantibodies, others) might further affect the CD risk in this clinical setting; unfortunately, no data are provided by the aforementioned studies in this regard.

3. Pediatric Systemic Lupus Erythematosus and Celiac Disease

Systemic lupus erythematosus (SLE) is an autoimmune disease with very variable expression, since all the organs and systems can be affected [39]. Pediatric SLE (pSLE) is diagnosed in patients younger than 18 years and represents 10–20% of all SLE cases [40]. The immunopathogenesis of SLE is extremely complex and involves both adaptive and innate immune mechanisms [41,42], but a large and heterogeneous production of autoantibodies can be considered a main feature, which is also consistent with its very variable clinical expression and organ/systemic involvement [43–45]. Among those, anti-dsDNA antibody is a hallmark of SLE, since it is a very specific and sensitive marker and even correlates with the disease activity [46,47].

Several case reports suggested a possible association between CD and SLE in adults [48–50]. An Israelian study based on a large medical database compared 5,018 patients with SLE and 25,090 age- and sex-matched controls and reported an association between SLE and CD with a multivariate OR of 3.92 [51]. Conversely, other studies found no association between SLE and CD [52,53] Very recently, a study by Soltani et al., including both adults and children (without any specific age-related analysis), reported a prevalence of 3% for biopsy-proven CD in patients with SLE and, thus, revamped this issue [54].

In this review, we focused on the pediatric population and, thus, pSLE. Based upon literature research in PubMed database ("children" AND "Celiac Disease" OR "[Juvenile] systemic lupus erythematosus") starting from 2000 until 2021 (31 December), we could retrieve only a few clinical studies (excluding case reports) assessing the presence of CD in pSLE patients, as summarized in Table 2 [26,55,56].

Unfortunately, these three pediatric studies included small cohorts of patients, and the screening approach was quite variable. Overall, none showed a potential increase in CD prevalence in pSLE patients [26,55,56].

However, a recent study by Shamseya et al., assessed CD serology in a group of 100 SLE adult patients (34.6 ± 9.6 years) who were actually diagnosed during the pediatric age (pSLE at their onset). These (p)SLE patients were compared with a sex- and age-matched control group ($n = 40$). All the study participants were tested for tTG IgA (or tTG IgG, if IgA deficiency was detected); moreover, if anyone was tTG-positive, this patient was tested for EmA IgA too. Briefly, 10 (p)SLE patients (10%) were both tTG and EmA IgA positive and all controls tested negative: such a difference was statistically significant. Upper gastrointestinal endoscopy was performed in all these 10 (p)SLE patients: the histopathological assessment confirmed CD in 6 patients, where 4 cases were labelled as latent CD at that moment [57]. Therefore, even though pSLE does not seem to be associated with CD during the pediatric age, these patients may be at increased risk later in their life.

Table 2. Clinical studies assessing CD in children affected with pSLE.

Author-1st-(Year) [Country]	Study Design	CD Tests	SLE Pts.	SLE M/F & Age *	SLE Duration	CD Pts.	CD Symptoms	Comments
Aikawa [55] (2012) [Brazil]	CROSS	EmA	79	33/67 10.3 ± 3.4	4.4 ± 3.7	1	No	Out of 79 pSLE pts. in follow-up, only 41 pts. accepted to participate in this study. CD: F; 12.6 yrs; Marsh: n/a.
Sahin [56] (2019) [Turkey]	CROSS	tTG IgA [EmA]	50	6/44 15.5 ± 3.4	n/a	0	n/a	Only tTG IgA+ patients were tested for EmA. 3 pts. resulted tTG IgA positive but were EmA- and did not undergo endoscopy.
AlEnzi [26] (2020) [Saudi Arabia]	CROSS	AGA (IgA + G) EmA tTG	34	6/28 10.3 ± 2.7	n/a	0	n/a	6 pts. had one or more positive CD markers. All underwent endoscopy, but all resulted Marsh negative.

* Age is expressed as mean and standard deviation. Abbreviations: M, male; F, female; pts., patients; AGA, anti-gliadin antibody; EmA, anti-endomysium antibody; tTG, anti-tissue transglutaminase antibody; CROSS, cross-sectional study.

4. Celiac Disease in Other Pediatric Rheumatic Disorders

In the aforementioned study by Aikawa et al., 41 patients with juvenile dermatomyositis (JDM) were included, in addition to those children affected with pSLE. Among them, only one JDM patient was diagnosed as CD [55]. The absence of additional clinical studies assessing CD in JDM patients precludes any conclusion in children. However, O'Callaghan et al. described 51 adult dermatomyositis patients who were tested by AGA IgA, EmA, and tTG IgA: 5 patients were positive for AGA, and 3 of them received histopathological confirmation for CD [58]. Similarly, Orbach et al. showed mildly but significantly higher levels of AGA IgA and anti-tTG IgA levels patients affected with idiopathic inflammatory myopathies (IIMs) compared with matched adult controls, but no histopathological data on duodenal biopsy were provided by these authors [59]. Therefore, further research may be advisable in patients affected with IIMs, including JDM, in order to assess the risk for CD.

In addition to JIA patients, the aforementioned study by Robazzi et al., also investigated 66 children affected with rheumatic fever. One patient was diagnosed with CD [19]. No studies are available in the adult population. Anyway, no plausible biological or medical link between rheumatic fever and CD can be highlighted.

Soylu et al. published a study on CD in children developing Henoch–Schoenlein purpura (IgA vasculitis): among 42 study participants tested by EmA, tTG IgA and anti-deamidated gliadin peptide (DGP) IgA/IgG, seropositivity was detected in 5 children, of whom 2 received histological confirmation for CD (one patient declined the duodenal biopsy) [60]. Further research may be appropriate in this specific clinical setting.

No studies assessed CD in children affected with systemic scleroderma (sSC). However, Nisihara et al. tested 60 adult patients affected with sSC for EmA and AGA IgA/IgG: all samples turned out negative [61]. Similarly, Forbess et al. screened 72 adult SSc patients by testing tTG IgA/IgG and DGP IgA/IgG: three patients tested positive for any markers, but no one was confirmed as being affected with CD [62]. Notably, these studies are in contrast with two previous reports by Luft et al. and Rosato et al., who estimated a CD prevalence of 7% and 8% in their respective cohorts of sSC patients; actually, the first study was not supported by any confirmatory duodenal biopsy [63,64]. Anyway, at the moment, there is no evidence to support any systematic CD screening in children affected with sSC.

5. Conclusions

The present literature analysis seems to support the indication of serological screening for CD in children affected with JIA, since the CD prevalence in JIA patients could be around threefold greater than in the pediatric general population, and all those patients diagnosed with CD after JIA onset were mostly asymptomatic. However, evidence-based policies and clear recommendations for CD screening are currently lacking in JIA patients; further research is needed to establish a cost-effective approach in terms of CD screening frequency and strategy over the follow-up for JIA patients. As regards other pediatric rheumatic disorders (including pSLE), at the moment, there is no evidence supporting a periodical CD screening.

Author Contributions: D.P. conceived and wrote the manuscript; K.D., D.A. and D.G. contributed to the literature research; M.R. and E.D. provided expert and intellectual contributions. All authors have read and agreed to the published version of the manuscript.

Funding: This review was supported by the Nazarbayev University Faculty Development Competitive Research Grant 2020-2022 (No. 240919FD3912), and the Nazarbayev University Social Policy Grant.

Institutional Review Board Statement: Not applicable.

Informed Consent Statement: Not applicable.

Data Availability Statement: Not applicable.

Conflicts of Interest: The authors declare no conflict of interest.

References

1. Lindfors, K.; Ciacci, C.; Kurppa, K.; Lundin, K.E.A.; Makharia, G.K.; Mearin, M.L.; Murray, J.A.; Verdu, E.F.; Kaukinen, K. Coeliac disease. *Nat. Rev. Dis. Primers* **2019**, *5*, 3. [CrossRef] [PubMed]
2. Poddighe, D.; Rebuffi, C.; De Silvestri, A.; Capittini, C. Carrier frequency of HLA-DQB1*02 allele in patients affected with celiac disease: A systematic review assessing the potential rationale of a targeted allelic genotyping as a first-line screening. *World J. Gastroenterol.* **2020**, *26*, 1365–1381. [CrossRef] [PubMed]
3. Oberhuber, G.; Granditsch, G.; Vogelsang, H. The histopathology of coeliac disease: Time for a standardized report scheme for pathologists. *Eur. J. Gastroenterol. Hepatol.* **1999**, *11*, 1185–1194. [CrossRef]
4. Therrien, A.; Kelly, C.P.; Silvester, J.A. Celiac Disease: Extraintestinal Manifestations and Associated Conditions. *J. Clin. Gastroenterol.* **2020**, *54*, 8–21. [CrossRef]
5. Poddighe, D.; Capittini, C.; Gaviglio, I.; Brambilla, I.; Marseglia, G.L. HLA-DQB1*02 allele in children with celiac disease: Potential usefulness for screening strategies. *Int. J. Immunogenet.* **2019**, *46*, 342–345. [CrossRef]
6. Zylberberg, H.M.; Lebwohl, B.; Green, P.H.R. Celiac Disease-Musculoskeletal Manifestations and Mechanisms in Children to Adults. *Curr. Osteoporos. Rep.* **2018**, *16*, 754–762. [CrossRef]
7. Sherman, Y.; Karanicolas, R.; DiMarco, B.; Pan, N.; Adams, A.B.; Barinstein, L.V.; Moorthy, L.N.; Lehman, T.J. Unrecognized Celiac Disease in Children Presenting for Rheumatology Evaluation. *Pediatrics* **2015**, *136*, e68–e75. [CrossRef]
8. Husby, S.; Koletzko, S.; Korponay-Szabó, I.R.; Mearin, M.L.; Phillips, A.; Shamir, R.; Troncone, R.; Giersiepen, K.; Branski, D.; Catassi, C.; et al. European Society for Pediatric Gastroenterology, Hepatology, and Nutrition guidelines for the diagnosis of coeliac disease. *J. Pediatr. Gastroenterol. Nutr.* **2012**, *54*, 136–160. [CrossRef]
9. George, D.K.; Evans, R.M.; Gunn, I.R. Familial chronic fatigue. *Postgrad. Med. J.* **1997**, *73*, 311–313. [CrossRef]
10. Lepore, L.; Martelossi, S.; Pennesi, M.; Falcini, F.; Ermini, M.L.; Ferrari, R.; Perticarari, S.; Presani, G.; Lucchesi, A.; Lapini, M.; et al. Prevalence of celiac disease in patients with juvenile chronic arthritis. *J. Pediatr.* **1996**, *129*, 311–313. [CrossRef]
11. Husby, S.; Koletzko, S.; Korponay-Szabó, I.; Kurppa, K.; Mearin, M.L.; Ribes-Koninckx, C.; Shamir, R.; Troncone, R.; Auricchio, R.; Castillejo, G.; et al. European Society Paediatric Gastroenterology, Hepatology and Nutrition Guidelines for Diagnosing Coeliac Disease 2020. *J. Pediatr. Gastroenterol. Nutr.* **2020**, *70*, 141–156. [CrossRef] [PubMed]
12. Prakken, B.; Albani, S.; Martini, A. Juvenile idiopathic arthritis. *Lancet* **2011**, *377*, 2138–2149. [CrossRef]
13. Hersh, A.O.; Prahalad, S. Immunogenetics of juvenile idiopathic arthritis: A comprehensive review. *J. Autoimmun.* **2015**, *64*, 113–124. [CrossRef] [PubMed]
14. De Silvestri, A.; Capittini, C.; Poddighe, D.; Marseglia, G.L.; Mascaretti, L.; Bevilacqua, E.; Scotti, V.; Rebuffi, C.; Pasi, A.; Martinetti, M.; et al. HLA-DRB1 alleles and juvenile idiopathic arthritis: Diagnostic clues emerging from a meta-analysis. *Autoimmun. Rev.* **2017**, *16*, 1230–1236. [CrossRef] [PubMed]
15. Stagi, S.; Giani, T.; Simonini, G.; Falcini, F. Thyroid function, autoimmune thyroiditis, and celiac disease in juvenile idiopathic arthritis. *Rheumatology* **2005**, *44*, 517–520. [CrossRef]
16. Alpigiani, M.G.; Haupt, R.; Parodi, S.; Calcagno, A.; Poggi, E.; Lorini, R. Coeliac disease in 108 patients with juvenile idiopathic arthritis: A 13-year follow-up study. *Clin. Exp. Rheumatol.* **2008**, *26*, 162.
17. Koehne Vde, B.; Bahia, M.; Lanna, C.C.; Pinto, M.R.; Bambirra, E.A.; Cunha, A.S. Prevalence of serological markers for celiac disease (IgA and IgG class antigliadin antibodies and IgA class antiendomysium antibodies) in patients with autoimmune rheumatologic diseases in Belo Horizonte, MG, Brazil. *Arq. Gastroenterol.* **2010**, *47*, 250–256. [CrossRef]
18. Stoll, M.L.; Patel, A.S.; Christadoss, M.L.; Punaro, M.; Olsen, N.J. IgA transglutaminase levels in children with Juvenile Idiopathic Arthritis. *Ann. Paediatr. Rheumatol.* **2012**, *1*, 31–35. [CrossRef]
19. Robazzi, T.C.; Adan, L.F.; Pimentel, K.; Guimarães, I.; Magalhães Filho, J.; Toralles, M.B.; Rolim, A.M. Autoimmune endocrine disorders and coeliac disease in children and adolescents with juvenile idiopathic arthritis and rheumatic fever. *Clin. Exp. Rheumatol.* **2013**, *31*, 310–317.
20. Moghtaderi, M.; Farjadian, S.; Aflaki, E.; Honar, N.; Alyasin, S.; Babaei, M. Screening of patients with juvenile idiopathic arthritis and those with rheumatoid arthritis for celiac disease in southwestern Iran. *Turk. J. Gastroenterol.* **2016**, *27*, 521–524. [CrossRef]
21. Nisihara, R.; Skare, T.; Jardim, A.C.; Utiyama, S.R. Celiac disease autoantibodies in juvenile idiopathic arthritis. *Rheumatol. Int.* **2017**, *37*, 323–324. [CrossRef]
22. Skrabl-Baumgartner, A.; Christine Hauer, A.; Erwa, W.; Jahnel, J. HLA genotyping as first-line screening tool for coeliac disease in children with juvenile idiopathic arthritis. *Arch. Dis. Child.* **2017**, *102*, 607–611. [CrossRef]
23. Tronconi, E.; Miniaci, A.; Pession, A. The autoimmune burden in juvenile idiopathic arthritis. *Ital. J. Pediatr.* **2017**, *43*, 56. [CrossRef]
24. Sahin, Y.; Sahin, S.; Barut, K.; Cokugras, F.C.; Erkan, T.; Adrovic, A.; Kutlu, T.; Kasapcopur, O. Serological screening for coeliac disease in patients with juvenile idiopathic arthritis. *Arab. J. Gastroenterol.* **2019**, *20*, 95–98. [CrossRef] [PubMed]
25. Öman, A.; Hansson, T.; Carlsson, M.; Berntson, L. Evaluation of screening for coeliac disease in children with juvenile idiopathic arthritis. *Acta Paediatr.* **2019**, *108*, 688–693. [CrossRef]
26. AlEnzi, F.; Yateem, M.; Shaikh, M.; AlSohaibani, F.; Alhaymouni, B.; Ahmed, A.; Al-Mayouf, S.M. The Value of Screening for Celiac Disease in Systemic Lupus Erythematosus: A Single Experience of a Tertiary Medical Center. *Rheumatol. Ther.* **2020**, *7*, 649–656. [CrossRef] [PubMed]

27. Pagnini, I.; Scavone, M.; Maccora, I.; Mastrolia, M.V.; Marrani, E.; Bertini, F.; Lamot, L.; Simonini, G. The Development of Extra-Articular Manifestations in Children with Enthesitis-Related Arthritis: Natural Course or Different Disease Entity? *Front. Med.* **2021**, *8*, 667305. [CrossRef]
28. Sadeghi, P.; Salari, K.; Ziaee, V.; Rezaei, N.; Eftekhari, K. Serological Screening of Celiac Disease in Patients with Juvenile Idiopathic Arthritis. *Arch. Iran. Med.* **2021**, *24*, 783–785. [CrossRef]
29. Lerner, A.; Ramesh, A.; Matthias, T. Serologic Diagnosis of Celiac Disease: New Biomarkers. *Gastroenterol. Clin. N. Am.* **2019**, *48*, 307–317. [CrossRef] [PubMed]
30. Abdukhakimova, D.; Dossybayeva, K.; Grechka, A.; Almukhamedova, Z.; Boltanova, A.; Kozina, L.; Nurgaliyeva, K.; Hasanova, L.; Tanko, M.N.; Poddighe, D. Reliability of the Multiplex CytoBead CeliAK Immunoassay to Assess Anti-tTG IgA for Celiac Disease Screening. *Front. Med.* **2021**, *8*, 731067. [CrossRef]
31. Roca, M.; Donat, E.; Marco-Maestud, N.; Masip, E.; Hervás-Marín, D.; Ramos, D.; Polo, B.; Ribes-Koninckx, C. Efficacy Study of Anti-Endomysium Antibodies for Celiac Disease Diagnosis: A Retrospective Study in a Spanish Pediatric Population. *J. Clin. Med.* **2019**, *8*, 2179. [CrossRef] [PubMed]
32. Kotze, L.M.; Utiyama, S.R.; Nisihara, R.M.; de Camargo, V.F.; Ioshii, S.O. IgA class anti-endomysial and anti-tissue transglutaminase antibodies in relation to duodenal mucosa changes in coeliac disease. *Pathology* **2003**, *35*, 56–60. [CrossRef]
33. Poddighe, D.; Capittini, C. The Role of HLA in the Association between IgA Deficiency and Celiac Disease. *Dis. Mark.* **2021**, *2021*, 8632861. [CrossRef]
34. Nazario, E.; Lasa, J.; Schill, A.; Duarte, B.; Berardi, D.; Paz, S.; Muryan, A.; Zubiaurre, I. IgA deficiency is not systematically ruled out in patients undergoing celiac disease testing. *Dig. Dis Sci.* 2021; *Online ahead of print*. [CrossRef]
35. Singh, K.; Chang, C.; Gershwin, M.E. IgA deficiency and autoimmunity. *Autoimmun. Rev.* **2014**, *13*, 163–177. [CrossRef]
36. Pelkonen, P.; Savilahti, E.; Mäkelä, A.L. Persistent and transient IgA deficiency in juvenile rheumatoid arthritis. *Scand. J. Rheumatol.* **1983**, *12*, 273–279. [CrossRef] [PubMed]
37. Singh, P.; Arora, A.; Strand, T.A.; Leffler, D.A.; Catassi, C.; Green, P.H.; Kelly, C.P.; Ahuja, V.; Makharia, G.K. Global Prevalence of Celiac Disease: Systematic Review and Meta-analysis. *Clin. Gastroenterol. Hepatol.* **2018**, *16*, 823–836. [CrossRef]
38. Saurenmann, R.K.; Rose, J.B.; Tyrrell, P.; Feldman, B.M.; Laxer, R.M.; Schneider, R.; Silverman, E.D. Epidemiology of juvenile idiopathic arthritis in a multiethnic cohort: Ethnicity as a risk factor. *Arthritis Rheum.* **2007**, *56*, 1974–1984. [CrossRef] [PubMed]
39. Kiriakidou, M.; Ching, C.L. systemic lupus erythematosus. *Ann. Intern. Med.* **2020**, *172*, 81–96. [CrossRef] [PubMed]
40. Kamphuis, S.; Silverman, E.D. Prevalence and burden of pediatric onset systemic lupus erythematosus. *Nat. Rev. Rheumatol.* **2010**, *6*, 538–546. [CrossRef]
41. Tsokos, G.C.; Lo, M.S.; Costa Reis, P.; Sullivan, K.E. New insights into the immunopathogenesis of systemic lupus erythematosus. *Nat. Rev. Rheumatol.* **2016**, *12*, 716–730. [CrossRef]
42. Dossybayeva, K.; Abdukhakimova, D.; Poddighe, D. Basophils and Systemic Lupus Erythematosus in Murine Models and Human Patients. *Biology* **2020**, *9*, 308. [CrossRef] [PubMed]
43. Bundhun, P.K.; Kumari, A.; Huang, F. Differences in clinical features observed between childhood-onset versus adult-onset systemic lupus erythematosus: A systematic review and meta-analysis. *Medicine* **2017**, *96*, 80–86. [CrossRef]
44. Smith, P.P.; Gordon, C. Systemic lupus erythematosus: Clinical presentations. *Autoimmun. Rev.* **2010**, *10*, 43–45. [CrossRef] [PubMed]
45. Abdirakhmanova, A.; Sazonov, V.; Mukusheva, Z.; Assylbekova, M.; Abdukhakimova, D.; Poddighe, D. Macrophage Activation Syndrome in Pediatric Systemic Lupus Erythematosus: A Systematic Review of the Diagnostic Aspects. *Front. Med.* **2021**, *8*, 681875. [CrossRef]
46. de Leeuw, K.; Bungener, L.; Roozendaal, C.; Bootsma, H.; Stegeman, C.A. Autoantibodies to double-stranded DNA as biomarker in systemic lupus erythematosus: Comparison of different assays during quiescent and active disease. *Rheumatology* **2017**, *56*, 698–703. [CrossRef]
47. Reveille, J.D. Predictive value of autoantibodies for activity of systemic lupus erythematosus. *Lupus* **2004**, *13*, 290–297. [CrossRef]
48. Ma, Y.; Zhuang, D.; Qiao, Z. Dual threat of comorbidity of celiac disease and systemic lupus erythematosus. *J. Int. Med. Res.* **2021**, *49*, 3000605211012258. [CrossRef]
49. Hrycek, A.; Siekiera, U. Coeliac disease in systemic lupus erythematosus: A case report. *Rheumatol. Int.* **2008**, *28*, 491–493. [CrossRef] [PubMed]
50. Mirza, N.; Bonilla, E.; Phillips, P.E. Celiac disease in a patient with systemic lupus erythematosus: A case report and review of literature. *Clin. Rheumatol.* **2007**, *26*, 827–828. [CrossRef] [PubMed]
51. Dahan, S.; Shor, D.B.; Comaneshter, D.; Tekes-Manova, D.; Shovman, O.; Amital, H.; Cohen, A.D. All disease begins in the gut: Celiac disease co-existence with SLE. *Autoimmun. Rev.* **2016**, *15*, 848–853. [CrossRef] [PubMed]
52. Picceli, V.F.; Skare, T.L.; Nisihara, R.; Kotze, L.; Messias-Reason, I.; Utiyama, S.R. Spectrum of autoantibodies for gastrointestinal autoimmune diseases in systemic lupus erythematosus patients. *Lupus* **2013**, *22*, 1150–1155. [CrossRef] [PubMed]
53. Elhami, E.; Zakeri, Z.; Sadeghi, A.; Rostami-Nejad, M.; Volta, U.; Zali, M.R. Prevalence of celiac disease in Iranian patients with rheumatologic disorders. *Gastroenterol. Hepatol. Bed Bench* **2018**, *11*, 239–243.
54. Soltani, Z.; Baghdadi, A.; Nejadhosseinian, M.; Faezi, S.T.; Shahbazkhani, B.; Mousavi, S.A.; Kazemi, K. Celiac disease in patients with systemic lupus erythematosus. *Reumatologia* **2021**, *59*, 85–89. [CrossRef]

55. Aikawa, N.E.; Jesus, A.A.; Liphaus, B.L.; Silva, C.A.; Carneiro-Sampaio, M.; Viana, V.S.; Sallum, A.M. Organ-specific autoantibodies and autoimmune diseases in juvenile systemic lupus erythematosus and juvenile dermatomyositis patients. *Clin. Exp. Rheumatol.* **2012**, *30*, 126–131. [CrossRef]
56. Şahin, Y.; Şahin, S.; Adrovic, A.; Kutlu, T.; Çokuğras, F.Ç.; Barut, K.; Erkan, T.; Kasapçopur, Ö. Serological screening for celiac disease in children with systemic lupus erythematosus. *Eur. J. Rheumatol.* **2019**, *6*, 142–145. [CrossRef]
57. Shamseya, A.M.; Elsayed, E.H.; Donia, H.M. Study of serology and genetics of celiac disease in patients with juvenile systemic lupus erythematosus 'celiac in juvenile systemic lupus'. *Eur. J. Gastroenterol. Hepatol.* **2020**, *32*, 1322–1327. [CrossRef]
58. Selva-O'Callaghan, A.; Casellas, F.; de Torres, I.; Palou, E.; Grau-Junyent, J.M.; Vilardell-Tarrés, M. Celiac disease and antibodies associated with celiac disease in patients with inflammatory myopathy. *Muscle Nerve.* **2007**, *35*, 49–54. [CrossRef]
59. Orbach, H.; Amitai, N.; Barzilai, O.; Boaz, M.; Ram, M.; Zandman-Goddard, G.; Shoenfeld, Y. Autoantibody screen in inflammatory myopathies high prevalence of antibodies to gliadin. *Ann. N. Y. Acad. Sci.* **2009**, *1173*, 174–179. [CrossRef]
60. Soylu, A.; Öztürk, Y.; Doğan, Y.; Özmen, D.; Yılmaz, Ö.; Kuyum, P.; Kavukçu, S. Screening of celiac disease in children with Henoch-Schoenlein purpura. *Rheumatol. Int.* **2016**, *36*, 713–717. [CrossRef]
61. Nisihara, R.; Aguiar Koubik, M.; Mateus, M.; da Silva Kotze, L.; Larocca Skare, T. Non-celiac gluten intolerance in patients with scleroderma. *Jt. Bone Spine* **2018**, *85*, 771–772. [CrossRef] [PubMed]
62. Forbess, L.J.; Gordon, J.K.; Doobay, K.; Bosworth, B.P.; Lyman, S.; Davids, M.L.; Spiera, R.F. Low prevalence of coeliac disease in patients with systemic sclerosis: A cross-sectional study of a registry cohort. *Rheumatology* **2013**, *52*, 939–943. [CrossRef] [PubMed]
63. Rosato, E.; De Nitto, D.; Rossi, C.; Libanori, V.; Donato, G.; Di Tola, M.; Pisarri, S.; Salsano, F.; Picarelli, A. High incidence of celiac disease in patients with systemic sclerosis. *J. Rheumatol.* **2009**, *36*, 965–969. [CrossRef] [PubMed]
64. Luft, L.M.; Barr, S.G.; Martin, L.O.; Chan, E.K.; Fritzler, M.J. Autoantibodies to tissue transglutaminase in Sjögren's syndrome and related rheumatic diseases. *J. Rheumatol.* **2003**, *30*, 2613–2619. [PubMed]

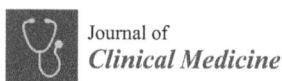

Protocol

New Strategy for the Detection and Treatment of *Helicobacter pylori* Infections in Primary Care Guided by a Non-Invasive PCR in Stool: Protocol of the French HepyPrim Study

Maxime Pichon [1,2,*,†], Bernard Freche [2,3,†] and Christophe Burucoa [1,2,*]

1. Bacteriology Laboratory, Infectious Agents Department, CHU Poitiers, 86021 Poitiers, France
2. INSERM U1070 Pharmacology of Antimicrobial Agents and Resistances, University of Poitiers, 86073 Poitiers, France; bernard.freche@univ-poitiers.fr
3. Department of General Medicine, Faculty of Medicine and Pharmacy, University of Poitiers, 86073 Poitiers, France
* Correspondence: maxime.pichon@chu-poitiers.fr (M.P.); christophe.burucoa@chu-poitiers.fr (C.B.); Tel.: +33-(0)5-49-44-41-43 (M.P.); +33-(0)5-49-44-64-68 (C.B.)
† These authors contributed equally to this work.

Abstract: *Helicobacter pylori* (Hp) infects half of the world population and is responsible for gastric, duodenal ulcers and gastric cancer. The eradication of Hp cures ulcers and prevents ulcer recurrences and gastric cancer. Antibiotic resistance of Hp, and particularly clarithromycin resistance, is the primary cause of treatment failure and is a major concern identified by the WHO as a high priority requiring research into new strategies. Treatments guided by the detection of antibiotic resistance have proven their medical and economical superiority. However, this strategy is severely hampered by the invasive nature of the fibroscopy, since antibiotic resistance detection requires gastric biopsies. The eradication of Hp involves primary care physicians. The objective of this study will be to evaluate the feasibility of a strategy for the management of Hp infection in primary care by a recently developed non-invasive procedure and its non-inferiority in eradication rates compared with the strategy recommended by the French National Authority of Health. The non-invasive procedure is a PCR on stool to detect Hp infection and mutations conferring resistance to clarithromycin allowing a treatment guided by the results of the PCR. We present the protocol of a prospective, multicenter, randomized, controlled interventional study in two arms.

Keywords: *Helicobacter pylori*; primary care physicians; antimicrobials; diagnosis

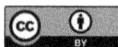

1. Introduction

Helicobacter pylori (Hp) infection is the most common chronic bacterial infection in the world (50% of the world population, 20 to 30% of the French population) [1–3]. Acquired in childhood, most often within the family, this infection persists throughout the individual's life in the absence of specific treatment [4]. Many infected persons present chronic gastritis, most of the time asymptomatic. Only 5–10% of infected people will develop a gastric or duodenal ulcer, 1–3% gastric cancer (adenocarcinoma or MALT lymphoma) [5]. This represents 80,000 cases of peptic ulcers and 6000 gastric cancers (5-year survival rate of 20%) in France each year [6,7]. Hp is recognized as a class 1 carcinogen by the WHO (800,000 deaths from gastric cancer worldwide each year) [7,8]. Treatment cures peptic ulcers and prevents their recurrence, prevents gastric adenocarcinoma and cures MALT lymphoma without associated translocation. Resistance to the antibiotics used in eradication therapy is the primary cause of treatment failure, followed by poor compliance [9,10].

In Europe *H. pylori* resistance rates in 2018 (on 1211 strains) were 21.4% for clarithromycin, 15.8% for levofloxacin and 38.9% for metronidazole. Prevalence was significantly higher in Central/Western and Southern than in the Northern European countries [11]. In the same year, 20.9% of Hp strains in France were resistant to clarithromycin, 17.6% to levofloxacin, and 58.6% to metronidazole [10,12,13]. The 2017 recommendations of the French National Authority for Health (Haute Autorité de Santé, HAS) placed "guided" and "empirical" treatment modalities at the heart of strategies for Hp eradication [14]. These "guided" treatments following the identification of resistance to certain antibiotics have proven their medico- economic superiority in the eradication of this bacterium [15]. This guided treatment strategy requires gastric biopsies and culture of this difficult-to-culture bacterium and/or a real-time PCR [16,17]. This strategy is severely hampered by the invasive nature of the gastroscopy, the difficulty of the culture and the cost of the PCR. It has been widely demonstrated that treatment guided by resistance detection is more effective, less expensive and better tolerated. The World Health Organization, WHO, has identified Hp resistance to clarithromycin as a high priority requiring research into new strategies. In France, guided treatment represents less than 1% of eradication treatments (Longitudinal Patient Data and French national Health information system, SNIIRAM), despite the recommendations of the HAS and the European and French Societies for Gastroenterology to favor treatment guided by the results of Antibiotic Susceptibility Testing, AST, or PCR.

Serology, a non-invasive test, easy-to-perform and inexpensive, has demonstrated good performances (sensitivity, Sen, over 96% and specificity, Spe, between 60 and 90%). However, it does not allow detection of antibiotic resistance and the active nature of the infection. Similarly, other non-invasive tests have been developed to detect Hp in other, less invasive specimens, such as respiratory specimens (for the urea breath test, used for eradication testing) or stool (stool antigen test) (described or reviewed in refs. [18–21]). The latter have the same limitations as serology, being limited to the presence/absence of Hp without any precision on the AST profile, crucial for disease management in many countries of the world. Several diagnostic companies have recently marketed PCR kits for the detection of Hp infection and clarithromycin resistance mutations in stool. The performances of the Amplidiag *H. pylori* + ClariR test (Mobidiag, Hologic Inc., Marlborough, MA, USA) for detection of Hp infection and detection of clarithromycin resistance by real-time PCR have been demonstrated [10]. These excellent performances (Sen 96.3% and Spe 98.7%) make it possible to consider using this non-invasive technique for diagnosis and treatment orientation and consequently to be able to carry out guided treatment without recourse to gastro-duodenal endoscopy and biopsies. PCR testing of stool for Hp infection and resistance to clarithromycin is simple and requires few trained personnel. Its non-invasive character may allow it to be used in patients with an indication for the detection and treatment of Hp infection and without an indication for gastro-duodenal endoscopy.

The eradication of Hp strongly involves primary care physicians (general practitioners, GPs). The diagnosis of Hp infections in the general population requires close collaboration between primary care physicians and other specialists (gastroenterologists, pathologists, bacteriologists...). In France, it has been estimated that GPs see almost the entire population of France in their offices at least once a year. Given the prevalence and incidence of Hp, their role is becoming increasingly important [22]. The present project is therefore related to a field problem. The GP's skills in the prevention of gastric cancer and pathologies of the upper digestive tract are an integral part of the discipline's professional reference system [23].

The main objective of this study will be to evaluate, in a real-life situation, the feasibility of a strategy for the management of Hp infection by a non-invasive procedure in primary care and its non-inferiority in eradication rate compared with the strategy recommended by the HAS using a combination of serology and endoscopy. The secondary objectives of this study will be: to evaluate the adherence of patients to the care pathway (compliance to endoscopy, treatment, stool collection, serology); to evaluate the follow-up of recommendations in the management of Hp infections by health professionals (GPs and gastroenterologists) (e.g., empirical/guided treatment, evaluation of pre-neoplastic lesions);

to validate, in real-life circumstances, real-time PCR in stool in comparison with serology in primary diagnosis and with urea breath test in eradication control.

2. Methods

2.1. Trial Design and Setting

This study will be a prospective, multicenter, randomized, controlled interventional study in two arms (Figure 1). Randomization will be carried out through a secure web-based randomization system and stratified by center (i.e., each investigator). The duration of the inclusion period will be 12 months. The participation period for each participant will be 4 months for a total study duration of 16 months (twelve months of inclusion plus four months of follow-up for the last included patient).

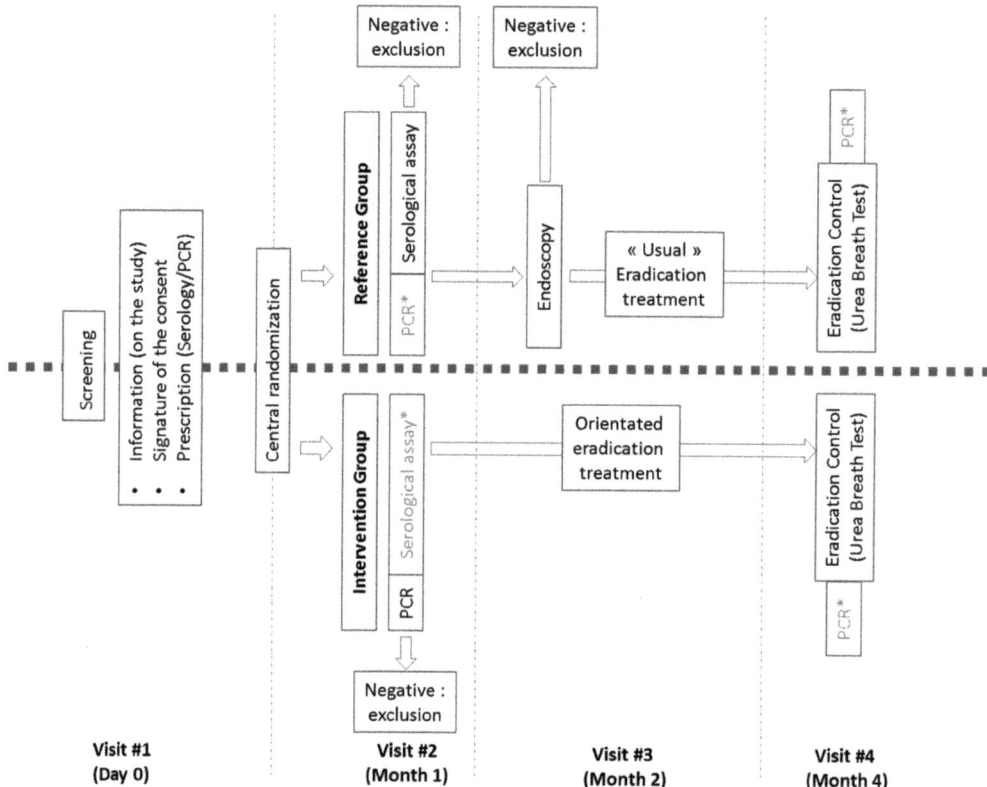

Figure 1. Trial design. *: Data collected for the study, the results of which will not be communicated to the patient and the physician before the end of the study.

A computer-generated block-randomization sequence using permuted-block randomization of varying block sizes will be performed by the statistician and will be carried out via Ennov System software. The statistician will not be involved in either screening the patients or assessing outcomes. The randomization process will be accessible to all physicians working in the emergency department through user personal identification logins to access the website (https://chu-poitiers.hugo-online.fr/CSOnline/, accessed on 27 December 2021). It will become effective following confirmation of inclusion and exclusion criteria. Thereafter, patients will be assigned to one of the two study groups (in a 1:1 randomization scheme) according to the strategy (described thereafter).

Intervention group. Patients randomized to the Intervention group (new strategy arm) will receive a prescription for Hp serology with instructions for the laboratory to limit the communication of the results to the physician alone and a stool self-sampling kit (containing instructions, biodegradable basket to be placed on the toilet, e-Nat tube (Copan, Italia), and stamped envelope for mailing to the laboratory). After centrifugation, 400 µL of the eNAT tube supernatant will be extracted using the NucliSENS easyMAG system (bioMérieux, Marcy-l'Étoile, France), according to the manufacturer's instructions, in 2 mL lysis buffer under the following conditions: the specific B 2.1 protocol with 140 µL of silica, after adding 1 µL of internal control (Amplidiag Easy Process Control I; Mobidiag, Hologic inc.), for a final volume of eluate of 70 µL. Nucleic acid will then be amplified using the Amplidiag *H. pylori* + ClariR test assay. This test, the only one that will be considered for this arm, consisting in a multiplex PCR, will obtain three different results (negative/absence of detection of *Helicobacter pylori* or detection of *Helicobacter pylori* or detection of *Helicobacter pylori* associated with mutation implicated in clarithromycin-resistance, i.e., A2142C, A2142G and A2143G). Originally developed for detection in gastric biopsy this kit may give appropriate results in stool samples [10,24]. According to the results of their biological assay, patients will be seen by their investigator within six weeks to either initiate or not initiate eradication therapy, i.e., a positive test will determine Hp infection and indication for treatment. The absence of detection of a clarithromycin-resistant strain will allow prescription of a guided treatment combining PPI, amoxicillin, and clarithromycin for 10 days according to the HAS recommendations. According to the same recommendations, the detection of a clarithromycin-resistant strain will allow prescription of a guided treatment combining PPI, amoxicillin, and metronidazole or quinolone for 10 days. At least 4 weeks after stopping antibiotics (and at least 2 weeks after stopping PPIs), an eradication control will be carried out using a respiratory test (urea breath test), concomitant to the collection of a stool sample for retrospective analysis by real-time PCR. A negative breath test will define the success of the treatment, while a positive test will define treatment failure. The latter will be managed in the usual manner by the GPs in charge of the patient. At the end of the follow-up, infected (positive for serology and/or PCR assays) and treated patients over 45 years of age will be referred to a gastroenterologist for gastric biopsies for histological analysis of the gastric mucosa for pre-neoplastic and cancerous lesions.

Control group. Patients randomized to the reference strategy control group (HAS strategy arm) will receive a prescription for Hp serology and a stool self-sampling kit (instructions, biodegradable basket to be placed on the toilet seat, E-Nat tube (Copan), swab, stamped envelope for mailing to the laboratory). Only the serology result will be considered for this arm (to avoid any deviation from the protocol, results of other tests will not be communicated before the end of the study). According to the results of their biological assay, patients will be seen by their investigator within six weeks. A positive serological test will lead to a gastroscopy with biopsies for histology/pathological and bacteriological analysis if available. Each person referred will be accompanied by the "request for gastroscopy in case of positive Hp serology" letter, according to the HAS model. These anatomopathological and/or bacteriological analyses will determine the presence of a Hp infection, if bacteria suggestive of Hp are observed in pathological examination and/or if the conventional and/or molecular biology are positive from gastric biopsies sent to bacteriology laboratories. An infection will determine the indication for treatment, either empirically, in the absence of an antibiogram or PCR result (bismuth or concomitant quadritherapy), or guided by the results of the AST or culture according to HAS recommendations (pertinence of care sheet). At least 4 weeks after stopping antibiotics (and at least 2 weeks after stopping PPIs), an eradication control will be carried out using a respiratory test (urea breath test), concomitant to collection of a stool sample for retrospective analysis by PCR. A negative breath test will define the success of the treatment, while a positive test will define treatment failure. The latter will be managed in the usual manner by the GPs in charge of the patient.

It should be noted that for ethical and regulatory considerations, it was decided, after the collection of results (at the end of the study for each patient), to give out the results of these analyses (urea breath test, serology, PCR before/after treatment) in order to allow the general practitioner to manage the patient in an appropriate manner.

2.2. Participant Eligibility and Consent

All consecutive patients will be considered candidates for inclusion in the study if they meet all inclusion criteria and none of the exclusion criteria (Figure 2.). Eligible patients will receive oral and written information and will be enrolled after giving written informed consent.

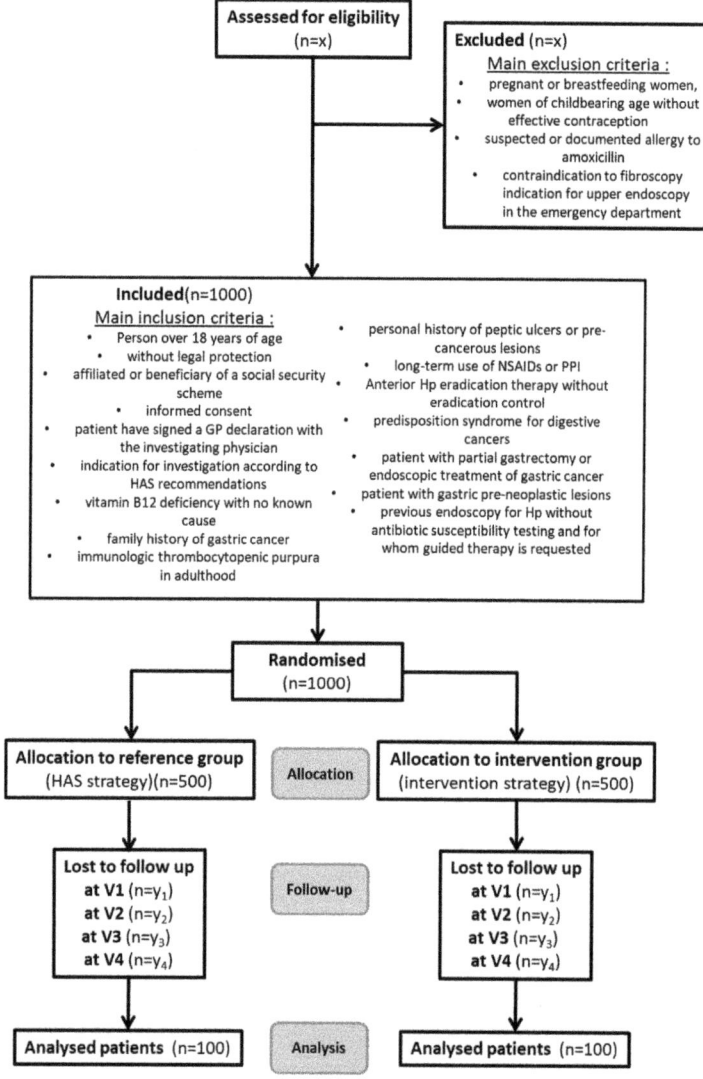

Figure 2. CONSORT Flow chart of the HepyPrim Study. X: data could not be predicted before the beginning of the screening. Y (= y1 + y2 + y3 + y4), corresponding to patients lost to follow-up, will be less than 50 patients per allocation group.

Inclusion criteria. Inclusion criteria will be: (i) over 18 years of age, (ii) affiliated to or beneficiary of a social security scheme, (iii) informed consent signed after clear and fair information about the study, (iv) patient having signed a GPs declaration with the investigating physician, (v) indication for investigation and treatment of Hp infection according to HAS recommendations (suffering from chronic dyspepsia, iron deficiency anemia with no known cause or resistant to iron supplementation, vitamin B12 deficiency with no known cause, family history of gastric cancer, immunologic thrombocytopenic purpura in adulthood, personal history of peptic ulcers or pre-cancerous lesions that have not been eradicated, long-term use of NSAIDs or PPI, patient who received Hp eradication therapy without eradication control, patient with a predisposition syndrome for digestive cancers (hereditary non-polyposis colorectal carcinoma cancer)), (vi) patient with partial gastrectomy or endoscopic treatment of gastric cancer, (vii) patient with gastric pre-neoplastic lesions (severe atrophy and/or intestinal metaplasia, dysplasia), and (viii) patient with previous endoscopy for Hp without antibiotic susceptibility testing (biopsy not referred to bacteriology) and for whom guided therapy is requested.

Non-inclusion criteria. Patients who will not be included are those who: (i) are legally protected; (ii) are pregnant or breastfeeding women or women of childbearing age without effective contraception; (iii) are suspected of or have a documented allergy to amoxicillin; (iv) have a contraindication to (or initial refusal of) esophageal endoscopy; and (v) have an indication for upper GI endoscopy in the emergency department according to the criteria of the European Panel on the Appropriateness of Gastrointestinal Endoscopy (i.e., upper GI bleeding, acute deglobulation without externalized GI bleeding, caustic ingestion, acute dysphagia or foreign body ingestion).

2.3. Study Outcomes

Primary endpoint. The primary endpoint will be an assessment of the cure rate through the results of a urea breath test performed 6 weeks after the end of treatment (proof of Hp eradication).

Secondary endpoints. The secondary endpoints will be assessment of: (i) the number of guided treatments (depending on the real-life application of the French authorities recommendations); (ii) the number of endoscopies (estimating the number of endoscopies avoided due to the optimized process); (iii) the number of biopsies at endoscopy; (iv) the number of patients who refused endoscopy after serology or positive PCR or did not follow-up after referral to the gastroenterologist; (v) the number of treatment side-effects and treatment dropouts; (vi) the discordance rate between real-time PCR tests in stool and serology in primary diagnosis; (vii) the discordance rate between real-time PCR tests in stool/breathing test in eradication control; and (viii) cure rate assessed by the result of a urea breath test performed 6 weeks after the end of treatment (proof of Hp eradication) depending on the antibiotic susceptibility testing identified at diagnostic.

2.4. Data Collection

Independent clinical research assistants will be available at each participating hospital to help in running the study and with data collection. Study documents will be deidentified and stored for 15 years, as per the protocol for non-clinical trial notification interventional studies. Data will be entered into the web-based eCRF (https://chu-poitiers.hugo-online.fr/CSOnline/, accessed on 27 December 2021) and electronically stored on double password-protected computers. Hard copies of data (clinical research files) will be stored in a secure locked office. All personnel involved in data analysis will be masked to study groups. Only the principal investigators and the statisticians will have access to the final data set.

The following data will be recorded:

Baseline characteristics. (i) Demographic data (age, gender, height, weight, and body mass index); (ii) comorbidities (active smoking, insulin-dependent or non-insulin-dependent diabetes, hypertension, hypercholesterolemia, chronic renal failure, COPD);

(iii) history of antimicrobial treatment for eradication of *H. pylori*; (iv) key laboratory findings (except for Hp); (v) familial history of cancer; and (vi) symptomatology (including clinical examination).

Biological data. Results of the following biological assays: (i) Results of the stool PCR searching for *H. pylori* (before and after eradication treatment); (ii) serological status of the patient regarding *H. pylori*; (iii) histopathological results (for HAS groups); and (iv) results of the urea breath test.

2.5. Statistical Analysis

Sample size calculation. Assuming 20% prevalence in source population, and based on a one-sided hypothesis, 100 patients will be included in each strategy arm to demonstrate a 15% difference between each strategy with statistical risks at 5% (type I error, α) and 15% (type II error, β). We are planning to enroll 1000 patients to consider a maximum patient loss of 10%. Considering that each investigator involved in the HepyPrim study follows more than 1200 patients each year, the inclusion objective was set to 50 patients per investigator and the number of investigators was set to 20. These investigators have been selected in the newly constituted "physicians' network for research in New Aquitaine".

Analysis. The data will be analyzed blindly on an intention-to-treat basis, assuming a non-inferiority hypothesis. No interim analysis is planned. A per protocol analysis will be performed as a secondary sensitivity analysis. Quantitative variables will be described by their mean and standard deviation or median and interquartile range according to the normality of the distribution. Categorical variables will be described by their number and percentage. Continuous variables will be compared by a Student's *t*-test or Mann–Whitney U-test according to the normality of the distribution. Categorical variables will be compared by a chi-square test or Fisher's exact test. The tests will be analyzed using GraphPad Prism version 9.0 (GraphPad Software, San Diego, CA, USA). A significant difference will be retained for a p-value < 0.05. All tests will be two-tailed, stratified by center and for multiple comparisons if appropriate.

2.6. Ethical Considerations

The clinical trial will be carried out in line with the principles of the Declaration of Helsinki, the guideline for Good Clinical Practice of the International Conference on Harmonization, in accordance with the French law No. 2012–300 of 5 March 2012 on research involving the human person and with the Clinical Trials Directives 2001/20/EC and 2005/28/EC of the European Parliament. All included patients will have consented to the protocol after an appropriate information session that includes processes of the study and the constitution of the biobank. As with all interventional studies in France and according to French legislation, the final protocol will be validated by a randomly selected ethical committee (Comité de Protection des Personnes, CPP).

The results of the study will be given to the participating GPs, referring physicians and medical community no later than 2 years after completion of the trial through presentation at scientific conferences and publication in peer-reviewed journals. The main manuscript will mention the name of the sponsor (French Ministry of Health), and all trial sites will be acknowledged. All investigators having included or followed participants in the study will appear with their names under 'the HepyPrim investigators' in an appendix to the final manuscript. Authorship will be completed in accordance with the guidelines of the International Committee of Medical Journal (ICMJ). No professional writer will be used.

3. Discussion

This study may be a major study to demonstrate the benefits of optimizing therapeutic management of Hp, through GP education and management. The patients included in the study may benefit from a reliable diagnosis without an invasive examination, use of a second diagnostic test (limiting the risk of false negative) with consideration of a possible positive result by the doctor and the systematic performance of a respiratory test to control eradication (underused in France despite recommendations).

This study may make it possible to assess the interest of a non-invasive procedure for the diagnosis of *Helicobacter pylori* infections that can be carried out in primary care practice in France, coordinated by general practitioners. This study may make it possible to achieve better efficiency in recourse to gastroenterologists and endoscopy by limiting it, in the indication of endoscopies of the upper digestive tract, to complex cases, thereby optimizing interdisciplinary collaboration. The aim of this study is to promote the appropriation of "guided" treatments in the care of Hp infection by primary care in future coordinated multidisciplinary practice, while also promoting the prevention of high-prevalence and potentially serious pathologies of the upper digestive system.

The main challenge in curing Hp is associated with the management of antimicrobial resistance, particularly to clarithromycin, a key component of triple therapy and impacted by increasing resistance (up to two-thirds of bacterial strains isolated) [13,25–27]. This situation justifies the crucial need for biological tests capable of determining the antimicrobial susceptibility profile [21]. To this end, detection by molecular analysis of Hp DNA on stools is crucial to develop Hp-guided therapeutic strategies. Its non-invasive nature would allow for easy sample acquisition (with improved compliance), thus optimizing the time-to-cost importance of the disease. With the exception of recent large studies, most of the few studies have used small numbers of patients, tests adapted to stool samples but designed for biopsies (GenoType HelicoDR (Hain Lifescience, Nehren, Germany) or *H. pylori* ClariRes (Ingenetix, Vienna, Austria) [28–35]. On the contrary, two recent studies demonstrated the very high performance of the stool test for the detection of Hp infection and clarithromycin resistance, in a process that takes little time [10,36].

Moreover, this is the first study to enable the structuring of a research network in primary care in Poitou-Charentes. This project is the first of this network, which will be made up of 20 co-investigators, all of whom are GPs. Others were identified during the recruitment phase carried out as part of a thesis on the practice of general medicine by two interns in general medicine. This project is therefore founding and structuring for a primary care research network.

This study may allow evaluation of the performance of PCR in stools in comparison with the combination of serology/pathology/bacteriology for the initial diagnosis, evaluation of the performance of PCR in stools in comparison to the respiratory test for the control of eradication. Moreover, it may lead to the constitution of a biobank of stools of infected patients, in view of further study of the development of in vitro diagnosis.

Author Contributions: Conceptualization, M.P., B.F. and C.B.; methodology, M.P., B.F. and C.B.; validation, M.P., B.F. and C.B.; resources, B.F.; data curation, M.P. formal analysis; M.P. and B.F.; writing—original draft preparation, M.P., B.F. and C.B.; writing—review and editing, M.P. and B.F.; supervision, M.P. and C.B.; project administration, C.B.; funding acquisition, B.F. All authors have read and agreed to the published version of the manuscript.

Funding: This research was funded by French Ministry of Health; grant ReSP-ir 2021.

Institutional Review Board Statement: The study will be conducted according to the guidelines of the Declaration of Helsinki and approved by the Institutional Review Board. The protocol was approved by Research Direction of the University Hospital of Poitiers.

Informed Consent Statement: Written informed consent of the patient will be requested prior to the enrolment. The investigators will provide clear and precise information about the protocol to the patient before requesting him/her for written informed consent.

Acknowledgments: The authors thank all the co-investigating physicians for agreeing to participate in the recruitment of patients and the patients for their participation in the study. The authors gratefully acknowledge Jeffrey Arsham for his help for the writing of the manuscript.

Conflicts of Interest: B.F. declares no conflict of interest. M.P. received travel grant for congresses from Pfizer and Genoscreen; and C.B. was the principal investigator of a study funded by the Mobidiag laboratory and sponsored by the Poitiers University Hospital. The funders had no role in the design of the study; in the collection, analyses, or interpretation of data; in the writing of the manuscript, or in the decision to publish the results.

References

1. Hooi, J.K.Y.; Lai, W.Y.; Ng, W.K.; Suen, M.M.Y.; Underwood, F.E.; Tanyingoh, D.; Malfertheiner, P.; Graham, D.Y.; Wong, V.W.S.; Wu, J.C.Y.; et al. Global Prevalence of Helicobacter Pylori Infection: Systematic Review and Meta-Analysis. *Gastroenterology* **2017**, *153*, 420–429. [CrossRef] [PubMed]
2. Guevara, B.; Cogdill, A.G. Helicobacter Pylori: A Review of Current Diagnostic and Management Strategies. *Dig. Dis. Sci.* **2020**, *65*, 1917–1931. [CrossRef] [PubMed]
3. Burucoa, C.; Axon, A. Epidemiology of Helicobacter Pylori Infection. *Helicobacter* **2017**, *22* (Suppl. 1), 42–59. [CrossRef] [PubMed]
4. Kalach, N.; Bontems, P.; Raymond, J. L'infection à Helicobacter pylori chez l'enfant. *Perfect. Pédiatrie* **2018**, *1*, 119–126. [CrossRef]
5. Kao, C.-Y.; Sheu, B.-S.; Wu, J.-J. Helicobacter Pylori Infection: An Overview of Bacterial Virulence Factors and Pathogenesis. *Biomed. J.* **2016**, *39*, 14–23. [CrossRef]
6. Muzaheed, M. Helicobacter Pylori Oncogenicity: Mechanism, Prevention, and Risk Factors. *Sci. World J.* **2020**, *2020*, 3018326. [CrossRef]
7. Mentis, A.-F.A.; Boziki, M.; Grigoriadis, N.; Papavassiliou, A.G. Helicobacter Pylori Infection and Gastric Cancer Biology: Tempering a Double-Edged Sword. *Cell Mol. Life Sci.* **2019**, *76*, 2477–2486. [CrossRef]
8. Haenszel, W.; Correa, P. Developments in the Epidemiology of Stomach Cancer over the Past Decade. *Cancer Res.* **1975**, *35*, 3452–3459.
9. Djennane-Hadibi, F.; Bachtarzi, M.; Layaida, K.; Ali Arous, N.; Nakmouche, M.; Saadi, B.; Tazir, M.; Ramdani-Bouguessa, N.; Burucoa, C. High-Level Primary Clarithromycin Resistance of Helicobacter Pylori in Algiers, Algeria: A Prospective Multicenter Molecular Study. *Microb. Drug Resist.* **2016**, *22*, 223–226. [CrossRef]
10. Pichon, M.; Pichard, B.; Barrioz, T.; Plouzeau, C.; Croquet, V.; Fotsing, G.; Chéron, A.; Vuillemin, É.; Wangermez, M.; Haineaux, P.-A.; et al. Diagnostic Accuracy of a Noninvasive Test for Detection of Helicobacter Pylori and Resistance to Clarithromycin in Stool by the Amplidiag H. Pylori+ClariR Real-Time PCR Assay. *J. Clin. Microbiol.* **2020**, *58*, e01787-19. [CrossRef]
11. Megraud, F.; Bruyndonckx, R.; Coenen, S.; Wittkop, L.; Huang, T.-D.; Hoebeke, M.; Bénéjat, L.; Lehours, P.; Goossens, H.; Glupczynski, Y. Helicobacter Pylori Resistance to Antibiotics in Europe in 2018 and Its Relationship to Antibiotic Consumption in the Community. *Gut* **2021**, *70*, 1815–1822. [CrossRef] [PubMed]
12. Mégraud, F.; Alix, C.; Charron, P.; Bénéjat, L.; Ducournau, A.; Bessède, E.; Lehours, P. Survey of the Antimicrobial Resistance of Helicobacter Pylori in France in 2018 and Evolution during the Previous 5 Years. *Helicobacter* **2021**, *26*, e12767. [CrossRef] [PubMed]
13. Megraud, F.; Coenen, S.; Versporten, A.; Kist, M.; Lopez-Brea, M.; Hirschl, A.M.; Andersen, L.P.; Goossens, H.; Glupczynski, Y. Study Group Participants Helicobacter Pylori Resistance to Antibiotics in Europe and Its Relationship to Antibiotic Consumption. *Gut* **2013**, *62*, 34–42. [CrossRef] [PubMed]
14. Malfertheiner, P.; Megraud, F.; O'Morain, C.A.; Gisbert, J.P.; Kuipers, E.J.; Axon, A.T.; Bazzoli, F.; Gasbarrini, A.; Atherton, J.; Graham, D.Y.; et al. Management of Helicobacter Pylori Infection-the Maastricht V/Florence Consensus Report. *Gut* **2017**, *66*, 6–30. [CrossRef] [PubMed]
15. Delchier, J.-C.; Bastuji-Garin, S.; Raymond, J.; Megraud, F.; Amiot, A.; Cambau, E.; Burucoa, C.; HELICOSTIC Study Group. Efficacy of a Tailored PCR-Guided Triple Therapy in the Treatment of Helicobacter Pylori Infection. *Med. Mal. Infect.* **2019**, *50*, 492–499. [CrossRef]
16. Pichon, M.; Burucoa, C. Impact of the Gastro-Intestinal Bacterial Microbiome on Helicobacter-Associated Diseases. *Healthcare* **2019**, *7*, 34. [CrossRef]
17. Pichon, M.; Tran, C.T.; Motillon, G.; Debiais, C.; Gautier, S.; Aballea, M.; Cremniter, J.; Vasseur, P.; Tougeron, D.; Garcia, M.; et al. Where to Biopsy to Detect Helicobacter Pylori and How Many Biopsies Are Needed to Detect Antibiotic Resistance in a Human Stomach. *JCM* **2020**, *9*, 2812. [CrossRef]
18. Monteiro, L.; De Mascarel, A.; Sarrasqueta, A.M.; Bergey, B.; Barberis, C.; Talby, P.; Roux, D.; Shouler, L.; Goldfain, D.; Lamouliatte, H.; et al. Diagnosis of Helicobacter Pylori Infection: Noninvasive Methods Compared to Invasive Methods and Evaluation of Two New Tests. *Am. J. Gastroenterol.* **2001**, *96*, 353–358. [CrossRef]
19. Ricci, C.; Holton, J.; Vaira, D. Diagnosis of Helicobacter Pylori: Invasive and Non-Invasive Tests. *Best Pract. Res. Clin. Gastroenterol.* **2007**, *21*, 299–313. [CrossRef]
20. Gatta, L.; Ricci, C.; Tampieri, A.; Vaira, D. Non-Invasive Techniques for the Diagnosis of Helicobacter Pylori Infection. *Clin. Microbiol. Infect.* **2003**, *9*, 489–496. [CrossRef]
21. Vaira, D.; Holton, J.; Menegatti, M.; Ricci, C.; Gatta, L.; Geminiani, A.; Miglioli, M. Review Article:Invasive and Non-Invasive Tests for Helicobacter Pylori Infection. *Aliment. Pharmacol. Ther.* **2000**, *14* (Suppl. 3), 13–22. [CrossRef] [PubMed]
22. Starfield, B. William Pickles Lecture. Primary and Specialty Care Interfaces: The Imperative of Disease Continuity. *Br. J. Gen. Pract.* **2003**, *53*, 723–729. [PubMed]

23. Aïm-Eusébi, A.; Cussac, F.; Aubin-Auger, I. Cancer prevention and screening: What french GPs could do? *Bull. Cancer* **2019**, *106*, 707–713. [CrossRef] [PubMed]
24. Hays, C.; Delerue, T.; Lamarque, D.; Burucoa, C.; Collobert, G.; Billöet, A.; Kalach, N.; Raymond, J. Molecular Diagnosis of Helicobacter Pylori Infection in Gastric Biopsies: Evaluation of the Amplidiag® H.Pylori + ClariR Assay. *Helicobacter* **2019**, *24*, e12560. [CrossRef]
25. Malfertheiner, P.; Megraud, F.; O'Morain, C.A.; Atherton, J.; Axon, A.T.R.; Bazzoli, F.; Gensini, G.F.; Gisbert, J.P.; Graham, D.Y.; Rokkas, T.; et al. Management of Helicobacter Pylori Infection—The Maastricht IV/Florence Consensus Report. *Gut* **2012**, *61*, 646–664. [CrossRef]
26. Savoldi, A.; Carrara, E.; Graham, D.Y.; Conti, M.; Tacconelli, E. Prevalence of Antibiotic Resistance in Helicobacter Pylori: A Systematic Review and Meta-Analysis in World Health Organization Regions. *Gastroenterology* **2018**, *155*, 1372–1382.e17. [CrossRef]
27. Raymond, J.; Lamarque, D.; Kalach, N.; Chaussade, S.; Burucoa, C. High Level of Antimicrobial Resistance in French Helicobacter Pylori Isolates. *Helicobacter* **2010**, *15*, 21–27. [CrossRef]
28. Brennan, D.E.; Omorogbe, J.; Hussey, M.; Tighe, D.; Holleran, G.; O'Morain, C.; Smith, S.M.; McNamara, D. Molecular Detection of Helicobacter Pylori Antibiotic Resistance in Stool vs Biopsy Samples. *World J. Gastroenterol.* **2016**, *22*, 9214–9221. [CrossRef]
29. Sun, L.; Talarico, S.; Yao, L.; He, L.; Self, S.; You, Y.; Zhang, H.; Zhang, Y.; Guo, Y.; Liu, G.; et al. Droplet Digital PCR-Based Detection of Clarithromycin Resistance in Helicobacter Pylori Isolates Reveals Frequent Heteroresistance. *J. Clin. Microbiol.* **2018**, *56*, e00019-18. [CrossRef]
30. Scaletsky, I.C.A.; Aranda, K.R.S.; Garcia, G.T.; Gonçalves, M.E.P.; Cardoso, S.R.; Iriya, K.; Silva, N.P. Application of Real-Time PCR Stool Assay for Helicobacter Pylori Detection and Clarithromycin Susceptibility Testing in Brazilian Children. *Helicobacter* **2011**, *16*, 311–315. [CrossRef]
31. Schabereiter-Gurtner, C.; Hirschl, A.M.; Dragosics, B.; Hufnagl, P.; Puz, S.; Kovách, Z.; Rotter, M.; Makristathis, A. Novel Real-Time PCR Assay for Detection of Helicobacter Pylori Infection and Simultaneous Clarithromycin Susceptibility Testing of Stool and Biopsy Specimens. *J. Clin. Microbiol.* **2004**, *42*, 4512–4518. [CrossRef]
32. Lottspeich, C.; Schwarzer, A.; Panthel, K.; Koletzko, S.; Rüssmann, H. Evaluation of the Novel Helicobacter Pylori ClariRes Real-Time PCR Assay for Detection and Clarithromycin Susceptibility Testing of H. Pylori in Stool Specimens from Symptomatic Children. *J. Clin. Microbiol.* **2007**, *45*, 1718–1722. [CrossRef] [PubMed]
33. Beer-Davidson, G.; Hindiyeh, M.; Muhsen, K. Detection of Helicobacter Pylori in Stool Samples of Young Children Using Real-Time Polymerase Chain Reaction. *Helicobacter* **2018**, *23*, e12450. [CrossRef] [PubMed]
34. Vécsei, A.; Innerhofer, A.; Binder, C.; Gizci, H.; Hammer, K.; Bruckdorfer, A.; Riedl, S.; Gadner, H.; Hirschl, A.M.; Makristathis, A. Stool Polymerase Chain Reaction for Helicobacter Pylori Detection and Clarithromycin Susceptibility Testing in Children. *Clin. Gastroenterol. Hepatol.* **2010**, *8*, 309–312. [CrossRef] [PubMed]
35. Noguchi, N.; Rimbara, E.; Kato, A.; Tanaka, A.; Tokunaga, K.; Kawai, T.; Takahashi, S.; Sasatsu, M. Detection of Mixed Clarithromycin-Resistant and -Susceptible Helicobacter Pylori Using Nested PCR and Direct Sequencing of DNA Extracted from Faeces. *J. Med. Microbiol.* **2007**, *56*, 1174–1180. [CrossRef]
36. Marrero Rolon, R.; Cunningham, S.A.; Mandrekar, J.N.; Polo, E.T.; Patel, R. Clinical Evaluation of a Real-Time PCR Assay for Simultaneous Detection of Helicobacter Pylori and Genotypic Markers of Clarithromycin Resistance Directly from Stool. *J. Clin. Microbiol.* **2021**, *59*, e03040-20. [CrossRef]

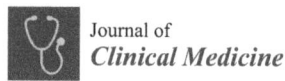

Review

The Coexistence of Nonalcoholic Fatty Liver Disease and Type 2 Diabetes Mellitus

Marcin Kosmalski [1,*], Sylwia Ziółkowska [2], Piotr Czarny [2], Janusz Szemraj [2] and Tadeusz Pietras [1]

[1] Department of Clinical Pharmacology, Medical University of Lodz, 90-153 Lodz, Poland; tadeusz.pietras@umed.lodz.pl
[2] Department of Medical Biochemistry, Medical University of Lodz, 92-215 Lodz, Poland; sylwia.ziolkowska@stud.umed.lodz.pl (S.Z.); piotr.czarny@umed.lodz.pl (P.C.); janusz.szemraj@umed.lodz.pl (J.S.)
* Correspondence: marcin.kosmalski@umed.lodz.pl

Abstract: The incidence of nonalcoholic fatty liver disease (NAFLD) is growing worldwide. Epidemiological data suggest a strong relationship between NAFLD and T2DM. This is associated with common risk factors and pathogenesis, where obesity, insulin resistance and dyslipidemia play pivotal roles. Expanding knowledge on the coexistence of NAFLD and T2DM could not only protect against liver damage and glucotoxicity, but may also theoretically prevent the subsequent occurrence of other diseases, such as cancer and cardiovascular disorders, as well as influence morbidity and mortality rates. In everyday clinical practice, underestimation of this problem is still observed. NAFLD is not looked for in T2DM patients; on the contrary, diagnosis for glucose metabolism disturbances is usually not performed in patients with NAFLD. However, simple and cost-effective methods of detection of fatty liver in T2DM patients are still needed, especially in outpatient settings. The treatment of NAFLD, especially where it coexists with T2DM, consists mainly of lifestyle modification. It is also suggested that some drugs, including hypoglycemic agents, may be used to treat NAFLD. Therefore, the aim of this review is to detail current knowledge of NAFLD and T2DM comorbidity, its prevalence, common pathogenesis, diagnostic procedures, complications and treatment, with special attention to outpatient clinics.

Keywords: nonalcoholic fatty liver disease; type 2 diabetes mellitus; epidemiology; diagnosis; treatment; insulin resistance; metabolic syndrome; obesity

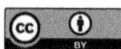

1. Introduction

The term nonalcoholic fatty liver disease (NAFLD) appeared more than 40 years ago, but neither its pathophysiology nor diagnostic criteria were established for many years [1]. In NAFLD, the buildup of excessive fat in the liver is not triggered by significant alcohol consumption. The American Association for the Study of Liver Diseases (AASLD) Practice Guidance of 2018 categorizes NAFLD into nonalcoholic fatty liver (NAFL) or nonalcoholic steatohepatitis (NASH) [2]. NAFL can be diagnosed in cases of at least 5% hepatic steatosis without appearance of hepatocellular injury, while NASH is defined as at least 5% steatosis but with inflammation and hepatocyte injury (e.g., ballooning). In both histological types, fibrosis may or may not be observed [2]. In 2020, the term metabolic-associated fatty liver disease (MAFLD) was coined, which more appropriately characterizes the nature of the disorder; in the definition of MAFLD, the excessive consumption of alcohol is not an excluding criterion [3].

With respect to the causes of excessive accumulation of triglycerides (TG) in the liver, there are two forms of NAFLD: primary and secondary, which have the same clinical and histological signs. The latter occurs in patients with metabolic syndrome (MetS), especially coexisting with type 2 diabetes mellitus (T2DM) [4]. The former is less common and should be suspected in patients with hepatic steatosis without conventional risk factors (Table 1) [5,6].

Table 1. Secondary causes of liver steatosis.

Medications	cART in HIV, chemotherapy, amiodarone, methotrexate, tamoxifen, corticosteroids, tetracyclines, valproic acid, amphetamines, acetylsalicylic acid
Genetic causes	haemochromatosis, alpha-1 antitrypsin deficiency, Wilson's disease, congenital lipodystrophy, abetalipoproteinaemia, hypobetalipoproteinaemia, familial hyperlipidaemia, lysosomal acid lipase deficiency, glycogen storage diseases, hereditary fructose intolerance, urea cycle disorders, citrin deficiency
Environmental causes	lead, arsenic, mercury, cadmium, herbicides, pesticides, polychlorinated biphenyls, chloroalkenes
Nutritional/gastroenterological causes	severe surgical weight loss, starvation, malnutrition, total parenteral nutrition, microbiome changes, coeliac disease, pancreatectomy, short bowel syndrome
Other causes	Chronic HCV infection, hypothyroidism, polycystic ovary syndrome, hypothalamic or pituitary dysfunction, growth hormone deficiency, HELLP syndrome, acute fatty liver of pregnancy, celiac disease, Wilson's disease, hepatitis C virus, *Amanita phalloides* mushrooms, phosphorous poisoning, petrochemicals, *Bacillus cereus* toxin

cART—combined antiretroviral therapy; HIV—human immunodeficiency virus; HELLP—hemolysis, elevated liver enzymes and low platelets.

It has been found that isolated ultrasonography (USS)-diagnosed NAFLD is not associated with increased mortality. However, in some cases it may progress to fibrosis, cirrhosis or hepatocellular carcinoma (HCC). It leads to increased liver-related and all-cause mortality, mainly due to cardiovascular causes, independent of other known factors [7]. Some data suggest that NAFLD is associated with damage to many organs and tissues, including the cardiovascular system [8].

Some data suggest that NAFLD may predict the development of T2DM in the future, and vice versa [9,10]. Additionally, the presence of NAFLD in diabetic patients is associated with poor glycemic control and other serious complications [11]. Similarly, the presence of T2DM in patients with excessive fatty liver infiltration can contribute to progress of NAFLD and damage of the organ [12].

To represent knowledge in the area of NAFLD and its association with T2DM, we searched PubMed papers focusing on common pathogenesis, diagnosis, complications and treatment. The following keywords were used: T2DM, insulin resistance, NAFLD, fatty liver, nonalcoholic fatty liver, nonalcoholic steatohepatitis, diagnosis, ultrasonography, transient elastography, complications, treatment, metformin, thiazolidinediones, GLP-1 agonists and DPP-4 inhibitors. The main aim of this review is to represent current knowledge on the coexistence of NAFLD and T2DM, its prevalence, common pathogenesis, diagnostic procedures and treatment, with special attention to outpatient clinics.

2. Epidemiology

The frequency of NAFLD differs in various parts of the world, but its prevalence is increasing worldwide [13]. Many studies suggest that its occurrence is determined by economic, genetic and ethnic risk factors [14]. Realistic assessment of the number of NAFLD cases is significantly affected by the diagnostic method used [15]. The problem with epidemiological data highlights the difficulty in distinguishing NAFLD from NASH, as well as the assessment of secondary causes of hepatic steatosis [16]. The proportion of patients with NAFLD in the world is 25.24% and is still increasing [17]. A higher prevalence is mostly observed in developed countries, with diets rich in saturated fats. For example, in Europe, NAFLD occurs in 23.17% of the population [18].

A meta-analysis published in 2021, comparing 32 studies, showed that the frequency of hepatic steatosis differs across populations, e.g., 31% in Asia [19]. Furthermore, data collected from the 2011–2014 National Health and Nutrition Examination Survey (NHANES) reported 21.9% (95% CI 20.6–23.3) cases of NAFLD among US adults [20].

Although the prevalence of NAFLD differs in various ethnic groups, it is more common among men and in patients older than 50 years [17]. Additionally, after adjustment for age, sex and race/ethnicity, it was found that NAFLD occurred significantly more often in overweight and obese individuals [21]. Similar observations have been found for other metabolic risk factors. A strong and independent correlation between NAFLD and insulin resistance (IR), in patients with or without diabetes, has been observed [22]. This problem also affects elderly patients. Data from the Rotterdam Study showed that NAFLD was present in 35.1% patients, but its prevalence decreased with advanced age [23].

NAFLD is an independent risk factor for MetS [24]. Furthermore, the criteria for MetS are similar to the symptoms of NAFLD [25]. Every component of MetS, as well as their number, increases the risk of NAFLD and its severity [26]. Furthermore, the great majority of NAFLD cases meet at least one MetS criterion, while 33% meet all five criteria [27]. Interestingly, in patients with MetS, fatty livers are diagnosed almost 10-fold more frequently than in patients without this disorder [28,29]. Nevertheless, T2DM is closely linked with MetS since it is considered to be a metabolic disorder. The key factor in the pathogenesis of NAFLD, T2DM and MetS is obesity. Although NAFLD can also occur in lean individuals, it has been found that the degree of steatosis increases with BMI [30]. Moreover, simple fatty liver will develop into NASH in 3% of non-obese patients, but in 20% of obese patients [31]. With respect to obesity and MetS, a European multi-cohort study of obese people found that MetS occurred in up to 78% of men and 65% of women [32]. Recent studies have suggested that MetS, obesity and T2DM may be associated with colonic diverticulosis [33,34]. Diverticula are structural changes in the wall of the colon that arise from a hernia of the colonic mucosa and submucosa as a result of defects in the muscle layers within the colonic wall [35]. Colonic diverticulosis is closely related to obesity. Excess visceral fat, which is important not only in obesity but also in NAFLD, T2DM, and MetS, is a significant risk factor in colonic diverticulosis. The development of the above diseases, as well as problems with gut microbiota, can contribute to the formation of diverticula [36]. It has been shown that the condition occurs more frequently in more severe cases of fatty liver. In patients with colonic diverticulosis and liver steatosis, hypertension, T2DM and hypothyroidism were observed more frequently. Moreover, fatty liver was more common in the more severe forms of colonic diverticulosis [37].

In some regions (e.g., the Asia-Pacific region), NAFLD is also diagnosed in patients with lower BMI [38]. In a Korean study of 29,994 adults, NAFLD was found in 12.6% of non-obese subjects and in 50.1% of obese subjects. Further, in non-obese NAFLD patients, especially women, significantly higher prevalence rates for other components of MetS than for obesity were observed [39]. Overall, studies show that NAFLD is found mostly in obese people, and the onset of hepatic steatosis in a lean person is a risk factor for expansion of fat mass [17,40]. An Indian study established a clinical association of NAFLD with dyslipidemia, hypertension and obesity. In this study, the T2DM population with these comorbidities had 38%, 17% and 14% higher risk for NAFLD, respectively. It should be emphasized that mean AST (aspartate aminotransferase) and ALT (alanine aminotransferase) levels in NAFLD patients were highest in those aged 25–40 and lowest in those aged 71–84 [41].

The prevalence of NAFLD in patients with abnormal glucose metabolism is very high, independently of diagnostic method. Ortiz-Lopez et al. found that patients with NAFLD had impaired fasting glucose (IFG) and/or impaired glucose tolerance (IGT) significantly more often than those without NAFLD [42]. Two major European studies reported NAFLD prevalence rates of 42.6–69.5% in large samples of T2DM patients [43]. A long term (5 years) Korean prospective cohort study, performed on 25,232 Korean men without T2DM, compared the incidence rate of T2DM according to the degree of NAFLD (normal, mild, and moderate to severe). The incidence of T2DM increased according to the degree of NAFLD (normal: 7.0%, mild: 9.8%, moderate to severe: 17.8%) [44]. The Ragama Health Study also revealed an increased risk of developing T2DM in patients with ultrasound-diagnosed NAFLD. Of 2984 subjects, 31% had NAFLD and 22.65% diabetes. After three years of observation, 19.7% patients with NAFLD and 10.5% without NAFLD developed T2DM. The frequency of diabetes was 64.2 and 34.0 per 1000 person-years for patients with and without NAFLD, respectively [9]. In a Polish study the frequency of ultrasound features of NAFLD in patients with newly diagnosed T2DM was 71% in patients with mean age 55.64 ± 13.42 years. Additionally, in patients with NAFLD, mean body weight, waist and hip circumferences, body mass index (BMI), liver enzyme activity, serum C-reactive protein, total cholesterol and TG were higher, while HDL-cholesterol was significantly lower. There were no statistical differences between parameters of glycemic control in groups with and without NAFLD [45]. On the other hand, Yan Y et al., by means of USS, found a high fatty liver (56.7%) in T2DM patients (69.6%) [46]. In the Edinburgh Type 2 Diabetes Study (ET2DS) (939 participants, aged 61–76 years with T2DM) ultrasound signs of fatty liver were present in 56.9% of participants. After excluding those with a secondary cause for steatosis, the prevalence of NAFLD in the study was 42.6%. Additionally, independent predictors of NAFLD were not only high BMI and TG, but also shorter duration of diabetes, HbA1c and metformin use [47]. In two meta-analyses from 2017 [48] and 2019 [49], 55.5–59.67% of T2DM cases had NAFLD, while 77.87% were simultaneously obese with fatty livers.

Despite the high prevalence of NAFLD and T2DM coexistence, AASLD guidelines do not recommend performing screening for NAFLD in diabetic patients. However, they suggest that screening tests for NAFLD are not cost–effective in relation to the long-term benefits [2].

3. Common Pathogenesis

The pathogenesis of T2DM and NAFLD is complex and not fully understood, but the presence of many common elements in the development of both diseases has been demonstrated. These include: alterations in glucose and lipid metabolism, IR, insulin secretion, genetic predisposition and environmental influences (such as endocrine disruptors), epigenetic factors and lifestyle changes [50]. Recently conducted studies indicate the complex interplay between carbohydrate metabolism and NAFLD and vice versa [51]. The development of NAFLD is strongly associated with hepatic IR. However, whether NAFLD is a consequence or cause of IR is a matter of debate. A number of studies conducted in NAFLD patients showed both an impaired ability of insulin to suppress endogenous glucose production (indicating the presence of hepatic IR) and approximately 50% reduction in glucose disposal (a measure of whole-body insulin-sensitivity) [52]. The associations between T2DM, NAFLD, IR are shown in Figure 1.

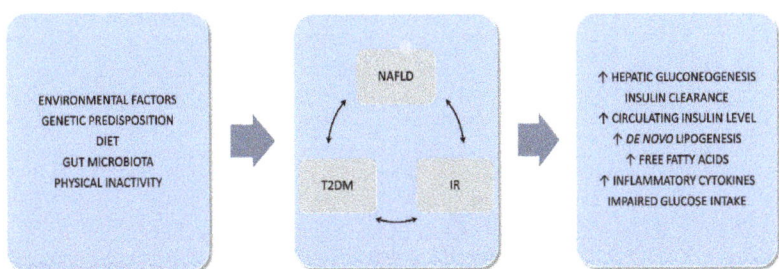

Figure 1. Common pathophysiologic mechanism in nonalcoholic fatty liver disease and type 2 diabetes mellitus. IR–insulin resistance; NAFLD–nonalcoholic fatty liver disease; T2DM–type 2 diabetes mellitus. The up arrow means height.

Chai et al. demonstrated that, in patients with similar levels of IR and hyperglycemia, NAFLD with T2DM was associated with higher serum insulin levels than T2DM alone. In these cases, hyperinsulinemia was caused mainly by beta-cell hypersecretion [53]. This observation was further confirmed in a study by Finucane et al., where healthy patients with NAFLD had higher insulin and C-peptide levels after oral glucose loading. However, in this group of patients, the C-peptide increment and adaptation index were significantly lower [54]. The association between NAFLD and IR can be explained by the "multiple-hit hypothesis". The "first hit" is associated with impaired cellular response to insulin and compensatory IR. In adipose tissue, this affects hormone-sensitive lipase (HSL) increasing the risk of lipolysis with consequent release of free fatty acids (FFA) to the liver. Glucose absorption decreases in the skeletal muscles, while, in hepatocytes, hyperinsulinemia increases gluconeogenesis, decreases glycogen synthesis, increases uptake of FFA, alters the transport of TG, such as very low-density lipoproteins (VLDL), and inhibits beta-oxidation. These alterations in the metabolism of fat are the basis of NAFLD development.

The changes referred to above result from a complex interplay between various factors, such as hepatic resistance to leptin, or the reduction of adiponectin levels. The "second hit" is a consequence of oxidative stress in hepatocytes, which is initially compensated by cellular antioxidant mechanisms. However, overload of the liver with FFA generates reactive oxygen species (ROS) in the mitochondrial chain, which act on the fatty acids of the cell membranes, causing lipid peroxidation. ROS induce proinflammatory cytokine synthesis in Kupffer cells and hepatocytes. This second phase explains the evaluation necroinflammatory phenomenon, fibrosis and liver cirrhosis. There are many other "hits" involved in the pathogenesis of NAFLD, including genetic and epigenetic factors, the intestinal microflora and the cannabinoid system [55]. In the case of hepatic steatosis, T2DM or dysregulation of fasting glucose is found in 18–33% of NAFLD cases [56]. Moreover, these patients, as well as those with advanced fibrosis, have a higher IR [57]. Furthermore, patients with T2DM usually present with dyslipidemia with an elevated plasma TG, small LDL and decreased HDL cholesterol. IR results in lipolysis and, hence, increased circulating FFA, which are later taken up and oxidized by the liver, leading to formation of free radicals. TNF alpha, which is a proinflammatory marker, is also elevated in patients who are insulin resistant, as opposed to adiponectin, an anti-lipogenic and anti-inflammatory factor, which is decreased.

The pathogenesis of T2DM or NAFLD is similar to the processes observed in obesity. In this condition, elevated levels of very low-density lipoproteins (VLDL) can be observed which act as TG carriers and play a role in hypertriglyceridemia [58]. Moreover, increase in TG concentration is also caused by enhanced FFA flow to the liver and other tissues, which may contribute to the development of IR present in NAFLD, T2DM and obesity [59]. Additionally, the accumulation of fat in adipose tissue leads to the development of inflammation by stimulating the production of cytokines, e.g., TNF-α and IL-6, and may result in hypertension [60].

All the changes referred to above may lead to NAFLD and NASH. TNF alpha increases mitochondrial generation of ROS and recruits inflammatory cells, which can lead to steatohepatitis [61]. Moreover, the presence of the *PNPLA3* single nucleotide polymorphism, that is common in individuals with fatty livers, links hepatic steatosis and diabetes. *PNPLA3* encodes adiponutrin, which is associated with TG metabolism in adipocytes. Unfortunately, its function is poorly understood. The occurrence of the I148M (polymorphism in 148 position; isoleucine to methionine) variant increases the risk of T2DM and IR in NAFLD patients [62,63].

Nevertheless, the border between NAFLD and NASH is very thin. It is difficult to differentiate simple fatty liver from steatohepatitis without using invasive diagnostic methods. In a study of T2DM patients, each of the 63 research participants had fatty liver, but 94.82% of them had NASH, which was confirmed by liver biopsy. This suggests that steatohepatitis may be associated with the early stages of T2DM development, perhaps due to the association of NASH with IR [64].

One of the "hits" in the multi-hit hypothesis is the gut microbiota, which play a role not only in NAFLD, but also in T2DM. The gut microbiota is found to be an important regulator of the host's energy metabolism [65,66]. Compounds are transported from the intestine to the liver through the portal vein, and the liver transfers antibodies back through the bile [67]. The permeability and composition of the mucus are dependent on the intestinal microflora, and its dysfunction results in the production of molecular patterns associated with pathogens (PAMP). Increased permeability results in enhanced liver inflammation [68,69]. Any changes that occur in its composition or its functioning may also affect metabolism in the liver, adipose tissue or muscles. Modulation of the intestinal microbiome may alleviate metabolic disorders by increasing the availability of fiber to microorganisms residing in the organism [70,71]. Moreover, less variability in the gut microflora was observed in NAFLD patients when compared to healthy controls [72,73].

Any disturbances in the gut-liver axis, including dysbiosis and increased gut permeability, may have an impact on NAFLD onset. Moreover, the impact of short-chain fatty acids (SCFAs) and succinate (microbial metabolites) on the microbiome promotes improvement in obesity-related insulin sensitivity in animals and influences mass control and glucose and lipid homeostasis in humans [74–76]. SCFAs, butyrate in particular, play a major role in maintaining the integrity of the intestinal wall, which prevents the migration of toxic and proinflammatory molecules into the liver [77]. Studies in rodent models of NAFLD fed a high-fat diet showed that sodium butyrate protected against the onset of fatty liver and decreased the IR [78,79]. Another well-known microbiome-derived compound is lipopolysaccharide, which is released in the colon from dead Gram-negative bacteria. Lipopolysaccharide plays a key role in the progression of metabolic diseases, such as NAFLD, insulin resistance and T2DM [80].

Obesity-induced IR is important in NAFLD and T2DM, and research findings show that IR may also be regulated by the gut microflora. The composition of the microbiome of obese individuals with T2DM is noticeably different from that of healthy people [81]. Men with MetS and IR, after receiving intestinal microbiota infusions from lean individuals, had a higher amount of butyrate produced and showed an improvement in insulin sensitivity [82]. Moreover, in patients with T2DM, a high-fat diet may lead to increased intestinal permeability and inflammation [83,84].

There is a significant link between NAFLD and cardiovascular disease. Fatty liver is associated with a high degree of calcification of the coronary arteries, regardless of the presence of metabolic syndrome, and risk factors for cardiovascular disorders and metabolic syndrome [85]. NAFLD patients have an increased risk of acute coronary syndrome and ischemic stroke due to endothelial dysfunction [86]. In the case of hepatic steatosis, an increase in arterial stiffness, a marker of cardiac hypertrophy and atherosclerotic lesions is also observed [87]. A meta-analysis involving 37 studies of metabolic syndrome confirmed the increased risk of cardiovascular events in this group of patients [88]. Another meta-analysis of 16 studies showed that a more severe course of NAFLD significantly increases the frequency of cardiovascular events [89]. Moreover, patients with fatty liver and coexistent T2DM have an almost four times higher risk of cardiovascular disease [85].

Moreover, recent studies have shown that treatment with direct-acting antivirals on HCV resulted in a reduction in HOMA-IR, an indicator that measures IR levels, in HCV patients [90]. Furthermore, the incidence of cardiovascular events was also reduced in both prediabetic and non-diabetic HCV patients treated with direct acting antivirals [91,92]. This suggests a link between liver disease and problems with the cardiovascular system.

An increase in fat content, which reduces insulin sensitivity, leads to increased lipolysis and an increase in FFA levels [93,94]. Moreover, skeletal muscle cells with IR have been shown to transfer stored glycogen to the de novo lipogenesis pathway in the liver [95,96]. Peripheral IR modifies lipid metabolism, which facilitates the generation of hepatic IR. Both visceral and peripheral fat content induce IR in hepatocytes [97]. Due to the hypertriglyceridemia present in fatty liver, visceral adipose tissue increases the production of leptin, which impairs insulin sensitivity, and reduces the level of adiponectin, which stimulates the action of insulin in peripheral tissues [98]. The decreased level of adiponectin leads to decreased antioxidant effects and the formation of hepatic fibrosis [99,100]. Recent studies showed an association between NAFLD and the incidence of fatty pancreas, also called nonalcoholic fatty pancreatic disease (NAFPD). NAFPD occurs in approximately 16% of the general adult population [101]. It is characterized by excessive accumulation of lipids in the pancreas [101,102]. Accumulated fat, and thus the presence of 12/15-lipoxygenase, lead to inflammation in pancreatic islet cells. Moreover, the accumulated fat may interfere with exocrine pancreatic function, which may lead to the development of pancreatic cancer [101]. There is also evidence of an association between fatty pancreatic and hepatic steatosis, and it can be argued that the presence of both conditions worsens the condition of NAFLD patients [103]. It has been shown that MetS risk factors are correlated with the risk of pancreatic steatosis, which may be a significant manifestation of MetS [104].

NAFPD is closely related, not only to MetS, but also to obesity, which is a risk factor for fatty pancreas. As for liver steatosis, there is also no approved treatment for pancreatic steatosis, but weight loss and bariatric surgery reduce the amount of fat in the pancreas [103]. Pancreatic steatosis occurs in approximately half of NAFLD patients, as confirmed by ultrasound, proton magnetic resonance spectroscopy and histopathological findings [105–107]. Human studies suggest that NAFPD also has an influence on the development of T2DM and prediabetic state [103]. Accumulated excess fat leads to loss of β-cell function, which may lead to diabetes [108]. In addition, NAFLD and NAFPD affect glucose metabolism and the function of β cells [102]. Prediabetic patients had a higher pancreatic fat content, but the relationship between insulin secretion and pancreatic fatty tissue has not been confirmed. However, there is evidence of the importance of IR in fatty pancreas [108]. Although a link with impaired sugar metabolism can be confirmed, the role of pancreatic fatty in the development of diabetes requires further clarification.

Mitochondria, responsible for beta-oxidation, are very important for metabolic disorders, NAFLD, and T2DM [109]. Mitochondrial dysfunction, and thus impaired fatty acid oxidation processes, leads to an increase in ROS levels and, consequently, to elevated oxidative stress [110]. ROS stimulate the activity of signaling pathways capable of inducing necroinflammation in liver cells. Impaired lipid beta-oxidation also leads to the accumulation of lipotoxic intermediates, which further increase inflammation and alter insulin signaling [111]. Insulin is important to mitochondria, due to their maintaining an appropriate NAD+/NADH ratio, while free radicals from mitochondria alter insulin sensitivity, disrupt insulin signaling and result in IR [112]. Molecules affecting the proper functioning of mitochondria include Slc25a1, associated with the metabolic processes of FFA and glycolytic pathways. Inhibition of Slc25a1 protects against NASH and reduces steatosis and steatohepatitis [113]. Another example is carnitine, which transports fatty acids into the mitochondrial matrix. It inhibits oxidative stress, enhances β-oxidation, and reduces IR. Carnitine supplementation improves both HOMA-IR and AST, ALT, and TG parameters in NAFLD patients [114].

4. Diagnosis

NAFLD is a common, often asymptomatic, liver disease. Therefore, its diagnosis requires the exclusion of other causes of steatosis, such as alcohol consumption [17]. Patients with NAFLD may report fatigue, daytime sleepiness, right upper quadrant abdominal pain or discomfort. On physical examination hepatomegaly and other signs of liver insufficiency are often present. In some cases, there are extrahepatic symptoms, such as joint and muscle pains [115].

Until now, steatosis required to be diagnosed by liver biopsy, which was considered the gold standard. Due to the fact that biopsy is an invasive method, transient elastography (TE), also known as FibroScan, is preferable. Unfortunately, biopsy is still considered the most accurate way to identify the stages of steatosis and fibrosis, despite the invasiveness of this method [116]. The most common method for identifying NAFLD is USS, because it is more widely available and cheaper than the other techniques. The USS diagnostic method has a sensitivity of 60–94% and a specificity of 66–95% [117]. However, this method does not reliably detect steatosis when it is below 20% in individuals with high BMI > 40 kg/m^2 and is operator dependent [118].

CT (computer tomography) is non-invasive, widely available and easy to perform, but it also has some disadvantages, including a potential ionizing radiation hazard and limited accuracy in diagnosing mild hepatic steatosis [119].

Magnetic resonance imaging has numerous advantages, including being unaffected by obesity, simple steatosis, inflammation or the presence of ascites. On the other hand, these imaging methods are limited by high cost and low accessibility. They are also dependent on patient factors, such as inability to perform breath-hold, and signal degradation in patients with severe iron overload [120]. Nevertheless, some studies have shown, that MRI-PDFF (magnetic resonance imaging–proton density fat fraction) can be as effective as liver biopsy in steatosis diagnostics [121,122]. Apart from this, a quantitative estimation of liver fat can only be obtained by magnetic resonance spectroscopy (MRS). Therefore, this technique is of value in clinical trials and experimental studies, but is expensive and not recommended for everyday clinical practice [123].

Another imaging technique, the controlled attenuation parameter (CAP) using TE, can diagnose steatosis and fibrosis, but has limited ability to discriminate histological grades [124]. CAP has shown excellent diagnostic accuracy for detecting hepatic steatosis, in comparison to liver biopsy [125–128] and MRI-PDFF [129,130], even in morbidly obese individuals [131].

Liver enzyme activity (ALT, AST, GGT), total bilirubin, lipids fractions, apolipoprotein A1 (ApoA1), α-2-macroglobulin (α2M), haptoglobin (Hp), fasting blood glucose, and fasting insulin are used to generate liver steatosis scores (Table 2.). The best-validated scores are the fatty liver index (FLI), the SteatoTest and the NAFLD liver fat score [132,133]. They predict metabolic, hepatic and cardiovascular outcomes/mortality. These scores are associated with IR and reliably predict the presence, but not the severity, of steatosis [120].

Table 2. Non-invasive scoring system to diagnose NAFLD progression.

Index	Factors
AST/ALT ratio	AST, ALT
APRI (AST to platelet ratio index)	AST, upper normal limit for ALT, PLT
FibroTest	Age, gender, total bilirubin, haptoglobin, GGT, α2-macroglobulin, apolipoprotein-A
FibroMax	Age, gender, total bilirubin, haptoglobin, GGT, α2-macroglobulin, apolipoprotein-A, ALT, AST, TCH, TG, fasting glucose, weight, height
FibroMeter	HA, PLT, prothrombin index, α2-macroglobulin
BARD	BMI, AST/ALT ratio, diabetes mellitus
NFS (NAFLD fibrosis score)	Age, hyperglycemia, BMI, PLT, albumin, AST/ALT ratio
FIB-4 (fibrosis 4 index)	Age, AST, ALT, PLT
HepatoScore	Age, gender, bilirubin, GGT, HA, α2-macroglobulin
OELF (Original European Liver Fibrosis panel)	Age, TIMP 1, HA, P3NP
ELF (European Liver Fibrosis panel)	HA, P3NP, TIMP-1
NIKEI (Noninvasive Koeln–Essen-index)	Age, AST, AST/ALT ratio, total bilirubin

ALT–alanine aminotransferase; AST–aspartate aminotransferase; BMI–body mass index; GGT–gammaglutamyltransferase; HA–hyaluronic acid P3NP–amino-terminal propeptide of type III procolagen; PLT–platelet count; TCH–total cholesterol; TG–trigycerides; TIMP-1–tissue inhibitor of metalloproteinase 1.

Attenuation coefficient (AC) measurements using ultrasound waves have shown the ability to differentiate the severity of hepatic steatosis [134]. Furthermore, AC measurements have been found to be as effective as MRI-PDFF, even in obese people. However, the accuracy of the AC is limited by the occurrence of fibrosis and inflammation [135]. A similar technique is use of the backscatter coefficient (BSC), which has shown similar effects to those of AC [136].

For every NAFLD patient, surrogate markers of fibrosis (NFS, FIB-4, ELF or FibroTest) should be calculated. If significant fibrosis cannot be ruled out, patients should be referred to a liver clinic for further diagnostic procedures, e.g., TE, or, less frequently, magnetic resonance elastography (MRE), acoustic resonance force impulse (AFRI), or supersonic shearwave imaging (SSI) [120].

The final diagnosis should be made by liver biopsy. Liver biopsy is the only procedure that reliably differentiates NAFLD from NASH. Liver biopsy is an expensive and invasive procedure and may cause numerous complications, such as pain, bleeding, infection and, in some rare cases, increases mortality risk [132]. Additionally, its interpretation is influenced by the subjective judgment of the pathologist. It explores only a small portion of the liver parenchyma, which is not always representative of the entire parenchyma [137].

The prevalence of NAFLD is higher in both T2DM and prediabetes patients. In both conditions, the severity of NAFLD, progression to NASH, advanced fibrosis, and the development of HCC, can be observed independently of the level of liver enzymes [9,10]. According to recommendations for patients with T2DM, routine screening for NAFLD is not advised at this time because of uncertainties surrounding diagnostic tests and treatment options, along with lack of knowledge related to the long-term benefit and cost-effectiveness of screening [2].

Conversely, USS-defined NAFLD is associated with a 2–5-fold risk of developing T2DM, after adjustment for several lifestyle and metabolic confounders [8]. In persons with NAFLD, screening for diabetes is mandatory, by fasting or random venous glucose concentration, HbA1c concentration, or standardized 75 g oral glucose tolerance test (OGTT) [138].

A diagram demonstrating non-invasive diagnostics methods of NAFLD is presented below (Figure 2).

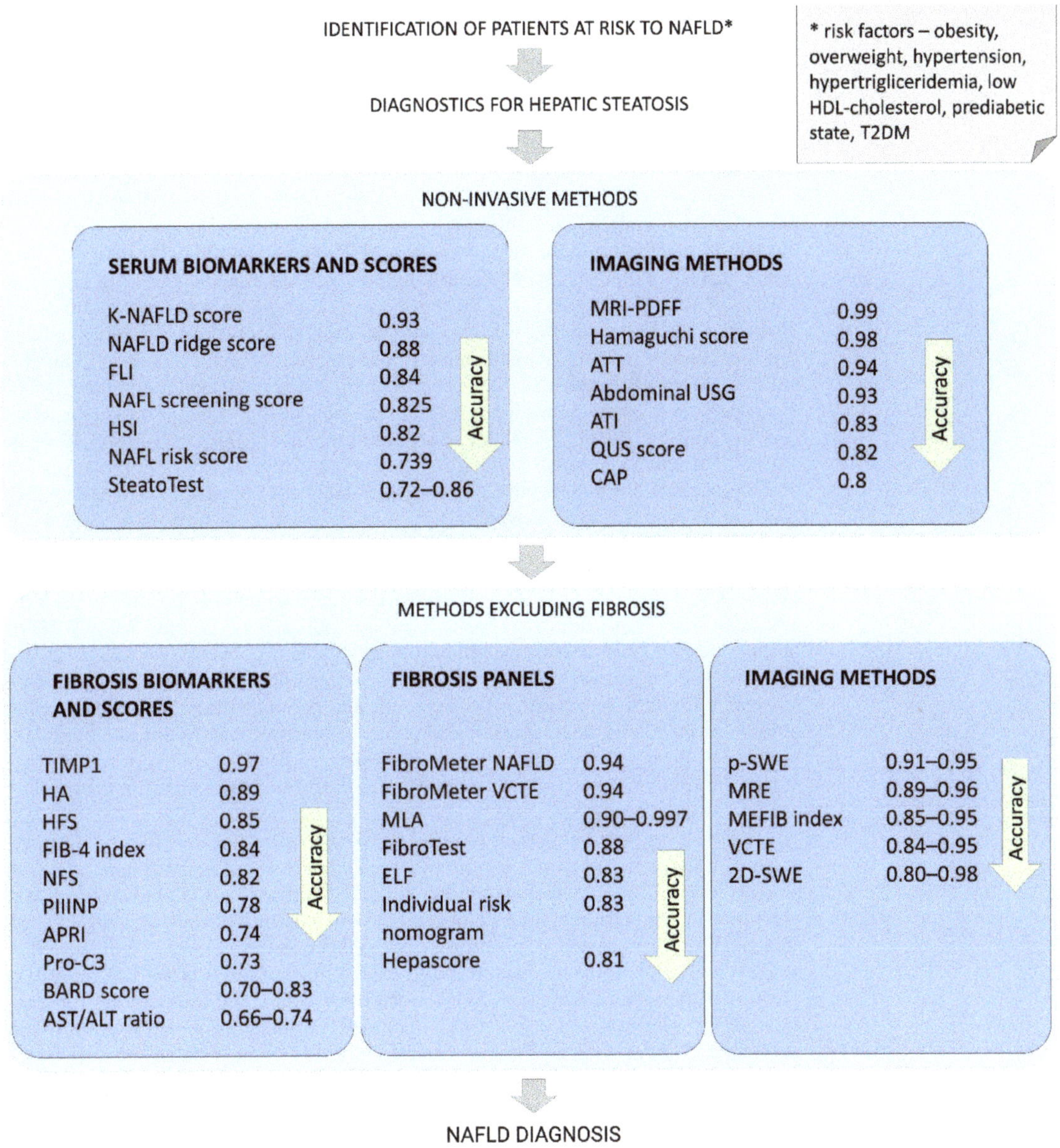

IDENTIFICATION OF PATIENTS AT RISK TO NAFLD*

*risk factors – obesity, overweight, hypertension, hypertriglyceridemia, low HDL-cholesterol, prediabetic state, T2DM

DIAGNOSTICS FOR HEPATIC STEATOSIS

NON-INVASIVE METHODS

SERUM BIOMARKERS AND SCORES

K-NAFLD score	0.93
NAFLD ridge score	0.88
FLI	0.84
NAFL screening score	0.825
HSI	0.82
NAFL risk score	0.739
SteatoTest	0.72–0.86

IMAGING METHODS

MRI-PDFF	0.99
Hamaguchi score	0.98
ATT	0.94
Abdominal USG	0.93
ATI	0.83
QUS score	0.82
CAP	0.8

METHODS EXCLUDING FIBROSIS

FIBROSIS BIOMARKERS AND SCORES

TIMP1	0.97
HA	0.89
HFS	0.85
FIB-4 index	0.84
NFS	0.82
PIIINP	0.78
APRI	0.74
Pro-C3	0.73
BARD score	0.70–0.83
AST/ALT ratio	0.66–0.74

FIBROSIS PANELS

FibroMeter NAFLD	0.94
FibroMeter VCTE	0.94
MLA	0.90–0.997
FibroTest	0.88
ELF	0.83
Individual risk nomogram	0.83
Hepascore	0.81

IMAGING METHODS

p-SWE	0.91–0.95
MRE	0.89–0.96
MEFIB index	0.85–0.95
VCTE	0.84–0.95
2D-SWE	0.80–0.98

NAFLD DIAGNOSIS

2D-SWE: Two-dimensional shear wave elastography; ALT: Alanine aminotransferase; APRI: Aspartate aminotransferase to platelet ratio index; AST: Aspartate aminotransferase; ATI: Attenuation imaging; ATT: Attenuation coefficient; BARD score: Calculated from BMI, AST:ALT ratio and DM presence; CAP: Controlled attenuation parameter; ELF: Enhanced liver fibrosis; FIB-4 index: Fibrosis-4 Index; FLI: Fatty liver index; HA: Hyaluronic acid; HDL: High-density lipoprotein; HFS: Hepamet fibrosis score; HSI: Hepatic steatosis index; MEFIB index: MRE combined with FIB-4 index; MLA: Machine learning algorithm; MRE: Magnetic resonance elastograph; MRI-PDFF: Magnetic resonance imaging proton density fat fraction; NAFL: Non-alcoholic fatty liver; NAFLD: Non-alcoholic fatty liver disease; NFS: NAFLD fibrosis score; PIIINP: Procollagen III amino-terminal peptide; Pro-C3: Neoepitope-specific competitive enzyme-linked immunosorbent assay for PIIINP; p-SWE: Point shear wave elastography; QUS: Quantitative ultrasound; T2DM: Type 2 diabetes mellitus; TIMP1: Tissue inhibitor of metalloproteinases 1; USG: Ultrasonography; VCTE: Vibration controlled transient elastography.

Figure 2. Diagram demonstrating the diagnosis methods of NAFLD in order of accuracy. Accuracy is presented as AUC (area under the receiver-operating characteristics curve) value. The figure does not include liver biopsy, which remains the gold standard procedure for the diagnosis of nonalcoholic steatohepatitis (NASH) and staging of nonalcoholic fatty liver disease (NAFLD) [139].

5. Complications

It seems that NAFLD is underdiagnosed in daily medical practice, even in patients with T2DM, even though coexistence of these pathologies increases the risk for patients. In subjects with NAFLD, T2DM appears to be a significant risk factor for advanced fibrosis. Additionally, not only T2DM, but also prediabetes are independently associated with portal inflammation, fibrosis, NASH and more severe histological findings in NAFLD patients [140].

Stepanova et al. found that patients with NAFLD and T2DM are at the highest risk for overall and liver-related mortality [141]. Of concern, T2DM is associated with a two-fold risk of chronic liver disease secondary to NAFLD, cirrhosis and HCC [17]. Moreover, family history of diabetes, especially among nondiabetics, is associated with NASH and fibrosis in NAFLD patients [142]. Furthermore, a diagnosis of NAFLD in patients with established T2DM is strongly associated with poor glycemic control, proliferative retinopathy, increased prevalence of cardiac/kidney disease and a 2.2-fold increase in all-cause mortality compared to subjects without NAFLD [8]. Hyperinsulinemia and hyperglycemia, and especially glycemic variability, are important predictive factors for the progression of hepatic fibrosis in NAFLD [143]. Lv et al. found that NAFLD was positively correlated with BMI, waist circumference (WC), TG, fasting blood glucose, diastolic blood pressure, and systolic blood pressure, but negatively correlated with the duration of diabetes, diabetic nephropathy, diabetic peripheral neuropathy and diabetic retinopathy and level of HDL-cholesterol [144].

The presence of NAFLD in T2DM patients may also increase the risk of cardiovascular disease (CVD) independently of MetS. Turkish researchers compared the CVD risk in T2DM and non-diabetic participants to evaluate the association between NASH and CVD risk. In this study 55 T2DM (study group) and 44 non-diabetic patients (control group) were included. Patients were also differentiated by the degree of hepatosteatosis. Hepatosteatosis rates were found to be similar in both diabetic and non-diabetic patients. Mean carotid intima–media thickness as cardiovascular risk assessment was found to be similar in both hepatosteatosis groups but substantially higher in diabetic patients, regardless of the degree of hepatosteatosis. Mean FPG and HbA1c were found to be higher in the grade ≥ 2 hepatosteatosis group [145].

A Polish study examined cardiovascular risk factors associated with NAFLD and the association between this pathology and macroangiopathy in T2DM patients. A total of 101 patients with T2DM were included in the study. Patients with NAFLD were significantly older but, surprisingly, the duration of diabetes was shorter. Patients with NAFLD had a statistically higher prevalence of coronary angioplasty, but there was no difference in the incidence of coronary heart disease and by-pass surgery. Significantly higher values of cardiovascular risk markers, such as HDL-cholesterol, ALT, and lower concentrations of creatinine were also found in this group of patients. Logistic regression analysis demonstrated that NAFLD was positively correlated with WC above normal and ALT activity but was negatively correlated with creatinine concentration. Further analysis showed that WC and total cholesterol were positive predictors of NAFLD and HDL-cholesterol was a negative prognostic parameter [146].

Targher et al. determined the prevalence of CVD and its risk factors between people diagnosed with T2DM with and without NAFLD. A total of 2839 patients with T2DM were screened. NAFLD was diagnosed by USS after exclusion of secondary causes of hepatic steatosis. To determine the risk of CVD, patients' history, electrocardiogram, echo-Doppler scanning of lower limb and carotid arteries were used. Nearly 70% of patients had NAFLD, and this pathology was the most common liver disease. Its incidence increased with age. It was found that NAFLD patients had a higher prevalence of coronary, cerebrovascular and peripheral vascular disease than their counterparts without NAFLD, after adjustment for age and sex. Additionally, statistical analysis showed that NAFLD was associated with incidence of CVD independently of classical risk factors (e.g., age, sex, smoking, BMI, duration of diabetes, HbA1c, LDL-cholesterol), and actual use of medications, such as, antihypertensive, lipid-lowering, hypoglycemic or antiplatelet drugs [147]. Idilman et al. used coronary computed tomography angiography (CTA) to diagnose coronary artery disease (CAD) in T2DM patients. They also found that tomography-diagnosed NAFLD was associated with significant CAD, even after adjusting for age, gender, obesity, hypertension, smoking status and serum LDL-levels [148].

Bonapace et al. evaluated 50 patients with T2DM (32 patients with NAFLD and 18 without USS signs of fatty liver). Neither ischemic nor valvular heart disease was previously recognized in these patients, who underwent detailed examination by Doppler echocardiography, 24-h Holter monitoring and bicycle ergometry. They showed that presence of NAFLD may impair active and passive left ventricular diastolic function. Additionally, early LV diastolic function impairment in this subgroup of patients was independent of diabetes duration, HbA1c and other cardiometabolic risk factors (including age and sex) [149]. The same main authors, with colleagues, found a positive and independent association between NAFLD and aortic valve sclerosis (AVS) in patients with T2DM [150].

Targher et al. observed 400 patients with T2DM with no history of atrial fibrillation (AF) prospectively for 10 years. A total of 70.2% of these patients had ultrasounds signs of NAFLD. Each year, for every patient, standard 12-lead electrocardiogram (ECG) was performed. During this time, they found 42 incidents of AF. It is important to highlight that 90% of the patients had NAFLD at baseline. Additionally, patients with NAFLD had higher systolic and diastolic blood pressures and pulse pressure. The incidence of AF substantially increased after six years of observation. Statistical analysis revealed that, after adjustment for sex, age, hypertension and ECG changes (PR interval and left ventricular hypertrophy), NAFLD was associated with higher incidence of AF interval [151].

NAFLD not accompanied by IR is not associated with carotid atherosclerosis burden. However, having both NAFLD and IR seems to be an independent predictor of increased C-IMT (carotid intima-media thickness test) [152]. Moreover, the presence of NAFLD in patients admitted for acute ischemic stroke does not appear to be associated with more severe stroke or with worse in-hospital outcomes [153].

In T2DM patients aged 60–74 years both sex (with and without secondary causes of hepatic steatosis), the presence of USS signs of hepatic steatosis was not associated with reduction in renal function based on glomerular filtration rate and albuminuria during a 4-year follow-up [154]. Kim et al. found that NAFLD is inversely associated with prevalence of diabetic retinopathy and nephropathy in Korean patients with T2DM [155].

T2DM that coexists with NAFLD elevates the risk of cirrhosis and HCC. These patients have dyslipidemia, as well as higher hepatic steatosis and inflammation. Moreover, they demonstrate increased blood pressure, LDL and TG, while their HDL level is lower. Thus, T2DM patients with NAFLD have more severe dyslipidemia, hyperinsulinemia and hepatic IR than those without fatty livers [156].

It seems that a diagnosis of NAFLD is associated with a low risk of complications. The risk of complications, mainly cardiovascular, dramatically increases when NAFLD is accompanied by T2DM.

6. NAFLD Pharmacotherapy with Hypoglycemic Agents

According to the recommendations of the AASLD, the management of patients with NAFLD requires not only treatment of liver disease, but also of comorbidities, such as obesity, IR, lipid disorders and T2DM. Although, NAFLD has been researched for decades, there is no approved pharmacological treatment for the disease. Due to this, proper diet and increased physical activity are recommended.

The basic form of treatment for patients with NAFLD and T2DM is lifestyle modification. A sedentary lifestyle is observed not only in patients with hepatic steatosis, but also in those with metabolic syndrome and T2DM [157]. Al-Jiffri et al. found that an approximate 15% reduction in BMI (aerobic exercise training and diet) is effective in improving liver condition and insulin resistance in T2DM patients with NAFLD (i.e., reduction in ALP, ALT, AST, GGT and HOMA-IR) [158]. In NAFLD patients, aerobic exercise improved markers of hepatocyte function and insulin sensitivity regardless of any change in body weight [159]. Generally, people with a healthy lifestyle are less prone to develop IR, impaired glucose tolerance and diabetes [160,161]. According to the AASLD guidance document, exercise can prevent or improve hepatic steatosis in NAFLD, and reduce the likelihood of NASH. Furthermore, vigorous activity has more benefits for NASH patients than moderate activity [2].

A special diet is an important part of treatment of NAFLD and T2DM. Bozzetto et al. suggest that an isocaloric diet enriched in monounsaturated fatty acids (MUFA) compared with a diet higher in carbohydrate and fiber was associated with a clinically significantly lower hepatic fat content in T2DM patients independently of pursuit of an aerobic training program. They suggest that this diet should be considered for nutritional management of hepatic steatosis in people with T2DM [162].

Time-restricted feeding (TRF) is a dietary approach in which access to food is available for 8 h and unavailable for 16 h per day. TRF significantly reduced weight in NAFLD patients [163] and the severity of hepatic steatosis and hyperinsulinemia in mice [164]. Unfortunately, nonpharmacological management of NAFLD and effective weight loss pose some problems, since Stewart K et al. demonstrated that only 10.4% of overweight/obese individuals with NAFLD changed their habits [165].

Clinical trials examining the pharmacotherapy of NAFLD have focused mainly on insulin sensitizers, however, the data is scarce, as the number of studies evaluating the efficacy of glucose lowering agents in patients with NAFLD is small [166].

6.1. Metformin

Data from clinical trials which assessed the usefulness of metformin in the treatment of NAFLD are not consistent. In some cases, metformin in T2DM patients reduced transaminase levels and histological damage [167]. According to the majority of studies, metformin leads to a significant loss in IR and weight reduction in patients with NAFLD [168]. In contrast, Haukeland et al., in a small randomized trial (n = 48), reported that metformin compared with placebo over six months of treatment did not improve liver histology in patients with NAFLD [169]. In animal models with hyperphagic OLETF, aerobic exercise training of rats was more effective than metformin administration in the management of T2DM and NAFLD outcomes. Combining therapies offered little additional benefit beyond exercise alone, and findings suggest that metformin potentially impairs exercise-induced hepatic mitochondrial adaptation [170].

6.2. Thiazolidinediones (TZDs)

TZDs are the most potent evidence-based drugs against NASH [171]. In a rat model, pioglitazone and rosiglitazone prevented activation of hepatic stellate cells in vitro and improved hepatic steatosis and fibrosis [172]. Shadid et al. showed, that pioglitazone improved liver function in obese volunteers with NAFLD [173]. In a Polish study, NAFLD treatment with rosiglitazone was associated with significant improvement in liver enzyme activity and insulin sensitivity. It should be underlined that this therapy was very safe and well tolerated by patients, without adverse effect on lipid metabolism [174]. A systematic review of the value of insulin sensitizers in patients with NAFLD showed that pioglitazone improves all parameters of liver histology [168]. However, after the discontinuation of treatment, transaminase levels may return to baseline values [175]. A meta-analysis evaluating the effects of pioglitazone treatment for patients with NAFLD combined with T2DM demonstrated significant improvement in steatosis, ballooning and inflammation but had no effect on fibrosis [176].

The efficacy of rosiglitazone on NAFLD was observed in a FLIRT study, which revealed a significant antiestrogenic effect in the first year of therapy, although there was no additional benefit with longer-term treatment [177]. In a study [178], 64 patients with both NAFLD and impaired glucose metabolism (impaired glucose tolerance or T2DM) were treated with metformin 1700 mg/day, rosiglitazone 4 mg/day or combined therapy for

12 months. After that time, BMI decreased for patients given metformin and a combination of drugs ($p = 0.002$, $p = 0.006$, respectively). Moreover, postprandial glucose was reduced in all three groups, and liver biopsy showed improved NAFLD activity scores after treatment with rosiglitazone ($p = 0.01$) and combined therapy ($p = 0.03$).

The second-generation insulin sensitizer, MSDC-0602K has been shown to reduce ballooning and inflammation with no fibrosis progression after 12-months of treatment. Moreover, treatment with MSDC-0602K did not show the side effects observed with first-generation insulin sensitizers [179].

6.3. GLP-1 Agonists and DPP-4 Inhibitors

Incretin-mimetics, such as exenatide and liraglutide, have generated great interest because of their potential to reduce hepatic steatosis in patients with NAFLD. The impact of exenatide and liraglutide therapy during six months treatment of obese, T2DM patients with hepatic steatosis on intrahepatic lipid (IHL) was explored by Cuthbertson et al. [180]. They determined the relationship between changes in IHL with HbA1c, body weight, volume of abdominal visceral and subcutaneous adipose tissue (VAT and SAT). IHL was measured by liver proton MRS (^{1}H MRS), while VAT and SAT were measured by whole body MRI. Patients were previously treated for at least three months with maximal tolerated doses of metformin, with either sulfonylureas (SU) or DPP-IV inhibitors. After conversion to GLP-1 agonists (exenatide, $n = 19$; liraglutide, $n = 6$), the following were observed: weight reduction (5.0 kg), 1.6% decrease in HbA1c, decrease in mean value of ALT activity (from 40 to 31 U/L) and GGT (from 69 to 43 U/L), 42% relative decrease in IHL and 7–11% in abdominal SAT or VAT. It should be emphasized that most of the patients had normal values of liver enzymes which significantly correlated with IHL. Compared with metformin, exenatide was not only found to better control blood glucose and body weight, but also to improve hepatic enzymes, attenuating hepatic steatosis in patients with T2DM concomitant with NAFLD [181].

Exenatide has a better hepatic-protective effect than intensive insulin therapy and, perhaps, represents a unique option for adjunctive therapy for patients with obesity, NAFLD with elevated liver enzymes and T2DM [182].

The LEAD-2 (Liraglutide Effect and Action in Diabetes) study examined the effect of liraglutide used for 24 weeks on liver function. In this placebo-controlled study, the effect of the drug was assessed by means of CT. It was found that 50.8% of patients with T2DM had an abnormal ALT at baseline. Application of 1.8 mg of liraglutide significantly decreased ALT activity and hepatic fat level compared to placebo, the effect being dose-dependent. Unfortunately, this effect was not observed after taking into account reduction in weight and HbA1c. In the liraglutide group, patients with and without baseline abnormal ALT did not differ in frequency of adverse effect. However, patients treated with liraglutide showed an improvement in hepatic steatosis—this trend also disappeared after adjusting for weight and HbA1c [183]

Sitagliptin used in T2DM coexisting with NAFLD was found to be safe and showed a similar antidiabetic effect as reported in patients with T2DM without NAFLD. It seems that tight glycemic control may contribute to the improvement of NAFLD. This observation was based on the correlation between changes in HbA1c and transaminases levels [184]. On the other hand, another study found no difference between various doses of sitagliptin (50–100 mg) on AST and ALT levels in comparison to physical activity and diet, although sitagliptin did decrease HbA1c after 1 year of treatment [185].

In a retrospective study of 82 patients with NAFLD and T2DM, Japanese researchers compared the efficacy of liraglutide, sitagliptin and pioglitazone. In all treatment groups they found significant improvements, not only in HbA1c level, but also in fasting blood glucose and ALT. Groups treated with liraglutide or pioglitazone had significantly lower AST to platelet ratios. Body weight was significantly lower in the liraglutide group (81.8 kg to 78.0 kg) and statistically higher in the pioglitazone group. This parameter did not change in the sitagliptin group. Multivariate regression analysis suggested that administration of liraglutide is an independent factor affecting body weight reduction of more than 5% [186]. In accordance with ADA or EASD statements, pioglitazone seems to be the preferred drug for patients with NAFLD and T2DM. Unfortunately, pioglitazone is not recommended by these institutions in cases of active liver disease and where liver enzymes are 2.5 times higher than the upper limit. It is emphasized that the use of PSU is rarely associated with an increase in liver enzymes, and their increase is not a contraindication to TZDs. The same prescribing guidelines are pertinent to meglitinides. In cases of severe liver damage, secretagogues should not be used because of the increased risk of hypoglycemia. Incretin-based drugs can be used safely in patients with NAFLD. EASD and ADA have emphasized that the limitations, particularly in patients with a history of pancreatitis, should be remembered. Fatty liver does not constitute a contraindication for insulin therapy, and for some patients with T2DM and NAFLD is the only therapeutic option [187].

6.4. Others

Lipid lowering medications (e.g., statins, fibrates, proprotein convertase subtilisin/kexin type 9), antioxidants (e.g., vitamin E, pentoxifylline and alpha lipoid acid), coleseve-lam, drugs that induce weight loss (e.g., orlistat and sibutramine), deferoxamina (an iron-chelating agent), antibiotics, probiotics, rimonabant, telimisartan, melatonin, betaina, aramchol, ursodeoxycholic acid, adenosine receptor agonists, nitro-aspirin, and omega-3 supplements, have all been considered in the treatment of NAFLD [137,174,188].

Bariatric surgery is an effective treatment for obesity and has been shown to markedly improve and even cure diabetes [89,90,189]. It also leads to improvement in histological features, ALT, AST and GGT levels, as well as lipid metabolism and inflammation [190–192]. The exact mechanisms that lead to improvement in NAFLD following bariatric surgery are not completely understood [193].

7. Summary

Coexistence of NAFLD and T2DM is common in everyday outpatient practice. NAFLD carries a low risk of complications, but the coexistence of NAFLD and T2DM significantly worsens prognosis. In persons with NAFLD, screening for diabetes is obligatory; on the other hand, in patients with diabetes, screening for NAFLD is not currently recommended. In treatment of NAFLD patients with diabetes, some hyperglycemic agents are useful, but lifestyle modification has the highest effectiveness. Further studies are needed because there is still a lack of adequate evidence-based methods for NAFLD screening. Assessment of the impact of newer anti-diabetic treatments, and identification of additional novel targets to treat NAFLD in diabetes patients, are also needed.

Author Contributions: Conceptualization, M.K. and S.Z.; methodology, M.K. and S.Z.; writing—original draft preparation, M.K. and S.Z.; writing—review and editing, P.C., J.S. and T.P.; visualization, S.Z.; supervision, J.S. and T.P. All authors have read and agreed to the published version of the manuscript.

Funding: This research was funded by Medical University of Lodz institutional grant no. 503/1-151-07/503-11-001-18 and 503/6-086-01/503-61-001-19-00.

Institutional Review Board Statement: Not applicable.

Informed Consent Statement: Not applicable.

Data Availability Statement: Not applicable.

Conflicts of Interest: The authors declare no conflict of interest.

References

1. Thaler, H. The fatty liver and its pathogenetic relation to liver cirrhosis. *Virchows Arch. Pathol. Anat. Physiol. Klin. Med.* **1962**, *335*, 180–210. [CrossRef] [PubMed]
2. Chalasani, N.; Younossi, Z.; Lavine, J.E.; Charlton, M.; Cusi, K.; Rinella, M.; Harrison, S.A.; Brunt, E.M.; Sanyal, A.J. The Diagnosis and Management of Nonalcoholic Fatty Liver Disease: Practice Guidance from the American Association for the Study of Liver Diseases. *Hepatology* **2018**, *67*, 328–357. [CrossRef] [PubMed]
3. Lin, S.; Huang, J.; Wang, M.; Kumar, R.; Liu, Y.; Liu, S.; Wu, Y.; Wang, X.; Zhu, Y. Comparison of MAFLD and NAFLD Diagnostic Criteria in Real World. *Liver Int. Off. J. Int. Assoc. Study Liver* **2020**, *40*, 2082–2089. [CrossRef]
4. Marchesini, G.; Brizi, M.; Morselli-Labate, A.M.; Bianchi, G.; Bugianesi, E.; McCullough, A.J.; Forlani, G.; Melchionda, N. Association of Nonalcoholic Fatty Liver Disease with Insulin Resistance. *Am. J. Med.* **1999**, *107*, 450–455. [CrossRef]
5. Liebe, R.; Esposito, I.; Bock, H.H.; Vom Dahl, S.; Stindt, J.; Baumann, U.; Luedde, T.; Keitel, V. Diagnosis and Management of Secondary Causes of Steatohepatitis. *J. Hepatol.* **2021**, *74*, 1455–1471. [CrossRef] [PubMed]
6. Kneeman, J.M.; Misdraji, J.; Corey, K.E. Secondary Causes of Nonalcoholic Fatty Liver Disease. *Ther. Adv. Gastroenterol.* **2012**, *5*, 199–207. [CrossRef] [PubMed]
7. Kim, D.; Kim, W.R.; Kim, H.J.; Therneau, T.M. Association between Noninvasive Fibrosis Markers and Mortality among Adults with Nonalcoholic Fatty Liver Disease in the United States. *Hepatology* **2013**, *57*, 1357–1365. [CrossRef]
8. Armstrong, M.J.; Adams, L.A.; Canbay, A.; Syn, W.-K. Extrahepatic Complications of Nonalcoholic Fatty Liver Disease. *Hepatology* **2014**, *59*, 1174–1197. [CrossRef]
9. Kasturiratne, A.; Weerasinghe, S.; Dassanayake, A.S.; Rajindrajith, S.; de Silva, A.P.; Kato, N.; Wickremasinghe, A.R.; de Silva, H.J. Influence of Non-Alcoholic Fatty Liver Disease on the Development of Diabetes Mellitus. *J. Gastroenterol. Hepatol.* **2013**, *28*, 142–147. [CrossRef]
10. El-Serag, H.B.; Tran, T.; Everhart, J.E. Diabetes Increases the Risk of Chronic Liver Disease and Hepatocellular Carcinoma. *Gastroenterology* **2004**, *126*, 460–468. [CrossRef]
11. Targher, G.; Bertolini, L.; Rodella, S.; Tessari, R.; Zenari, L.; Lippi, G.; Arcaro, G. Nonalcoholic Fatty Liver Disease Is Independently Associated with an Increased Incidence of Cardiovascular Events in Type 2 Diabetic Patients. *Diabetes Care* **2007**, *30*, 2119–2121. [CrossRef] [PubMed]
12. Leite, N.C.; Villela-Nogueira, C.A.; Pannain, V.L.N.; Bottino, A.C.; Rezende, G.F.M.; Cardoso, C.R.L.; Salles, G.F. Histopathological Stages of Nonalcoholic Fatty Liver Disease in Type 2 Diabetes: Prevalences and Correlated Factors. *Liver Int. Off. J. Int. Assoc. Study Liver* **2011**, *31*, 700–706. [CrossRef] [PubMed]
13. Loomba, R.; Sanyal, A.J. The Global NAFLD Epidemic. *Nat. Rev. Gastroenterol. Hepatol.* **2013**, *10*, 686–690. [CrossRef]
14. Bambha, K.; Belt, P.; Abraham, M.; Wilson, L.A.; Pabst, M.; Ferrell, L.; Unalp-Arida, A.; Bass, N. Ethnicity and Nonalcoholic Fatty Liver Disease. *Hepatology* **2012**, *55*, 769–780. [CrossRef] [PubMed]
15. Lazo, M.; Clark, J.M. The Epidemiology of Nonalcoholic Fatty Liver Disease: A Global Perspective. *Semin. Liver Dis.* **2008**, *28*, 339–350. [CrossRef] [PubMed]
16. Castera, L.; Vilgrain, V.; Angulo, P. Noninvasive Evaluation of NAFLD. *Nat. Rev. Gastroenterol. Hepatol.* **2013**, *10*, 666–675. [CrossRef]
17. Mitra, S.; De, A.; Chowdhury, A. Epidemiology of Non-Alcoholic and Alcoholic Fatty Liver Diseases. *Transl. Gastroenterol. Hepatol.* **2020**, *5*, 16. [CrossRef]
18. Chen, Y.-Y.; Yeh, M.M. Non-Alcoholic Fatty Liver Disease: A Review with Clinical and Pathological Correlation. *J. Formos. Med. Assoc.* **2021**, *120*, 68–77. [CrossRef]
19. Dufour, J.-F.; Scherer, R.; Balp, M.-M.; McKenna, S.J.; Janssens, N.; Lopez, P.; Pedrosa, M. The Global Epidemiology of Nonalcoholic Steatohepatitis (NASH) and Associated Risk Factors—A Targeted Literature Review. *Endocr. Metab. Sci.* **2021**, *3*, 100089. [CrossRef]
20. Wong, R.J.; Liu, B.; Bhuket, T. Significant Burden of Nonalcoholic Fatty Liver Disease with Advanced Fibrosis in the US: A Cross-Sectional Analysis of 2011–2014 National Health and Nutrition Examination Survey. *Aliment. Pharmacol. Ther.* **2017**, *46*, 974–980. [CrossRef]
21. Rinella, M.; Charlton, M. The Globalization of Nonalcoholic Fatty Liver Disease: Prevalence and Impact on World Health. *Hepatology* **2016**, *64*, 19–22. [CrossRef] [PubMed]
22. Lazo, M.; Hernaez, R.; Eberhardt, M.S.; Bonekamp, S.; Kamel, I.; Guallar, E.; Koteish, A.; Brancati, F.L.; Clark, J.M. Prevalence of Nonalcoholic Fatty Liver Disease in the United States: The Third National Health and Nutrition Examination Survey, 1988–1994. *Am. J. Epidemiol.* **2013**, *178*, 38–45. [CrossRef]
23. Koehler, E.M.; Schouten, J.N.L.; Hansen, B.E.; van Rooij, F.J.A.; Hofman, A.; Stricker, B.H.; Janssen, H.L.A. Prevalence and Risk Factors of Non-Alcoholic Fatty Liver Disease in the Elderly: Results from the Rotterdam Study. *J. Hepatol.* **2012**, *57*, 1305–1311. [CrossRef] [PubMed]
24. Ryoo, J.-H.; Choi, J.-M.; Moon, S.Y.; Suh, Y.J.; Shin, J.-Y.; Shin, H.C.; Park, S.K. The Clinical Availability of Non Alcoholic Fatty Liver Disease as an Early Predictor of the Metabolic Syndrome in Korean Men: 5-Year's Prospective Cohort Study. *Atherosclerosis* **2013**, *227*, 398–403. [CrossRef] [PubMed]
25. Yasutake, K.; Kohjima, M.; Kotoh, K.; Nakashima, M.; Nakamuta, M.; Enjoji, M. Dietary Habits and Behaviors Associated with Nonalcoholic Fatty Liver Disease. *World J. Gastroenterol.* **2014**, *20*, 1756–1767. [CrossRef]

26. Zeb, I.; Katz, R.; Nasir, K.; Ding, J.; Rezaeian, P.; Budoff, M.J. Relation of Nonalcoholic Fatty Liver Disease to the Metabolic Syndrome: The Multi-Ethnic Study of Atherosclerosis. *J. Cardiovasc. Comput. Tomogr.* **2013**, *7*, 311–318. [CrossRef] [PubMed]
27. Paschos, P.; Paletas, K. Non Alcoholic Fatty Liver Disease and Metabolic Syndrome. *Hippokratia* **2009**, *13*, 9–19.
28. Kotronen, A.; Westerbacka, J.; Bergholm, R.; Pietiläinen, K.H.; Yki-Järvinen, H. Liver Fat in the Metabolic Syndrome. *J. Clin. Endocrinol. Metab.* **2007**, *92*, 3490–3497. [CrossRef] [PubMed]
29. Hamaguchi, M.; Kojima, T.; Takeda, N.; Nakagawa, T.; Taniguchi, H.; Fujii, K.; Omatsu, T.; Nakajima, T.; Sarui, H.; Shimazaki, M.; et al. The Metabolic Syndrome as a Predictor of Nonalcoholic Fatty Liver Disease. *Ann. Intern. Med.* **2005**, *143*, 722–728. [CrossRef]
30. Moretto, M.; Kupski, C.; Mottin, C.C.; Repetto, G.; Garcia Toneto, M.; Rizzolli, J.; Berleze, D.; de Souza Brito, C.L.; Casagrande, D.; Colossi, F. Hepatic Steatosis in Patients Undergoing Bariatric Surgery and Its Relationship to Body Mass Index and Co-Morbidities. *Obes. Surg.* **2003**, *13*, 622–624. [CrossRef]
31. Basaranoglu, M.; Neuschwander-Tetri, B.A. Nonalcoholic Fatty Liver Disease: Clinical Features and Pathogenesis. *Gastroenterol. Hepatol.* **2006**, *2*, 282–291.
32. Van Vliet-Ostaptchouk, J.V.; Nuotio, M.-L.; Slagter, S.N.; Doiron, D.; Fischer, K.; Foco, L.; Gaye, A.; Gögele, M.; Heier, M.; Hiekkalinna, T.; et al. The Prevalence of Metabolic Syndrome and Metabolically Healthy Obesity in Europe: A Collaborative Analysis of Ten Large Cohort Studies. *BMC Endocr. Disord.* **2014**, *14*, 9. [CrossRef]
33. Kopylov, U.; Ben-Horin, S.; Lahat, A.; Segev, S.; Avidan, B.; Carter, D. Obesity, Metabolic Syndrome and the Risk of Development of Colonic Diverticulosis. *Digestion* **2012**, *86*, 201–205. [CrossRef] [PubMed]
34. Lin, X.; Li, J.; Ying, M.; Wei, F.; Xie, X. Diabetes Increases Morbidities of Colonic Diverticular Disease and Colonic Diverticular Hemorrhage: A Systematic Review and Meta-Analysis. *Am. J. Ther.* **2017**, *24*, e213–e221. [CrossRef] [PubMed]
35. Feuerstein, J.D.; Falchuk, K.R. Diverticulosis and Diverticulitis. *Mayo Clin. Proc.* **2016**, *91*, 1094–1104. [CrossRef]
36. Pantic, I.; Lugonja, S.; Rajovic, N.; Dumic, I.; Milovanovic, T. Colonic Diverticulosis and Non-Alcoholic Fatty Liver Disease: Is There a Connection? *Medicina* **2021**, *58*, 38. [CrossRef]
37. Milovanovic, T.; Pantic, I.; Dragasevic, S.; Lugonja, S.; Dumic, I.; Rajilic-Stojanovic, M. The Interrelationship Among Non-Alcoholic Fatty Liver Disease, Colonic Diverticulosis and Metabolic Syndrome. *J. Gastrointestin. Liver Dis.* **2021**, *30*, 274–282. [CrossRef]
38. Wah-Kheong, C.; Khean-Lee, G. Epidemiology of a Fast Emerging Disease in the Asia-Pacific Region: Non-Alcoholic Fatty Liver Disease. *Hepatol. Int.* **2013**, *7*, 65–71. [CrossRef]
39. Kwon, Y.-M.; Oh, S.-W.; Hwang, S.; Lee, C.; Kwon, H.; Chung, G.E. Association of Nonalcoholic Fatty Liver Disease with Components of Metabolic Syndrome According to Body Mass Index in Korean Adults. *Am. J. Gastroenterol.* **2012**, *107*, 1852–1858. [CrossRef]
40. Wong, V.W.-S.; Wong, G.L.-H.; Yeung, D.K.-W.; Lau, T.K.-T.; Chan, C.K.-M.; Chim, A.M.-L.; Abrigo, J.M.; Chan, R.S.-M.; Woo, J.; Tse, Y.-K.; et al. Incidence of Non-Alcoholic Fatty Liver Disease in Hong Kong: A Population Study with Paired Proton-Magnetic Resonance Spectroscopy. *J. Hepatol.* **2015**, *62*, 182–189. [CrossRef]
41. Kalra, S.; Vithalani, M.; Gulati, G.; Kulkarni, C.M.; Kadam, Y.; Pallivathukkal, J.; Das, B.; Sahay, R.; Modi, K.D. Study of Prevalence of Nonalcoholic Fatty Liver Disease (NAFLD) in Type 2 Diabetes Patients in India (SPRINT). *J. Assoc. Physicians India* **2013**, *61*, 448–453. [PubMed]
42. Ortiz-Lopez, C.; Lomonaco, R.; Orsak, B.; Finch, J.; Chang, Z.; Kochunov, V.G.; Hardies, J.; Cusi, K. Prevalence of Prediabetes and Diabetes and Metabolic Profile of Patients with Nonalcoholic Fatty Liver Disease (NAFLD). *Diabetes Care* **2012**, *35*, 873–878. [CrossRef] [PubMed]
43. Blachier, M.; Leleu, H.; Peck-Radosavljevic, M.; Valla, D.-C.; Roudot-Thoraval, F. The Burden of Liver Disease in Europe: A Review of Available Epidemiological Data. *J. Hepatol.* **2013**, *58*, 593–608. [CrossRef] [PubMed]
44. Park, S.K.; Seo, M.H.; Shin, H.C.; Ryoo, J.-H. Clinical Availability of Nonalcoholic Fatty Liver Disease as an Early Predictor of Type 2 Diabetes Mellitus in Korean Men: 5-Year Prospective Cohort Study. *Hepatology* **2013**, *57*, 1378–1383. [CrossRef]
45. Kosmalski, M.; Kasznicki, J.; Drzewoski, J. Relationship between Ultrasound Features of Nonalcoholic Fatty Liver Disease and Cardiometabolic Risk Factors in Patients with Newly Diagnosed Type 2 Diabetes. *Pol. Arch. Med. Wewn.* **2013**, *123*, 436–442. [CrossRef] [PubMed]
46. Yan, Y.; Bian, H.; Xia, M.; Yan, H.; Chang, X.; Yao, X.; Rao, S.; Zeng, M.; Gao, X. Liver disease spectrum in hospitalized type 2 diabetes and related risk factors analysis of non-alcoholic fatty liver disease. *Zhonghua Yi Xue Za Zhi* **2013**, *93*, 270–274.
47. Williamson, R.M.; Price, J.F.; Glancy, S.; Perry, E.; Nee, L.D.; Hayes, P.C.; Frier, B.M.; Van Look, L.A.F.; Johnston, G.I.; Reynolds, R.M.; et al. Prevalence of and Risk Factors for Hepatic Steatosis and Nonalcoholic Fatty Liver Disease in People with Type 2 Diabetes: The Edinburgh Type 2 Diabetes Study. *Diabetes Care* **2011**, *34*, 1139–1144. [CrossRef] [PubMed]
48. Dai, W.; Ye, L.; Liu, A.; Wen, S.W.; Deng, J.; Wu, X.; Lai, Z. Prevalence of Nonalcoholic Fatty Liver Disease in Patients with Type 2 Diabetes Mellitus: A Meta-Analysis. *Medicine* **2017**, *96*, e8179. [CrossRef]
49. Younossi, Z.M.; Golabi, P.; de Avila, L.; Paik, J.M.; Srishord, M.; Fukui, N.; Qiu, Y.; Burns, L.; Afendy, A.; Nader, F. The Global Epidemiology of NAFLD and NASH in Patients with Type 2 Diabetes: A Systematic Review and Meta-Analysis. *J. Hepatol.* **2019**, *71*, 793–801. [CrossRef]
50. Saponaro, C.; Gaggini, M.; Gastaldelli, A. Nonalcoholic Fatty Liver Disease and Type 2 Diabetes: Common Pathophysiologic Mechanisms. *Curr. Diabetes Rep.* **2015**, *15*, 607. [CrossRef]

51. Williams, K.H.; Shackel, N.A.; Gorrell, M.D.; McLennan, S.V.; Twigg, S.M. Diabetes and Nonalcoholic Fatty Liver Disease: A Pathogenic Duo. *Endocr. Rev.* **2013**, *34*, 84–129. [CrossRef] [PubMed]
52. Fruci, B.; Giuliano, S.; Mazza, A.; Malaguarnera, R.; Belfiore, A. Nonalcoholic Fatty Liver: A Possible New Target for Type 2 Diabetes Prevention and Treatment. *Int. J. Mol. Sci.* **2013**, *14*, 22933–22966. [CrossRef] [PubMed]
53. Chai, S.-Y.; Pan, X.-Y.; Song, K.-X.; Huang, Y.-Y.; Li, F.; Cheng, X.-Y.; Qu, S. Differential Patterns of Insulin Secretion and Sensitivity in Patients with Type 2 Diabetes Mellitus and Nonalcoholic Fatty Liver Disease versus Patients with Type 2 Diabetes Mellitus Alone. *Lipids Health Dis.* **2014**, *13*, 7. [CrossRef] [PubMed]
54. Finucane, F.M.; Sharp, S.J.; Hatunic, M.; Sleigh, A.; De Lucia Rolfe, E.; Aihie Sayer, A.; Cooper, C.; Griffin, S.J.; Wareham, N.J. Liver Fat Accumulation Is Associated with Reduced Hepatic Insulin Extraction and Beta Cell Dysfunction in Healthy Older Individuals. *Diabetol. Metab. Syndr.* **2014**, *6*, 43. [CrossRef]
55. Buzzetti, E.; Pinzani, M.; Tsochatzis, E.A. The Multiple-Hit Pathogenesis of Non-Alcoholic Fatty Liver Disease (NAFLD). *Metabolism* **2016**, *65*, 1038–1048. [CrossRef]
56. Browning, J.D.; Szczepaniak, L.S.; Dobbins, R.; Nuremberg, P.; Horton, J.D.; Cohen, J.C.; Grundy, S.M.; Hobbs, H.H. Prevalence of Hepatic Steatosis in an Urban Population in the United States: Impact of Ethnicity. *Hepatology* **2004**, *40*, 1387–1395. [CrossRef]
57. Ekstedt, M.; Franzén, L.E.; Mathiesen, U.L.; Thorelius, L.; Holmqvist, M.; Bodemar, G.; Kechagias, S. Long-Term Follow-up of Patients with NAFLD and Elevated Liver Enzymes. *Hepatology* **2006**, *44*, 865–873. [CrossRef]
58. Kashyap, S.R.; Defronzo, R.A. The Insulin Resistance Syndrome: Physiological Considerations. *Diabetes Vasc. Dis. Res.* **2007**, *4*, 13–19. [CrossRef]
59. Kahn, B.B.; Flier, J.S. Obesity and Insulin Resistance. *J. Clin. Investig.* **2000**, *106*, 473–481. [CrossRef]
60. Katagiri, H.; Yamada, T.; Oka, Y. Adiposity and Cardiovascular Disorders: Disturbance of the Regulatory System Consisting of Humoral and Neuronal Signals. *Circ. Res.* **2007**, *101*, 27–39. [CrossRef]
61. Ahmadieh, H.; Azar, S.T. Liver Disease and Diabetes: Association, Pathophysiology, and Management. *Diabetes Res. Clin. Pract.* **2014**, *104*, 53–62. [CrossRef] [PubMed]
62. Palmer, C.N.A.; Maglio, C.; Pirazzi, C.; Burza, M.A.; Adiels, M.; Burch, L.; Donnelly, L.A.; Colhoun, H.; Doney, A.S.; Dillon, J.F.; et al. Paradoxical Lower Serum Triglyceride Levels and Higher Type 2 Diabetes Mellitus Susceptibility in Obese Individuals with the PNPLA3 148M Variant. *PLoS ONE* **2012**, *7*, e39362. [CrossRef] [PubMed]
63. Dubuquoy, C.; Burnol, A.-F.; Moldes, M. PNPLA3, a Genetic Marker of Progressive Liver Disease, Still Hiding Its Metabolic Function? *Clin. Res. Hepatol. Gastroenterol.* **2013**, *37*, 30–35. [CrossRef] [PubMed]
64. Masarone, M.; Rosato, V.; Aglitti, A.; Bucci, T.; Caruso, R.; Salvatore, T.; Sasso, F.C.; Tripodi, M.F.; Persico, M. Liver Biopsy in Type 2 Diabetes Mellitus: Steatohepatitis Represents the Sole Feature of Liver Damage. *PLoS ONE* **2017**, *12*, e0178473. [CrossRef] [PubMed]
65. Le Chatelier, E.; Nielsen, T.; Qin, J.; Prifti, E.; Hildebrand, F.; Falony, G.; Almeida, M.; Arumugam, M.; Batto, J.-M.; Kennedy, S.; et al. Richness of Human Gut Microbiome Correlates with Metabolic Markers. *Nature* **2013**, *500*, 541–546. [CrossRef]
66. Dao, M.C.; Everard, A.; Aron-Wisnewsky, J.; Sokolovska, N.; Prifti, E.; Verger, E.O.; Kayser, B.D.; Levenez, F.; Chilloux, J.; Hoyles, L.; et al. Akkermansia Muciniphila and Improved Metabolic Health during a Dietary Intervention in Obesity: Relationship with Gut Microbiome Richness and Ecology. *Gut* **2016**, *65*, 426–436. [CrossRef]
67. Albillos, A.; de Gottardi, A.; Rescigno, M. The Gut-Liver Axis in Liver Disease: Pathophysiological Basis for Therapy. *J. Hepatol.* **2020**, *72*, 558–577. [CrossRef]
68. Hu, H.; Lin, A.; Kong, M.; Yao, X.; Yin, M.; Xia, H.; Ma, J.; Liu, H. Intestinal Microbiome and NAFLD: Molecular Insights and Therapeutic Perspectives. *J. Gastroenterol.* **2020**, *55*, 142–158. [CrossRef]
69. Dong, T.S.; Jacobs, J.P. Nonalcoholic Fatty Liver Disease and the Gut Microbiome: Are Bacteria Responsible for Fatty Liver? *Exp. Biol. Med.* **2019**, *244*, 408–418. [CrossRef]
70. Menni, C.; Jackson, M.A.; Pallister, T.; Steves, C.J.; Spector, T.D.; Valdes, A.M. Gut Microbiome Diversity and High-Fibre Intake Are Related to Lower Long-Term Weight Gain. *Int. J. Obes.* **2017**, *41*, 1099–1105. [CrossRef]
71. Zhao, L.; Zhang, F.; Ding, X.; Wu, G.; Lam, Y.Y.; Wang, X.; Fu, H.; Xue, X.; Lu, C.; Ma, J.; et al. Gut Bacteria Selectively Promoted by Dietary Fibers Alleviate Type 2 Diabetes. *Science* **2018**, *359*, 1151–1156. [CrossRef]
72. Wang, B.; Jiang, X.; Cao, M.; Ge, J.; Bao, Q.; Tang, L.; Chen, Y.; Li, L. Altered Fecal Microbiota Correlates with Liver Biochemistry in Nonobese Patients with Non-Alcoholic Fatty Liver Disease. *Sci. Rep.* **2016**, *6*, 32002. [CrossRef] [PubMed]
73. Shen, F.; Zheng, R.-D.; Sun, X.-Q.; Ding, W.-J.; Wang, X.-Y.; Fan, J.-G. Gut Microbiota Dysbiosis in Patients with Non-Alcoholic Fatty Liver Disease. *Hepatobiliary Pancreat. Dis. Int* **2017**, *16*, 375–381. [CrossRef]
74. Mollica, M.P.; Mattace Raso, G.; Cavaliere, G.; Trinchese, G.; De Filippo, C.; Aceto, S.; Prisco, M.; Pirozzi, C.; Di Guida, F.; Lama, A.; et al. Butyrate Regulates Liver Mitochondrial Function, Efficiency, and Dynamics in Insulin-Resistant Obese Mice. *Diabetes* **2017**, *66*, 1405–1418. [CrossRef] [PubMed]
75. De Vadder, F.; Kovatcheva-Datchary, P.; Zitoun, C.; Duchampt, A.; Bäckhed, F.; Mithieux, G. Microbiota-Produced Succinate Improves Glucose Homeostasis via Intestinal Gluconeogenesis. *Cell Metab.* **2016**, *24*, 151–157. [CrossRef]
76. Lu, Y.; Fan, C.; Li, P.; Lu, Y.; Chang, X.; Qi, K. Short Chain Fatty Acids Prevent High-Fat-Diet-Induced Obesity in Mice by Regulating G Protein-Coupled Receptors and Gut Microbiota. *Sci. Rep.* **2016**, *6*, 37589. [CrossRef]

77. Kelly, C.J.; Zheng, L.; Campbell, E.L.; Saeedi, B.; Scholz, C.C.; Bayless, A.J.; Wilson, K.E.; Glover, L.E.; Kominsky, D.J.; Magnuson, A.; et al. Crosstalk between Microbiota-Derived Short-Chain Fatty Acids and Intestinal Epithelial HIF Augments Tissue Barrier Function. *Cell Host Microbe* **2015**, *17*, 662–671. [CrossRef]
78. Gao, Z.; Yin, J.; Zhang, J.; Ward, R.E.; Martin, R.J.; Lefevre, M.; Cefalu, W.T.; Ye, J. Butyrate Improves Insulin Sensitivity and Increases Energy Expenditure in Mice. *Diabetes* **2009**, *58*, 1509–1517. [CrossRef]
79. Mattace Raso, G.; Simeoli, R.; Russo, R.; Iacono, A.; Santoro, A.; Paciello, O.; Ferrante, M.C.; Canani, R.B.; Calignano, A.; Meli, R. Effects of Sodium Butyrate and Its Synthetic Amide Derivative on Liver Inflammation and Glucose Tolerance in an Animal Model of Steatosis Induced by High Fat Diet. *PLoS ONE* **2013**, *8*, e68626. [CrossRef]
80. Canfora, E.E.; Meex, R.C.R.; Venema, K.; Blaak, E.E. Gut Microbial Metabolites in Obesity, NAFLD and T2DM. *Nat. Rev. Endocrinol.* **2019**, *15*, 261–273. [CrossRef]
81. Palermo, A.; Maggi, D.; Maurizi, A.R.; Pozzilli, P.; Buzzetti, R. Prevention of Type 2 Diabetes Mellitus: Is It Feasible? *Diabetes Metab. Res. Rev.* **2014**, *30* (Suppl. S1), 4–12. [CrossRef] [PubMed]
82. Vrieze, A.; Van Nood, E.; Holleman, F.; Salojärvi, J.; Kootte, R.S.; Bartelsman, J.F.W.M.; Dallinga-Thie, G.M.; Ackermans, M.T.; Serlie, M.J.; Oozeer, R.; et al. Transfer of Intestinal Microbiota from Lean Donors Increases Insulin Sensitivity in Individuals with Metabolic Syndrome. *Gastroenterology* **2012**, *143*, 913–916.e7. [CrossRef]
83. Erridge, C. Diet, Commensals and the Intestine as Sources of Pathogen-Associated Molecular Patterns in Atherosclerosis, Type 2 Diabetes and Non-Alcoholic Fatty Liver Disease. *Atherosclerosis* **2011**, *216*, 1–6. [CrossRef] [PubMed]
84. Firneisz, G. Non-Alcoholic Fatty Liver Disease and Type 2 Diabetes Mellitus: The Liver Disease of Our Age? *World J. Gastroenterol.* **2014**, *20*, 9072–9089.
85. Wójcik-Cichy, K.; Koślińska-Berkan, E.; Piekarska, A. The Influence of NAFLD on the Risk of Atherosclerosis and Cardiovascular Diseases. *Clin. Exp. Hepatol.* **2018**, *4*, 1–6. [CrossRef] [PubMed]
86. Colak, Y.; Senates, E.; Yesil, A.; Yilmaz, Y.; Ozturk, O.; Doganay, L.; Coskunpinar, E.; Kahraman, O.T.; Mesci, B.; Ulasoglu, C.; et al. Assessment of Endothelial Function in Patients with Nonalcoholic Fatty Liver Disease. *Endocrine* **2013**, *43*, 100–107. [CrossRef] [PubMed]
87. Salvi, P.; Ruffini, R.; Agnoletti, D.; Magnani, E.; Pagliarani, G.; Comandini, G.; Praticò, A.; Borghi, C.; Benetos, A.; Pazzi, P. Increased Arterial Stiffness in Nonalcoholic Fatty Liver Disease: The Cardio-GOOSE Study. *J. Hypertens.* **2010**, *28*, 1699–1707. [CrossRef]
88. Gami, A.S.; Witt, B.J.; Howard, D.E.; Erwin, P.J.; Gami, L.A.; Somers, V.K.; Montori, V.M. Metabolic Syndrome and Risk of Incident Cardiovascular Events and Death: A Systematic Review and Meta-Analysis of Longitudinal Studies. *J. Am. Coll. Cardiol.* **2007**, *49*, 403–414. [CrossRef]
89. Targher, G.; Byrne, C.D.; Lonardo, A.; Zoppini, G.; Barbui, C. Non-Alcoholic Fatty Liver Disease and Risk of Incident Cardiovascular Disease: A Meta-Analysis. *J. Hepatol.* **2016**, *65*, 589–600. [CrossRef]
90. Adinolfi, L.E.; Petta, S.; Fracanzani, A.L.; Nevola, R.; Coppola, C.; Narciso, V.; Rinaldi, L.; Calvaruso, V.; Pafundi, P.C.; Lombardi, R.; et al. Reduced Incidence of Type 2 Diabetes in Patients with Chronic Hepatitis C Virus Infection Cleared by Direct-Acting Antiviral Therapy: A Prospective Study. *Diabetes Obes. Metab.* **2020**, *22*, 2408–2416. [CrossRef]
91. Adinolfi, L.E.; Petta, S.; Fracanzani, A.L.; Coppola, C.; Narciso, V.; Nevola, R.; Rinaldi, L.; Calvaruso, V.; Staiano, L.; Di Marco, V.; et al. Impact of Hepatitis C Virus Clearance by Direct-Acting Antiviral Treatment on the Incidence of Major Cardiovascular Events: A Prospective Multicentre Study. *Atherosclerosis* **2020**, *296*, 40–47. [CrossRef]
92. Sasso, F.C.; Pafundi, P.C.; Caturano, A.; Galiero, R.; Vetrano, E.; Nevola, R.; Petta, S.; Fracanzani, A.L.; Coppola, C.; Di Marco, V.; et al. Impact of Direct Acting Antivirals (DAAs) on Cardiovascular Events in HCV Cohort with Pre-Diabetes. *Nutr. Metab. Cardiovasc. Dis.* **2021**, *31*, 2345–2353. [CrossRef] [PubMed]
93. Donnelly, K.L.; Smith, C.I.; Schwarzenberg, S.J.; Jessurun, J.; Boldt, M.D.; Parks, E.J. Sources of Fatty Acids Stored in Liver and Secreted via Lipoproteins in Patients with Nonalcoholic Fatty Liver Disease. *J. Clin. Investig.* **2005**, *115*, 1343–1351. [CrossRef] [PubMed]
94. Eguchi, Y.; Eguchi, T.; Mizuta, T.; Ide, Y.; Yasutake, T.; Iwakiri, R.; Hisatomi, A.; Ozaki, I.; Yamamoto, K.; Kitajima, Y.; et al. Visceral Fat Accumulation and Insulin Resistance Are Important Factors in Nonalcoholic Fatty Liver Disease. *J. Gastroenterol.* **2006**, *41*, 462–469. [CrossRef] [PubMed]
95. Perry, R.J.; Samuel, V.T.; Petersen, K.F.; Shulman, G.I. The Role of Hepatic Lipids in Hepatic Insulin Resistance and Type 2 Diabetes. *Nature* **2014**, *510*, 84–91. [CrossRef] [PubMed]
96. Petersen, K.F.; Dufour, S.; Savage, D.B.; Bilz, S.; Solomon, G.; Yonemitsu, S.; Cline, G.W.; Befroy, D.; Zemany, L.; Kahn, B.B.; et al. The Role of Skeletal Muscle Insulin Resistance in the Pathogenesis of the Metabolic Syndrome. *Proc. Natl. Acad. Sci. USA* **2007**, *104*, 12587–12594. [CrossRef]
97. Asrih, M.; Jornayvaz, F.R. Metabolic Syndrome and Nonalcoholic Fatty Liver Disease: Is Insulin Resistance the Link? *Mol. Cell. Endocrinol.* **2015**, *418 Pt 1*, 55–65. [CrossRef] [PubMed]
98. Ahima, R.S.; Lazar, M.A. Adipokines and the Peripheral and Neural Control of Energy Balance. *Mol. Endocrinol.* **2008**, *22*, 1023–1031. [CrossRef]
99. Rinaldi, L.; Pafundi, P.C.; Galiero, R.; Caturano, A.; Morone, M.V.; Silvestri, C.; Giordano, M.; Salvatore, T.; Sasso, F.C. Mechanisms of Non-Alcoholic Fatty Liver Disease in the Metabolic Syndrome. A Narrative Review. *Antioxidants* **2021**, *10*, 270. [CrossRef]

100. Caturano, A.; Acierno, C.; Nevola, R.; Pafundi, P.C.; Galiero, R.; Rinaldi, L.; Salvatore, T.; Adinolfi, L.E.; Sasso, F.C. Non-Alcoholic Fatty Liver Disease: From Pathogenesis to Clinical Impact. *Processes* **2021**, *9*, 135. [CrossRef]
101. Della Corte, C.; Mosca, A.; Majo, F.; Lucidi, V.; Panera, N.; Giglioni, E.; Monti, L.; Stronati, L.; Alisi, A.; Nobili, V. Nonalcoholic Fatty Pancreas Disease and Nonalcoholic Fatty Liver Disease: More than Ectopic Fat. *Clin. Endocrinol.* **2015**, *83*, 656–662. [CrossRef] [PubMed]
102. Alempijevic, T.; Dragasevic, S.; Zec, S.; Popovic, D.; Milosavljevic, T. Non-Alcoholic Fatty Pancreas Disease. *Postgrad. Med. J.* **2017**, *93*, 226–230. [CrossRef] [PubMed]
103. Filippatos, T.D.; Alexakis, K.; Mavrikaki, V.; Mikhailidis, D.P. Nonalcoholic Fatty Pancreas Disease: Role in Metabolic Syndrome, "Prediabetes" Diabetes and Atherosclerosis. *Dig. Dis. Sci.* **2022**, *67*, 26–41. [CrossRef] [PubMed]
104. Wang, C.-Y.; Ou, H.-Y.; Chen, M.-F.; Chang, T.-C.; Chang, C.-J. Enigmatic Ectopic Fat: Prevalence of Nonalcoholic Fatty Pancreas Disease and Its Associated Factors in a Chinese Population. *J. Am. Heart Assoc.* **2014**, *3*, e000297. [CrossRef]
105. Lee, J.S.; Kim, S.H.; Jun, D.W.; Han, J.H.; Jang, E.C.; Park, J.Y.; Son, B.K.; Kim, S.H.; Jo, Y.J.; Park, Y.S.; et al. Clinical Implications of Fatty Pancreas: Correlations between Fatty Pancreas and Metabolic Syndrome. *World J. Gastroenterol.* **2009**, *15*, 1869–1875. [CrossRef]
106. Van Geenen, E.-J.M.; Smits, M.M.; Schreuder, T.C.M.A.; van der Peet, D.L.; Bloemena, E.; Mulder, C.J.J. Nonalcoholic Fatty Liver Disease Is Related to Nonalcoholic Fatty Pancreas Disease. *Pancreas* **2010**, *39*, 1185–1190. [CrossRef]
107. Uygun, A.; Kadayifci, A.; Demirci, H.; Saglam, M.; Sakin, Y.S.; Ozturk, K.; Polat, Z.; Karslioglu, Y.; Bolu, E. The Effect of Fatty Pancreas on Serum Glucose Parameters in Patients with Nonalcoholic Steatohepatitis. *Eur. J. Intern. Med.* **2015**, *26*, 37–41. [CrossRef]
108. Ou, H.-Y.; Wang, C.-Y.; Yang, Y.-C.; Chen, M.-F.; Chang, C.-J. The Association between Nonalcoholic Fatty Pancreas Disease and Diabetes. *PLoS ONE* **2013**, *8*, e62561. [CrossRef]
109. Prasun, P. Mitochondrial Dysfunction in Metabolic Syndrome. *Biochim. Biophys. Acta-Mol. Basis Dis.* **2020**, *1866*, 165838. [CrossRef]
110. Begriche, K.; Massart, J.; Robin, M.-A.; Bonnet, F.; Fromenty, B. Mitochondrial Adaptations and Dysfunctions in Nonalcoholic Fatty Liver Disease. *Hepatology* **2013**, *58*, 1497–1507. [CrossRef]
111. Patterson, R.E.; Kalavalapalli, S.; Williams, C.M.; Nautiyal, M.; Mathew, J.T.; Martinez, J.; Reinhard, M.K.; McDougall, D.J.; Rocca, J.R.; Yost, R.A.; et al. Lipotoxicity in Steatohepatitis Occurs despite an Increase in Tricarboxylic Acid Cycle Activity. *Am. J. Physiol. Endocrinol. Metab.* **2016**, *310*, E484–E494. [CrossRef] [PubMed]
112. Cheng, Z.; Tseng, Y.; White, M.F. Insulin Signaling Meets Mitochondria in Metabolism. *Trends Endocrinol. Metab.* **2010**, *21*, 589–598. [CrossRef] [PubMed]
113. Tan, M.; Mosaoa, R.; Graham, G.T.; Kasprzyk-Pawelec, A.; Gadre, S.; Parasido, E.; Catalina-Rodriguez, O.; Foley, P.; Giaccone, G.; Cheema, A.; et al. Inhibition of the Mitochondrial Citrate Carrier, Slc25a1, Reverts Steatosis, Glucose Intolerance, and Inflammation in Preclinical Models of NAFLD/NASH. *Cell Death Differ.* **2020**, *27*, 2143–2157. [CrossRef]
114. Li, N.; Zhao, H. Role of Carnitine in Non-Alcoholic Fatty Liver Disease and Other Related Diseases: An Update. *Front. Med.* **2021**, *8*, 689042. [CrossRef]
115. Harrison, S.A.; Di Bisceglie, A.M. Advances in the Understanding and Treatment of Nonalcoholic Fatty Liver Disease. *Drugs* **2003**, *63*, 2379–2394. [CrossRef] [PubMed]
116. Hsu, C.; Caussy, C.; Imajo, K.; Chen, J.; Singh, S.; Kaulback, K.; Le, M.-D.; Hooker, J.; Tu, X.; Bettencourt, R.; et al. Magnetic Resonance vs. Transient Elastography Analysis of Patients with Nonalcoholic Fatty Liver Disease: A Systematic Review and Pooled Analysis of Individual Participants. *Clin. Gastroenterol. Hepatol. Off. Clin. Pract. J. Am. Gastroenterol. Assoc.* **2019**, *17*, 630–637.e8. [CrossRef] [PubMed]
117. Schwenzer, N.F.; Springer, F.; Schraml, C.; Stefan, N.; Machann, J.; Schick, F. Non-Invasive Assessment and Quantification of Liver Steatosis by Ultrasound, Computed Tomography and Magnetic Resonance. *J. Hepatol.* **2009**, *51*, 433–445. [CrossRef]
118. Lomonaco, R.; Sunny, N.E.; Bril, F.; Cusi, K. Nonalcoholic Fatty Liver Disease: Current Issues and Novel Treatment Approaches. *Drugs* **2013**, *73*, 1–14. [CrossRef]
119. Bohte, A.E.; van Werven, J.R.; Bipat, S.; Stoker, J. The Diagnostic Accuracy of US, CT, MRI and 1H-MRS for the Evaluation of Hepatic Steatosis Compared with Liver Biopsy: A Meta-Analysis. *Eur. Radiol.* **2011**, *21*, 87–97. [CrossRef]
120. Cheah, M.C.; McCullough, A.J.; Goh, G.B.-B. Current Modalities of Fibrosis Assessment in Non-Alcoholic Fatty Liver Disease. *J. Clin. Transl. Hepatol.* **2017**, *5*, 261–271. [CrossRef]
121. Yokoo, T.; Shiehmorteza, M.; Hamilton, G.; Wolfson, T.; Schroeder, M.E.; Middleton, M.S.; Bydder, M.; Gamst, A.C.; Kono, Y.; Kuo, A.; et al. Estimation of Hepatic Proton-Density Fat Fraction by Using MR Imaging at 3.0 T. *Radiology* **2011**, *258*, 749–759. [CrossRef] [PubMed]
122. Tang, A.; Tan, J.; Sun, M.; Hamilton, G.; Bydder, M.; Wolfson, T.; Gamst, A.C.; Middleton, M.; Brunt, E.M.; Loomba, R.; et al. Nonalcoholic Fatty Liver Disease: MR Imaging of Liver Proton Density Fat Fraction to Assess Hepatic Steatosis. *Radiology* **2013**, *267*, 422–431. [CrossRef] [PubMed]
123. Graffy, P.M.; Pickhardt, P.J. Quantification of Hepatic and Visceral Fat by CT and MR Imaging: Relevance to the Obesity Epidemic, Metabolic Syndrome and NAFLD. *Br. J. Radiol.* **2016**, *89*, 20151024. [CrossRef]
124. Petroff, D.; Blank, V.; Newsome, P.N.; Shalimar; Voican, C.S.; Thiele, M.; de Lédinghen, V.; Baumeler, S.; Chan, W.K.; Perlemuter, G.; et al. Assessment of Hepatic Steatosis by Controlled Attenuation Parameter Using the M and XL Probes: An Individual Patient Data Meta-Analysis. *Lancet Gastroenterol. Hepatol.* **2021**, *6*, 185–198. [CrossRef]

125. De Lédinghen, V.; Wong, G.L.-H.; Vergniol, J.; Chan, H.L.-Y.; Hiriart, J.-B.; Chan, A.W.-H.; Chermak, F.; Choi, P.C.-L.; Foucher, J.; Chan, C.K.-M.; et al. Controlled Attenuation Parameter for the Diagnosis of Steatosis in Non-Alcoholic Fatty Liver Disease. *J. Gastroenterol. Hepatol.* **2016**, *31*, 848–855. [CrossRef]
126. Lee, H.W.; Park, S.Y.; Kim, S.U.; Jang, J.Y.; Park, H.; Kim, J.K.; Lee, C.K.; Chon, Y.E.; Han, K.-H. Discrimination of Nonalcoholic Steatohepatitis Using Transient Elastography in Patients with Nonalcoholic Fatty Liver Disease. *PLoS ONE* **2016**, *11*, e0157358. [CrossRef] [PubMed]
127. Newsome, P.N.; Sasso, M.; Deeks, J.J.; Paredes, A.; Boursier, J.; Chan, W.-K.; Yilmaz, Y.; Czernichow, S.; Zheng, M.-H.; Wong, V.W.-S.; et al. FibroScan-AST (FAST) Score for the Non-Invasive Identification of Patients with Non-Alcoholic Steatohepatitis with Significant Activity and Fibrosis: A Prospective Derivation and Global Validation Study. *Lancet Gastroenterol. Hepatol.* **2020**, *5*, 362–373. [CrossRef]
128. Agarwal, L.; Aggarwal, S.; Shalimar; Yadav, R.; Dattagupta, S.; Garg, H.; Agarwal, S. Bariatric Surgery in Nonalcoholic Fatty Liver Disease (NAFLD): Impact Assessment Using Paired Liver Biopsy and Fibroscan. *Obes. Surg.* **2021**, *31*, 617–626. [CrossRef]
129. Caussy, C.; Alquiraish, M.H.; Nguyen, P.; Hernandez, C.; Cepin, S.; Fortney, L.E.; Ajmera, V.; Bettencourt, R.; Collier, S.; Hooker, J.; et al. Optimal Threshold of Controlled Attenuation Parameter with MRI-PDFF as the Gold Standard for the Detection of Hepatic Steatosis. *Hepatology* **2018**, *67*, 1348–1359. [CrossRef]
130. Sasso, M.; Audière, S.; Kemgang, A.; Gaouar, F.; Corpechot, C.; Chazouillères, O.; Fournier, C.; Golsztejn, O.; Prince, S.; Menu, Y.; et al. Liver Steatosis Assessed by Controlled Attenuation Parameter (CAP) Measured with the XL Probe of the FibroScan: A Pilot Study Assessing Diagnostic Accuracy. *Ultrasound Med. Biol.* **2016**, *42*, 92–103. [CrossRef]
131. Garg, H.; Aggarwal, S.; Shalimar; Yadav, R.; Datta Gupta, S.; Agarwal, L.; Agarwal, S. Utility of Transient Elastography (Fibroscan) and Impact of Bariatric Surgery on Nonalcoholic Fatty Liver Disease (NAFLD) in Morbidly Obese Patients. *Surg. Obes. Relat. Dis. Off. J. Am. Soc. Bariatr. Surg.* **2018**, *14*, 81–91. [CrossRef] [PubMed]
132. Festi, D.; Schiumerini, R.; Marzi, L.; Di Biase, A.R.; Mandolesi, D.; Montrone, L.; Scaioli, E.; Bonato, G.; Marchesini-Reggiani, G.; Colecchia, A. Review Article: The Diagnosis of Non-Alcoholic Fatty Liver Disease—Availability and Accuracy of Non-Invasive Methods. *Aliment. Pharmacol. Ther.* **2013**, *37*, 392–400. [CrossRef]
133. Miyake, T.; Kumagi, T.; Furukawa, S.; Tokumoto, Y.; Hirooka, M.; Abe, M.; Hiasa, Y.; Matsuura, B.; Onji, M. Non-Alcoholic Fatty Liver Disease: Factors Associated with Its Presence and Onset. *J. Gastroenterol. Hepatol.* **2013**, *28* (Suppl. S4), 71–78. [CrossRef] [PubMed]
134. Ahlman, H.; Ahlund, L.; Dahlström, A.; Nilsson, O.; Skolnik, G.; Tisell, L.E.; Tylén, U. Use of a Somatostatin Analogue in Association with Surgery and Hepatic Arterial Embolisation in the Treatment of the Carcinoid Syndrome. *Br. J. Cancer* **1987**, *56*, 840–842. [CrossRef]
135. Tada, T.; Kumada, T.; Toyoda, H.; Kobayashi, N.; Sone, Y.; Oguri, T.; Kamiyama, N. Utility of Attenuation Coefficient Measurement Using an Ultrasound-Guided Attenuation Parameter for Evaluation of Hepatic Steatosis: Comparison with MRI-Determined Proton Density Fat Fraction. *Am. J. Roentgenol.* **2019**, *212*, 332–341. [CrossRef]
136. Pirmoazen, A.M.; Khurana, A.; El Kaffas, A.; Kamaya, A. Quantitative Ultrasound Approaches for Diagnosis and Monitoring Hepatic Steatosis in Nonalcoholic Fatty Liver Disease. *Theranostics* **2020**, *10*, 4277–4289. [CrossRef]
137. Janes, C.H.; Lindor, K.D. Outcome of Patients Hospitalized for Complications after Outpatient Liver Biopsy. *Ann. Intern. Med.* **1993**, *118*, 96–98. [CrossRef]
138. Oki, Y.; Ono, M.; Hyogo, H.; Ochi, T.; Munekage, K.; Nozaki, Y.; Hirose, A.; Masuda, K.; Mizuta, H.; Okamoto, N.; et al. Evaluation of Postprandial Hypoglycemia in Patients with Nonalcoholic Fatty Liver Disease by Oral Glucose Tolerance Testing and Continuous Glucose Monitoring. *Eur. J. Gastroenterol. Hepatol.* **2018**, *30*, 797–805. [CrossRef] [PubMed]
139. Li, G.; Zhang, X.; Lin, H.; Liang, L.Y.; Wong, G.L.; Wong, V.W. Non-Invasive Tests of Non-Alcoholic Fatty Liver Disease. *Chin. Med. J.* **2022**. [CrossRef]
140. Nakahara, T.; Hyogo, H.; Yoneda, M.; Sumida, Y.; Eguchi, Y.; Fujii, H.; Ono, M.; Kawaguchi, T.; Imajo, K.; Aikata, H.; et al. Type 2 Diabetes Mellitus Is Associated with the Fibrosis Severity in Patients with Nonalcoholic Fatty Liver Disease in a Large Retrospective Cohort of Japanese Patients. *J. Gastroenterol.* **2014**, *49*, 1477–1484. [CrossRef]
141. Stepanova, M.; Rafiq, N.; Makhlouf, H.; Agrawal, R.; Kaur, I.; Younoszai, Z.; McCullough, A.; Goodman, Z.; Younossi, Z.M. Predictors of All-Cause Mortality and Liver-Related Mortality in Patients with Non-Alcoholic Fatty Liver Disease (NAFLD). *Dig. Dis. Sci.* **2013**, *58*, 3017–3023. [CrossRef] [PubMed]
142. Loomba, R.; Abraham, M.; Unalp, A.; Wilson, L.; Lavine, J.; Doo, E.; Bass, N.M. Association between Diabetes, Family History of Diabetes, and Risk of Nonalcoholic Steatohepatitis and Fibrosis. *Hepatology* **2012**, *56*, 943–951. [CrossRef] [PubMed]
143. Hashiba, M.; Ono, M.; Hyogo, H.; Ikeda, Y.; Masuda, K.; Yoshioka, R.; Ishikawa, Y.; Nagata, Y.; Munekage, K.; Ochi, T.; et al. Glycemic Variability Is an Independent Predictive Factor for Development of Hepatic Fibrosis in Nonalcoholic Fatty Liver Disease. *PLoS ONE* **2013**, *8*, e76161. [CrossRef]
144. Lv, W.-S.; Sun, R.-X.; Gao, Y.-Y.; Wen, J.-P.; Pan, R.-F.; Li, L.; Wang, J.; Xian, Y.-X.; Cao, C.-X.; Zheng, M. Nonalcoholic Fatty Liver Disease and Microvascular Complications in Type 2 Diabetes. *World J. Gastroenterol.* **2013**, *19*, 3134–3142. [CrossRef]
145. Cakır, E.; Ozbek, M.; Colak, N.; Cakal, E.; Delıbaşi, T. Is NAFLD an Independent Risk Factor for Increased IMT in T2DM? *Minerva Endocrinol.* **2012**, *37*, 187–193. [PubMed]
146. Trojak, A.; Waluś-Miarka, M.; Woźniakiewicz, E.; Małecki, M.T.; Idzior-Waluś, B. Nonalcoholic Fatty Liver Disease Is Associated with Low HDL Cholesterol and Coronary Angioplasty in Patients with Type 2 Diabetes. *Med. Sci. Monit.* **2013**, *19*, 1167–1172.

147. Targher, G.; Bertolini, L.; Padovani, R.; Rodella, S.; Tessari, R.; Zenari, L.; Day, C.; Arcaro, G. Prevalence of Nonalcoholic Fatty Liver Disease and Its Association with Cardiovascular Disease among Type 2 Diabetic Patients. *Diabetes Care* **2007**, *30*, 1212–1218. [CrossRef]
148. Idilman, I.S.; Akata, D.; Hazirolan, T.; Doganay Erdogan, B.; Aytemir, K.; Karcaaltincaba, M. Nonalcoholic Fatty Liver Disease Is Associated with Significant Coronary Artery Disease in Type 2 Diabetic Patients: A Computed Tomography Angiography Study 2. *J. Diabetes* **2015**, *7*, 279–286. [CrossRef]
149. Bonapace, S.; Perseghin, G.; Molon, G.; Canali, G.; Bertolini, L.; Zoppini, G.; Barbieri, E.; Targher, G. Nonalcoholic Fatty Liver Disease Is Associated with Left Ventricular Diastolic Dysfunction in Patients with Type 2 Diabetes. *Diabetes Care* **2012**, *35*, 389–395. [CrossRef]
150. Bonapace, S.; Valbusa, F.; Bertolini, L.; Pichiri, I.; Mantovani, A.; Rossi, A.; Zenari, L.; Barbieri, E.; Targher, G. Nonalcoholic Fatty Liver Disease Is Associated with Aortic Valve Sclerosis in Patients with Type 2 Diabetes Mellitus. *PLoS ONE* **2014**, *9*, e88371. [CrossRef]
151. Targher, G.; Valbusa, F.; Bonapace, S.; Bertolini, L.; Zenari, L.; Rodella, S.; Zoppini, G.; Mantovani, W.; Barbieri, E.; Byrne, C.D. Non-Alcoholic Fatty Liver Disease Is Associated with an Increased Incidence of Atrial Fibrillation in Patients with Type 2 Diabetes. *PLoS ONE* **2013**, *8*, e57183. [CrossRef] [PubMed]
152. Kim, S.; Jeon, M.; Lee, J.; Han, J.; Oh, S.J.; Jung, T.; Nam, S.J.; Kil, W.H.; Lee, J.E. Induction of Fibronectin in Response to Epidermal Growth Factor Is Suppressed by Silibinin through the Inhibition of STAT3 in Triple Negative Breast Cancer Cells. *Oncol. Rep.* **2014**, *32*, 2230–2236. [CrossRef] [PubMed]
153. Tziomalos, K.; Giampatzis, V.; Bouziana, S.D.; Spanou, M.; Papadopoulou, M.; Pavlidis, A.; Kostaki, S.; Bozikas, A.; Savopoulos, C.; Hatzitolios, A.I. Association between Nonalcoholic Fatty Liver Disease and Acute Ischemic Stroke Severity and Outcome. *World J. Hepatol.* **2013**, *5*, 621–626. [CrossRef]
154. Jenks, S.J.; Conway, B.R.; Hor, T.J.; Williamson, R.M.; McLachlan, S.; Robertson, C.; Morling, J.R.; Strachan, M.W.J.; Price, J.F. Hepatic Steatosis and Non-Alcoholic Fatty Liver Disease Are Not Associated with Decline in Renal Function in People with Type 2 Diabetes. *Diabet. Med.* **2014**, *31*, 1039–1046. [CrossRef]
155. Kim, B.-Y.; Jung, C.-H.; Mok, J.-O.; Kang, S.K.; Kim, C.-H. Prevalences of Diabetic Retinopathy and Nephropathy Are Lower in Korean Type 2 Diabetic Patients with Non-Alcoholic Fatty Liver Disease. *J. Diabetes Investig.* **2014**, *5*, 170–175. [CrossRef] [PubMed]
156. Ziolkowska, S.; Binienda, A.; Jabłkowski, M.; Szemraj, J.; Czarny, P. The Interplay between Insulin Resistance, Inflammation, Oxidative Stress, Base Excision Repair and Metabolic Syndrome in Nonalcoholic Fatty Liver Disease. *Int. J. Mol. Sci.* **2021**, *22*, 11128. [CrossRef]
157. Dunstan, D.W.; Salmon, J.; Healy, G.N.; Shaw, J.E.; Jolley, D.; Zimmet, P.Z.; Owen, N. Association of Television Viewing with Fasting and 2-h Postchallenge Plasma Glucose Levels in Adults without Diagnosed Diabetes. *Diabetes Care* **2007**, *30*, 516–522. [CrossRef]
158. Al-Jiffri, O.; Al-Sharif, F.M.; Abd El-Kader, S.M.; Ashmawy, E.M. Weight Reduction Improves Markers of Hepatic Function and Insulin Resistance in Type-2 Diabetic Patients with Non-Alcoholic Fatty Liver. *Afr. Health Sci.* **2013**, *13*, 667–672. [CrossRef]
159. Kistler, K.D.; Brunt, E.M.; Clark, J.M.; Diehl, A.M.; Sallis, J.F.; Schwimmer, J.B. Physical Activity Recommendations, Exercise Intensity, and Histological Severity of Nonalcoholic Fatty Liver Disease. *Am. J. Gastroenterol.* **2011**, *106*, 460–468. [CrossRef]
160. Thomas, D.E.; Elliott, E.J.; Naughton, G.A. Exercise for Type 2 Diabetes Mellitus. *Cochrane Database Syst. Rev.* **2006**, *3*, CD002968. [CrossRef]
161. Snowling, N.J.; Hopkins, W.G. Effects of Different Modes of Exercise Training on Glucose Control and Risk Factors for Complications in Type 2 Diabetic Patients: A Meta-Analysis. *Diabetes Care* **2006**, *29*, 2518–2527. [CrossRef] [PubMed]
162. Bozzetto, L.; Prinster, A.; Annuzzi, G.; Costagliola, L.; Mangione, A.; Vitelli, A.; Mazzarella, R.; Longobardo, M.; Mancini, M.; Vigorito, C.; et al. Liver Fat Is Reduced by an Isoenergetic MUFA Diet in a Controlled Randomized Study in Type 2 Diabetic Patients. *Diabetes Care* **2012**, *35*, 1429–1435. [CrossRef] [PubMed]
163. Cai, H.; Qin, Y.-L.; Shi, Z.-Y.; Chen, J.-H.; Zeng, M.-J.; Zhou, W.; Chen, R.-Q.; Chen, Z.-Y. Effects of Alternate-Day Fasting on Body Weight and Dyslipidaemia in Patients with Non-Alcoholic Fatty Liver Disease: A Randomised Controlled Trial. *BMC Gastroenterol.* **2019**, *19*, 219. [CrossRef] [PubMed]
164. Chung, H.; Chou, W.; Sears, D.D.; Patterson, R.E.; Webster, N.J.G.; Ellies, L.G. Time-Restricted Feeding Improves Insulin Resistance and Hepatic Steatosis in a Mouse Model of Postmenopausal Obesity. *Metabolism* **2016**, *65*, 1743–1754. [CrossRef] [PubMed]
165. Stewart, K.E.; Haller, D.L.; Sargeant, C.; Levenson, J.L.; Puri, P.; Sanyal, A.J. Readiness for Behaviour Change in Non-Alcoholic Fatty Liver Disease: Implications for Multidisciplinary Care Models. *Liver Int. Off. J. Int. Assoc. Study Liver* **2015**, *35*, 936–943. [CrossRef]
166. Ibrahim, M.A.; Kelleni, M.; Geddawy, A. Nonalcoholic Fatty Liver Disease: Current and Potential Therapies. *Life Sci.* **2013**, *92*, 114–118. [CrossRef]
167. Duseja, A.; Das, A.; Dhiman, R.K.; Chawla, Y.K.; Thumburu, K.T.; Bhadada, S.; Bhansali, A. Metformin Is Effective in Achieving Biochemical Response in Patients with Nonalcoholic Fatty Liver Disease (NAFLD) Not Responding to Lifestyle Interventions. *Ann. Hepatol.* **2007**, *6*, 222–226. [CrossRef]

168. Shyangdan, D.; Clar, C.; Ghouri, N.; Henderson, R.; Gurung, T.; Preiss, D.; Sattar, N.; Fraser, A.; Waugh, N. Insulin Sensitisers in the Treatment of Non-Alcoholic Fatty Liver Disease: A Systematic Review. *Health Technol. Assess.* **2011**, *15*, 1–110. [CrossRef]
169. Haukeland, J.W.; Konopski, Z.; Eggesbø, H.B.; von Volkmann, H.L.; Raschpichler, G.; Bjøro, K.; Haaland, T.; Løberg, E.M.; Birkeland, K. Metformin in Patients with Non-Alcoholic Fatty Liver Disease: A Randomized, Controlled Trial. *Scand. J. Gastroenterol.* **2009**, *44*, 853–860. [CrossRef]
170. Linden, M.A.; Fletcher, J.A.; Morris, E.M.; Meers, G.M.; Kearney, M.L.; Crissey, J.M.; Laughlin, M.H.; Booth, F.W.; Sowers, J.R.; Ibdah, J.A.; et al. Combining Metformin and Aerobic Exercise Training in the Treatment of Type 2 Diabetes and NAFLD in OLETF Rats. *Am. J. Physiol. Endocrinol. Metab.* **2014**, *306*, E300–E310. [CrossRef]
171. Vuppalanchi, R.; Chalasani, N. Nonalcoholic Fatty Liver Disease and Nonalcoholic Steatohepatitis: Selected Practical Issues in Their Evaluation and Management. *Hepatology* **2009**, *49*, 306–317. [CrossRef] [PubMed]
172. Duvnjak, M.; Tomasic, V.; Gomercic, M.; Smircic Duvnjak, L.; Barsic, N.; Lerotic, I. Therapy of Nonalcoholic Fatty Liver Disease: Current Status. *J. Physiol. Pharmacol.* **2009**, *60* (Suppl. S7), 57–66.
173. Shadid, S.; Jensen, M.D. Effect of Pioglitazone on Biochemical Indices of Non-Alcoholic Fatty Liver Disease in Upper Body Obesity. *Clin. Gastroenterol. Hepatol.* **2003**, *1*, 384–387. [CrossRef]
174. Saryusz-Wolska, M.; Szymańska-Garbacz, E.; Jabłkowski, M.; Białkowska, J.; Pawłowski, M.; Kwiecińska, E.; Omulecka, A.; Borkowska, A.; Ignaczak, A.; Loba, J.; et al. Rosiglitazone Treatment in Nondiabetic Subjects with Nonalcoholic Fatty Liver Disease. *Pol. Arch. Med. Wewn.* **2011**, *121*, 61–66. [CrossRef]
175. Lutchman, G.; Modi, A.; Kleiner, D.E.; Promrat, K.; Heller, T.; Ghany, M.; Borg, B.; Loomba, R.; Liang, T.J.; Premkumar, A.; et al. The Effects of Discontinuing Pioglitazone in Patients with Nonalcoholic Steatohepatitis. *Hepatology* **2007**, *46*, 424–429. [CrossRef] [PubMed]
176. Lian, J.; Fu, J. Pioglitazone for NAFLD Patients with Prediabetes or Type 2 Diabetes Mellitus: A Meta-Analysis. *Front. Endocrinol.* **2021**, *12*, 428. [CrossRef] [PubMed]
177. Ratziu, V.; Charlotte, F.; Bernhardt, C.; Giral, P.; Halbron, M.; Lenaour, G.; Hartmann-Heurtier, A.; Bruckert, E.; Poynard, T. Long-Term Efficacy of Rosiglitazone in Nonalcoholic Steatohepatitis: Results of the Fatty Liver Improvement by Rosiglitazone Therapy (FLIRT 2) Extension Trial. *Hepatology* **2010**, *51*, 445–453. [CrossRef] [PubMed]
178. Omer, Z.; Cetinkalp, S.; Akyildiz, M.; Yilmaz, F.; Batur, Y.; Yilmaz, C.; Akarca, U. Efficacy of Insulin-Sensitizing Agents in Nonalcoholic Fatty Liver Disease. *Eur. J. Gastroenterol. Hepatol.* **2010**, *22*, 18–23. [CrossRef]
179. Colca, J.R.; McDonald, W.G.; Adams, W.J. MSDC-0602K, a Metabolic Modulator Directed at the Core Pathology of Non-Alcoholic Steatohepatitis. *Expert Opin. Investig. Drugs* **2018**, *27*, 631–636. [CrossRef]
180. Cuthbertson, D.J.; Irwin, A.; Gardner, C.J.; Daousi, C.; Purewal, T.; Furlong, N.; Goenka, N.; Thomas, E.L.; Adams, V.L.; Pushpakom, S.P.; et al. Improved Glycaemia Correlates with Liver Fat Reduction in Obese, Type 2 Diabetes, Patients given Glucagon-like Peptide-1 (GLP-1) Receptor Agonists. *PLoS ONE* **2012**, *7*, e50117. [CrossRef]
181. Fan, H.; Pan, Q.; Xu, Y.; Yang, X. Exenatide Improves Type 2 Diabetes Concomitant with Non-Alcoholic Fatty Liver Disease. *Arq. Bras. Endocrinol. Metabol.* **2013**, *57*, 702–708. [CrossRef] [PubMed]
182. Shao, N.; Kuang, H.Y.; Hao, M.; Gao, X.Y.; Lin, W.J.; Zou, W. Benefits of Exenatide on Obesity and Non-Alcoholic Fatty Liver Disease with Elevated Liver Enzymes in Patients with Type 2 Diabetes. *Diabetes Metab. Res. Rev.* **2014**, *30*, 521–529. [CrossRef] [PubMed]
183. Armstrong, M.J.; Houlihan, D.D.; Rowe, I.A.; Clausen, W.H.O.; Elbrønd, B.; Gough, S.C.L.; Tomlinson, J.W.; Newsome, P.N. Safety and Efficacy of Liraglutide in Patients with Type 2 Diabetes and Elevated Liver Enzymes: Individual Patient Data Meta-Analysis of the LEAD Program. *Aliment. Pharmacol. Ther.* **2013**, *37*, 234–242. [CrossRef] [PubMed]
184. Fukuhara, T.; Hyogo, H.; Ochi, H.; Fujino, H.; Kan, H.; Naeshiro, N.; Honda, Y.; Miyaki, D.; Kawaoka, T.; Tsuge, M.; et al. Efficacy and Safety of Sitagliptin for the Treatment of Nonalcoholic Fatty Liver Disease with Type 2 Diabetes Mellitus. *Hepatogastroenterology* **2014**, *61*, 323–328.
185. Deng, X.-L.; Ma, R.; Zhu, H.-X.; Zhu, J. Short Article: A Randomized-Controlled Study of Sitagliptin for Treating Diabetes Mellitus Complicated by Nonalcoholic Fatty Liver Disease. *Eur. J. Gastroenterol. Hepatol.* **2017**, *29*, 297–301. [CrossRef] [PubMed]
186. Ohki, T.; Isogawa, A.; Iwamoto, M.; Ohsugi, M.; Yoshida, H.; Toda, N.; Tagawa, K.; Omata, M.; Koike, K. The Effectiveness of Liraglutide in Nonalcoholic Fatty Liver Disease Patients with Type 2 Diabetes Mellitus Compared to Sitagliptin and Pioglitazone. *Sci. World J.* **2012**, *2012*, 496453. [CrossRef]
187. Inzucchi, S.E.; Bergenstal, R.M.; Buse, J.B.; Diamant, M.; Ferrannini, E.; Nauck, M.; Peters, A.L.; Tsapas, A.; Wender, R.; Matthews, D.R. Management of Hyperglycaemia in Type 2 Diabetes: A Patient-Centered Approach. Position Statement of the American Diabetes Association (ADA) and the European Association for the Study of Diabetes (EASD). *Diabetologia* **2012**, *55*, 1577–1596. [CrossRef]
188. Chatran, M.; Pilehvar-Soltanahmadi, Y.; Dadashpour, M.; Faramarzi, L.; Rasouli, S.; Jafari-gharabaghlou, D.; Asbaghi, N.; Zarghami, N.; Zarghami, N.; Street, G.; et al. Synergistic Anti-Proliferative Effects of Metformin and Silibinin Combination on T47D Breast Cancer Cells via HTERT and Cyclin D1 Inhibition. *Drug Res.* **2018**, *68*, 710–716. [CrossRef]
189. Fraser, A.; Harris, R.; Sattar, N.; Ebrahim, S.; Davey Smith, G.; Lawlor, D.A. Alanine Aminotransferase, Gamma-Glutamyltransferase, and Incident Diabetes: The British Women's Heart and Health Study and Meta-Analysis. *Diabetes Care* **2009**, *32*, 741–750. [CrossRef]

190. Klein, S.; Mittendorfer, B.; Eagon, J.C.; Patterson, B.; Grant, L.; Feirt, N.; Seki, E.; Brenner, D.; Korenblat, K.; McCrea, J. Gastric Bypass Surgery Improves Metabolic and Hepatic Abnormalities Associated with Nonalcoholic Fatty Liver Disease. *Gastroenterology* **2006**, *130*, 1564–1572. [CrossRef]
191. Viana, E.C.; Araujo-Dasilio, K.L.; Miguel, G.P.S.; Bressan, J.; Lemos, E.M.; Moyses, M.R.; de Abreu, G.R.; de Azevedo, J.L.M.C.; Carvalho, P.S.; Passos-Bueno, M.R.S.; et al. Gastric Bypass and Sleeve Gastrectomy: The Same Impact on IL-6 and TNF-α. Prospective Clinical Trial. *Obes. Surg.* **2013**, *23*, 1252–1261. [CrossRef] [PubMed]
192. Bower, G.; Toma, T.; Harling, L.; Jiao, L.R.; Efthimiou, E.; Darzi, A.; Athanasiou, T.; Ashrafian, H. Bariatric Surgery and Non-Alcoholic Fatty Liver Disease: A Systematic Review of Liver Biochemistry and Histology. *Obes. Surg.* **2015**, *25*, 2280–2289. [CrossRef] [PubMed]
193. Praveen Raj, P.; Gomes, R.M.; Kumar, S.; Senthilnathan, P.; Karthikeyan, P.; Shankar, A.; Palanivelu, C. The Effect of Surgically Induced Weight Loss on Nonalcoholic Fatty Liver Disease in Morbidly Obese Indians: "NASHOST" Prospective Observational Trial. *Surg. Obes. Relat. Dis.* **2015**, *11*, 1315–1322. [CrossRef] [PubMed]

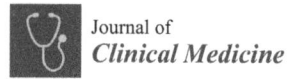

Article

Paracrine Interaction of Cholangiocellular Carcinoma with Cancer-Associated Fibroblasts and Schwann Cells Impact Cell Migration

Jan-Paul Gundlach [1,2,*,†], Jannik Kerber [1,2,†], Alexander Hendricks [3], Alexander Bernsmeier [1], Christine Halske [4], Christian Röder [2], Thomas Becker [1], Christoph Röcken [4], Felix Braun [1], Susanne Sebens [2,‡] and Nils Heits [1,5,‡]

[1] Department of General, Visceral-, Thoracic-, Transplantation- and Pediatric Surgery, University Medical Center Schleswig-Holstein (UKSH), Campus Kiel, Arnold-Heller-Str. 3, Building C, 24105 Kiel, Germany; jannik-kerber@t-online.de (J.K.); alexander.bernsmeier@uksh.de (A.B.); thomas.becker@uksh.de (T.B.); felix.braun@uksh.de (F.B.); nheits@web.de (N.H.)

[2] Institute for Experimental Cancer Research, Kiel University and University Medical Center Schleswig-Holstein (UKSH), Campus Kiel, Arnold-Heller-Str. 3, Building U30, 24105 Kiel, Germany; christian.Roeder@email.uni-kiel.de (C.R.); susanne.sebens@email.uni-kiel.de (S.S.)

[3] Department of General, Visceral-, Vascular-, and Transplantation Surgery, Medical University Rostock, Schillingallee 35, 18057 Rostock, Germany; alexander.hendricks@med.uni-rostock.de

[4] Institute of Pathology, University Medical Center Schleswig-Holstein (UKSH), Campus Kiel, Arnold-Heller-Str. 3, Building U33, 24105 Kiel, Germany; christine.halske@uksh.de (C.H.); christoph.roecken@uksh.de (C.R.)

[5] Gesundheitszentrum Kiel-Mitte, Prüner Gang 15, 24103 Kiel, Germany

* Correspondence: jan-paul.gundlach@uksh.de

† These authors contributed equally to this work.

‡ These authors contributed equally to this work.

Abstract: Although the Mitogen-activated protein kinase (MAPK) pathway is enriched in cholangiocarcinoma (CCA), treatment with the multityrosine kinase-inhibitor Sorafenib is disappointing. While cancer-associated fibroblasts (CAF) are known to contribute to treatment resistance in CCA, knowledge is lacking for Schwann cells (SC). We investigated the impact of stromal cells on CCA cells and whether this is affected by Sorafenib. Immunohistochemistry revealed elevated expression of CAF and SC markers significantly correlating with reduced tumor-free survival. In co-culture with CAF, CCA cells mostly migrated, which could be diminished by Sorafenib, while in SC co-cultures, SC predominantly migrated towards CCA cells, unaffected by Sorafenib. Moreover, increased secretion of pro-inflammatory cytokines MCP-1, CXCL-1, IL-6 and IL-8 was determined in CAF mono- and co-cultures, which could be reduced by Sorafenib. Corresponding to migration results, an increased expression of phospho-AKT was measured in CAF co-cultured HuCCT-1 cells, although was unaffected by Sorafenib. Intriguingly, CAF co-cultured TFK-1 cells showed increased activation of STAT3, JNK, ERK and AKT pathways, which was partly reduced by Sorafenib. This study indicates that CAF and SC differentially impact CCA cells and Sorafenib partially reverts these stroma-mediated effects. These findings contribute to a better understanding of the paracrine interplay of CAF and SC with CCA cells.

Keywords: cholangiocellular carcinoma; cancer-associated fibroblasts; Schwann cells; tumor stroma; CCA; Sorafenib

Citation: Gundlach, J.-P.; Kerber, J.; Hendricks, A.; Bernsmeier, A.; Halske, C.; Röder, C.; Becker, T.; Röcken, C.; Braun, F.; Sebens, S.; et al. Paracrine Interaction of Cholangiocellular Carcinoma with Cancer-Associated Fibroblasts and Schwann Cells Impact Cell Migration. *J. Clin. Med.* 2022, 11, 2785. https://doi.org/10.3390/jcm11102785

Academic Editors: Gian Paolo Caviglia and Davide Giuseppe Ribaldone

Received: 13 April 2022
Accepted: 13 May 2022
Published: 15 May 2022

Publisher's Note: MDPI stays neutral with regard to jurisdictional claims in published maps and institutional affiliations.

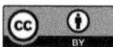

Copyright: © 2022 by the authors. Licensee MDPI, Basel, Switzerland. This article is an open access article distributed under the terms and conditions of the Creative Commons Attribution (CC BY) license (https://creativecommons.org/licenses/by/4.0/).

1. Introduction

Cholangiocarcinoma (CCA) is the most common malignancy of the biliary tract and the second most common primary hepatic malignancy [1]. Its incidence in Western countries is increasing [2], which particularly applies to intrahepatic CCA [3]. Treatment options for CCA are limited. Until now, the only curative therapy is resection of the primary tumor.

Cisplatin and Gemcitabine are used as standard practice chemotherapeutics [4], though due to a lack of qualified data, a lively debate on well-established and broadly accepted therapeutic regime is ongoing [5]. Furthermore, CCA patients may benefit from concomitant radiotherapy, and also liver transplantation can be an option in selected cases [5]. Other current treatment regimens for CCA patients imply transarterial chemoembolization (TACE), intra-arterial chemotherapy and radiofrequency ablation (RFA) approaches [1,5].

Whereas targeted therapies have become effective therapeutic options in different tumor entities, biological treatments for CCA are still scarce [6]. Genetic and microarray data analysis revealed that genes of the Mitogen-activated protein kinase (MAPK) pathway are enriched in CCA as similarly seen in hepatocellular carcinoma (HCC) [7] and the Mitogen-Activated Protein Kinase (MAPK) pathway was demonstrated to be activated in CCA tissue compared to non-tumorous tissue [8]. Since, in advanced HCC, the multityrosine kinase inhibitor Sorafenib was the first drug to significantly improve overall survival [9], Sorafenib was proposed to be advantageous in CCA treatment too [7]. In vitro studies with Sorafenib treatment revealed contrasting results [10,11]: Huether et al. were able to demonstrate the inhibition of cell growth in CCA cell lines by showing that a combined treatment of Sorafenib with Doxorubicin or insulin-like growth factor-1 receptor (IGF-1R)-inhibition resulted in additive antiproliferative effects. However, co-application of Sorafenib and the antimetabolites 5-Fluoruracil (5-FU) or Gemcitabine diminished the antineoplastic effects of cytostatic drugs [10]. Overall, these data indicate that Sorafenib may exert its effects in a context-dependent manner.

As in other solid tumors, CCA cells are embedded in a tumor microenvironment consisting of extracellular matrix (ECM) and a variety of inflammatory stromal cells. Thus, tumor and stromal cells reciprocally interact and impact each other, thereby essentially driving malignant progression and also affecting therapy responses [12]. Interestingly, apart from the MAPK pathway, the above-mentioned genetic analysis also revealed genes encoding for ECM proteins to be significantly enriched [7]. In the tumor stroma, myofibroblasts, also termed cancer-associated fibroblasts (CAF), are of particular interest [13] because they often represent one major stroma cell population. CAF are characterized—amongst others—by high expression of α-smooth muscle actin (α-SMA) and fibroblast specific protein-1 (FSP-1) and produce a plethora of inflammatory mediators, growth factors and ECM molecules by which they promote malignant progression of different tumor entities [14,15]. Even though a high abundance of CAF was correlated with poor survival of CCA patients [16] and CAF are known to contribute to treatment resistance in CCA [13], detailed analyses on the impact of CAF on CCA cells are still missing.

Apart from CAF, Schwann cells (SC) are also an important part of the tumor microenvironment of CCA, though their contribution to tumor progression is not yet fully understood [17]. SC represent a major component of the peripheral nervous system in their function in myelination, axonal maintenance and repair [17]. SC are commonly detected in tumor tissues by staining of the protein S100, which is a calcium binding protein [18]. Several studies indicate that nerves have a stimulatory role in cancer progression [19–21], e.g., in promoting tumor cell (perineural) invasion [21].

Since knowledge on the role of CAF and SC in CCA progression is still very poor, the present study aimed to better understand the impact of either stromal cell population on CCA migratory abilities and to analyze whether treatment with Sorafenib might be effective in inhibiting CCA migration.

2. Results

2.1. High Abundance of CAF and SC Is Associated with Reduced Survival of CCA Patients

First, tumor sections of 14 CCA patients (5 intrahepatic and 9 extrahepatic) were immunohistochemically analyzed for the abundance of CAF (by staining of α-SMA and FSP-1) and SC (by staining of S100). Of these cases, three patients were operated in TNM-stadium T1, nine patients in stadium T2 and two patients in T3. Representative stainings of CAF and SC in a T1 tumor and a T3 tumor are shown in Figure 1A, indicating that the accumulation of either stromal cell population already starts in early stage CCA. Overall, a moderate to strong staining of either α-SMA or FSP-1 was detected in 10/14 tissues as well as a weak to moderately positive S100 staining in 5/14 tissues. Moreover, elevated expression of either marker showed a reduced tumor-free survival of the patients (Figure 1C–E). Although obtained from a small cohort, these findings support previous studies [14] and underscore that a high abundance of CAF and SC is associated with reduced survival of CCA patients.

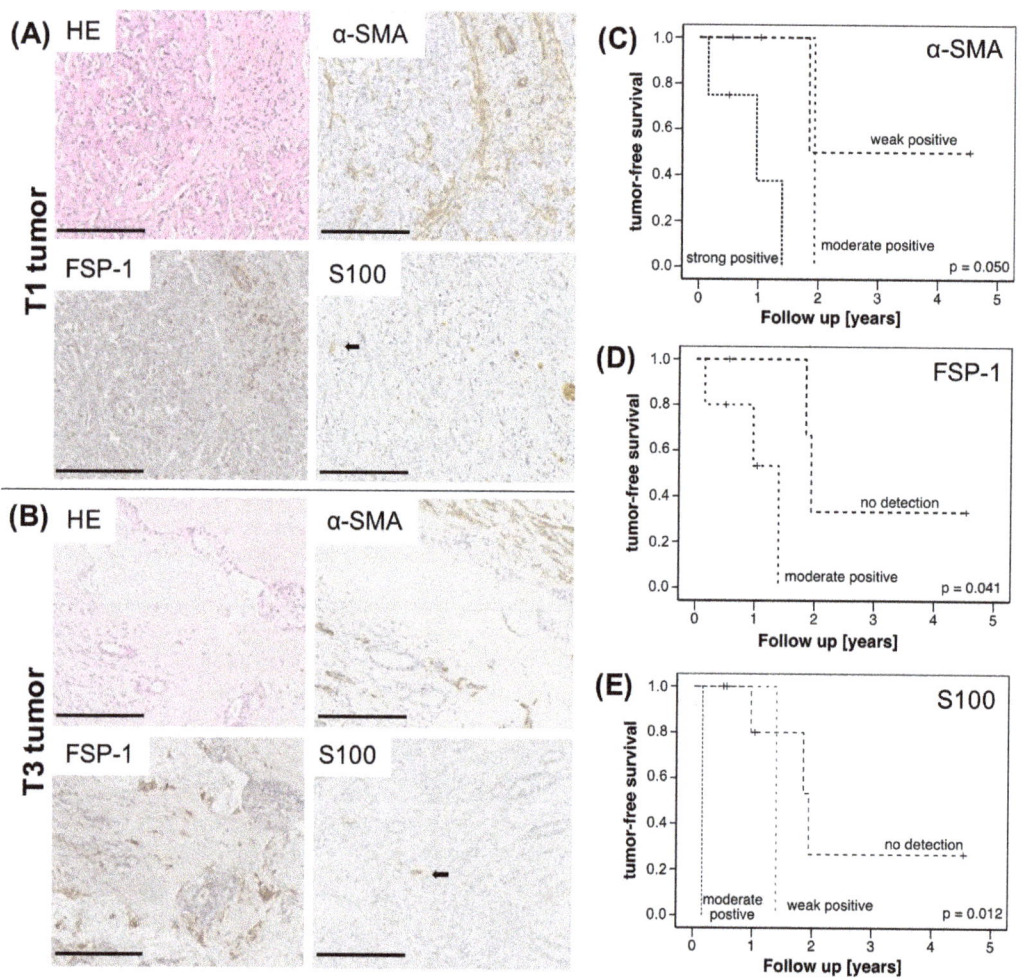

Figure 1. Immunohistochemical analysis of CCA specimens and correlation with survival of CCA patients. (**A**) Representative HE stainings and stainings for α-SMA, FSP-1 and S100 in pT1 N0 (scale bar = 250 µm) and (**B**) pT3 N0 (scale bar = 500 µm) CCA specimens. Kaplan–Meier plots for tumor-free survival of CCA patients depending on (**C**) α-SMA, (**D**) FSP-1- and (**E**) S100-expression; (n = 14 CCA, thereof 5 with intrahepatic and 9 with extrahepatic tumors). Statistical significances are indicated in the figure.

2.2. Impact of CAF and SC on Cell Migration of CCA Cells

To elucidate the impact of CAF and SC on the migratory behavior of CCA cells, HuCCT-1 and TFK-1 cells as well as both stromal cell populations were cultured either alone (mono-culture) or CCA cell lines were co-cultured with CAF or SC in four chamber ibidi slides. Cell migration was assessed by measuring the gap closure by determining cell confluence (Figure 2). Figure 2A–C show representative images of one experiment (out of three independent experiments). Mono-cultured CCA cell lines as well as stromal cells only led to a gap closure of 5.4% (mono-cultured CAF) to 17.5% (mono-cultured HuCCT-1) after 18 h (Figure 2D–G). Since HuCCT-1 cells showed a higher basal migratory potential than TFK-1 cells (17.5% versus 1.4% TFK-1 cells after 18 h), gap closure was analyzed after 18 h in HuCCT-1 (Figure 2D,F) and in TFK-1 cells after 18 (not shown) and 68 h (Figure 2E,G). Moreover, while gap closure by mono-cultured CAF was only marginally increased from 18 h to 68 h (5.4 to 10.5%), gap closure by mono-cultured SC increased from 6.8% after 18 h to 49.2% after 68 h, indicating a higher basal migratory potential of SC (Figure 2F,G).

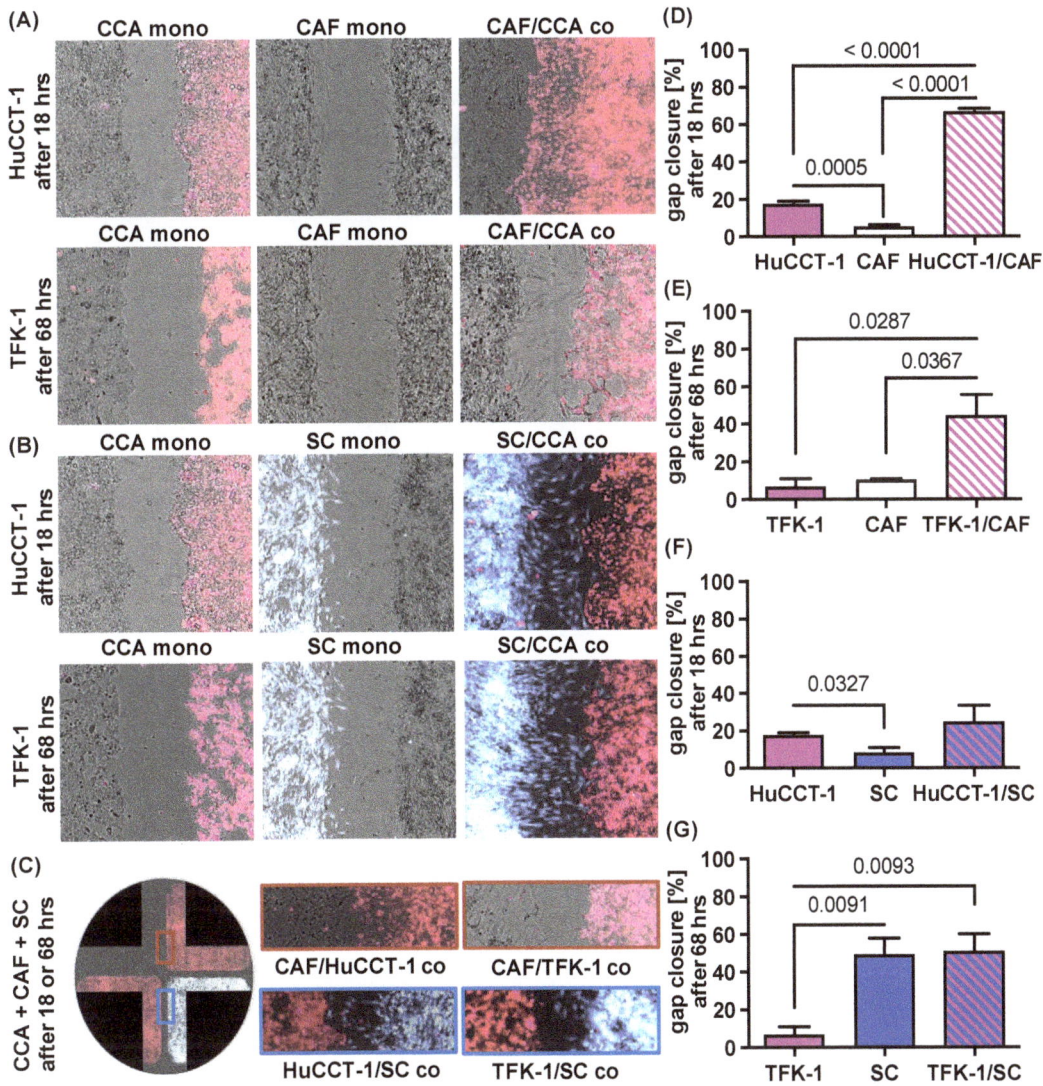

Figure 2. Paracrine impact of CAF and SC on cell migration of CCA cells. HuCCT-1 and TFK-1 cells were cultured either alone (CCA mono) or together with CAF (CAF/CCA co) or SC (SC/CCA co) in

4 chamber ibidi slides. Mono-cultured CAF (CAF mono) and SC (SC mono) were cultured in parallel as control. Mono- and co-cultures with HuCCT-1 cells were analyzed after 18 h and those of TFK-1 cells after 18 h and 68 h (representative pictures at 10-fold magnification). CCA cells were stained with CellTracker Deep Red, SC were stained with CellTracker CMAC blue and CAF were not stained. (**A,B**) Representative pictures of gap closure of the different mono- and co-cultured cell populations. (**C**) Representative images of co-cultured CCA cells, CAF and SC in a 4 chamber ibidi slide showing gap closure after 18 h (HuCCT-1) and 68 h (TFK-1). (**D–G**) Quantification of cell migration of the depicted cell populations after 18 h (HuCCT-1) and 68 h (TFK-1) were performed with the Wound healing beta 2F-Operator (Synentec). Data are presented as % gap closure normalized to t = 0 h and as mean and standard deviation of 3 independent experiments. Statistical significances are indicated in the figure.

Importantly, gap closure was most pronounced when either CCA cell line was co-cultured with stromal cells, albeit clear differences were observed in dependence on the stromal cells (Figure 2A,B,D–G). While in the co-culture of CCA cells and CAF, the gap was closed predominantly by migration of CCA cells (Figure 2A), gap closure during co-culture of CCA cells and SC was predominantly mediated by the migration of SC cells towards CCA cells (Figure 2B). This migratory behavior was also not changed when CCA cells were concomitantly exposed to CAF and SC (Figure 2C). In HuCCT-1 co-cultures, gap closure was significantly more pronounced in the presence of CAF ($p < 0.0001$) than SC ($p = 0.4489$; 66.9% gap closure after CAF co-culture versus 24.8% after SC co-culture, Figure 2D,F), while in TFK-1 co-cultures, gap closure was slightly more pronounced in the presence of SC after 18 h ($p = 0.0083$) but comparable in the presence of CAF ($p = 0.0287$; 44.7%) and SC ($p = 0.0093$; 50.1%) after 68 h (Figure 2E,G). Overall, these data indicate that cell migration of CCA cells is enhanced in the presence of CAF, while the presence of CCA cells, in turn, increases cell migration of SC.

2.3. Sorafenib Inhibits Migration of CCA and Stromal Cells in a Context Dependent Manner

Since the multityrosine kinase inhibitor Sorafenib has already shown growth inhibitory effects on CCA cells [7], we next investigated whether Sorafenib might be also able to inhibit cell migration of CCA cells and different stromal cells. Since a dosage of 1 µM has been shown to hardly impact the cell growth of neither CCA cells nor both stromal cell populations (data not shown), mono- and co-cultures of CCA cells, CAF and SC, respectively, in the absence or presence of 1 µM Sorafenib were conducted to analyze gap closure. As seen in Figure 3A, Sorafenib treatment even intensified cell migration of mono-cultured HuCCT-1 cells, leading to an increased gap closure from 17.5% to 28.2%, while cell migration of mono-cultured CAF was clearly diminished after 18 h (from 5.4% to 2.9%, $p = 0.0668$, Figure 3A,B) and even more pronounced after 68 h (from 10.5% to 3.8%, $p = 0.0005$, Figure 3C). Furthermore, a clear reduction in cell migration was observed in co-cultures from HuCCT-1 cells and CAF (from 66.9% to 38.0%, $p = 0.0548$). In contrast, gap closure by mono-cultured SC after 18 h (8.2% versus 8.6%, Figure 3A,B) and after 68 h (49.3% versus 45.2%, Figure 3C) as well as HuCCT-1 co-cultures with SC (from 24.8% to 28.5%; Figure 3A) remained nearly unaffected. Similar observations could be made with TFK-1 cells. Here, Sorafenib treatment also did not impact cell migration of mono- and co-cultured CCA cells with SC (Figure 3B,C). In line with the results described for HuCCT-1 cells and mono-cultured CAF, a clear inhibitory effect on cell migration could only be observed on co-cultures of CAF and TFK-1 cells, leading to a reduced gap closure from 8.9% to 4.5% ($p = 0.0145$) and from 44.5% to 23.4% ($p = 0.1489$) after 18 h and 68 h, respectively (Figure 3B,C). Overall, these data indicate that Sorafenib treatment impairs the migratory abilities of CAF and CCA cells but not SC. The fact that particularly the co-culture increased cell migration of CAF and CCA cells was affected point to a Sorafenib-mediated inhibition of paracrine interactions between tumor cells and CAF.

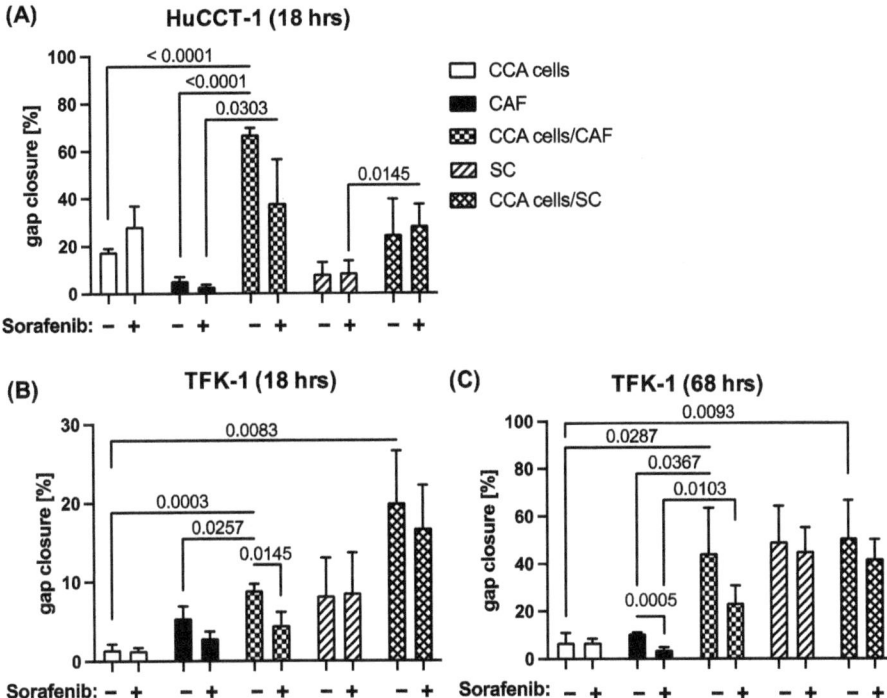

Figure 3. Sorafenib reduces migration of CAF and CAF co-cultivated CCA cells. HuCCT-1 and TFK-1 cells were cultured either alone or together with CAF or SC in 4 chamber ibidi slides. Mono-cultured CAF and SC were cultured in parallel as control. Additionally, cells were either left untreated or treated with 1 µM Sorafenib. (**A**) Gap closure of mono- and co-cultures with HuCCT-1 cells was analyzed after 18 h and those with TFK-1 cells after (**B**) 18 h and (**C**) 68 h. Data are presented as % gap closure normalized to t = 0 h and as mean and standard deviation of 3 independent experiments. Statistical significances are indicated in the figure.

2.4. Analysis of Potential Migratory Inducing Factors in Co-Culture with CAF or SC

In order to better understand the paracrine interactions between CCA cells and stromal cell populations, which might impact cell migration and might be affected by Sorafenib treatment, Proteome Profiler Human Cytokine Array Kit Panel A was used to determine the release of cytokines and chemokines during the different mono- and co-cultures in the absence or presence of 1 µM Sorafenib. No differences in the release of C5a, CD40 Ligand/TNFSF5, G-CSF, GM-CSF, CXCL1/GROα, CCL1/I-309, ICAM-1, IFN-µ, Interleukin (IL)-1α /IL-1F1, IL-1ß/IL-1F2, IL-1ra/IL-1F3, IL-2, IL-4, IL-5, IL-6, IL-8, IL-10, IL-12 p70, IL-13, IL-16, IL-17, IL-17E, IL-23, IL-27, IL-32α, CXCL10/IP-10, CXCL11/I-TAC, CCL2/MCP-1, MIF, CCL3/MIP-1α, CCL4/MIP-1ß, CCL5/RANTES, CXCL12/SDF-1, serpin E1/PAI-1, TNF-α and TREM-1 could be observed in supernatants of the different co-cultures compared to respective mono-cultures as well as after treatment with Sorafenib (data not shown). In contrast, clearly detectable levels of Monocyte Chemoattractant Protein-1 (MCP-1), Chemokine (C-X-C motif) ligand 1 (CXCL-1), IL-6 and IL-8 could be determined in supernatants of CAF as well as in supernatants of co-cultures of CAF and either CCA cell line (Figure 4A). Moreover, after Sorafenib treatment, the levels of all factors were strongly reduced compared to the respective untreated samples (Figure 4A).

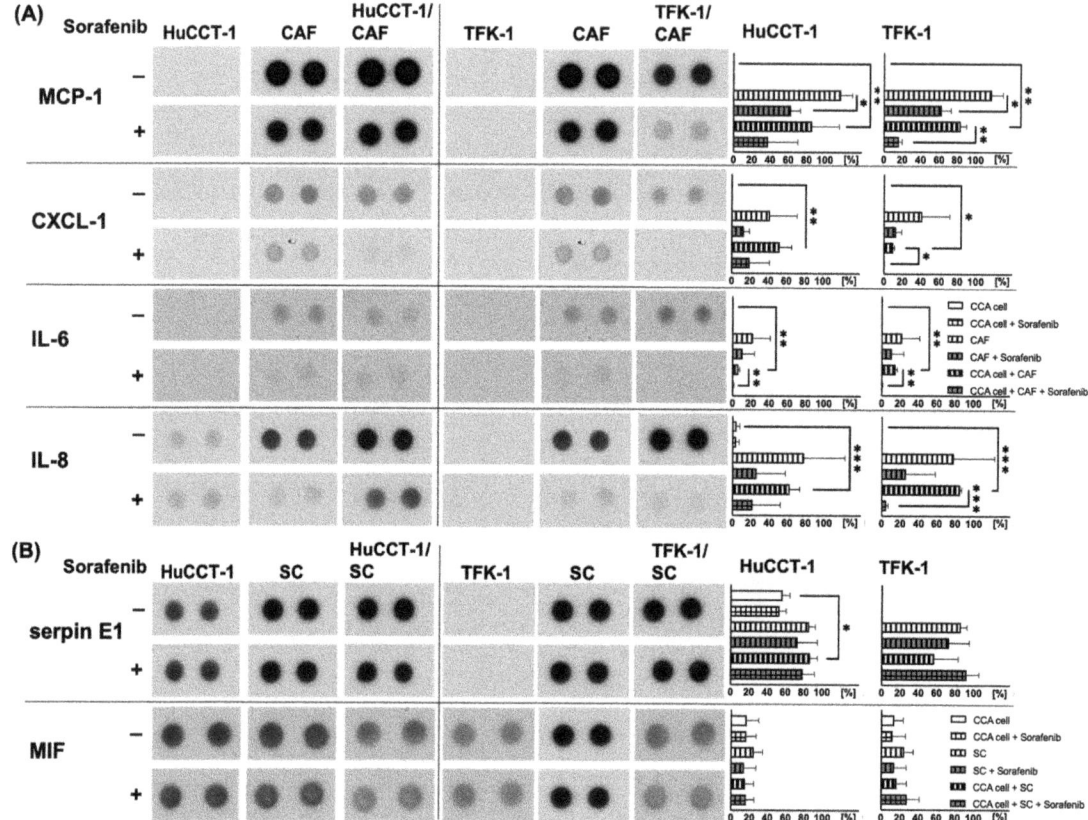

Figure 4. Detection of human cytokines and chemokines in supernatants of mono- and co-cultured CCA and stromal cells. HuCCT-1 and TFK-1 cells were cultured either alone or together with CAF or SC in transwell systems. Mono-cultured CAF and SC were cultured in parallel as control. Additionally, cells were either left untreated or treated with 1 µM Sorafenib for 72 h. Cell culture supernatants were analyzed using the Proteome Profiler Human Cytokine Array Kit, Panel A. Shown are representative results of mono- and co-cultures of CCA cells with (**A**) CAF and (**B**) SC. Pictures are taken from one experiment out of three independent biological replicates. Right to each blot, mean spot densitometries of all replicates ± standard deviation are shown. Significances were defined using asterisks: * $p < 0.05$, ** $p < 0.01$, *** $p < 0.001$.

Furthermore, considerable amounts of serpin E1 and Macrophage migration inhibitory factor (MIF) could be determined in supernatants of mono-cultured HuCCT-1 and SC as well as in co-cultures of both CCA lines and SC (Figure 4B), while in supernatants of mono-cultured TFK-1 cells, no serpin E1 could be detected. However, Sorafenib treatment did not impact serpin E1 and MIF levels in supernatants of either condition. Overall, these data indicate that Sorafenib mostly inhibited the release of CAF-derived factors.

2.5. Altered Signal Transduction in CAF and SC Stimulated CCA Cells

To elucidate whether the paracrine interactions with stromal cells led to an altered signal transduction in CCA cells, Western blot analyses of CCA cells exposed to medium or conditioned medium from either stromal cell line in the absence or presence of 1 µM Sorafenib were conducted to detect activated (phosphorylated) forms of STAT3, JNK, ERK and AKT (Figure 5A).

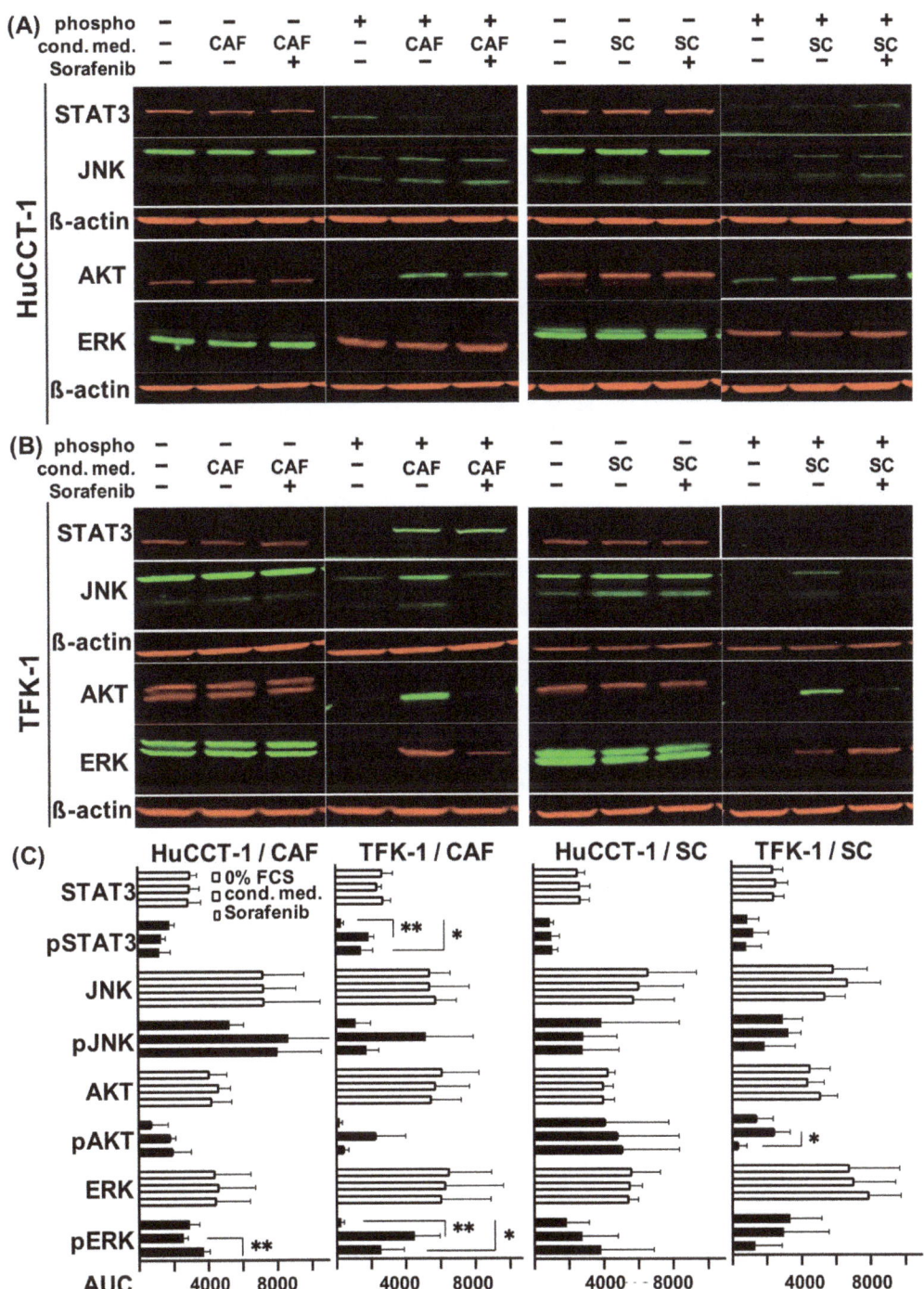

Figure 5. Impact of CAF and SC on signaling pathways in CCA cells in the absence or presence of Sorafenib. (**A**) HuCCT-1 cells and (**B**) TFK-1 cells were initially cultured in 0% FCS medium for 24 h

with additional Sorafenib treatment for another 24 h where appropriate. The following day, cells were treated for 15 min in unconditioned medium or in conditioned medium from CAF or SC, which was either left untreated or supplemented with 1 µM Sorafenib beforehand. Shown are representative blots out of three replicates demonstrating expression levels of the phosphorylated and total forms of STAT3, JNK, AKT and ERK. ß-actin was determined in parallel as control. (C) Quantifications of fluorescence signals of the detected total and phosphorylated signaling proteins are demonstrated as area under the curve (AUC). Bars represent from top to bottom unconditioned medium, treatment with conditioned medium and Sorafenib treatment. Significances were defined using asterisks: * $p < 0.05$, ** $p < 0.01$.

In HuCCT-1 cells, expression levels of phospho-STAT3 and phospho-JNK were not altered, while increased expression of phospho-JNK and phospho-AKT could be determined when CCA cells were cultured in CAF conditioned medium. However, treatment with Sorafenib showed no effect on activation of either protein and even increased expression of phospho-ERK ($p = 0.0084$; Figure 5A,C). Intriguingly, CAF-conditioned TFK-1 cells showed increased activation of all four signaling mediators (highly significantly for phospho-STAT3 and phospho-ERK with $p = 0.0011$ and $p = 0.0072$, respectively) and Sorafenib treatment reduced it (Figure 5B,C).

HuCCT-1 cells cultured in SC-conditioned medium showed almost no changes in the expression of activated forms of the MAPK and JAK-STAT signaling pathway. Again, a slight increase in phospho-ERK expression after Sorafenib treatment could be observed (Figure 5A,C). In contrast, TFK-1 cells exposed to SC-conditioned medium exhibited an increased activation of STAT3, JNK and AKT (Figure 5B,C), whereas no SC-mediated effects could be observed on the expression level of phospho-ERK. Treatment with Sorafenib resulted in a reduced phosphorylation of JNK and AKT, but also in an increased phosphorylation of ERK in TFK-1 cells. Again, no synergistic effect of the CCA cell lines in co-cultivation with both stromal cell lines was detected on signal transduction (data not shown).

To rule out a direct inhibition of activation of the above-mentioned pathways in the CCA cells by Sorafenib, Western blot analysis was carried out in Sorafenib-treated mono-cultured TFK-1 and HuCCT-1 cells. For the TFK-1 cells, a light activation of ERK and JNK was observed after Sorafenib treatment (AUC in phospho-ERK from 201 to 8490 and in phospho-JNK from 331 to 5941). This finding in the mono-culture contrasted to the inhibition of the different pathways after Sorafenib treatment of the cancer cell-SC and -CAF co-cultures. For the AKT and JAK-STAT pathway, no difference in activation was observed after treatment with Sorafenib. In mono-cultured HuCCT-1 cells, no difference in activation of the different pathways was observed after treatment with Sorafenib either (phospho-STAT3 from 6625 to 5992; phospho-JNK from 7925 to 7627; phospho-AKT from 5278 to 2302 and phospho-ERK from 9109 to 8432 AUC, respectively).

Altogether, these findings indicate that CAF and SC impact signaling pathways in CCA cells in a paracrine manner. Moreover, Sorafenib treatment inhibited only the activation of JNK, AKT and ERK in TFK-1 cells.

3. Discussion

Although CCA is less frequent than other gastrointestinal malignancies, its incidence is rapidly increasing [2]. Additionally, CCA treatment remains challenging because of its often late diagnosis, limiting surgical resection, poor response to standard chemotherapy, missing standardized second-line chemotherapeutic approaches and difficulty for targeted therapies due to tumor heterogeneity without established molecular-targeted therapeutic regimens [5,22]. Thus, this underscores the urgent need to develop more effective treatment options. While the tumor microenvironment and, particularly, CAF have been already shown to essentially determine the progression and therapy response of many tumor entities [23], knowledge on the role of CAF on CCA cells and CCA progression is still poor [13]. Chuaysri et al. could already demonstrate that the occurrence of CAF is correlated with poor survival of CCA patients [16]. This finding was confirmed by the immunohistochemical analysis of a small cohort of CCA patients in our study, which requires further validation in larger cohorts. Even though the impact of SC on tumor cell migration, invasion and metastasis has been reported in different malignancies (e.g., pancreatic ductal adenocarcinoma) [24], their role in CCA progression and metastatic spread has not yet been investigated.

Since the role of CAF and SC on CCA progression is poorly understood and the effects of treatment with the multityrosine kinase inhibitor Sorafenib are rather disappointing in CCA [25,26], our study aimed at elucidating the paracrine impact of CAF and SC on CCA cells with a particular focus on cell migration and whether this can be targeted by Sorafenib.

Using four chamber ibidi slides and cell tracing of distinct cell populations for gap closure experiments, we were able to demonstrate that cell migration of CCA cells is significantly enhanced in the presence of CAF. One possible explanation could be the paracrine interaction with tumor cells as CAF are known to produce ECM and release inflammatory cytokines such as IL-6 and IL-8 and several chemokines, among them CCL2/MCP1, CXCL12/SDF1, CCL5 and 7 as well as CXCL16, by which they can promote cancer cell migration [27]. In contrast, in co-cultures of CCA cells with SC, gap closure was also increased but this was predominantly mediated by enhanced cell migration of SC towards CCA cells. These data are in line with a study demonstrating that SC migrate towards cancer cells in pancreatic ductal adenocarcinoma as well as in colon carcinoma cell lines but not towards benign cells [19]. Thus, the study by Demir et al. and our study provide evidence that not tumor cells but, instead, SC migrate during neural invasion which might contribute to tumor cell dissemination.

We were also able to demonstrate that Sorafenib could reduce migration of CAF as well as of CAF co-cultivated CCA cells but not that of SC and SC co-cultivated CCA cells, supporting the view that Sorafenib exerts its effects in a context-dependent manner.

However, the findings that Sorafenib reduced the migratory abilities of CAF and CAF co-cultured CCA cells are in line with other studies demonstrating the antimigratory effects of Sorafenib [26,27]. Accordingly, Sorafenib was found to suppress the Epithelial–Mesenchymal Transition (EMT) and cell migration by reducing matrix metalloproteinase (MMP) expression in HCC cells. This in turn led to suppressed c-MET and reduced activation of the Mitogen-activated protein kinase (MEK)/ERK pathway [28]. In line with these findings, Sorafenib reduced phospho-ERK levels and migration of breast cancer cells [29]. Considering the effects of Sorafenib in HCC, the inhibited ERK pathway highlights one possibility by which Sorafenib treatment was able to inhibit migration in CAF and CAF co-culture-treated CCA cells. SC dedifferentiation is known to be activated through the Ras/Raf/ERK signaling pathway [30] and it was demonstrated that ERK1/2 and AKT signals were involved in the migratory potential of SC [31]; however, ERK1/2 activity inhibition did not show a reduction in SC migration [31]. In line with this, migration of mono- and co-cultured SC could not be inhibited by Sorafenib. The observed resistance of SC and SC co-culture to the treatment with Sorafenib might be caused either by a shorter and weaker ERK1/2 activity in SC or a possible requirement for additional factors, such as insulin-like growth factor to stimulate the ERK1/2 pathway [32]. Future studies are needed to explore these findings more in detail.

To further elucidate the paracrine impact of CAF and SC, respectively, on CCA cells and whether this is impacted by Sorafenib treatment, we determined a spectrum of cytokines and chemokines in supernatants of mono- and co-cultures of CCA cells and the different stromal cell populations. From the series of investigated cytokines, the following have been shown to be of particular importance for tumor cell migration: IL5 [33], IL6 [34], IL8 [35], IL17 [36], IL23 [37], CXCL-1, CXCL11 [38], CXCL12 [39], CCL5 [40], MCP-1 [41], MIF [42], serpin E1 [43] and TNFα [44]. While MCP-1, CXCL-1, IL-6 and IL-8 could not be detected in supernatants of mono-cultured CCA cells, a strong release of MCP-1 and IL-8 was measured in supernatants of mono-cultured CAF as well as of CCA cells co-cultured with CAF. Both factors are known for their pro-inflammatory [45] and migratory capacity [27]. Of note, MCP-1 (also known as CCL2) has been reported to be secreted by CAF at elevated levels, promoting cancer progression and migration in HCC [46] as well as in oral cancer [47]. Additionally, CXCL-1 and IL-6 could also be detected at elevated levels in supernatants of mono-cultured CAF, both factors being reported to be highly expressed in CCA [48]. Our findings are in line with studies demonstrating a role of CXCL-1, IL-6 and IL-8 in tumor cell migration and metastasis in other tumor entities [49,50]. Importantly, Sorafenib treatment effectively reduced levels of MCP-1, CXCL-1, IL-6 and IL-8 in supernatants of mono-cultured CAF and CAF co-cultured with either CCA cell line, which is in line with the observation that Sorafenib efficiently reduced cell migration of mono-cultured CAF as well as those of CAF co-cultured CCA cells. Overall, these findings indicate that Sorafenib is able to efficiently interfere with the paracrine tumor stroma interplay in CCA.

Furthermore, supernatants of mono-cultured HuCCT-1 cells as well as of mono- and co-cultured SC contained considerably higher amounts of serpin E1 and MIF. High MIF levels are found in almost all type of cancers exerting multifunctional effects contributing to cancer development and progression such as promoting migration and reducing apoptosis [51]. In addition, it is known to inhibit the tumor suppressor gene p53 and its stimulatory function of pro-inflammatory cytokines such as TNFα, INF γ, IL-1ß, IL-6, and IL-8 in a positive feedback loop [52]. It appears possible that SC migration is enhanced by MIF. In this study, we analyzed the secretion of the cytokines in mono- and co-culture of CCA cells, SC and CAF and examined whether paracrine interaction of the above mentioned cell types and Sorafenib treatment impact this cytokine and chemokine secretion. Based on these results, it can be speculated whether enhanced factors under co-culture conditions are responsible for enhanced migratory abilities of CCA cells or SC migration. Thus, future studies involving experiments with blocking antibodies will have to examine whether these inflammatory factors (such as MCP-1, CXCL-1, IL-6 or IL-8) are responsible for enhanced migration of CCA cells and SC, respectively. As an overrepresentation of the MAPK/ERK signaling pathway was already described in CCA [7], Sorafenib has been postulated to be an effective treatment option like in HCC. Having shown that Sorafenib reduced cell migration of CAF and CAF co-cultured CCA cells, we elucidated the paracrine influence of CAF on signal transduction in the two CCA cell lines as well as whether this is impacted by Sorafenib treatment. In addition, we investigated activation of the PI3K-AKT and JAK-STAT signaling pathways, which are both known to be possible targeting structures for CCA treatment [53]. First of all, HuCCT-1 cells already showed a stroma-independent higher expression of activated signaling mediators, particularly of phospho-AKT and phospho-ERK compared to TKF-1 cells. Moreover, in HuCCT-1 cells, only phospho-AKT expression was increased in response to CAF, while the presence of SC did not impact the expression of either phosphorylated form of the analyzed signaling proteins. Interestingly, Sorafenib treatment did not alter the expression of the activated forms of the four signaling mediators in HuCCT-1 cells under either culture condition, though a clear reducing effect was observed on cell migration in CAF co-cultivated cells, possibly due to decreased levels of CXCL-1, IL-6 or IL-8 leading to reduced migration of HuCCT-1 cells. In contrast, low basal expression levels of phospho-JNK, phospho-AKT and phospho-ERK in TFK-1 cells were increased in a stroma-dependent manner by CAF, which could be clearly reduced by Sorafenib treatment.

Of note, while Sorafenib seemed to have little to no effects on cytokine levels in SC co-cultured cells, SC co-cultured TFK-1 cells showed an increased activation of ERK, which was even enhanced by Sorafenib treatment. A reason for the stronger migration of SC in co-culture with extrahepatic TFK-1 cells might be explained by the fact that extrahepatic CCA disseminate into the liver via perineural guidance [21], while intrahepatic carcinomas (such as the HuCCT-1 cells) are more surrounded by CAF and hepatic stellate cells in the tumoral environment [13]. Therefore, intrahepatic CCA (cells) might be primarily activated by a paracrine stimulation from stellate cells/CAF and less by SC. Thus, there are apparent differences in the activation and migration of SC and tumor cells, respectively, which might be caused by the different paracrine interplay of CCA cells and surrounding stromal cells. Furthermore, the antitumoral efficacy of Sorafenib seems to be dependent on the tumoral context as, predominantly, the interplay between CAF and CCA cells could be impaired by Sorafenib but not those of SC and CCA cells. Thus, it can be speculated that Sorafenib treatment might be more effective and suitable for treatment of CCA lacking neural invasion.

In line with other studies, the results of our study showed lower survival rates in CCA patients with an increased immunohistochemical staining of α-SMA in CAF in surgically resected intrahepatic CCA [16,54,55]. Prospective risk assessment regarding survival after surgery could favor patients with a low density of α-SMA in CAF. Therefore, tumor biopsies in the evaluation process before surgery could add to a better selection of patients who might benefit from surgery with a better tumor-free survival for CCA. Furthermore, the results of the study suggest that a suppression of the crosstalk between CAF and CCA tumor cells leads to an impaired tumor invasion. Therefore, future research should focus on identifying targets by which deregulated expression and release of tumor-stimulating cytokines by CAF are reversed. Of note, since CAF have been demonstrated to be heterogeneous in different tumor entities, especially in pancreatic and breast cancer [13], future research should also focus on CAF heterogeneity in CCA in order to elucidate whether different CAF subtypes might exert pro- and antitumorigenic effects in CCA cells. Moreover, owing to the fact that our results are based on the use of two CCA cell lines that differ in their origin (intrahepatic vs. extrahepatic) and therefore generalization is difficult in the presence of inconsistent findings observed, the use of additional CCA cell lines as well as CAF populations is planned for further studies. For extrahepatic CCA, a migration of SC towards the tumor cells was seen. Extrahepatic CCA cells need SC for perineural invasion to invade in the liver [21]. Since the results of this study demonstrate migration of SC towards CCA cells and a synergistic effect of SC and CCA cells in co-culture, future research should investigate the mechanisms of the migration of SC towards CCA cells in more detail and targets should be identified to block this malignancy, promoting crosstalk.

4. Materials and Methods

4.1. Immunohistochemical Stainings of CCA Tissues

Formalin-fixed and paraffin-embedded tumor specimens of 14 CCA patients were analyzed for the presence of CAF and SC and correlated with survival rates. All patients signed the informed consent. The study was approved by the local institutional review board of the Medical Faculty of the Kiel University (A 110/99). For immunohistochemistry, 5 μm paraffin sections were used. Antigen retrieval was not necessary. Slides were incubated with primary antibodies for α-SMA (1:400, clone 1A4, mouse, NeoMarkers, Fremont, CA, USA), FSP-1 (1:200, abcam ab93283, Cambridge, UK) and S100 (1:400, Z0311, polyclonal, rabbit, Dako, Glostrup, Denmark). Bound antibodies were detected by EnVision+System-HRP anti-mouse antibody (Dako, Glostrup, Denmark). Color development was performed with the DAB substrate kit (Dako, Glostrup, Denmark). All slides were counterstained with hemalum and cover slipped. Evaluation of the stainings was performed on a Leica DM 1000 microscope (Leica, Wetzlar, Germany). The intensity of the staining was judged on an arbitrary scale of 0 to 3 with 0: no staining; 1: weak staining; 2: moderate staining and 3: strong staining by two independent pathologists.

4.2. Cell Lines and Generation of CAF

CAF were prepared from two different human CCA tissues and pooled after in vitro selection as previously described and tested by positive staining for α-SMA and Vimentin as well as negative staining for the pan-cytokeratin marker KL-1 [56]. Patients gave their consent for use of their tumor tissue and the procedure was approved by the ethics committee of Kiel University (A 110/99). In brief, immediately after resection, the tissue was cultivated with DMEM low glucose (Gibco Invitrogen, Grand Island, NY, USA), 10% FCS (PAN Biotech, Aidenbach, Germany), 1% GlutaMAX, 1% sodium pyruvate (both Gibco Invitrogen, Grand Island, NY, USA) and 1% penicillin/streptomycin (Biochrom, Berlin, Germany), sliced into 1 mm^3 pieces and cultivated in 6-well plates in DMEM low glucose medium (10% FCS, 1% GlutaMAX, 1% sodium pyruvate, as described above). After 2 days, pieces were transferred into new 6-well plates. The medium was changed three times per week. After 2 weeks, when sufficient CAF were migrated out of the tissues, the tumor blocks were removed. At a confluency of 80%, CAF were detached with accutase (Gibco Invitrogen, Grand Island, NY, USA) and the cells were stored in FCS with 10% DMSO (Sigma-Aldrich Chemie GmbH, Steinheim, Germany) in liquid nitrogen for further studies.

The human CCA cell lines HuCCT-1 and TFK-1 (Cell Bank RIKEN Bio Resource Centre, Koyadai Tsukuba, Japan) as well as CAF were cultured in DMEM low glucose medium supplemented with 10% FCS, 1 mM GlutaMAX and 1 mM sodium-pyruvate (culture medium), as described before. SC were purchased from ScienCell Research Laboratories (San Diego, CA, USA) and kept in SC culture medium of the distributor.

4.3. Paracrine Interaction Model to Analyze Cell Migration

To analyze the influence of SC and CAF on growth behavior and cell migration of CCA cell lines, HuCCT-1 and TFK-1 cells were resuspended in culture medium without FCS but supplemented with 25 µM CellTracker Deep Red. SC were resuspended in culture medium without FCS and supplemented with 25 µM CellTracker CMAC blue (both dyes from Molecular Probes by Life Technologies, Waltham, MA, USA). They were stained for 45 min at 37 °C and subsequently resuspended in cell culture medium containing FCS. CAF remained unlabeled. Each cell population was seeded at a cell density of 0.35×10^5 cells in each well of the ibidi plate (Culture-Insert 4 well in µ-Dish, ibidi, Munich, Germany) in 75 µL DMEM low glucose with 10% FCS. For mono-culture, CCA cell lines as well as CAF and SC were seeded in all 4 wells of the ibidi dish, while for co-culture experiments, either CCA cell line was seeded in 2 wells and in the other two wells either CAF or SC were seeded. The next day, the medium was removed from all wells and replaced by 75 µL DMEM FluoroBrite high-glucose (Gibco Invitrogen) lacking FCS. In the case of Sorafenib treatment, medium was replaced by 75 µL DMEM FluoroBrite (-FCS) containing 1 µM Sorafenib. After 4 h, the stamp was removed and the ibidi plates were washed with DMEM FluoroBrite (-FCS) in order to remove detached cells or cellular debris that had arisen after removal of the stamp. The ibidi plates were then refilled with DMEM FluoroBrite (-FCS) for the control and DMEM FluoroBrite (-FCS) with 1 µM Sorafenib for the treatment. Subsequently, selected regions of the well containing the gaps were imaged in all four channels (brightfield: Ex: BF, Em: Blue (452/45); CellTracker CMAC Blue: Ex: UV (377/50), Em: Blue (452/45); CellTracker Deep Red: Ex: Red (632/22), Em: Red (685/40)) using the 10x objective of a NYONE cell imager (Synentec GmbH, Elmshorn, Germany). To analyze the cell confluence in the brightfield channel, the 'Wound healing beta 2F' application of YT-Software (SYNENTEC GmbH) was used. In this application, four regions of interest (ROIs) could be placed into the four gaps of each well and the confluency within this ROI was determined. To determine gap closure, cellular confluency was measured directly after removal of the stamp (=t0) as well as after 18 h and 68 h. As cellular debris or detached cells could interfere with the analysis, after 18 h and 68 h, the medium was collected, filtered (0.45 µm) and directly re-applied. After 72 h, supernatants were centrifuged, aliquoted and stored in −20 °C for further experiments (cytokine assay).

4.4. Human Cytokine Array

To further characterize the impact of CAF and SC on tumor cell lines, supernatants of mono- and co-cultures were analyzed after 72 h for cytokine release using the Proteome Profiler Human Cytokine Array Kit (Panel A, R&D SYSTEMS, Minneapolis, MN, USA) following the manufacturer's specifications. For detection of cytokines, the substrate was catalyzed with peroxidase into a luminescent product, which was detected on a Curix-60 developer (AGFA, Mortsel, Belgium).

4.5. Generation of Conditioned Medium of Stromal Cells

Conditioned medium of mono-cultured stromal cells was prepared as follows in T75 cm^2 cell culture flasks: 80–90% confluent CAF or SC were cultured with 10 mL 0% FCS medium (CAF in DMEM low glucose (Gibco Invitrogen, Grand Island, NY, USA), SC in SC medium (ScienCell Research Laboratories, San Diego, CA, USA)) without or with 1 µM Sorafenib (Nexavar, Bayer, Leverkusen, Germany) for 24 h. Supernatants (=conditioned medium) were centrifuged, aliquoted and stored at −20 °C for analyzing the impact of CAF and SC on signaling pathways in CCA cell lines.

4.6. Western Blot to Analyze Activation of Signaling Pathways

To analyze the impact of CAF and SC on distinct signaling pathways in the CCA cell lines, 3×10^5 HuCCT-1 and TFK-1 cells were seeded per well in a 6-well plate. The following day, the medium was removed, cells were washed twice with PBS and cells were cultured in culture medium of CAF (DMEM) or SC (SC medium) without FCS for 24 h.

The next day, cells were either left untreated or treated with 1 µM Sorafenib. After another 24 h, the medium was removed and cells were cultured for 15 min in conditioned medium from CAF or SC (see above) supplemented with or without 1 µM Sorafenib. As the control, cells were cultured in culture medium without FCS and without preconditioning by SC and CAF to rule out a direct inhibition of the signaling pathways in the cancer cells by Sorafenib.

Cell lysates were generated from the differentially cultured cells by lysing the cells in 80 µL RIPA buffer inclusive PhosSTOP and Complete Protease Inhibitor Cocktail (both Roche, Penzberg, Germany) according to established protocols [57]. SDS-gel electrophoresis as well as Western blotting was conducted as described previously [56] using the following antibodies (all Cell Signalling Technology, Leiden, Holland; diluted in BSA, Carl Roth GmbH, Karlsruhe, Germany): STAT3 (mouse 124H6, 1:1000, 5% BSA in TBS-T), Phospho-STAT3 (rabbit 1:300, 5% BSA in TBS-T), SAPK/JNK (both rabbit 1:500, 0.5% BSA in TBS-T) and Phospho-SAPK/JNK antibody (rabbit 1:500, 0.5% BSA in TBS-T), AKT (mouse, 1:1000, 5% BSA in TBS-T) Phospho-AKT (rabbit 1:1000, 5% BSA in TBS-T), p44/42 MAPK (ERK1/2) (rabbit 1:1000, 5% BSA in TBS-T) and Phospho-p44/42 MAPK (ERK1/2) (rabbit 1:300, 5% BSA in TBS-T). ß-actin was used in a concentration of 1:10,000 (Sigma Aldrich Chemie GmbH, Steinheim, Germany, 0.5% milk in TBS-T).

4.7. Statistical Analyses

Statistical analyses were carried out using SPSS 23.0 (SPSS, IBM Corporation, Armonk, NY, USA). Represented are mean values ± standard deviation. The data were tested for normal distribution and equal variances using the Shapiro–Wilk test. Non-parametric datasets of different groups were analyzed using the Kruskal–Wallis one-way ANOVA on ranks. Statistical significance was defined at a p-value of <0.05, according to the Dunn method for non-parametric data. Survival analyses were performed by Kaplan–Meier estimates and statistical evaluations were performed using log-rank tests. Significances were defined using asterisks: * $p < 0.05$, ** $p < 0.01$, *** $p < 0.001$.

5. Conclusions

Overall, this study contributes toward a better understanding of the paracrine interplay of CAF and SC, respectively, with CCA cells and provides explanations on how these cells may impact cell migration, with this being an important metastasis-associated process. Co-cultivation of the two CCA cell lines HuCCT-1 and TFK-1 with CAF increased tumor cell migration and secretion of the pro-inflammatory cytokines MCP-1, CXCL-1, IL-6 and IL-8, which could be clearly diminished by Sorafenib treatment. In contrast, co-culture of CCA cells with SC predominantly increased the cell migration of SC, which could not be inhibited by Sorafenib. The fact that Sorafenib treatment inhibited the cell migration of CAF and CAF co-cultured CCA but not those of SC, along with the observation that signaling pathways that are important for malignant progression are also not impacted by

Sorafenib in both CCA cell lines, underscores that the therapeutic efficacy of Sorafenib is highly context-dependent and provides an explanation as to why Sorafenib failed in the treatment of CCA patients in some clinical studies [25,26]. Thus, further studies are needed to elucidate the conditions determining the efficacy of Sorafenib for treatment of CCA.

Author Contributions: J.K. performed the majority of the experiments. J.-P.G. helped with analyzing the data and generated the figures. A.H. and A.B. carried out the statistics. C.H. performed immunohistochemical stainings. J.K., J.-P.G. and S.S. wrote the manuscript. C.R. (Christian Röder) helped in the review process. S.S., J.-P.G., T.B., C.R. (Christoph Röcken) and F.B. provided resources. N.H. conceived the study. All authors have read and agreed to the published version of the manuscript.

Funding: This work was supported by the Medical Faculty of Kiel University.

Institutional Review Board Statement: The study was conducted according to the guidelines of the Declaration of Helsinki, and approved by the local institutional review board of the Medical Faculty of the Kiel University (A-110/99).

Informed Consent Statement: Informed consent was obtained from all subjects involved in the study.

Data Availability Statement: The clinical datasets supporting the conclusions of this study were derived from patient files (paper and electronic form). Therefore, restrictions to availability apply due to data protection regulations. Anonymized data are, however, available from the corresponding author on reasonable request and with permission of the University Hospital Schleswig-Holstein and the local review board.

Acknowledgments: We thank Reinhild Geisen (SYNENTEC GmbH) for the idea of using NYONE to analyze the wound healing assays and for her support with imaging and analysis. We thank SYNENTEC GmbH, especially Martin Stoehr, for the possibility to use their NYONE imager and for customizing the image analysis application. We thank Björn Konukiewitz and Katharina Hess for their courteous help in revising the immunohistological images. The authors thank Julia Wilking for excellent technical support. We acknowledge financial support by DFG within the funding programme Open Access-Publikationskosten.

Conflicts of Interest: The authors declare no conflict of interest.

References

1. Rizvi, S.; Khan, S.A.; Hallemeier, C.L.; Kelley, R.K.; Gores, G.J. Cholangiocarcinoma—Evolving concepts and therapeutic strategies. *Nat. Rev. Clin. Oncol.* **2018**, *15*, 95–111. [CrossRef] [PubMed]
2. Khan, A.S.; Dageforde, L.A. Cholangiocarcinoma. *Surg. Clin. N. Am.* **2019**, *99*, 315–335. [CrossRef] [PubMed]
3. Khan, S.A.; Emadossadaty, S.; Ladep, N.G.; Thomas, H.C.; Elliott, P.; Taylor-Robinson, S.D.; Toledano, M.B. Rising trends in cholangiocarcinoma: Is the ICD classification system misleading us? *J. Hepatol.* **2012**, *56*, 848–854. [CrossRef] [PubMed]
4. Bridgewater, J.; Galle, P.R.; Khan, S.A.; Llovet, J.M.; Park, J.W.; Patel, T.; Pawlik, T.M.; Gores, G.J. Guidelines for the diagnosis and management of intrahepatic cholangiocarcinoma. *J. Hepatol.* **2014**, *60*, 1268–1289. [CrossRef]
5. Squadroni, M.; Tondulli, L.; Gatta, G.; Mosconi, S.; Beretta, G.; Labianca, R. Cholangiocarcinoma. *Crit. Rev. Oncol. Hematol.* **2017**, *116*, 11–31. [CrossRef]
6. Labib, P.L.; Goodchild, G.; Pereira, S.P. Molecular Pathogenesis of Cholangiocarcinoma. *BMC Cancer* **2019**, *19*, 185. [CrossRef]
7. Wang, C.; Maass, T.; Krupp, M.; Thieringer, F.; Strand, S.; Worns, M.A.; Barreiros, A.P.; Galle, P.R.; Teufel, A. A systems biology perspective on cholangiocellular carcinoma development: Focus on MAPK-signaling and the extracellular environment. *J. Hepatol.* **2009**, *50*, 1122–1131. [CrossRef]
8. Dokduang, H.; Juntana, S.; Techasen, A.; Namwat, N.; Yongvanit, P.; Khuntikeo, N.; Riggins, G.J.; Loilome, W. Survey of activated kinase proteins reveals potential targets for cholangiocarcinoma treatment. *Tumour Biol.* **2013**, *34*, 3519–3528. [CrossRef]
9. Pang, R.W.; Poon, R.T. From molecular biology to targeted therapies for hepatocellular carcinoma: The future is now. *Oncology* **2007**, *72* (Suppl. S1), 30–44. [CrossRef]
10. Huether, A.; Hopfner, M.; Baradari, V.; Schuppan, D.; Scherubl, H. Sorafenib alone or as combination therapy for growth control of cholangiocarcinoma. *Biochem. Pharmacol.* **2007**, *73*, 1308–1317. [CrossRef]
11. Yokoi, K.; Kobayashi, A.; Motoyama, H.; Kitazawa, M.; Shimizu, A.; Notake, T.; Yokoyama, T.; Matsumura, T.; Takeoka, M.; Miyagawa, S.I. Survival pathway of cholangiocarcinoma via AKT/mTOR signaling to escape RAF/MEK/ERK pathway inhibition by sorafenib. *Oncol. Rep.* **2018**, *39*, 843–850. [CrossRef] [PubMed]
12. Wu, P.; Gao, W.; Su, M.; Nice, E.C.; Zhang, W.; Lin, J.; Xie, N. Adaptive Mechanisms of Tumor Therapy Resistance Driven by Tumor Microenvironment. *Front. Cell Dev. Biol.* **2021**, *9*, 641469. [CrossRef] [PubMed]

13. Vaquero, J.; Aoudjehane, L.; Fouassier, L. Cancer-associated fibroblasts in cholangiocarcinoma. *Curr. Opin. Gastroenterol.* **2020**, *36*, 63–69. [CrossRef] [PubMed]
14. Shimoda, M.; Mellody, K.T.; Orimo, A. Carcinoma-associated fibroblasts are a rate-limiting determinant for tumour progression. *Semin. Cell Dev. Biol.* **2010**, *21*, 19–25. [CrossRef] [PubMed]
15. Huang, L.; Xu, A.M.; Liu, S.; Liu, W.; Li, T.J. Cancer-associated fibroblasts in digestive tumors. *World J. Gastroenterol.* **2014**, *20*, 17804–17818. [CrossRef] [PubMed]
16. Chuaysri, C.; Thuwajit, P.; Paupairoj, A.; Chau-In, S.; Suthiphongchai, T.; Thuwajit, C. Alpha-smooth muscle actin-positive fibroblasts promote biliary cell proliferation and correlate with poor survival in cholangiocarcinoma. *Oncol. Rep.* **2009**, *21*, 957–969. [PubMed]
17. Bunimovich, Y.L.; Keskinov, A.A.; Shurin, G.V.; Shurin, M.R. Schwann cells: A new player in the tumor microenvironment. *Cancer Immunol. Immunother.* **2017**, *66*, 959–968. [CrossRef]
18. Liu, Z.; Jin, Y.Q.; Chen, L.; Wang, Y.; Yang, X.; Cheng, J.; Wu, W.; Qi, Z.; Shen, Z. Specific marker expression and cell state of Schwann cells during culture in vitro. *PLoS ONE* **2015**, *10*, e0123278. [CrossRef]
19. Demir, I.E.; Boldis, A.; Pfitzinger, P.L.; Teller, S.; Brunner, E.; Klose, N.; Kehl, T.; Maak, M.; Lesina, M.; Laschinger, M.; et al. Investigation of Schwann cells at neoplastic cell sites before the onset of cancer invasion. *J. Natl. Cancer Inst.* **2014**, *106*, dju184. [CrossRef]
20. Boilly, B.; Faulkner, S.; Jobling, P.; Hondermarck, H. Nerve Dependence: From Regeneration to Cancer. *Cancer Cell* **2017**, *31*, 342–354. [CrossRef]
21. Deborde, S.; Omelchenko, T.; Lyubchik, A.; Zhou, Y.; He, S.; McNamara, W.F.; Chernichenko, N.; Lee, S.Y.; Barajas, F.; Chen, C.H.; et al. Schwann cells induce cancer cell dispersion and invasion. *J. Clin. Investig.* **2016**, *126*, 1538–1554. [CrossRef] [PubMed]
22. Wang, M.; Chen, Z.; Guo, P.; Wang, Y.; Chen, G. Therapy for advanced cholangiocarcinoma: Current knowledge and future potential. *J. Cell. Mol. Med.* **2021**, *25*, 618–628. [CrossRef] [PubMed]
23. Fiori, M.E.; Di Franco, S.; Villanova, L.; Bianca, P.; Stassi, G.; De Maria, R. Cancer-associated fibroblasts as abettors of tumor progression at the crossroads of EMT and therapy resistance. *Mol. Cancer* **2019**, *18*, 70. [CrossRef] [PubMed]
24. Su, D.; Guo, X.; Huang, L.; Ye, H.; Li, Z.; Lin, L.; Chen, R.; Zhou, Q. Tumor-neuroglia interaction promotes pancreatic cancer metastasis. *Theranostics* **2020**, *10*, 5029–5047. [CrossRef] [PubMed]
25. Lee, J.K.; Capanu, M.; O'Reilly, E.M.; Ma, J.; Chou, J.F.; Shia, J.; Katz, S.S.; Gansukh, B.; Reidy-Lagunes, D.; Segal, N.H.; et al. A phase II study of gemcitabine and cisplatin plus sorafenib in patients with advanced biliary adenocarcinomas. *Br. J. Cancer* **2013**, *109*, 915–919. [CrossRef]
26. Moehler, M.; Maderer, A.; Schimanski, C.; Kanzler, S.; Denzer, U.; Kolligs, F.T.; Ebert, M.P.; Distelrath, A.; Geissler, M.; Trojan, J.; et al. Gemcitabine plus sorafenib versus gemcitabine alone in advanced biliary tract cancer: A double-blind placebo-controlled multicentre phase II AIO study with biomarker and serum programme. *Eur. J. Cancer* **2014**, *50*, 3125–3135. [CrossRef]
27. Erdogan, B.; Webb, D.J. Cancer-associated fibroblasts modulate growth factor signaling and extracellular matrix remodeling to regulate tumor metastasis. *Biochem. Soc. Trans.* **2017**, *45*, 229–236. [CrossRef]
28. Ha, T.Y.; Hwang, S.; Moon, K.M.; Won, Y.J.; Song, G.W.; Kim, N.; Tak, E.; Ryoo, B.Y.; Hong, H.N. Sorafenib inhibits migration and invasion of hepatocellular carcinoma cells through suppression of matrix metalloproteinase expression. *Anticancer Res.* **2015**, *35*, 1967–1976.
29. Dattachoudhury, S.; Sharma, R.; Kumar, A.; Jaganathan, B.G. Sorafenib Inhibits Proliferation, Migration and Invasion of Breast Cancer Cells. *Oncology* **2020**, *98*, 478–486. [CrossRef]
30. Harrisingh, M.C.; Perez-Nadales, E.; Parkinson, D.B.; Malcolm, D.S.; Mudge, A.W.; Lloyd, A.C. The Ras/Raf/ERK signalling pathway drives Schwann cell dedifferentiation. *EMBO J.* **2004**, *23*, 3061–3071. [CrossRef]
31. Yu, H.; Zhu, L.; Li, C.; Sha, D.; Pan, H.; Wang, N.; Ma, S. ERK1/2 and AKT are vital factors in regulation of the migration of rat Schwann cells. *J. Vet. Med. Sci.* **2015**, *77*, 427–432. [CrossRef] [PubMed]
32. Ammoun, S.; Flaiz, C.; Ristic, N.; Schuldt, J.; Hanemann, C.O. Dissecting and targeting the growth factor-dependent and growth factor-independent extracellular signal-regulated kinase pathway in human schwannoma. *Cancer Res.* **2008**, *68*, 5236–5245. [CrossRef] [PubMed]
33. Lee, E.J.; Lee, S.J.; Kim, S.; Cho, S.C.; Choi, Y.H.; Kim, W.J.; Moon, S.K. Interleukin-5 enhances the migration and invasion of bladder cancer cells via ERK1/2-mediated MMP-9/NF-kappaB/AP-1 pathway: Involvement of the p21WAF1 expression. *Cell. Signal.* **2013**, *25*, 2025–2038. [CrossRef] [PubMed]
34. Zhou, S.; Du, X.; Xie, J.; Wang, J. Interleukin-6 regulates iron-related proteins through c-Jun N-terminal kinase activation in BV2 microglial cell lines. *PLoS ONE* **2017**, *12*, e0180464. [CrossRef]
35. Fu, S.; Lin, J. Blocking Interleukin-6 and Interleukin-8 Signaling Inhibits Cell Viability, Colony-forming Activity, and Cell Migration in Human Triple-negative Breast Cancer and Pancreatic Cancer Cells. *Anticancer Res.* **2018**, *38*, 6271–6279. [CrossRef]
36. Guo, N.; Shen, G.; Zhang, Y.; Moustafa, A.A.; Ge, D.; You, Z. Interleukin-17 Promotes Migration and Invasion of Human Cancer Cells through Upregulation of MTA1 Expression. *Front. Oncol.* **2019**, *9*, 546. [CrossRef]
37. Xu, X.; Yang, C.; Chen, J.; Liu, J.; Li, P.; Shi, Y.; Yu, P. Interleukin-23 promotes the migration and invasion of gastric cancer cells by inducing epithelial-to-mesenchymal transition via the STAT3 pathway. *Biochem. Biophys. Res. Commun.* **2018**, *499*, 273–278. [CrossRef]

38. Wang, Y.; Xu, H.; Si, L.; Li, Q.; Zhu, X.; Yu, T.; Gang, X. MiR-206 inhibits proliferation and migration of prostate cancer cells by targeting CXCL11. *Prostate* **2018**, *78*, 479–490. [CrossRef]
39. Arya, M.; Ahmed, H.; Silhi, N.; Williamson, M.; Patel, H.R. Clinical importance and therapeutic implications of the pivotal CXCL12-CXCR4 (chemokine ligand-receptor) interaction in cancer cell migration. *Tumour Biol.* **2007**, *28*, 123–131. [CrossRef]
40. Huang, C.Y.; Fong, Y.C.; Lee, C.Y.; Chen, M.Y.; Tsai, H.C.; Hsu, H.C.; Tang, C.H. CCL5 increases lung cancer migration via PI3K, Akt and NF-kappaB pathways. *Biochem. Pharmacol.* **2009**, *77*, 794–803. [CrossRef]
41. Johrer, K.; Janke, K.; Krugmann, J.; Fiegl, M.; Greil, R. Transendothelial migration of myeloma cells is increased by tumor necrosis factor (TNF)-alpha via TNF receptor 2 and autocrine up-regulation of MCP-1. *Clin. Cancer Res.* **2004**, *10*, 1901–1910. [CrossRef] [PubMed]
42. Mitchell, R.A.; Bucala, R. Tumor growth-promoting properties of macrophage migration inhibitory factor (MIF). *Semin. Cancer Biol.* **2000**, *10*, 359–366. [CrossRef] [PubMed]
43. Yang, J.D.; Ma, L.; Zhu, Z. SERPINE1 as a cancer-promoting gene in gastric adenocarcinoma: Facilitates tumour cell proliferation, migration, and invasion by regulating EMT. *J. Chemother.* **2019**, *31*, 408–418. [CrossRef] [PubMed]
44. Zhao, P.; Zhang, Z. TNF-alpha promotes colon cancer cell migration and invasion by upregulating TROP-2. *Oncol. Lett.* **2018**, *15*, 3820–3827. [PubMed]
45. Yoshimura, T. The production of monocyte chemoattractant protein-1 (MCP-1)/CCL2 in tumor microenvironments. *Cytokine* **2017**, *98*, 71–78. [CrossRef] [PubMed]
46. Liu, J.; Chen, S.; Wang, W.; Ning, B.F.; Chen, F.; Shen, W.; Ding, J.; Chen, W.; Xie, W.F.; Zhang, X. Cancer-associated fibroblasts promote hepatocellular carcinoma metastasis through chemokine-activated hedgehog and TGF-beta pathways. *Cancer Lett.* **2016**, *379*, 49–59. [CrossRef] [PubMed]
47. Min, A.; Zhu, C.; Wang, J.; Peng, S.; Shuai, C.; Gao, S.; Tang, Z.; Su, T. Focal adhesion kinase knockdown in carcinoma-associated fibroblasts inhibits oral squamous cell carcinoma metastasis via downregulating MCP-1/CCL2 expression. *J. Biochem. Mol. Toxicol.* **2015**, *29*, 70–76. [CrossRef]
48. Haga, H.; Yan, I.K.; Takahashi, K.; Wood, J.; Zubair, A.; Patel, T. Tumour cell-derived extracellular vesicles interact with mesenchymal stem cells to modulate the microenvironment and enhance cholangiocarcinoma growth. *J. Extracell. Vesicles* **2015**, *4*, 24900. [CrossRef]
49. Hwang, H.J.; Oh, M.S.; Lee, D.W.; Kuh, H.J. Multiplex quantitative analysis of stroma-mediated cancer cell invasion, matrix remodeling, and drug response in a 3D co-culture model of pancreatic tumor spheroids and stellate cells. *J. Exp. Clin. Cancer Res.* **2019**, *38*, 258. [CrossRef]
50. Prieto-Garcia, E.; Diaz-Garcia, C.V.; Agudo-Lopez, A.; Pardo-Marques, V.; Garcia-Consuegra, I.; Asensio-Pena, S.; Alonso-Riano, M.; Perez, C.; Gomez, J.; Adeva, J.; et al. Tumor-Stromal Interactions in a Co-Culture Model of Human Pancreatic Adenocarcinoma Cells and Fibroblasts and Their Connection with Tumor Spread. *Biomedicines* **2021**, *9*, 364. [CrossRef]
51. Nobre, C.C.; de Araujo, J.M.; Fernandes, T.A.; Cobucci, R.N.; Lanza, D.C.; Andrade, V.S.; Fernandes, J.V. Macrophage Migration Inhibitory Factor (MIF): Biological Activities and Relation with Cancer. *Pathol. Oncol. Res.* **2017**, *23*, 235–244. [CrossRef] [PubMed]
52. Conroy, H.; Mawhinney, L.; Donnelly, S.C. Inflammation and cancer: Macrophage migration inhibitory factor (MIF)—The potential missing link. *QJM* **2010**, *103*, 831–836. [CrossRef] [PubMed]
53. Zhu, B.; Wei, Y. Antitumor activity of celastrol by inhibition of proliferation, invasion, and migration in cholangiocarcinoma via PTEN/PI3K/Akt pathway. *Cancer Med.* **2020**, *9*, 783–796. [CrossRef] [PubMed]
54. Okabe, H.; Beppu, T.; Hayashi, H.; Horino, K.; Masuda, T.; Komori, H.; Ishikawa, S.; Watanabe, M.; Takamori, H.; Iyama, K.; et al. Hepatic stellate cells may relate to progression of intrahepatic cholangiocarcinoma. *Ann. Surg. Oncol.* **2009**, *16*, 2555–2564. [CrossRef]
55. Nakamura, T.; Matsumoto, K.; Kiritoshi, A.; Tano, Y.; Nakamura, T. Induction of hepatocyte growth factor in fibroblasts by tumor-derived factors affects invasive growth of tumor cells: In vitro analysis of tumor-stromal interactions. *Cancer Res.* **1997**, *57*, 3305–3313.
56. Heits, N.; Heinze, T.; Bernsmeier, A.; Kerber, J.; Hauser, C.; Becker, T.; Kalthoff, H.; Egberts, J.H.; Braun, F. Influence of mTOR-inhibitors and mycophenolic acid on human cholangiocellular carcinoma and cancer associated fibroblasts. *BMC Cancer* **2016**, *16*, 322. [CrossRef]
57. Tawfik, D.; Groth, C.; Gundlach, J.P.; Peipp, M.; Kabelitz, D.; Becker, T.; Oberg, H.H.; Trauzold, A.; Wesch, D. TRAIL-Receptor 4 Modulates gammadelta T Cell-Cytotoxicity toward Cancer Cells. *Front. Immunol.* **2019**, *10*, 2044. [CrossRef]

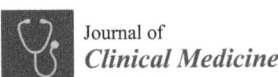

Article

The Clinical Dilemma of Esophagogastroduodenoscopy for Gastrointestinal Bleeding in Cardiovascular Disease Patients: A Nationwide-Based Retrospective Study

Chao-Feng Chang [1], Wu-Chien Chien [2,3], Chi-Hsiang Chung [3,4], Hsuan-Hwai Lin [1], Tien-Yu Huang [1], Peng-Jen Chen [1], Wei-Kuo Chang [1] and Hsin-Hung Huang [5,*]

[1] Division of Gastroenterology and Hepatology, Department of Internal Medicine, Tri-Service General Hospital, National Defense Medical Center, Taipei City 114, Taiwan; taiwanvincent777@gmail.com (C.-F.C.); redstone120@gmail.com (H.-H.L.); teinyu.chun@msa.hinet.net (T.-Y.H.); pjc.taiwan@gmail.com (P.-J.C.); weikuohouse@hotmail.com (W.-K.C.)
[2] Department of Medical Research, Tri-Service General Hospital, National Defense Medical Center, Taipei City 114, Taiwan; chienwu@mail.ndmctsgh.edu.tw
[3] School of Public Health, Tri-Service General Hospital, National Defense Medical Center, Taipei City 114, Taiwan; g694810042@gmail.com
[4] Taiwanese Injury Prevention and Safety Promotion Association, Tri-Service General Hospital, National Defense Medical Center, Taipei City 114, Taiwan
[5] Division of Gastroenterology, Department of Internal Medicine, Cheng Hsin General Hospital, National Defense Medical Center, Taipei City 114, Taiwan
* Correspondence: xinhung@gmail.com

Abstract: Performing esophagogastroduodenoscopy (EGD) in recently occurring peri-coronary artery disease (CAD) accident settings is always a dilemma. This study used the Taiwan National Health Insurance Research Database to identify patients with CAD and gastrointestinal bleeding who had received EGD or not between 2000 and 2013.The final population included in this study was 15,147 individuals, with 3801 individuals having received EGD (study cohort group) and 11,346 individuals not having received EGD (comparison cohort group). We initially performed a sensitivity test for CAD recurrence-related factors using multivariable Cox regression during the tracking period. A relatively earlier EGD intervention within one week demonstrated a lower risk of CAD recurrence (adjusted HR = 0.712). Although there were no significant differences in the overall tracking period, the adjusted HR of CAD recurrence was still lower in patients in the EGD group. Furthermore, our findings revealed that there were no remarkably short intervals to CAD recurrence in the study group. The Kaplan–Meier survival curve demonstrated that individuals who underwent EGD were not associated with a significantly increased CAD recurrence rate compared with the control (Log-rank test, $p = 0.255$). CAD recurrence is always an issue in recent episodes of peri-CAD accident settings while receiving EGD. However, there is not a higher risk in comparison with the normal population in our study, and waiting periods may not be required.

Keywords: esophagogastroduodenoscopy; gastrointestinal bleeding; cardiovascular disease

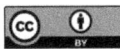

1. Introduction

Patients suffering from coronary artery disease (CAD) have significantly high mortality rates within a period of one month. Antithrombotic agents are a common method of treating CAD as they can decrease the incidence of subsequent CAD events; however, these drugs are more likely to increase bleeding tendency, especially upper gastrointestinal bleeding (UGIB). Approximately 1–4% of patients have concurrent CAD and UGIB, and up to 7% of patients develop sustained nosocomial GI bleeding following a PCI condition [1].

It is always important to consider the indications and contraindications when performing an endoscopic procedure so as to decide the exact timing of the endoscopy. A common dilemma is when patients have unstable hemodynamic status and a serious concurrent comorbidity, especially when it comes to cardiopulmonary problems. In clinical practice, perivascular accident settings with EGD are always more alarming to clinicians. This is because there are no guidelines to clearly define indications and contraindications in these cases. Cardiopulmonary side effects account for more than 50% of all complications and causes of death. Among endoscopic procedures, esophagogastroduodenoscopy (EGD) induces significant stress on the cardiopulmonary system, and the associated complications include hypertension and hypoxia. Fluctuations in blood pressure in approximately 40% of patients and unstable oxygenation with an oxygen saturation reduction in up to 70% of patients have been noted. Additionally, stress related to arrhythmias may result in cardiac ischemia in which the ECG shows ST-segment depression [2–4]. Furthermore, with the above urgent condition and possible unstable vital signs, analgesic agents for conscious sedation to relieve patient stress are far from appropriate.

Several studies in the current literature have investigated the utility of EGD in patients with concurrent vascular accident problems. Manifestations of severe complications while performing EGD are relatively infrequent [5]. However, peri-procedural complications are a great concern. Therefore, the purpose of our study was to use a national, large-population data sample to analyze CAD recurrence, mortality rates, and associated parameters in patients with CAD who received or did not receive EGD.

2. Methods

2.1. Data

The Taiwan National Health Insurance Research Database (NHIRD) was established in 1995, and the Taiwan National Health Insurance Administration Ministry of Health and Welfare (Taipei, Taiwan, China) provides a number of medical services, including inpatient, outpatient, and emergency services to >99% of the population in Taiwan. In the present study, data from the NHIRD were used. The investigation protocols were approved by the official peer review committee of the Tri-Service General Hospital (Taipei, Taiwan, China). The diagnoses were made according to the International Classification of Diseases, 9th Revision, Clinical Modification (ICD-9-CM) [6].

2.2. Study Cohort

A retrospective cohort design was used, and we selected outpatient and inpatient data between 1 January 2000 and 31 December 2013 from the NHIRD in Taiwan. The selected patient cases had concurrent health problems such as cardiovascular accident (CAD) and (UGIB). The included case group defined CAD by ICD-9-CM 410–414 and UGIB by ICD-9-CM 53X.0, 53X.2, 53X.4, 53X.6 (X = 1–4), 535.X1. We excluded patients for whom CAD/UGIB diagnosis was performed before the index date and patients under 20 years old. We also excluded cases where diagnosis of CAD/UGIB was performed before 1 January 2000. Furthermore, we excluded cases with unknown gender.

Initially, data from 16,482 patients were collected, of which 1335 individuals were excluded. Finally, our study included data from 15,147 patients. A total of 3801 individuals had received EGD as opposed to 11,346 individuals who had not. Next, we used a 4-fold propensity-score matching by gender, age, and index date. The 218 individuals who had received EGD within one month were defined as the study cohort group. In contrast, the 872 individuals without EGD were defined as the comparison cohort group (Figure 1). Notable variables included age, sex, and comorbidities of diabetes mellitus (DM) type II (ICD-9-CM 250), hypertension (ICD-9-CM 401-405), chronic obstructive pulmonary disease (COPD) (ICD-9-CM 491-493, 406), dyslipidemia (ICD-9-CM 272.0, 272.2, 272.4), and cancer (ICD-9-CM-140-208). The outcomes between these two groups were compared by balancing the above characteristics, follow-up durations, and survival status at the end of the tracking period, 31 December 2013. Thirteen individuals in the study cohort group and sixty-four individuals in the comparison cohort group experienced CAD recurrence within one month. When evaluating follow-up duration and survival status, we further analyzed other parameters, including urbanization level and level of care. In addition to CAD recurrence as the primary end point, we analyzed the severity by other factors: whether patients were admitted to an intensive care unit or were under mechanical ventilation or for the use of vasoconstrictors.

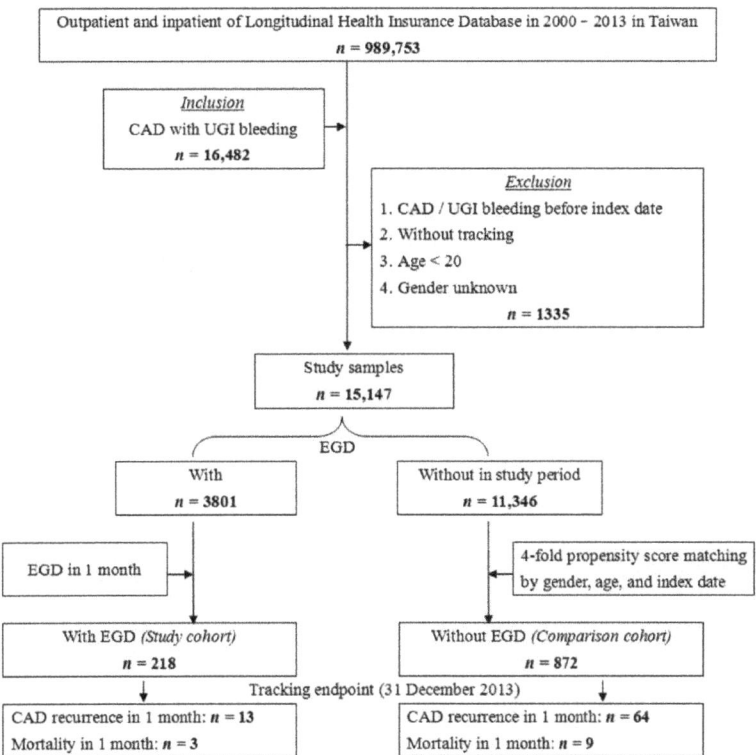

Figure 1. Flowchart of the study. The abbreviations: coronary artery disease (CAD); esophagogastroduodenoscopy (EGD); upper gastrointestinal (UGI).

2.3. Statistical Analysis

We conducted all analyses by SPSS software (version 18; SPSS, Inc., Chicago, IL, USA). The χ^2 and Fisher's exact test were used for analysis of categorical variables, such as sex and comorbidities. The Student's *t*-test was used for continuous variables, such as age, and the data are presented as mean ± standard error of the mean. Multivariate Cox regression was used to adjust the independent variables and to determine the association between each variable and CAD recurrence in one month. Additionally, CAD recurrence with different tracking periods and other covariates of outcomes were further analyzed by multivariable Cox regression stratified by EGD. Hazard ratios (HR) and 95% confidence intervals (CI) were used to evaluate the relative risks between each variable. Mean ± standard error of days to CAD recurrence were further investigated between the two groups. The Kaplan–Meier test was conducted to identify the cumulative survival of CAD with UGI bleeding to determine the statistical significance between groups.

3. Results

The clinical characteristics of the patients included in the present study are shown in Table 1. A total of 218 (20.00%) underwent EGD in the study cohort group, and 872 (80.00%) patients without EGD comprised the comparison cohort group. Following adjustment of variables, there were no statistical differences in the clinical characteristics between the study cohort group and the comparison cohort group. The distribution of gender, age, insurance premium, DM type II, HTN, COPD, dyslipidemia, and cancer between the two groups (with and without EGD) were similar. The mean age was 70.28 ± 12.08 years in patients with EGD and 71.12 ± 10.81 in patients without EGD. Males outnumbered females in both groups at the end of follow-up (58.26%). We identified that the insurance premiums were mostly less than New Taiwan dollar (NTD) 18,000, but this finding did not reach statistical significance ($p = 0.328$). There was no statistical difference in therapeutic variables hemostasis and endoscopic varices ligation ($p = 0.560$ and 0.844, respectively). Antiplatelet agent use between the two groups (with and without EGD) showed no significance ($p = 0.172$ and 0.221). Similarly, the urbanization level (from the highest to the lowest) was also not significant ($p = 0.012$). In contrast, the characteristic level of care was statistically different between the two groups (with more patients without receiving EGD). A greater number of patients with CAD received EGD in regional and local hospitals (Table 1). Additionally, our findings revealed that initial characteristics, including CAD recurrence and mortality rates within one month ($p = 0.556$ and 0.715, respectively) and length of days ($p = 0.664$), were not significantly different between the two groups. The average length of hospitalization was 70.30 ± 98.71 days (70.95 ± 95.10 and 67.70 ± 112.21 with and without EGD, respectively). Other factors included whether patients were admitted to an intensive care unit, underwent mechanical ventilation, or were administered vasoconstrictors, and these factors were further analyzed in our study and no significant difference was found in initial characteristics ($p = 0.867$, 0.867, and 0.727, respectively).

Table 1. Characteristics of study.

EGD Variables	Total n	%	With n	%	Without n	%	p
Total	1090		218	20.00	872	80.00	
Gender							0.999
Male	635	58.26	127	58.26	508	58.26	
Female	455	41.74	91	41.74	364	41.74	
Age (yrs)	70.45 ± 11.84		70.28 ± 12.08		71.12 ± 10.81		0.349
Insured premium (NTD)							0.328
<18,000	1075	98.62	217	99.54	858	98.39	
18,000–34,999	15	1.38	1	0.46	14	1.61	
≥35,000	0	0.00	0	0.00	0	0.00	
DM type II							0.055
Without	719	65.96	156	71.56	563	64.56	
With	371	34.04	62	28.44	309	35.44	
HTN							0.024
Without	667	61.19	148	67.89	519	59.52	
With	423	38.81	70	32.11	353	40.48	
COPD							0.341
Without	1045	95.87	212	97.25	833	95.53	
With	45	4.13	6	2.75	39	4.47	
Dyslipidemia							0.081
Without	1047	96.06	214	98.17	833	95.53	
With	43	3.94	4	1.83	39	4.47	
Cancer							0.010
Without	985	90.37	207	94.95	778	89.22	
With	105	9.63	11	5.05	94	10.78	
Hemostasis							0.560
Without	919	84.31	181	83.03	738	84.63	
With	171	15.69	37	16.97	134	15.37	
EVL							0.844
Without	1028	94.31	205	94.04	823	94.38	
With	62	5.69	13	5.96	49	5.62	
Clopidogrel							0.172
Without	857	78.62	164	75.23	693	79.47	
With	233	21.38	54	24.77	179	20.53	
Aspirin							0.221
Without	689	63.21	130	59.63	559	64.11	
With	401	36.79	88	40.37	313	35.89	
Urbanization level							0.012
1 (Highest)	347	31.83	74	33.94	273	31.31	
2	507	46.51	86	39.45	421	48.28	

Table 1. Cont.

EGD Variables	Total n	Total %	With n	With %	Without n	Without %	p
Total	1090		218	20.00	872	80.00	
3	62	5.69	21	9.63	41	4.70	
4 (Lowest)	174	15.96	37	16.97	137	15.71	
Level of care							<0.001
Hospital center	402	36.88	56	25.69	346	39.68	
Regional hospital	486	44.59	99	45.41	387	44.38	
Local hospital	202	18.53	63	28.90	139	15.94	
CAD recurrence in 1 month							0.556
Without	1013	92.94	205	94.04	808	92.66	
With	77	7.06	13	5.96	64	7.34	
Mortality in 1 month							0.715
Without	1078	98.90	215	98.62	863	98.97	
With	12	1.10	3	1.38	9	1.03	
Length of days	70.30 ± 98.71	70.95 ± 95.10	67.70 ± 112.21	0.664			
ICU in 1 month							0.867
Without	1081	99.17	216	99.08	865	99.20	
With	9	0.83	2	0.92	7	0.80	
Mechanical ventilation in 1 month							0.867
Without	1081	99.17	216	99.08	865	99.20	
With	9	0.83	2	0.92	7	0.80	
Vasoconstrictors in 1 month							0.727
Without	1036	95.05	206	94.50	830	95.18	
With	54	4.95	12	5.50	42	4.82	

p: Chi-square/Fisher exact test on category variables and t-test on continue variables. The abbreviations: esophagoduodenoscopy (EGD); New Taiwan dollar (NTD); diabetes mellitus (DM); hypertension (HTN); chronic obstructive pulmonary disease (COPD); endoscopic variceal ligation (EVL); coronary artery disease (CAD); intensive care unit (ICU).

Multivariable Cox regression analysis on CAD recurrence within one month revealed no statistical significance in all variables examined, namely EGD, gender, age group, DM type II, HTN, COPD, CKD, dyslipidemia, cancer, urbanization level, and level of care. Patients in the EGD group were relatively less likely to experience recurrent CAD (adjusted HR = 0.855, p = 0.411). Furthermore, male patients had a relatively higher risk of CAD recurrence than female patients (adjusted HR = 1.052, p = 0.382). The elderly group of patients had an average higher risk of CAD recurrence; however, there were no significant differences among different age groups. With respect to variables of comorbidity (DM type II, HTN, COPD, dyslipidemia, and cancer), HTN and COPD were more likely to induce CAD recurrence (adjusted HR = 1.172 and 1.653, p = 0.424 and 0.598, respectively) as was the relatively higher urbanization level (adjusted HR = 1.503); however, there were no significant differences among different levels of urbanization. Furthermore, hospital centers and regional hospitals were more likely to be associated with CAD recurrence (adjusted HR = 2.986 and 1.872, respectively), but there were no significant differences among different levels of care (Table 2).

A sensitivity test was then performed pertaining to the factors of CAD recurrence by using multivariable Cox regression during the tracking period. Compared to patients without EGD, a lower adjusted HR was found in patients in the EGD group. EGD intervention within one month was the reference time point, and we observed that relatively earlier EGD intervention within one week had a lower risk of CAD recurrence (adjusted HR = 0.712). Moreover, we observed that when the intervention occurred at a later time, the adjusted HR became relatively higher. For instance, the adjusted HR of EGD interventions at 2 weeks, 3 weeks, and 1 month were 0.775, 0.834, and 0.855, respectively. Although there were no significant differences in the overall tracking period, the adjusted HR of CAD recurrence was still lower in patients in the EGD group (Table 3). In addition to CAD recurrence, other covariates that may associate with outcome were further analyzed by multivariable Cox regression, and increased adjusted HRs for ICU, mechanical ventilation, and vasoconstrictor use were found in EGD-receiving groups (adjusted HR = 1.298, 1.134, and 1.560, respectively). However, there was no statistical significance (p = 0.303, 0.486, and 0.762, respectively) (Table 4).

Table 2. Factors of CAD recurrence in one month by using multivariable Cox regression.

Variables	Adjusted HR	95% CI	95% CI	p
EGD				
Without	Reference			
With	0.855	0.793	1.352	0.411
Gender				
Male	1.052	0.599	4.578	0.382
Female	Reference			
Age group (yrs)	1.372	0.956	1.981	0.392
Insured premium (NTD)				
<18,000	Reference			
18,000–34,999	0.000	-	-	0.999
≥35,000	-	-	-	-
DM type II				
Without	Reference			
With	0.952	0.446	2.240	0.789
HTN				
Without	Reference			
With	1.172	0.420	3.052	0.424
COPD				
Without	Reference			
With	1.653	0.222	9.762	0.598
Dyslipidemia				
Without	Reference			
With	0.965	0.242	3.802	0.755
Cancer				
Without	Reference			
With	0.000	-	-	0.744
Hemostasis				
Without	Reference			
With	1.113	0.520	1.973	0.497
EVL				
Without	Reference			
With	1.253	0.635	1.997	0.386
Clopidogrel				
Without	Reference			
With	0.825	0.562	1.342	0.489
Aspirin				
Without	Reference			
With	0.777	0.357	1.241	0.635
Urbanization level				
1 (Highest)	Reference			
2	1.503	0.552	4.097	0.435
3	0.000	-	-	0.999
4 (Lowest)	0.000	-	-	0.999
Level of care				
Hospital center	2.986	0.411	19.560	0.268
Regional hospital	1.872	0.184	11.435	0.562
Local hospital	Reference			

The abbreviations: hazard ratio (HR); confidence interval (CI); esophagogastroduodenoscopy (EGD); New Taiwan dollar (NTD); diabetes mellitus (DM); hypertension (HTN); chronic obstructive pulmonary disease (COPD); endoscopic variceal ligation (EVL).

The days to CAD recurrence in one month between the two groups with and without EGD were 19.00 and 14.00, respectively, and the total average days to CAD recurrence in one month were 15.44. There were no remarkably short intervals to CAD recurrence in the study group (Table 5).

Table 3. CAD recurrence by using multivariable Cox regression during the tracking period.

Tracking Period	EGD	Adjusted HR	95% CI	95% CI	p
Overall (in 1 month)	Without	Reference			
	With	0.855	0.793	1.352	0.411
In 3 weeks	Without	Reference			
	With	0.834	0.693	2.111	0.653
In 2 weeks	Without	Reference			
	With	0.775	0.601	3.075	0.751
In 1 week	Without	Reference			
	With	0.712	0.567	4.235	0.850

The abbreviations: coronary artery disease (CAD); esophagogastroduodenoscopy (EGD); hazard ratio (HR); confidence interval (CI).

Table 4. Other covariates of outcomes in 1 month by using multivariable Cox regression.

	EGD	Adjusted HR	95% CI	95% CI	p
ICU	Without	Reference			
	With	1.298	0.796	1.896	0.303
Mechanical ventilation	Without	Reference			
	With	1.134	0.675	1.813	0.486
Vasoconstrictors	Without	Reference			
	With	1.560	0.865	2.204	0.762

The abbreviations: esophagogastroduodenoscopy (EGD); hazard ratio (HR); confidence interval (CI); intensive care unit (ICU).

Table 5. Days to CAD recurrence in one month.

EGD	Min	Median	Max	Mean ± SD
With	1.00	19.50	21.00	19.50 ± 2.12
Without	1.00	14.00	29.44	14.93 ± 9.96
Total	1.00	15.44	29.44	15.47 ± 9.45

The abbreviations: coronary artery disease (CAD); esophagogastroduodenoscopy (EGD); standard deviation (SD).

The Kaplan–Meier survival curve was used to analyze the cumulative survival of CAD recurrence. It was demonstrated that patients who underwent EGD were not associated with a significantly increased CAD recurrence rate compared with the control (Log-rank test, $p = 0.255$) (Figure 2).

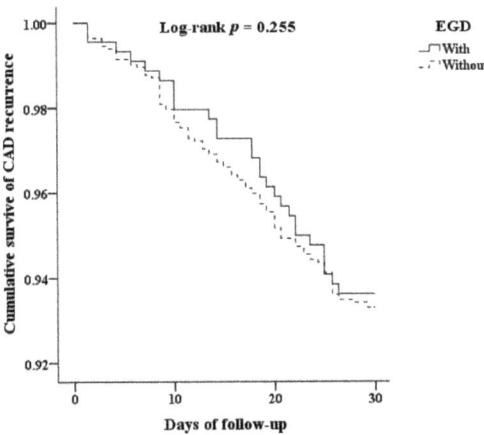

Figure 2. Kaplan–Meier for cumulative survival among CAD with UGI bleeding, aged 20 and over stratified by EGD with log-rank test. The abbreviations: coronary artery disease (CAD); upper gastrointestinal (UGI); esophagogastroduodenoscopy (EGD).

4. Discussion

Most CAD cases showed improvement in the 28-day mortality and incidence rates of recurrent CAD episodes after increased use of fibrinolytic agents. Use of antiplatelet agents and heparin increased the risk of bleeding, especially UGI bleeding, which is usually caused by antiplatelet agents. However, discontinuation of these agents in UGIB is a significant concern for the development of CAD recurrence; hence, these drugs should be re-prescribed as soon as possible [7]. Clinically, UGIB can be divided into overt and occult bleeding. Patients with overt UGI bleeding commonly present with hematemesis and melena and are prone to developing signs of active bleeding. Hence, EGD results in remarkably positive effects and outcomes. In contrast, patients with occult bleeding may not be confronted with high-risk conditions. Cases with occult bleeding are at a relatively lower risk of requiring urgent endoscopy and discontinuation of anticoagulant therapy. As EGD is believed to be liable to lead to CAD development, gastroenterologists may be reluctant to perform EGD in the urgent situation of UGIB [8,9]. Whether CAD patients, who are prone to experiencing cardiopulmonary complications, should receive EGD or not depends on their clinical status. Among patients with epicardial coronary disease undergoing UGD, up to 16% are bound to show electrocardiographic evidence of periprocedural CAD events [10]. Endoscopic evaluation carries a higher-than-average risk in patients with recent CAD [11]. The severe endoscopic complications rate when performing EGD in acute myocardial infraction is approximately 1%, which is 10 times higher than routine EGD [1]. It was postulated that approximately 42% of patients may suffer from silent ischemia, which has been correlated to heartrate during EGD; thus, administration of β-blockers may be beneficial in this condition [9].

To our knowledge, this is the first large-scale study to explore the EGD procedure in recently-diagnosed CAD patients. We observed that EGD is a safe and beneficial procedure in relatively stable patients without unnecessary delays. The latest randomized controlled trial of early endoscopy for UGIB in CAD patients postulated that there was not a higher complication rate for EGD as compared with medication alone [12]. However, being different from other common severe complications such as gastrointestinal perforation or hemorrhage, cardiopulmonary conditions are a major concern, especially in CAD patients with decreased cardiopulmonary tolerance. The complication rate of EGD when performed on day 0 was higher than that performed after 24 h in the hospital setting, but endoscopy is more likely to be required sooner in sicker patients. Early endoscopy (more than 6 h and less than 24 h) provides superior timing compared to emergent EGD (less than 6 h), especially in nonvariceal bleeding conditions [8,13]. Rather than urgent UGD, a waiting period for later UGD is rarely mentioned and depends on patient condition. However, some studies suggest that it may be reasonable to wait up to a week after MI before performing EGD. Moreover, clinicians may have adequate time to perform fluid resuscitation, blood transfusion, and provide effective medication [14]. In our study, we performed a sensitivity test for different timings (weekly intervals) to analyze CAD recurrence using multivariable Cox regression. Our findings revealed that there was no significant difference between different timings using "weeks" as the unit for the waiting period. However, we did observe that the adjusted HR when performing UGD within one month was 0.855, which is slightly higher compared to 1, 2, and 3 weeks (Table 3). CAD recurrence events were not correlated with a waiting period for observation in clinical practice. Furthermore, we analyzed days to CAD recurrence: the number of days to CAD recurrence for the total population was 15.47 ± 9.45 days; with EGD and without EGD the figures were 19.50 ± 2.12 days and 14.93 ± 9.96 days, respectively (Table 5). In the CAD study group, CAD events occurred the most within 2 and 3 weeks, and there was no significant difference between the two groups. Unstable hemodynamic conditions a few weeks after CAD recurrence may deteriorate the cardiopulmonary condition of the patient. An observation period of 14–21 days after CAD recurrence is still important when performing EGD in CAD patients. Hence, a comprehensive evaluation before EGD is more important than performing endoscopy immediately. In our observation, there were increased risks with other covariates such as intensive care unit admission, mechanical ventilation, or the use of vasoconstrictors, but no statistical significance was observed. Although EGD was an important tool in UGIB diagnosis, the sicker patients with EGD intervention led to more complications, especially with multiple comorbidities. Risk stratification and gastrointestinal pathology confirmation were essential for selection of the patients to receive EGD [15].

International consensus recommendations on the management of patients with non-variceal upper GI bleeding indicate that EGD should not be delayed for more than 24 h except in certain high-risk patients, such as those with acute coronary syndrome or a perforation [7]. With the recent advances in endoscopic techniques, the overall complication rates of EGD in clinical practice have been reduced from 0.13% to 0.08% [16–20]. However, performing endoscopy in peri-CAD accident settings, such as those related to insurance premium, urbanization level, and level of care, remains worrisome. In our study case, insurance premiums mostly ranged between NTD 18,000–34,999. However, this parameter was not found to be significant when performing endoscopy in the peri-CAD accident settings. Urgent endoscopic intervention was not correlated with increasing the cost of patient's care among CAD patients. The ratio of CAD patients receiving EGD in hospital centers was relatively lower than those for regional and local hospitals. It was thought that CAD patients in hospital centers may suffer from multiple morbidities, and criteria for performing EGD would be stricter in consideration of the respective risk.

Despite efforts to control confounding factors, there is a number of limitations in the present study. Firstly, the information obtained from the NHIRD regarding patient characteristics was lacking in terms of detailed severity of CAD, medications used, and treatment modalities. Secondly, thorough information regarding the diagnosis of patients with CAD with UGIB was not disclosed in detail (e.g., hemoglobulin, coagulability). Thirdly, despite review from a specialist, there was potential bias due complicated comorbidities being missed. Further prospective studies may be required due to the retrospective nature of this observational study.

5. Conclusions

Comprehensive studies before the investigation of EGD in concurrent UGIB patients remain important. Different from common complications, cardiopulmonary complications should be more alarming to endoscopists. When EGD is performed, CAD recurrence is always an issue in recent episodes of peri-CAD accident settings while receiving care management. However, our retrospective study reveals that there this condition is not associated with an increased risk compared to normal populations, and a waiting period may not be required. EGD investigations should be based on an individual basis.

Author Contributions: Conceptualization, C.-F.C. and H.-H.H.; data curation, C.-H.C.; formal analysis, C.-H.C.; investigation, C.-H.C.; methodology, W.-C.C.; resources, C.-F.C. and W.-C.C.; software, C.-H.C.; supervision, C.-F.C. and H.-H.H.; validation, W.-C.C. and C.-H.C.; visualization, H.-H.L., T.-Y.H., P.-J.C. and W.-K.C.; Writing—original draft, C.-F.C.; Writing—review and editing, C.-F.C. All authors have read and agreed to the published version of the manuscript.

Funding: This research received no external funding.

Institutional Review Board Statement: The study was conducted in accordance with the Declaration of Helsinki and approved by the Institutional Review Board of Tri-service General Hospital, Taiwan, Republic of China (approval no. TSGH-IRB No. B-111-06) for studies involving humans.

Informed Consent Statement: Not applicable and personal information included in the NHIRD is encrypted to protect individual patient privacy.

Data Availability Statement: All data generated or analyzed during this study are included in this published article.

Conflicts of Interest: The authors declare no conflict of interest.

References

1. Lin, S.; Konstance, R.; Jollis, J.; Fisher, D.A. The utility of upper endoscopy in patients with concomitant upper gastrointestinal bleeding and acute myocardial infarction. *Dig. Dis. Sci.* **2006**, *51*, 2377–2383. [CrossRef] [PubMed]
2. Cappell, M.S. A study of the syndrome of simultaneous acute upper gastrointestinal bleeding and myocardial infarction in 36 patients. *Am. J. Gastroenterol.* **1995**, *90*, 1444–1449. [PubMed]
3. Fujita, R.; Kumura, F. Arrythmias and ischemic changes of the heart induced by gastric endoscopic procedures. *Am. J. Gastroenterol.* **1975**, *64*, 44–48. [PubMed]
4. Levy, N.; Abinader, E. Continuous electrocardiographic monitoring with Holter electrocardiocorder throughout all stages of gastroscopy. *Am. J. Dig. Dis.* **1977**, *22*, 1091–1096. [CrossRef] [PubMed]
5. Hoffman, G.R.; Stein, D.J.; Moore, M.B.; Feuerstein, J.D. Safety of endoscopy for hospitalized patients with acute myocardial infarction: A national analysis. *Off. J. Am. Coll. Gastroenterol. ACG* **2020**, *115*, 376–380. [CrossRef] [PubMed]
6. Slee, V.N. The International classification of diseases: Ninth revision (ICD-9). *Ann. Intern. Med.* **1978**, *88*, 424–426. [CrossRef] [PubMed]
7. Barkun, A.N.; Bardou, M.; Kuipers, E.J.; Sung, J.; Hunt, R.H.; Martel, M.; Sinclair, P. International consensus recommendations on the management of patients with nonvariceal upper gastrointestinal bleeding. *Ann. Intern. Med.* **2010**, *152*, 101–113. [CrossRef]
8. Hoffman, G.R.; Stein, D.J.; Moore, M.B.; Feuerstein, J.D. Safety of endoscopic procedures after acute myocardial infarction: A systematic review. *Cardiol. J.* **2012**, *19*, 447–452.
9. Mumtaz, K.; Wasim, F.; Jafri, W.; Abid, S.; Hamid, S.; Shah, H.; Dhakam, S. Safety and utility of oesophago-gastro-duodenoscopy in acute myocardial infarction. *Eur. J. Gastroenterol. Hepatol.* **2008**, *20*, 51–55. [CrossRef]
10. Lee, J.G.; Krucoff, M.W.; Brazer, S.R. Periprocedural myocardial ischemia in patients with severe symptomatic coronary artery disease undergoing endoscopy: Prevalence and risk factors. *Am. J. Med.* **1995**, *99*, 270–275. [PubMed]
11. Yachimski, P.; Hur, C. Upper endoscopy in patients with acute myocardial infarction and upper gastrointestinal bleeding: Results of a decision analysis. *Dig. Dis. Sci.* **2009**, *54*, 701–711. [CrossRef] [PubMed]
12. Chung, C.; Chen, C.; Chen, K.; Fang, Y.; Hsu, W.; Chen, Y.; Tseng, W.; Lin, C.; Lee, T.; Wang, H.; et al. Randomized controlled trial of early endoscopy for upper gastrointestinal bleeding in acute coronary syndrome patients. *Sci. Rep.* **2022**, *12*, 1–9. [CrossRef] [PubMed]
13. Guo, C.L.; Wong, S.H.; Lau, L.H.; Lui, R.N.; Mak, J.W.; Tang, R.S.; Yip, T.C.; Wu, W.K.; Wong, G.L.; Chan, F.K.; et al. Timing of endoscopy for acute upper gastrointestinal bleeding: A territory-wide cohort study. *Gut* **2021**, *0*, 1–7. [CrossRef] [PubMed]
14. Hoffman, G.R.; Stein, D.J.; Moore, M.B.; Feuerstein, J.D. Safety of endoscopy after myocardial infarction based on cardiovascular risk categories: A retrospective analysis of 135 patients at a tertiary referral medical center. *J. Clin. Gastroenterol.* **2007**, *41*, 462–467.
15. Al-Ebrahim, F.; Khan, K.J.; Alhazzani, W.; Alnemer, A.; Alzahrani, A.; Marshall, J.; Armstrong, D. Safety of esophagogastroduodenoscopy within 30 days of myocardial infarction: A retrospective cohort study from a Canadian tertiary centre. *Can. J. Gastroenterol.* **2012**, *26*, 151–154. [CrossRef] [PubMed]
16. Katz, D. Cardiac arrest during gastroscopy. *Gastroenterology* **1957**, *33*, 650–654. [CrossRef]
17. Silvis, S.E.; Nebel, O.; Rogers, G.; Sugawa, C.; Mandelstam, P. Endoscopic complications: Results of the 1974 American Society for Gastrointestinal Endoscopy survey. *JAMA* **1976**, *235*, 928–930. [CrossRef] [PubMed]
18. Lieberman, D.A.; Wuerker, C.K.; Katon, R.M. Cardiopulmonary risk of esophagogastroduodenoscopy: Role of endoscope diameter and systemic sedation. *Gastroenterology* **1985**, *88*, 468–472. [CrossRef]
19. Hart, R.; Classen, M. Complications of diagnostic gastrointestinal endoscopy. *Endoscopy* **1990**, *22*, 229–233. [CrossRef] [PubMed]
20. Mergener, K.; Baillie, J. Complications of endoscopy. *Endoscopy* **1998**, *30*, 230–243. [CrossRef]

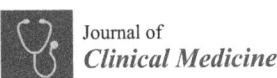

Article

The Combining of Tyrosine Kinase Inhibitors and Immune Checkpoint Inhibitors as First-Line Treatment for Advanced Stage Hepatocellular Carcinoma

Shou-Wu Lee [1,2,3,4], Sheng-Shun Yang [1,2,3,5,6], Han-Chung Lien [1,3,4], Yen-Chun Peng [1,3], Chun-Fang Tung [1,3] and Teng-Yu Lee [1,2,*]

1. Division of Gastroenterology, Department of Internal Medicine, Taichung Veterans General Hospital, Taichung 40705, Taiwan
2. Department of Internal Medicine, Chung Shan Medical University, Taichung 40201, Taiwan
3. Department of Internal Medicine, Yang Ming Chiao Tung University, Taipei 112304, Taiwan
4. Department of Post-Baccalaureate Medicine, College of Medicine, Chung Hsing University, Taichung 40227, Taiwan
5. Ph.D. Program in Translational Medicine, Chung Hsing University, Taichung 40227, Taiwan
6. Institute of Biomedical Sciences, Chung Hsing University, Taichung 40227, Taiwan
* Correspondence: ericest429@yahoo.com.tw; Tel.: +886-4-23592525 (ext. 3306); Fax: +886-4-23595046

Abstract: Aim: Hepatocellular carcinoma (HCC) is one of the most common cancers. Tyrosine kinase inhibitors (TKIs), including sorafenib (SOR) and lenvatinib (LEN), as well as immune checkpoint inhibitors (ICIs), including nivolumab (NIVO) and pembrolizumab (PEMBRO), have been approved for the treatment of advanced HCC. The aim of the study is to determine whether advanced-stage HCC patients should receive a combination of TKI and ICI as first-line therapy. Methods: Data for subjects with BCLC stage C HCC, who were receiving combining TKI and ICI as first-line therapy at Taichung Veterans General Hospital from April 2019 to July 2021, were evaluated. The general and therapeutic outcome data were collected and analyzed. Results: A total of 33 patients were enrolled (8 SOR/NIVO, 4 SOR/PEMBRO, 11 LEN/NIVO, and 10 LEN/PEMBRO). All cases belonged to Child-Pugh class A. The objective response rate was 48.5%, and disease control rate was 72.7%. The average progression-free survival (PFS) and overall survival (OS) of all patients was 9.2 and 17.0 months, respectively. The use of PEMBRO, when compared with NIVO, had a significantly positive impact towards achieving an objective response, defined as either complete response or partial response (OR 5.54, $p = 0.045$). PFS and OS between the different TKIs or ICIs had no differences. The most adverse event was fatigue (36.4%), and most cases were mild and manageable. Conclusion: Combining TKI and ICI provides an acceptable antitumor efficacy in first-line therapy for advanced-stage HCC patients. The survival outcomes between different TKIs or ICIs display no differences.

Keywords: hepatocellular carcinoma; immune checkpoint inhibitor; tyrosine kinase inhibitor

1. Introduction

Liver cancer, mainly hepatocellular carcinoma (HCC), is the most common liver cancer, as well as a leading cause of cancer death globally [1]. For those with newly diagnosed HCC, many patients are presented with an intermediate (Barcelona Clinic of Liver Cancer stage B) or advanced stage (BCLC stage C) of the disease at their time of initial diagnosis [2]. Regarding the advanced stage (BCLC stage C) HCC, tyrosine kinase inhibitor (TKI) therapies play an essential role in the patient's overall systematic therapy. Currently, approved first-line TKI therapies include sorafenib (SOR) and lenvatinib (LEN), according to meaningful phase 3 trials [3–5].

In the last few days, immune checkpoint inhibitor (ICI) therapies, including programmed cell death protein 1 (PD-1), programmed cell death protein ligand 1 (PD-L1), and cytotoxic T lymphocyte antigen 4 (CTLA-4), were approved for the treatment of

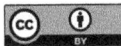

several human cancers [6]. Currently, anti-PD-1 agents, including nivolumab (NIVO) or pembrolizumab (PEMBRO), are approved for treatment in unresectable HCC [7–10].

Lately, the IMbrave150 study, the combination of atezolizumab (anti-PD-L1 antibody) and bevacizumab (anti-VEGF monoclonal antibody), was accepted as a promising first-line treatment for advanced HCC [11]. These better results also suggest that there is a promising future for combining TKI and ICI therapies in the treatment of advanced HCC. However, the cost of atezolizumab and bevacizumab is high. Alternatively, another combination therapy involving TKIs, including SOR and LEN, plus ICIs, including NIVO and PEMBRO, have been better adapted in clinical practices.

The aim of the present study is to generate real-world data on patients with advanced-stage HCC that have received a combination of TKIs and ICIs as first-line therapy.

2. Methods

Data for patients with BCLC stage C HCC, and who were receiving a combination of TKIs and ICIs as first-line therapy at Taichung Veterans General Hospital from April 2019 to July 2021, were evaluated. HCC was diagnosed according to the American Association for the Study of Liver Disease (AASLD) guidelines [12]. All enrolled patients were categorized as Child-Pugh class A. The exclusion criteria included those patients diagnosed with Child-Pugh stage B or C, had an intolerance to combining therapy, a poor performance status (Eastern Cooperative Oncology Group performance score ≥ 2), a survival period of less than 2 months, and absence of a radiological images within the following day. The characteristics of the enrolled patients, including age, gender, presence of chronic hepatitis B (HBV), hepatitis C (HCV) infection, macroscopic vascular invasion (MVI), or extrahepatic spread (EHS), were all collected. Their laboratory data, including serum level of bilirubin, alanine aminotransferase (ALT), and alpha-fetoprotein (AFP), were also recorded for each individual.

After administering combination therapy, the patients received regular follow-up in the outpatient clinic every 2 weeks. The treatment of TKIs and ICIs usage was determined by each patient's hepatologist. The mean dosage of TKIs and ICIs for each enrolled subject patient was also determined by each patient's hepatologist according to each patient's clinical condition.

Tumor response, as seen on radiological dynamic images, was assessed every 8 weeks by experienced radiologists. Treatment of TKI and ICI was discontinued once obvious tumor progression was disclosed through subsequent imaging studies. The mean dosage and therapeutic duration of TKIs and ICIs for each enrolled subject patient were subsequently recorded.

The best tumor response was assessed according to the modified RECIST (mRECIST) criteria [13], which included complete response (CR), partial response (PR), stable disease (SD), and progressive disease (PD). The patients showing either CR or PR were categorized into the objective response group. The objective response rate (ORR) and disease control rate (DCR) of patients' tumors treated using combination therapy were calculated.

Adverse events were recorded as the appearance of hand-foot skin reaction (HFSR), hypertension, diarrhea, or fatigue after administration of combination therapy. The associations between different TKIs; ICIs; clinical parameters, including age, gender, serum level of AFP; presence of HBV, HCV, MVI, and EHS; and the efficacy of combination therapy were analyzed. Progression-free survival (PFS) was defined as the time from start of combination therapy administration to either radiological confirmation of tumor progression or death, and presented as median value with a 95% confidence interval (CI). Overall survival (OS) was defined as the time from start of combination therapy until death and also presented as a median value with a 95% CI.

Data are expressed as median and interquartile range (IQR) for each continuous variable and a percentage of the total patient number for each category variable. Statistical comparisons were made using Pearson's chi-square test in order to compare category variable parameters. Mann–Whitney test was adapted to analyze continuous variable parameters. A p-value below 0.05 was defined as statistically significant. Survival analysis was applied using the Kaplan–Meier method for univariate and multivariate analysis and comparisons were subsequently performed with the log-rank test.

3. Results

3.1. Patient Characteristics

A total of 33 patients being treated with combination therapy were enrolled, with 8, 4, 11, and 10 cases receiving SOR/NIVO, SOR/PEMBRO, LEN/NIVO, and LEN/PEMBRO respectively. The general data of these patients are shown in Table 1. Overall, the median age was 66 years, with a male predominance (78.8%) being noted. The prevalence of chronic HBV and HCV infection was 57.6% and 24.2% respectively. All cases belonged to Child-Pugh class A and BCLC stage C. Sixteen (48.2%) and 19 patients (57.6%) had MVI and EHS, respectively. The median value of AFP was 130 ng/mL, with 13 patients (39.4%) having AFP $\geq$ 400 ng/mL at the baseline value prior to the administration of combination therapy. There were 10 patients (30.8%) who experienced an AFP decrease over 10% from the baseline value during the course of their combination therapy.

The mean oral daily doses of SOR and LEN were 366 mg and 7 mg respectively, while the mean intravenous doses given every 2 to 3 weeks of NIVO and PEMBRO were 120 mg and 158 mg, respectively. The mean usage duration periods of SOR, LEN, NIVO, and PEMBRO were 7.1, 7.8, 10.8, and 7.9 months, respectively.

3.2. Best Radiological Response

The outcomes for the enrolled patients are listed in Table 2. The numbers of patients with CR, PR, SD, and PD were 2 (6.1%), 14 (42.4%), 8 (24.2%), and 9 (27.3%), respectively. Overall, the ORR was 48.5%, and the DCR was 72.7%. Regarding the individuals treated with different combination therapy regimens, the patients receiving SOR/PEMBRO (75.0%) had the highest ORR, followed by LEN/PEMBRO (70.0%), LEN/NIVO (51.8%), and SOR/NIVO (25.0%).

Logistic analysis of the patients who achieved tumor objective response through combination therapy is shown in Table 3. Clinical parameters including age, gender, viral hepatitis; presence of MVI, EHS, and adverse effects; values of AFP; and different TKIs had non-significant effects. In contrast, the use of PEMBRO, when compared with NIVO, had a significantly positive impact (OR 5.42, 95% CI 1.19–24.52, p = 0.028), with the significance still existing after being adjusted through multivariable analysis (OR 5.54, 95% CI 1.06–28.91, p = 0.045).

3.3. Progression-Free Survival and Overall Survival

As shown in Figure 1, the PFS of all patients was 9.2 $\pm$ 6.4 months, and the OS 17.0 $\pm$ 6.3 months. Further analysis of both PFS and OS when stratified by different TKIs or ICIs is shown in Figure 2. PFS was 9.1 $\pm$ 6.8 months and 9.3 $\pm$ 6.4 months, and OS 17.0 $\pm$ 7.1 months and 17.0 $\pm$ 6.2 months, in patients with SOR and LEN, respectively. These differences were non-significant (p = 0.963 and 0.987). PFS was 9.6 $\pm$ 7.4 and 8.5 $\pm$ 4.4 months, and OS 17.4 $\pm$ 7.2 and 16.2 $\pm$ 4.6 months, in patients with NIVO and PEMBRO, respectively. Similarly, these differences were insignificant (p = 0.214 and 0.197).

Table 1. General characteristics of patients.

		All (N = 33)				SOR/NIVO (N = 8)				SOR/PEMBRO (N = 4)				LEN/NIVO (N = 11)				LEN/PEMBRO (N = 10)				p-Value
		M	(IQR)	N	%	M	(IQR)	N	%	M	(IQR)	N	%	M	(IQR)	N	%	M	(IQR)	N	%	
Age (years)		66	(14)			68	(9)			70	(4)			60	(18)			56	(15)			0.090 [a]
Gender (male)				26	(78.8%)			6	(75.0%)			2	(50.0%)			8	(72.7%)			10	(100%)	0.173 [b]
Hepatitis infection	HBV			19	(57.6%)			4	(50.0%)			0				8	(72.7%)			7	(70.0%)	0.063 [b]
	HCV			8	(24.2%)			0				4	(100%)			2	(18.2%)			2	(25.0%)	0.062 [b]
Child-Pugh stage	A			33	(100%)			8	(100%)			4	(100%)			11	(100%)			10	(100%)	1.000 [b]
BCLC stage	C			33	(100%)			8	(100%)			4	(100%)			11	(100%)			10	(100%)	1.000 [b]
MVI				16	(48.2%)			4	(50.0%)							6	(54.5%)			6	(60.0%)	0.215 [b]
EHS				19	(57.6%)			4	(50.0%)			4	(100%)			6	(54.5%)			5	(50.0%)	0.332 [b]
Bilirubin (U/L)		0.7	(0.9)			1.4	(1.9)			0.5	(0.2)			0.7	(0.5)			0.9	(0.8)			0.281 [a]
ALT (U/L)		36	(34)			34	(25)			15	(15)			51	(45)			40	(19)			0.206 [a]
Abnormal ALT (male > 50 U/L or female > 35 U/L)				10	(30.3%)			2	(25.0%)			0				6	(54.5%)			2	(20.0%)	0.144 [b]
AFP (ng/mL)		130	(3115)			227	(3408)			1036	(2067)			132	(3916)			34	(7502)			0.575 [a]
Abnormal AFP (AFP > 7 ng/mL)				22	(66.7%)			6	(75.0%)			2	(50.0%)			9	(81.8%)			5	(50.0%)	0.371 [b]
AFP (ng/mL)	≥400			13	(39.4%)			2	(25.0%)			2	(50.0%)			5	(45.5%)			4	(40.0%)	0.788 [b]
	<400			20	(60.6%)			6	(75.0%)			2	(50.0%)			6	(54.5%)			6	(60.0%)	
AFP decreased > 10%				10	(30.3%)			4	(50.0%)			0				4	(36.4%)			2	(20.0%)	0.272 [b]

All p-values were analyzed with Mann–Whitney test [a] and Pearson's Chi-square test [b]. Abbreviations: AFP, alpha-fetoprotein; ALT, alanine aminotransferase; EHS, extrahepatic spread; HBV, Hepatitis B; HCV, Hepatitis C; IQR, interquartile range; LEN, lenvatinib; M, median; MVI, macroscopic vascular invasion; N, number of patients; NIVO, nivolumab; PEMBRO, pembrolizumab; SOR, sorafenib.

Table 2. Best radiological responses.

		All (N = 33)		SOR/NIVO (N = 8)		SOR/PEMBRO (N = 4)		LEN/NIVO (N = 11)		LEN/PEMBRO (N = 10)		p-Value
		N	%	N	%	N	%	N	%	N	%	
mRECIST												0.279
	CR	2	(6.1%)	0		1	(25.0%)	1	(7.4%)	0		
	PR	14	(42.4%)	2	(25.0%)	2	(50.0%)	3	(44.4%)	7	(70.0%)	
	SD	8	(24.2%)	2	(25.0%)	1	(25.0%)	4	(22.3%)	1	(10.0%)	
	PD	9	(27.3%)	4	(50.0%)	0		3	(25.9%)	2	(20.0%)	
ORR		16	(48.5%)	2	(25.0%)	3	(75.0%)	4	(51.8%)	7	(70.0%)	0.145
DCR		24	(72.7%)	4	(50.0%)	4	(100%)	8	(74.1%)	8	(80.0%)	0.278

All p-values were analyzed with Pearson's Chi-square test. Abbreviations: CR, complete response; DCR, disease control rate; LEN, lenvatinib; N, number of patients; NIVO, nivolumab; ORR, objective response rate; PD, progressive disease; PEMBRO, pembrolizumab; PR, partial response; SD, stable disease; SOR, sorafenib.

Table 3. Logistic analysis of each item to achieve objective response.

	Univariate Analysis			Multivariate Analysis		
	HR	(95% CI)	p-Value	HR	(95% CI)	p-Value
Age (≤65 vs. >65 years)	1.87	(0.44–7.85)	0.395	1.07	(0.13–8.96)	0.948
Gender (male vs. female)	8.17	(0.85–77.97)	0.068	8.69	(0.66–114.26)	0.100
HBV (HBsAg + vs. −)	0.90	(0.23–3.58)	0.881			
HCV (anti-HCV + vs. −)	4.50	(0.75–26.93)	0.099			
AFP (≤400 vs. >400 ng/mL)	1.96	(0.47–8.11)	0.356			
AFP decreased > 10% (yes vs. no)	1.64	(0.36–7.38)	0.521			
MVI (yes vs. no)	0.42	(0.10–1.70)	0.224			
EHS (yes vs. no)	0.55	(0.14–2.20)	0.394			
TKI (LEN vs. SOR)	1.54	(0.37–6.45)	0.554	1.27	(0.15–11.09)	0.826
ICI (PEMBRO vs. NIVO)	5.42	(1.19–24.52)	0.028	5.54	(1.06–28.91)	0.042
HFRS (yes vs. no)	1.95	(0.43–8.82)	0.386			
Hypertension (yes vs. no)	1.29	(0.10–3.27)	0.849			
Diarrhea (yes vs. no)	1.09	(0.25–4.81)	0.908			
Fatigue (yes vs. no)	3.00	(0.92–23.45)	0.057			

Abbreviations: AFP, alpha-fetoprotein; CI, confidence interval; EHS, extrahepatic spread; HBV, Hepatitis B; HCV, Hepatitis C; HR, hazard ratio; ICI, immune checkpoint inhibitor; LEN, lenvatinib; MVI, microscopic vascular invasion; N, number of patients; NIVO, nivolumab; PEMBRO, pembrolizumab; SOR, sorafenib; TKI, tyrosine kinase inhibitor.

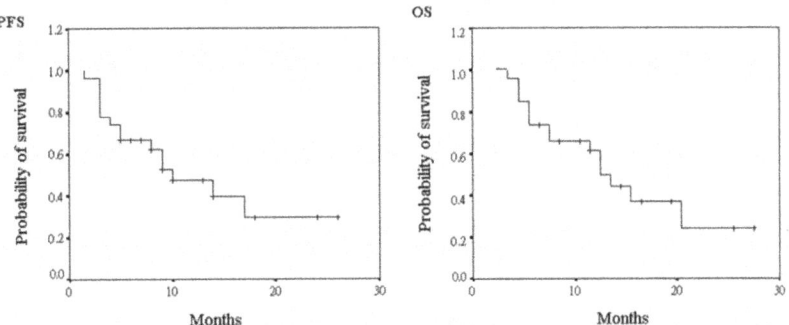

Figure 1. The survival time of hepatocellular carcinoma patients receiving combination therapy. (PFS, progress free survival; OS, overall survival).

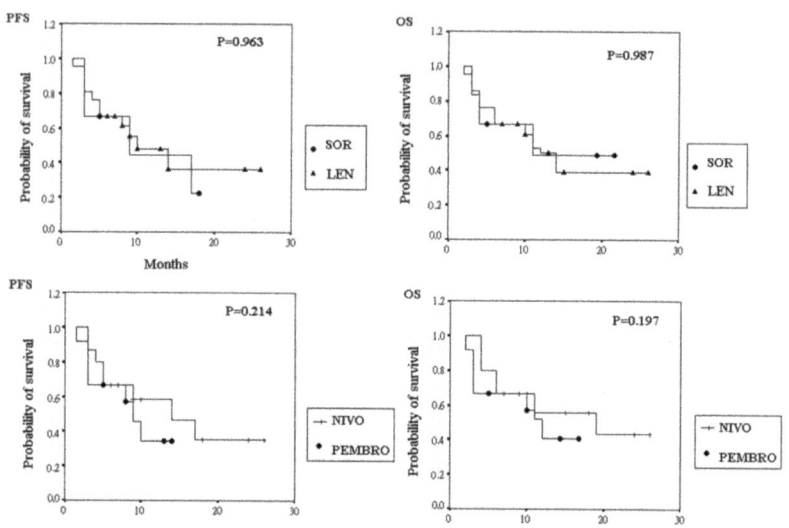

Figure 2. The survival time of hepatocellular carcinoma patients receiving different tyrosine kinase inhibitors and immune checkpoint inhibitors. (LEN, lenvatinib; NIVO, nivolumab; OS, overall survival; PEMBRO, pembrolizumab; PFS, progression free survival; SOR, sorafenib).

3.4. Adverse Events

The adverse events detected in each group are shown in Table 4. Overall, the prevalences of HFRS, hypertension, diarrhea, and fatigue were 30.3%, 18.2%, 30.3%, and 36.4% respectively. All instances of hypertension occurred in the patients receiving LEN, while the cases receiving SOR had a higher prevalence of HFSR.

Table 4. Adverse events of combination therapy.

	All (N = 33)		SOR/NIVO (N = 8)		SOR/PEMBRO (N = 4)		LEN/NIVO (N = 11)		LEN/PEMBRO (N = 10)		p-Value
	N	%	N	%	N	%	N	%	N	%	
HFRS	10	(30.3%)	4	(50.0%)	2	(50.0%)	1	(16.7%)	3	(30.0%)	0.208
Hypertension	6	(18.2%)	0		0		2	(18.2%)	4	(40.0%)	0.118
Diarrhea	10	(30.3%)	2	(25.0%)	2	(50.0%)	3	(27.3%)	3	(30.0%)	0.828
Fatigue	12	(36.4%)	2	(25.0%)	2	(50.0%)	5	(45.5%)	3	(30.0%)	0.721

All p-values were analyzed with Pearson's Chi-square test. Abbreviations: HFRS, hand foot syndrome reaction; LEN, lenvatinib; N, number of patients. NIVO, nivolumab; PEMBRO, pembrolizumab; SOR, sorafenib.

4. Discussion

HCC represents the most common type of cancer worldwide, with its incidence rate continuously increasing. However, although screening programs diagnose numerous HCCs at an early stage, still more than half of patients will be diagnosed at an advanced stage [2]. SOR is a TKI, targeting mainly VEGFR2, PDGFR, and KIT [14]. In the SHARP trial, SOR was associated with a significantly increased OS compared with patients receiving a placebo (10.7 vs. 7.9 months; $p < 0.001$). Additionally, PFS was shown to be significantly longer with SOR (5.5 vs. 2.8 months; $p < 0.001$) [3]. Similar efficacy was reported from the Asia-Pacific trial (OS: 6.5 vs. 4.2 months; HR: 0.68; $p = 0.014$) [4]. Therefore, when treating unresectable HCC, SOR has been used as the first systemic standard treatment since back in 2007.

LEN is another available TKI, targeting VEGFR1–3, FGFR1–4, PDGFR, RET, and KIT [15]. LEN was tested within the REFLECT trial, which acted as an open-label, multicenter, noninferiority trial comparing SOR with LEN in previously untreated patients. Although the study showed no significant improvements in median survival in the LEN arm (13.6 vs. 12.3 months), there was still a significant improvement seen in tumor response (ORR: 24.1 vs. 9.2%; $p = 0.001$) and time to progression (8.9 vs. 3.7 months; $p < 0.0001$) [5]. Currently, LEN has also been approved as a first-line treatment for patients with intermediate or advanced-stage HCC who have not received prior systemic therapy.

Unfortunately, regarding the current first-line TKIs for treating HCC, their disadvantages include a low ORR, easier to tumor progression, and a lack of long-term survival.

ICI therapy, particularly antibodies targeting the programmed cell death-1 (PD-1)/programmed cell death ligand-1 (PD-L1) pathway, represented a major breakthrough in drug development for oncologists during the past decade. Anti-PD-1 or anti-PD-L1 monotherapy has been approved for the treatment of more than 10 cancer types, with ORRs of 15–20% and good safety profiles being seen [6]. In the context of HCC, the CheckMate-040 study, a nonrandomized Phase I/II study that included 56 therapy-naive patients, suggested that NIVO may be meaningfully effective as first-line therapy for patients with advanced HCC (ORR 13%; with 6- and 9-month survival rates of 89 and 82%) [7]. However, the phase III randomized CheckMate-459 study involving a total of 743 patients who were receiving NIVO or SOR, disclosed no differences in either OS (16.4 vs. 14.7 months; $p = 0.0752$) or PFS (3.7 vs. 3.8 months), although tumor response was slightly better for NIVO (ORR: 15 vs. 7%) [10].

Similarly, for PEMBRO, the results of the Phase III randomized double-blind keynote-240 trial involving a total of 413 patients receiving either PEMBRO or a placebo, noted a non-significant OS (13.9 vs. 10.6 months; $p = 0.0238$, it did not meet the prespecified boundaries of $p = 0.0174$) and PFS periods (3.0 vs. 2.8 months; $p = 0.0022$, it did not meet the prespecified boundaries of $p = 0.002$) [9]. Based on the above studies, ICIs should not be used in the routine care of patients with untreated advanced HCC. However, the combining of TKIs and ICIs may be an alternative choice in the first-line treatment of advanced HCC.

Interstitial cells, including Kupffer cells; dendritic cells; liver endothelial cells; liver stellate cells; and immunosuppressive cytokines, including IL-10 or TGF-β, may play an important role in the development of the immunosuppressive environment of HCC. Combining TKI and IO is expected to improve this immunosuppressive microenvironment [16]. Regarding experimental models for HCC, SOR, in combination with NIVO, showed a stronger tumor growth inhibition as opposed to SOR or NIVO monotherapy [17]. In a phase 1b trial, LEN plus NIVO in patients with unresectable HCC revealed a high ORR of 76.7% and an ability to manage adverse events [18]. A phase 1b trial involving LEN plus PEMBRO as a first-line treatment for advanced HCC, reported an ORR as high as 36.0% (95% CI 26.6–46.2%) with a tolerable safety profile [19]. Furthermore, a phase 3 trial for the purpose of assessing the efficacy of the combination of LEN and PEMBRO as first-line treatment for HCC is now also underway.

This open-label phase 3 IMbrave150 trial compared the combination of atezolizumab and bevacizumab with SOR in untreated patients diagnosed with advanced unresectable HCC. The ORR between the two approaches was 27.3% vs. 11.9%, with a 5.5% complete response seen in the atezolizumab and bevacizumab group. The PFS was 6.8 months (95% CI 5.7–8.3) for the atezolizumab/bevacizumab group, with the HR for mortality being 0.58 (95% CI 0.42–0.79; $p = 0.001$) in favor of atezolizumab/bevacizumab [11].

For our 33 patients receiving combination therapy as first-line treatment for advanced stage HCC, the ORR and DCR were 48.5% and 72.7%, respectively, with the average PFS and OS being 9.2 and 17.0 months, respectively. Radiological CR occurred in two patients (6.1%). The antitumor results of our study were shown to be better than previous trials involving monotherapy with TKI or ICI, and similar to studies using combination regimens. The average dose of TKI (SOR 366 mg and LEN 7 mg per day) and ICI (NIVO 120 mg and PEMBRO 158 mg every 2–3 weeks) administered to our patients was low, with the reasons for that possibly being concern over drug-associated adverse effects and economic factors, as ICI treatment is not currently covered by national health insurance in Taiwan. Certainly, the low doses of TKI and ICI may cause a negative impact on treatment efficacy for HCC.

Further analysis of our data determined that achieving an objective response was significantly associated with different ICIs. The prescription of PEMBRO, when compared with NIVO, had a significantly positive impact towards achieving tumor objective response (OR 5.54, p = 0.045). This may be due to a relatively acceptable average dose of PEMBRO (158 mg every 3 weeks) when compared with NIVO (120 mg every 2 weeks). The patients receiving NIVO and those receiving PEMBRO showed no differences in PFS (9.6 vs. 8.5 months; p = 0.214) or OS (17.4 vs. 16.2 months; p = 0.197). As for the different TKIs, the antitumor responses were similar both in the radiological responses and survival time.

The most adverse events our patients experienced were fatigue (36.4%), followed by HFSR (30.3%), diarrhea (30.3%) and hypertension (18.2%). Not surprisingly, HFRS usually occurred in the patients receiving SOR, with all hypertension happening in the patients receiving LEN. The incidences of adverse events in our patients are similar with previous trials, with most being mild and manageable. However, the rate of adverse events in our study may be underestimated due to its retrospective design. Additionally, our enrolled patients followed good compliance to combination therapy, so because certain individuals who experienced severe adverse events were excluded, their data may have been excluded. Besides, some data about immune-related adverse events (IRAEs), such as pneumonitis, thyroiditis, or hepatitis, may be missed in our study.

There were several limitations to our study. First, this study was designed as being retrospective and was conducted at a single tertiary care center. Selection bias may therefore have existed. Second, only subjects diagnosed with Child–Pugh class A and BCLC stage C HCC were enrolled in our study. Third, our sample size was small and the follow-up period was short. Four, alcohol consumption or other underlying diseases, such as immune diseases and non-alcoholic fatty liver disease (NAFLD), may influence the therapeutic response of the enrolled patients, and these data were unavailable in our study. Lastly, no sufficient data surrounding the regimen of atezolizumab/bevacizumab was obtained and compared. Further prospective research involving the analysis of more variables is therefore warranted.

5. Conclusions

Combining TKIs and ICIs provides an acceptable antitumor efficacy in first-line therapy for advanced-stage HCC. The use of PEMBRO, as compared with NIVO, makes it easier to achieve a tumor-objective response. The survival outcomes seen between either different TKIs or ICIs show no differences.

Author Contributions: Conceptualization, T.-Y.L. and S.-S.Y.; methodology, S.-W.L. and T.-Y.L.; formal analysis, S.-W.L. and S.-S.Y.; investigation, S.-W.L., T.-Y.L., and S.-S.Y.; data curation, H.-C.L., Y.-C.P., and C.-F.T.; writing—original draft preparation, S.-W.L., H.-C.L., and C.-F.T.; writing—review and editing, S.-W.L. and H.-C.L.; supervision, T.-Y.L. and S.-S.Y. All authors have read and agreed to the published version of the manuscript.

Funding: This research received no external funding.

Institutional Review Board Statement: The study was conducted in accordance with the Declaration of Helsinki and approved by the Institutional Review Board of Taichung Veterans General Hospital (CF21236B).

Informed Consent Statement: Written informed consent has been obtained from the patients to publish this paper.

Data Availability Statement: Not applicable.

Acknowledgments: Not applicable.

Conflicts of Interest: The authors declare no conflict of interest.

References

1. Kulik, L.; El-Serag, H.B. Epidemiology and Management of Hepatocellular Carcinoma. *Gastroenterology* **2019**, *156*, 477–491. [CrossRef] [PubMed]
2. Marrero, J.A.; Kulik, L.M.; Sirlin, C.B.; Zhu, A.X.; Finn, R.S.; Abecassis, M.M.; Roberts, L.R.; Heimbach, J.K. Diagnosis, staging, and management of hepatocellular carcinoma: 2018 practice guidance by the American Association for the Study of Liver Diseases. *Hepatology* **2018**, *68*, 723–750. [CrossRef] [PubMed]
3. Llovet, J.M.; Ricci, S.; Mazzaferro, V.; Hilgard, P.; Gane, E.; Blanc, J.F.; de Oliveira, A.C.; Santoro, A.; Raoul, J.L.; Forner, A.; et al. Sorafenib in Advanced Hepatocellular Carcinoma. *N. Engl. J. Med.* **2008**, *359*, 378–390. [CrossRef]
4. Cheng, A.L.; Kang, Y.K.; Chen, Z.; Tsao, C.J.; Qin, S.; Kim, J.S.; Luo, R.; Feng, J.; Ye, S.; Yang, T.S.; et al. Efficacy and safety of sorafenib in patients in the Asia-Pacific region with advanced hepatocellular carcinoma: A Phase III randomised, double-blind, placebo-controlled trial. *Lancet Oncol.* **2009**, *10*, 25–34. [CrossRef]
5. Kudo, M.; Finn, R.S.; Qin, S.; Han, K.-H.; Ikeda, K.; Piscaglia, F.; Baron, A.; Park, J.W.; Han, G.; Jassem, J.; et al. Lenvatinib versus Sorafenib in First-Line Treatment of Patients with Unresectable Hepatocellular Carcinoma: A Randomised Phase 3 Non-Inferiority Trial. *Lancet* **2018**, *391*, 1163–1173. [CrossRef]
6. Callahan, M.K.; Postow, M.A.; Wolchok, J.D. Targeting T cell co-receptors for cancer therapy. *Immunity* **2016**, *44*, 1069–1078. [CrossRef] [PubMed]
7. El-Khoueiry, A.B.; Sangro, B.; Yau, T.; Crocenzi, T.S.; Kudo, M.; Hsu, C.; Kim, T.Y.; Choo, S.P.; Trojan, J.; Welling, T.H.; et al. Nivolumab in patients with advanced hepatocellular carcinoma (CheckMate 040): An open-label, non-comparative, phase 1/2 dose escalation and expansion trial. *Lancet* **2017**, *389*, 2492–2502. [CrossRef]
8. Zhu, A.X.; Finn, R.S.; Edeline, J.; Cattan, S.; Ogasawara, S.; Palmar, D.; Verslype, C.; Zagonel, V.; Fartoux, L.; Vogel, A.; et al. Pembrolizumab in patients with advanced hepatocellular carcinoma previously treated with sorafenib (KEYNOTE-224): A non-randomised, open-label phase 2 trial. *Lancet Oncol.* **2018**, *19*, 940–952. [CrossRef]
9. Finn, R.S.; Ryoo, B.Y.; Merle, P.; Kudo, M.; Bouattour, M.; Lim, H.Y.; Breder, V.; Edeline, J.; Chao, Y.; Ogasawara, S.; et al. Pembrolizumab as second-line therapy in patients with advanced hepatocellular carcinoma in KEYNOTE-240: A randomized, double-blind, phase III trial. *J. Clin. Oncol.* **2020**, *38*, 193–202. [CrossRef] [PubMed]
10. Sangro, B.; Park, J.; Finn, R.; Cheng, A.; Mathurin, P.; Edeline, J.; Kudo, M.; Han, K.; Harding, J.; Merle, P.; et al. LBA-3 CheckMate 459: Long-term (minimum follow-up 33.6 months) survival outcomes with nivolumab versus sorafenib as first-line treatment in patients. *Ann. Oncol.* **2020**, *31*, S241–S242. [CrossRef]
11. Finn, R.S.; Qin, S.; Ikeda, M.; Galle, P.R.; Ducreux, M.; Kim, T.Y.; Kudo, M.; Breder, V.; Merle, P.; Kaseb, A.O.; et al. Atezolizumab plus bevacizumab in unresectable hepatocellular carcinoma. *N. Engl. J. Med.* **2020**, *382*, 1894–1905. [CrossRef] [PubMed]
12. Heimbach, J.K.; Kulik, L.M.; Finn, R.S.; Sirlin, C.B.; Abecassis, M.M.; Roberts, L.R.; Zhu, A.X.; Murad, M.H.; Marrero, J.A. AASLD guidelines for the treatment of hepatocellular carcinoma. *Hepatology* **2018**, *67*, 358–380. [CrossRef]
13. Lencioni, R.; Llovet, J.M. Modified RECIST (mRECIST) assessment for hepatocellular carcinoma. *Semin. Liver Dis.* **2010**, *30*, 52–60. [CrossRef]
14. Clark, J.W.; Eder, J.P.; Ryan, D.; Lathia, C.; Lenz, H.J. Safety and pharmacokinetics of the dual action Raf kinase and vascular endothelial growth factor receptor inhibitor, BAY 43-9006, in patients with advanced, refractory solid tumors. *Clin. Cancer Res.* **2005**, *11*, 5472–5480. [CrossRef] [PubMed]
15. Kudo, M. Lenvatinib in advanced hepatocellular carcinoma. *Liver Cancer* **2017**, *6*, 253–263. [CrossRef] [PubMed]
16. Kudo, M. Combination cancer immunotherapy in hepatocellular carcinoma. *Liver Cancer* **2018**, *7*, 20–27. [CrossRef] [PubMed]
17. Wang, Y.; Li, H.; Liang, Q.; Liu, B.; Mei, X.; Ma, Y. Combinatorial immunotherapy of sorafenib and blockade of programmed death-ligand 1 induces effective natural killer cell responses against hepatocellular carcinoma. *Tumor Biol.* **2015**, *36*, 1561–1566. [CrossRef] [PubMed]
18. Kudo, M.; Ikeda, M.; Motomura, K.; Okusaka, T.; Kato, N.; Dutcus, C.E.; Hisai, T.; Suzuki, M.; Ikezawa, H.; Iwatam, T.; et al. A phase Ib study of lenvatinib (LEN) plus nivolumab (NIV) in patients (pts) with unresectable hepatocellular carcinoma (uHCC): Study 117. *J. Clin. Oncol.* **2020**, *38*, 513. [CrossRef]
19. Finn, R.S.; Ikeda, M.; Zhu, A.X.; Sung, M.W.; Baron, A.D.; Kudo, M.; Okusaka, T.; Kobayashi, M.; Kumada, H.; Kaneko, S.; et al. Phase Ib study of lenvatinib plus pembrolizumab in patients with unresectable hepatocellular carcinoma. *J. Clin. Oncol.* **2020**, *38*, 2960–2970. [CrossRef] [PubMed]

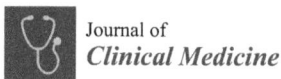

Communication

Predictive Factors of Surgical Recurrence in Patients with Crohn's Disease on Long-Term Follow-Up: A Focus on Histology

Gian Paolo Caviglia [1], Chiara Angela Mineo [1], Chiara Rosso [1], Angelo Armandi [1], Marco Astegiano [2], Gabriella Canavese [3], Andrea Resegotti [4], Giorgio Maria Saracco [1,2] and Davide Giuseppe Ribaldone [1,2,*]

[1] Department of Medical Sciences, University of Turin, 10126 Turin, Italy
[2] Division of Gastroenterology, AOU Città della Salute e della Scienza–Molinette Hospital, 10126 Turin, Italy
[3] General Surgery 1U, Città della Salute e della Scienza–Molinette Hospital, 10126 Turin, Italy
[4] Department of Pathology, AOU Città della Salute e della Scienza–Molinette Hospital, 10126 Turin, Italy
* Correspondence: davidegiuseppe.ribaldone@unito.it; Tel.: +39-011-6333710

Abstract: In patients with Crohn's disease (CD) that underwent surgery, predictive factors of surgical recurrence have been only partially identified. The aim of our study was to identify potential factors associated with an increased risk of surgical recurrence. A monocentric retrospective observational study was conducted including patients diagnosed with CD, according to ECCO criteria who received their first ileocolic resection. Overall, 162 patients were enrolled in our study; 54 of them were excluded due to a lack of sufficient data. The median follow-up was 136.5 months, IQR 91.5–176.5, and the surgical recurrence rate after the median follow-up was 21.3%. In the multivariate analysis, an age ≤ 28 years at the first surgical resection (aHR = 16.44, $p < 0.001$), current smoking (aHR = 15.84, $p < 0.001$), female sex (aHR = 7.58, $p < 0.001$), presence of granulomas at local lymph nodes (aHR = 12.19, $p < 0.001$), and treatment with systemic corticosteroids after the first surgical resection (aHR = 7.52, $p = 0.002$) were factors significantly associated with a risk of surgical recurrence, while cryptitis resulted in a protective factor (aHR = 0.02, $p < 0.001$). In conclusion, the heterogeneous spectrum of factors associated to the risk of surgical recurrence in patients with CD that underwent ileocolic resection supports the need of a personalized follow-up taking into account different clinical, surgical, and histologic features.

Keywords: cryptitis; granulomas; inflammatory bowel diseases; IBD

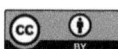

1. Introduction

Crohn's disease (CD) is a chronic inflammatory disorder that can affect any segment of the gastrointestinal tract, from the mouth to the anus [1]. The etiopathogenesis of CD is still largely unknown; likely, the disease is the result of the interaction between genetic susceptibility, environmental factors, and intestinal microbiome, which lead to an abnormal mucosal immune response and to an impairment of the intestinal barrier function [2–4].

Despite recent advances in the medical therapy of CD, approximately 70% patients will undergo surgery, and more than 20% of them will experience surgical recurrence after 10 years [5,6]. Worthy of mention is the risk of developing short bowel syndrome in patients with CD undergoing multiple resections; approximately 60% of CD patients with short bowel syndrome are permanently dependent on parenteral nutrition [7].

An early study published in 1981 already reported a 50% reoperation rate in 146 patients with CD at 14 years after first surgery [8]. Subsequently, in a larger cohort of 639 patients that required surgical intervention for their CD, a recurrence rate of 34% at 10 years has been reported; the number of intestinal sites involved was associated with the intra-abdominal recurrence rate, while the perineal disease was associated with the risk of local recurrence [9]. Though recurrence usually affects the site of the original surgery, one-third of recurrences occur elsewhere in the bowel according to the intervention site and operative technique [10].

To date, several studies investigated factors associated with surgical recurrence, mainly focusing on clinical and surgical features. Despite being controversial, data such as family history, smoking habit, age at surgery, type of surgical intervention, and subsequent type of medication have been suggested as risk factor for reoperation [11–14]. However, to the best of our knowledge, data on the association between histopathological features and the risk of surgical recurrence are scanty.

The purpose of our study was to identify potential predictive factors, related to the clinical characteristics of the patient, the characteristics of the disease, the anatomopathological characteristics of the resected intestinal tract and the surgical technique, associated with an increased risk of long-term surgical recurrence in patients with CD that underwent ileocolic resection.

2. Materials and Methods

2.1. Patients

In this single-center study, we retrospectively enrolled patients with CD in follow-up (FU) at the outpatients clinic of the Unit of Gastroenterology of "Città della Salute e della Scienza di Torino–Molinette" Hospital, Turin, Italy, that underwent first ileocolic resection between 2000 and 2013.

The study inclusion criteria were: diagnosis of CD according to the criteria of the European Crohn's and Colitis Organization (ECCO) [15,16] and first surgery for right ileocolic resection performed at the General Surgery of the "Città della Salute e della Scienza di Torino–Molinette" Hospital. Exclusion criteria were: lack of data on post-surgery FU, lack of data concerning anatomopathological examination, lack of data on type of surgical procedure, and surgery other than right ileo-colic resection.

For all patients included, we collected the following data: age, sex, smoking habit, family history of IBD, clinical history (i.e., age at diagnosis, age at first resection, disease location, and behavior), medical therapy administered after the first surgery (i.e., mesalamine, thiopurine, systemic steroids, and biologics), features related to the surgical intervention (i.e., length of bowel resection, type of surgical intervention, type of anastomosis performed, and temporary or permanent ostomy), and anatomopathological characteristics (i.e., stenosis, fistulas, pseudopiloric metaplasia, basal plasmacytosis, granulomas at loco-regional lymph nodes, surgical margin, degree of inflammation, hyper-eosinophilia, colonic microscopic inflammation, reactive lymphoid hyperplasia, cryptitis, serositis, perivisceritis, and inflammatory pseudopolyps). Hematoxylin eosin saffron stain was applied to full-thickness 3-mm sections of paraffin blocks of the ileal border. An experienced pathologist examined each part (G. C.). To evaluate CD-related lesions affecting each layer of the intestinal wall, an analytical grid was created (mucosa, submucosa, and subserosa or muscularis). We measured the length of the ileal resection for each patient (in centimeters) and the separation between the ileal margin and the first CD mucosal ulceration seen by the pathologist on the opened material for macroscopic inspection (in centimeters). If CD's mucosal ulcerations were seen on the ileal margin, the margin was considered to be "macroscopically impacted".

2.2. Statistical Analysis

All data were collected in a dedicated Microsoft Excel® database. Statistical analysis was performed using MedCalc Statistical Software version 18.9.1 (MedCalc Software bvba, Ostend, Belgium).

The distribution of continuous variables was checked by D'agostino–Perason test ($p < 0.05$ = reject normality). According to data normality, continuous variables were reported as mean ± standard deviation (SD) or as median and interquartile range (IQR). Categorical variables were expressed as frequencies (n) and percentage (%). Survival curves were calculated according to the Kaplan–Meier method; differences between survival curves were assessed by the Log-rank test. Univariate and multivariate analysis for variables associated to the risk of surgical recurrence was performed by Cox proportional-hazard regression; the strength of association was reported as Hazard Ratio (HR) with the corresponding 95% confidence interval (CI). In order to check for potential interaction among variables, all variables were tested at multivariate Cox regression, irrespectively from the statistical significance at univariate analysis; by a backward approach, we first entered all variables into the model and next removed the non-significant variables sequentially.

For all analyses, a p value < 0.05 was considered statistically significant.

3. Results

A total of 162 medical records from patients with CD that underwent ileocolic resection between 2000 and 2013 were evaluated. Overall, 54 patients were excluded due to the lack of data (n = 52) or lost to FU (n = 2). Of the 108 patients included in the study, 36 of them had at least one surgical recurrence (33.3%); the baseline characteristics are reported in Table 1.

Table 1. Baseline characteristics of the patients included in the study.

Characteristics	n = 108
Age at first surgery (years), mean ± SD	38.8 ± 13.8
Age at CD diagnosis (years), median (IQR)	28.5 (22.0–45.0)
Sex (M/F), n	60/48
Smoking habit (current/ex/never), n (%)	54 (50.0%)/22 (20.4%)/32 (29.6%)
Family history of CD, n (%)	20 (18.5%)
Colonic involvement, n (%)	54 (50.0%)
Upper gastrointestinal tract involvement (L4), n (%) [1]	13 (12.0%)

[1] L4, any location proximal to the terminal ileum, except the mouth. Abbreviations: Crohn's disease (CD), interquartile range (IQR), female (F), male (M), number (n), standard deviation (SD).

The median FU was 136.5 (91.5–176.5) months; at 137 months, 23 (21.3%) patients had surgical recurrence (Figure 1). To note, among the thirty-six patients with surgical recurrence, ten (27.8%) experienced more than one recurrence: six (16.7%) patients underwent two ileocolic resections, two (5.6%) underwent three ileocolic resections, and two (5.6%) patients underwent four ileocolic resections.

In the univariate analysis, we observed different cumulative incidences of surgical recurrence according to age at CD diagnosis $\leq$ 27 years (Log-rank test, p = 0.040), age at first surgery $\leq$ 28 years (Log-rank test, p = 0.001), current smoking status (Log-rank test, p = 0.001), and administration of systemic steroids after surgery (Log-rank test, p = 0.002) (Figure 2). Interestingly, in the multivariate Cox regression analysis, we observed that an age $\leq$ 28 years at the first surgical resection (aHR = 16.44, p < 0.001), current smoking (aHR = 15.84, p < 0.001), female sex (aHR = 7.58, p < 0.001), cryptitis (aHR = 0.02, p < 0.001), presence of granulomas at the local lymph nodes (aHR = 12.19, p < 0.001), and treatment with systemic corticosteroids after the first surgical resection (aHR = 7.52, p = 0.002) were factors significantly associated with the risk of surgical recurrence (Table 2).

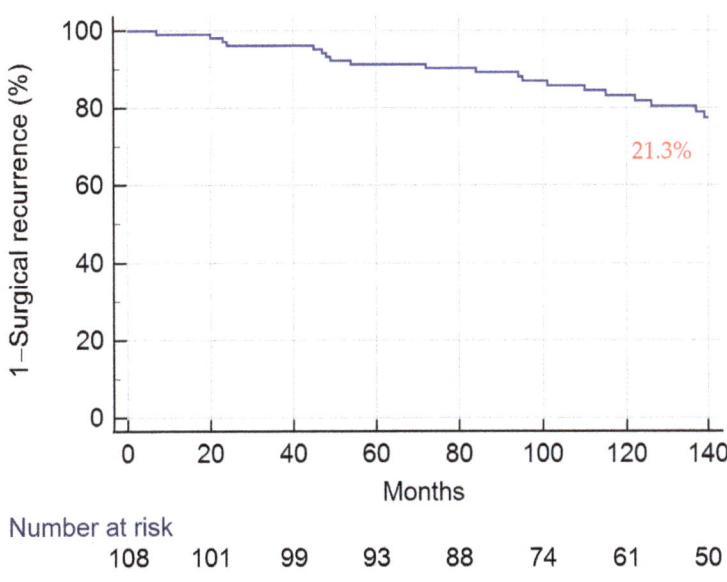

Figure 1. Cumulative surgical recurrence rates calculated using the Kaplan–Meier method.

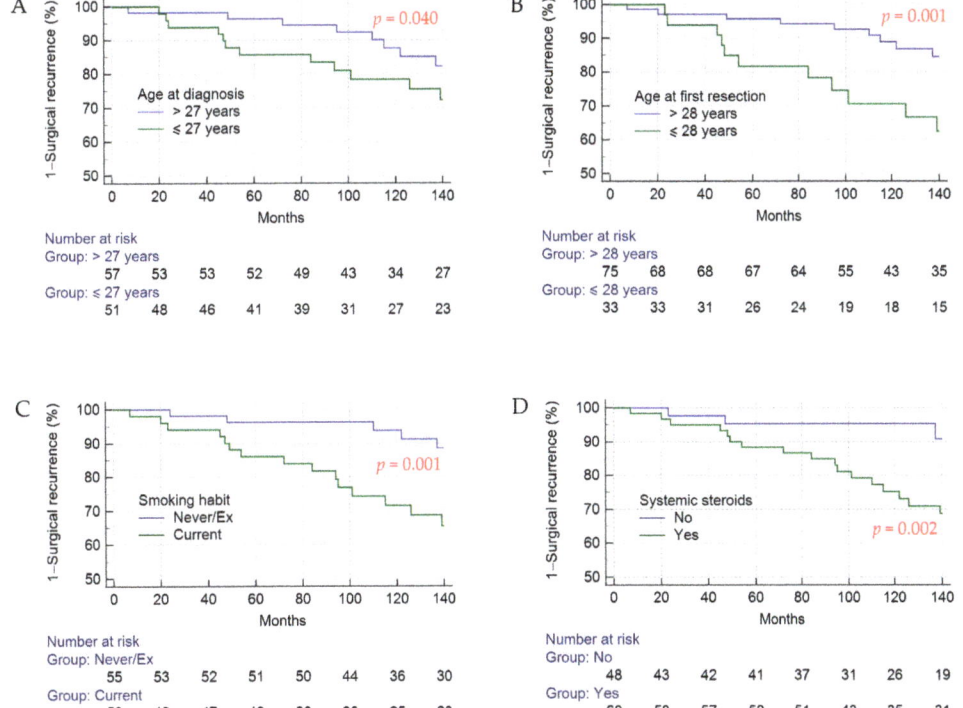

Figure 2. Cumulative surgical recurrence rates calculated using the Kaplan–Meier method. At the median FU of 136.5 months, the 82.2% of patients with age > 27 years at CD diagnosis was surgical

recurrence-free, compared to the 75.5% of patients with age ≤ 27 years at CD diagnosis (**A**), the 84.6% of patients with age > 28 years at first surgery was surgical recurrence-free as compared to the 66.7% of patients with age ≤ 28 years at first surgery (**B**), the 90.1% of former/never smokers was surgical recurrence-free as compared to the 68.7% of current smokers (**C**), and the 92.7% of patients that did not receive systemic steroid therapy was surgical recurrence-free as compared to the 70.9% of patients administered with systemic steroid therapy (**D**).

Table 2. Univariate and multivariate Cox regression analysis of factors associated to surgical recurrence.

Variables	Univariate (HR; 95% CI)	p Value	Multivariate * (aHR; 95%CI)	p Value
Age at first surgery ≤ 28 years	2.95 (1.52–5.76)	0.001	16.44 (4.63–58.34)	<0.001
Age at CD diagnosis ≤ 27 years	1.98 (1.01–3.90)	0.048	/	/
Female sex	1.24 (0.64–2.40)	0.530	7.58 (2.50–22.99)	<0.001
Current smoker	3.28 (1.59–6.78)	0.001	15.84 (4.80–52.23)	<0.001
Family history of CD	0.84 (0.36–1.96)	0.840	/	/
Colonic involvement	0.57 (0.29–1.12)	0.100	/	/
Upper gastrointestinal tract involvement (L4)	1.63 (0.63–4.27)	0.310	/	/
Perianal lesions	1.29 (0.60–2.76)	0.510	/	/
Fistulas	0.68 (0.34–1.34)	0.260	/	/
Stenosis	0.70 (0.29–1.72)	0.440	/	/
Laparoscopic resection	1.14 (0.27–4.78)	0.860	/	/
Length of bowel resection (cm)	1.01 (0.99–1.02)	0.500	/	/
Surgical margins involvement	1.11 (0.49–2.50)	0.800	/	/
Temporary ostomy	0.52 (0.20–1.34)	0.180	/	/
Cryptitis	0.49 (0.17–1.38)	0.180	0.02 (0.00–0.11)	<0.001
Plexitis	2.06 (0.62–6.82)	0.240	/	/
Sierositis	0.97 (0.46–2.02)	0.930	/	/
Perivisceritis	0.23 (0.03–1.68)	0.150	/	/
Colonic microscopic inflammation	0.56 (0.28–1.13)	0.110	/	/
Granulomas at loco-regional lymph nodes	2.16 (0.98–4.77)	0.056	12.19 (3.27–45.46)	<0.001
Reactive lymphoid hyperplasia	1.44 (0.69–3.00)	0.330	/	/
Hyper-eosinophilia	2.68 (0.36–19.90)	0.330	/	/
Pseudopiloric metaplasia	0.23 (0.03–1.68)	0.150	/	/
Inflammatory pseudopolyps	0.64 (0.19–2.09)	0.460	/	/
Anti-TNF administration	0.63 (0.29–1.36)	0.240	/	/
Thiopurine administration	0.55 (0.27–1.12)	0.100	/	/
Corticosteroid administration	4.07 (1.57–10.55)	0.002	7.52 (2.15–26.22)	0.002

* Multivariate Cox regression analysis was performed with a backward approach. Abbreviations: adjusted hazard ratio (aHR), Crohn's disease (CD), confidence interval (CI), hazard ratio (HR), tumor necrosis factor (TNF).

4. Discussion

In the present study, we investigated the surgical recurrence rate in patients with CD and potential predictors of surgical recurrence. In agreement with the literature data, we observed that the 21.3% of our patients had surgical recurrence during a median FU of 136.5 months; the age at first surgery, female sex, smoking habit, cryptitis, presence of granulomas at loco-regional lymph nodes, and systemic corticosteroid administration after the first surgery resulted in independent predictors of surgical recurrence. As a matter of fact, our results are somehow consistent with those reported in a seminal study published in 2006, where the authors observed that the requirement for steroid use, an age < 40 years at CD diagnosis, and the presence of a perianal disease were all independent factors associated with a disabling disease course, whose definition included intestinal resection [17].

Among patients-related variables, a smoking habit is a well-known risk factor associated to CD development, with a four-fold higher risk of CD development in current smokers in comparison to subjects that had never smoked [18]. Here, we observed that current smoking was one of the strongest predictors of surgical recurrence; our results agree with the study of Unkart and colleagues [11], that reported a higher risk of second ileo-colectomy for current smokers at the time of first surgical intervention (HR = 2.08, $p = 0.023$). Taken together, these results highlight that smoking not only has a significant impact on CD development, but also on the progression of the disease, increasing the risk of further surgery. Additionally, a younger age at first surgery, probably as a surrogate of a more aggressive disease, was associated with an increased risk of surgical recurrence; our results agree with the study of Wang and colleagues where it was reported that an early age at first CD surgery (OR = 1.12, $p < 0.001$) predicted a higher surgical recurrence risk [19]. Finally, we found that the female sex was associated to surgical recurrence; to date, sex has been evaluated in several studies, but most found no difference between the sexes [20].

Among histology-related factors, we observed that cryptitis was associated with a reduced risk of surgical recurrence. A previous French study investigated the association between histologic features of the ileal margin with disease recurrence in a cohort of 211 patients with ileal or ileocolonic CD; contrarily to our findings, the authors pointed out that transmural lesions were associated with an increased risk of post-operative recurrence (endoscopic recurrence, OR = 3.83, $p = 0.008$; clinical recurrence, OR = 2.04, $p = 0.026$) [21]. Together with the paucity of the available evidence, it is likely that the differences in the clinical characteristics among the study cohorts and the different study endpoints could have led to conflicting results. Further studies are needed to better elucidate this aspect. Concerning the presence of intestinal granulomas in tissue specimens, a 2010 meta-analysis of 22 studies (2236 patients) reported an association between granulomatous CD and an increased risk of recurrence and reoperation [22]. In addition, a subsequent study found that the presence of granulomas in the mesenteric lymph node was a significant risk factor for both postoperative endoscopic ($p = 0.015$) and surgical recurrence ($p = 0.035$) [23]. These results are consistent with our findings, where the presence of granulomas at loco-regional lymph nodes was independently associated with an increased risk of surgical recurrence (aHR = 12.19, $p < 0.001$). Furthermore, the presence of granulomas in resection specimens has been recognized as a risk factor for post-operative recurrence by the ECCO guidelines, together with smoking, the absence of prophylactic treatment, a penetrating disease at index surgery, a perianal location, and myenteric plexitis [24]. However, it must be acknowledged that the definition of post-operative recurrence varies greatly among studies. Indeed, CD recurrence could be considered clinical, endoscopic, radiological or surgical; our study was focused on surgical recurrence only, thus contributing to explain the discrepancies between our results and those from previous studies.

Finally, concerning medications, we observed that patients treated with systemic corticosteroids after surgery were those with a higher incidence of surgical recurrence (aHR = 7.52, $p = 0.002$). This result could be explained by the fact that patients receiving systemic corticosteroids had a more aggressive post-surgical disease phenotype, thus being intrinsically at risk of disease progression, including surgical recurrence.

Our study has some limitations that should be acknowledged. Firstly, given the retrospective nature of the study, we cannot rule out possible biases related to data loss; furthermore, the wide observation period (2000–2013) may have led to non-homogeneous data collection over time. In addition, data on extraintestinal manifestations were not systematically available for all patients; though CD patients with liver involvement (such as primary sclerosing cholangitis) could have a phenotypical and clinical pattern that sharply differs from patients with CD alone [25]. For the abovementioned reason, we were not able to investigate this aspect in our series. Secondly, the number of patients included in the study was relatively small, which may have had an impact on the lack of statistical significance for variables such as perianal diseases and the presence of fistulas, which have been consistently identified as risk factors for surgical recurrence by previous studies.

Lastly, the single-center study design may represent an additional limitation. Nevertheless, all patients included in the study were followed with regular scheduling by the same gastroenterologist (M.A.), surgical procedures were performed by the same surgeon (A.R.), and histologic examination was performed by the same pathologist (G.C.), thus allowing to avoid any potential operator-dependent bias.

5. Conclusions

In conclusion, we observed a heterogeneous spectrum of factors associated to the risk of surgical recurrence in CD patients that underwent ileocolic resection. In particular, other than patient- and surgical-related factors, the presence of granulomas in loco-regional lymph nodes could represent an additional risk factor for surgical recurrence. In patients with CD with past surgical history, a personalized follow-up taking into account different clinical, surgical, and histologic features is mandatory to identify patients at the highest risk of surgical recurrence.

Author Contributions: Conceptualization, M.A. and D.G.R.; methodology, D.G.R.; software, G.P.C., C.R. and A.A; validation, M.A., G.C., A.R. and G.M.S.; formal analysis, D.G.R.; investigation, C.A.M., M.A., G.C., A.R. and D.G.R.; resources, D.G.R.; data curation, C.A.M. and D.G.R.; writing—original draft preparation, G.P.C.; writing—review and editing, D.G.R.; visualization, C.R., A.A. and D.G.R.; supervision, G.M.S.; project administration, D.G.R. All authors have read and agreed to the published version of the manuscript.

Funding: This research received no external funding.

Institutional Review Board Statement: The study was conducted according to the guidelines of the Declaration of Helsinki and approved by the Ethics Committee of the Città della Salute e della Scienza—University Hospital of Turin (approval code 0056924, 8 June 2016).

Informed Consent Statement: Informed consent was obtained from all subjects involved in the study.

Data Availability Statement: The data presented in this study are available upon request from the corresponding author.

Conflicts of Interest: The authors declare no conflict of interest.

References

1. Ye, Y.; Manne, S.; Treem, W.R.; Bennett, D. Prevalence of Inflammatory Bowel Disease in Pediatric and Adult Populations: Recent Estimates From Large National Databases in the United States, 2007–2016. *Inflamm. Bowel. Dis.* **2020**, *26*, 619–625. [CrossRef] [PubMed]
2. Momozawa, Y.; Dmitrieva, J.; Théâtre, E.; Deffontaine, V.; Rahmouni, S.; Charloteaux, B.; Crins, F.; Docampo, E.; Elansary, M.; Gori, A.S.; et al. IBD risk loci are enriched in multigenic regulatory modules encompassing putative causative genes. *Nat. Commun.* **2018**, *9*, 2427. [CrossRef] [PubMed]
3. Caviglia, G.P.; Rosso, C.; Ribaldone, D.G.; Dughera, F.; Fagoonee, S.; Astegiano, M.; Pellicano, R. Physiopathology of intestinal barrier and the role of zonulin. *Minerva Biotecnol.* **2019**, *31*, 83–92. [CrossRef]
4. Holleran, G.; Lopetuso, L.R.; Ianiro, G.; Pecere, S.; Pizzoferrato, M.; Petito, V.; Graziani, C.; McNamara, D.; Gasbarrini, A.; Scaldaferri, F. Gut microbiota and inflammatory bowel disease: So far so gut! *Minerva Gastroenterol. Dietol.* **2017**, *63*, 373–384. [CrossRef]
5. Shaffer, V.O.; Wexner, S.D. Surgical management of Crohn's disease. *Langenbecks Arch. Surg.* **2013**, *398*, 13–27. [CrossRef]
6. Valibouze, C.; Desreumaux, P.; Zerbib, P. Post-surgical recurrence of Crohn's disease: Situational analysis and future prospects. *J. Visc. Surg.* **2021**, *158*, 401–410. [CrossRef]
7. Aksan, A.; Farrag, K.; Blumenstein, I.; Schröder, O.; Dignass, A.U.; Stein, J. Chronic intestinal failure and short bowel syndrome in Crohn's disease. *World J. Gastroenterol.* **2021**, *27*, 3440–3465. [CrossRef]
8. Lock, M.R.; Farmer, R.G.; Fazio, V.W.; Jagelman, D.G.; Lavery, I.C.; Weakley, F.L. Recurrence and reoperation for Crohn's disease: The role of disease location in prognosis. *N. Engl. J. Med.* **1981**, *304*, 1586–1588. [CrossRef]
9. Michelassi, F.; Balestracci, T.; Chappell, R.; Block, G.E. Primary and recurrent Crohn's disease. Experience with 1379 patients. *Ann. Surg.* **1991**, *214*, 230–238. [CrossRef]
10. Fichera, A.; Lovadina, S.; Rubin, M.; Cimino, F.; Hurst, R.D.; Michelassi, F. Patterns and operative treatment of recurrent Crohn's disease: A prospective longitudinal study. *Surgery* **2006**, *140*, 649–654. [CrossRef]
11. Unkart, J.T.; Anderson, L.; Li, E.; Miller, C.; Yan, Y.; Gu, C.C.; Chen, J.; Stone, C.D.; Hunt, S.; Dietz, D.W. Risk factors for surgical recurrence after ileocolic resection of Crohn's disease. *Dis. Colon Rectum* **2008**, *51*, 1211–1216. [CrossRef] [PubMed]

12. Zhou, J.; Li, Y.; Gong, J.; Zhu, W. Frequency and risk factors of surgical recurrence of Crohn's disease after primary bowel resection. *Turk. J. Gastroenterol.* **2018**, *29*, 655–663. [CrossRef] [PubMed]
13. Aaltonen, G.; Carpelan-Holmström, M.; Keränen, I.; Lepistö, A. Surgical recurrence in Crohn's disease: A comparison between different types of bowel resections. *Int. J. Colorectal Dis.* **2018**, *33*, 473–477. [CrossRef]
14. Kim, S.B.; Cheon, J.H.; Park, J.J.; Kim, E.S.; Jeon, S.W.; Jung, S.A.; Park, D.I.; Lee, C.K.; Im, J.P.; Kim, Y.S.; et al. Risk Factors for Postoperative Recurrence in Korean Patients with Crohn's Disease. *Gut Liver* **2020**, *14*, 331–337. [CrossRef]
15. Maaser, C.; Sturm, A.; Vavricka, S.R.; Kucharzik, T.; Fiorino, G.; Annese, V.; Calabrese, E.; Baumgart, D.C.; Bettenworth, D.; Borralho Nunes, P.; et al. ECCO-ESGAR Guideline for Diagnostic Assessment in IBD Part 1: Initial diagnosis, monitoring of known IBD, detection of complications. *J. Crohns Colitis* **2019**, *13*, 144–164. [CrossRef] [PubMed]
16. Sturm, A.; Maaser, C.; Calabrese, E.; Annese, V.; Fiorino, G.; Kucharzik, T.; Vavricka, S.R.; Verstockt, B.; van Rheenen, P.; Tolan, D.; et al. ECCO-ESGAR Guideline for Diagnostic Assessment in IBD Part 2: IBD scores and general principles and technical aspects. *J. Crohns Colitis* **2019**, *13*, 273–284. [CrossRef] [PubMed]
17. Beaugerie, L.; Seksik, P.; Nion-Larmurier, I.; Gendre, J.P.; Cosnes, J. Predictors of Crohn's disease. *Gastroenterology* **2006**, *130*, 650–656. [CrossRef]
18. Maaser, C.; Langholz, E.; Gordon, H.; Burisch, J.; Ellul, P.; Ramirez, V.H.; Karakan, T.; Katsanos, K.H.; Krustins, E.; Levine, A.; et al. European Crohn's and Colitis Organisation Topical Review on Environmental Factors in IBD. *J. Crohns Colitis* **2017**, *11*, 905–920. [CrossRef]
19. Wang, M.H.; Friton, J.J.; Raffals, L.E.; Leighton, J.A.; Pasha, S.F.; Picco, M.F.; Monroe, K.; Nix, B.D.; Newberry, R.D.; Faubion, W.A. Novel Genetic Variant Predicts Surgical Recurrence Risk in Crohn's Disease Patients. *Inflamm. Bowel Dis.* **2021**, *27*, 1968–1974. [CrossRef]
20. Gklavas, A.; Dellaportas, D.; Papaconstantinou, I. Risk factors for postoperative recurrence of Crohn's disease with emphasis on surgical predictors. *Ann. Gastroenterol.* **2017**, *30*, 598–612. [CrossRef]
21. Hammoudi, N.; Cazals-Hatem, D.; Auzolle, C.; Gardair, C.; Ngollo, M.; Bottois, H.; Nancey, S.; Pariente, B.; Buisson, A.; Treton, X.; et al. Association between Microscopic Lesions at Ileal Resection Margin and Recurrence After Surgery in Patients With Crohn's Disease. *Clin. Gastroenterol. Hepatol.* **2020**, *18*, 141–149.e2. [CrossRef] [PubMed]
22. Simillis, C.; Jacovides, M.; Reese, G.E.; Yamamoto, T.; Tekkis, P.P. Meta-analysis of the role of granulomas in the recurrence of Crohn disease. *Dis. Colon Rectum* **2010**, *53*, 177–185. [CrossRef] [PubMed]
23. Li, Y.; Stocchi, L.; Liu, X.; Rui, Y.; Liu, G.; Remzi, F.H.; Shen, B. Presence of Granulomas in Mesenteric Lymph Nodes Is Associated with Postoperative Recurrence in Crohn's Disease. *Inflamm. Bowel Dis.* **2015**, *21*, 2613–2618. [CrossRef]
24. Gionchetti, P.; Dignass, A.; Danese, S.; Magro Dias, F.J.; Rogler, G.; Lakatos, P.L.; Adamina, M.; Ardizzone, S.; Buskens, C.J.; Sebastian, S.; et al. 3rd European Evidence-based Consensus on the Diagnosis and Management of Crohn's Disease 2016: Part 2: Surgical Management and Special Situations. *J. Crohns Colitis* **2017**, *11*, 135–149. [CrossRef]
25. Losurdo, G.; Brescia, I.V.; Lillo, C.; Mezzapesa, M.; Barone, M.; Principi, M.; Ierardi, E.; Di Leo, A.; Rendina, M. Liver involvement in inflammatory bowel disease: What should the clinician know? *World J. Hepatol.* **2021**, *13*, 1534–1551. [CrossRef] [PubMed]

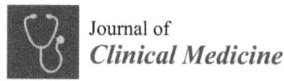

Review

Inflammatory Bowel Disease: Role of Vagus Nerve Stimulation

Riccardo Fornaro [1], Giovanni Clemente Actis [2], Gian Paolo Caviglia [3], Demis Pitoni [3] and Davide Giuseppe Ribaldone [3],*

1. Department of Neurosurgery, University Hospital "Maggiore Della Carità", 28100 Novara, Italy
2. The Medical Center Practice Office, 10100 Turin, Italy
3. Department of Medical Sciences, Division of Gastroenterology, University of Torino, 10126 Torino, Italy
* Correspondence: davidegiuseppe.ribaldone@unito.it; Tel.: +39-011-6333710

Abstract: Vagus nerve stimulation (VNS) is an accepted therapy for the treatment of refractory forms of epilepsy and depression. The brain–gut axis is increasingly being studied as a possible etiological factor of chronic inflammatory diseases, including inflammatory bowel diseases (IBD). A significant percentage of IBD patients lose response to treatments or experience side effects. In this perspective, VNS has shown the first efficacy data. The aim of this narrative review is to underline the biological plausibility of the use of VNS in patients affected by IBD, collect all clinical data in the literature, and hypothesize a target IBD population on which to focus the next clinical study.

Keywords: ulcerative colitis; Crohn's disease; acetyl-choline; IL-1β; corticotropin-releasing factor; central autonomic network; cholinergic anti-inflammatory pathway; α7 nicotinic ACh receptor; Cyberonics

Citation: Fornaro, R.; Actis, G.C.; Caviglia, G.P.; Pitoni, D.; Ribaldone, D.G. Inflammatory Bowel Disease: Role of Vagus Nerve Stimulation. J. Clin. Med. 2022, 11, 5690. https://doi.org/10.3390/jcm11195690

Academic Editors: Faming Zhang and John F. Mayberry

Received: 16 August 2022
Accepted: 24 September 2022
Published: 26 September 2022

Publisher's Note: MDPI stays neutral with regard to jurisdictional claims in published maps and institutional affiliations.

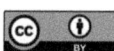

Copyright: © 2022 by the authors. Licensee MDPI, Basel, Switzerland. This article is an open access article distributed under the terms and conditions of the Creative Commons Attribution (CC BY) license (https://creativecommons.org/licenses/by/4.0/).

1. Introduction

Inflammatory bowel disease (IBD) is an organic disorder that is typically categorized into CD and UC. While UC exclusively affects the rectum and the colon, CD can affect the entire digestive tract, from the mouth to the anus. IBD begins early in life (between 15 and 30 years) and progresses through flare-ups alternated with remissions of varying lengths. Genetic, immunologic, viral, and environmental variables all play a role in the complex pathophysiology of IBD [1]. Despite the presence of more and more new mechanisms of action, we are far from being able to cure these diseases. Furthermore, such drugs must be taken for a long time (if not for life), leading many patients to search for non-drug alternatives. In this review, we want to explore the potential of the vagus nerve (VN) and its stimulation as a possible new therapeutic weapon in IBD.

The vagus nerve (VN), an X pair of cranial nerves (also called the pneumogastric nerve), arises from the brain stem (including the pons, medulla oblongata, and midbrain), leaves the medulla oblongata, and travels down the chest and abdomen, passing through the jugular foramen.

The VN provides parasympathetic nerves to the digestive tract and pancreas, including 70–80% of sensory fibers; it is defined as a mixed sensory–motor nerve [2]. The system mainly recognizes two ganglia: the superior (jugular), which provides general sensation, and the inferior, which sorts the visceral and special sensation. In simplified anatomical–functional terms, the system recognizes efferent and afferent fibers. The former originates from the medullary dorsal motor nucleus and innervates the digestive tract from the esophagus to the splenic flexure, opposing the left colon and rectum, innervated by the S2-S4 sacral parasympathetic nucleus. This second-order neuron, a true "second brain" or "gut brain", is a crucial component of the enteric (or intrinsic) neural system in the digestive tract, ensuring the motor and secretory autonomy of the digestive tract [3], with direct interaction with mast cells in the gut mucosa [4]. Notably, these efferent fibers are not anatomically connected with the intestinal lamina propria but are so with enteric neurons; these, in turn, can release acetyl-choline (ACh), a swinging modulator of muscarinic and/or nicotinic receptors. The afferent fibers originate from the mucosa and the muscular masses of the digestive tract: the relevant cells belong to the nodose ganglia, conveying information to the nucleus of the solitary tract and the postrema area in close relationship with the dorsal motor nucleus, giving rise to the complex dorsal vagal. Autonomic, endocrine, and limbic responses all depend on this complex relationship. Relevant information is extended to the amygdala, hypothalamus, and cortex through the main hypothalamic–pituitary–adrenal arm (discussed below) [5].

2. The Afferent Vagus and the Hypothalamic–Pituitary–Adrenal Anti-Inflammatory Pathway

For the purpose of maintaining homeostasis, research from the 20th and 21st centuries has identified the neuroendocrine route as the activation signal for endocrine, neural, and behavioral responses, allowing varying levels of innate defense (e.g., non-acquired immunity as opposed to acquired immunity). The VN, a key node in the defensive path, is now considered a cytokine receptor, including interleukin (IL)-1, IL-6, and tumor necrosis factor (TNF)-α. The protagonists, in the last decades, of the most typical pictures of experimental and spontaneous septic shock, IL-1, IL-6, and TNF-α are the cytokines that are the protagonists of translational research.

In extreme analysis, the afferent vagal tracts exert a specific anti-inflammatory action based on the following points:

1. The vagal afferents are equipped with IL-1β receptors at the paraganglia level [6].
2. From here, the information is conveyed to the core of the solitary tract.
3. Through the paraventricular nucleus of the hypothalamus, the information is then extended to populations of specific neurons that release CRF (corticotropin-releasing factor) [7].
4. The final task of these neurons is, therefore, to favor the release of the pituitaryadrenocorticotropic hormone (ACTH), which, as known, can, in turn, mediate the production and release of adrenocorticoids from the adrenal gland, having established anti-inflammatory effects (hypothalamic–pituitary–adrenal axis, HPA) (Figure 1).

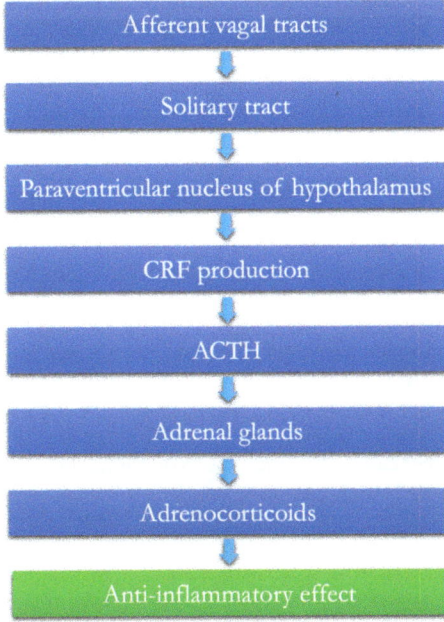

Figure 1. The afferent vagus and the hypothalamic–pituitary–adrenal anti-inflammatory pathway.

The in-vivo importance of this anti-inflammatory vagal pathway is demonstrated by the distorted response to inflammogenic stimuli exhibited by vagotomized animals. Through its afferents, the VN may identify microbial metabolites and transmit this information to the central autonomic network (CAN), which can subsequently respond appropriately or inappropriately to the intestinal input and the microbiota [8].

The Vagus Nerve at the Microbiota–Gut–Brain Axis Interconnection

The human gut is home to 10^{13} to 10^{14} bacteria; it has 100 times more genes than our genome and much more than our body's cells. The microbiota weighs roughly 1 kg in humans, which is equivalent to the weight of the human brain. The microbiota–gut–brain axis has been proven to be a communication pathway between the gut, the microbiota, and the brain [9,10]. Different gastrointestinal pathogenic disorders, such as IBD, are characterized by dysbiosis [11]. A crucial part of this microbiota–gut–brain axis is the VN. The microbiota's interactions with digestive endocrine cells, which release serotonin and act on vagal afferents' 5-HT3 receptors, can indirectly activate it [8]. By detecting small-chain fatty acids (SCFAs) and/or gut hormones, vagal chemoreceptors are likely engaged in the communication between the microbiota and the brain [12]. In fact, *Lactobacillus johnsonii* intraduodenal injections increased stomach VN activity [13]. Chronic *Lactobacillus rhamnosus* treatment in healthy mice caused changes in GABA brain expression that were greater in the cingulate cortex and smaller in the hippocampus, amygdala, and locus coeruleus. These mice also showed a decrease in stress-related corticosterone levels as well as anxiety- and depression-related behavior. After vagotomy, these effects were not seen [14].

3. The Anti-Inflammatory Cholinergic Vagal Pathway (CAIP: Cholinergic Anti-Inflammatory Pathway)

If the previously mentioned hypothalamic–pituitary pathway inhibits inflammation by an afferent mechanism, it might be balanced by an efferent pathway, described by Tracey's group in 2003 and reappraised in 2015. In this model, we speak of an "inflammatory reflex", a sort of diastaltic arch where afferent vagal fibers activate their corresponding efferent ways. The following concepts were derived from an animal model of septic shock after intravenous injections of lipopolysaccharide: the shock was inhibited by stimulation of a dissected vagal terminal. Subsequent studies then identified ACh as the mediator released by the dissected terminal, demonstrating, in this context, the property of ACh to inhibit the release of shock effectors (IL-1, TNF-α, etc.) through the binding of ACh itself with the α7 nicotinic ACh receptor (α-7-nAchR) on macrophages [15]. Through the activation of α-7-nAchR, parasympathetic innervation of the gut contributes to the neuroimmune control of the intestinal barrier. It interacts with innate immune cells, myenteric neurons, and resident macrophages that express α7nAChR while acting on enteroglial cells [16].

Incidentally, these data can have an important translational value for gastroenterologists. In fact, the known protective effect of smoking on ulcerative colitis (UC) and, by contrast, the serious relapses in ex-smokers can be explained by the anti-inflammatory effect resulting from the link between vagal ACh and intestinal macrophages [17]; on the other hand, the lack of this effect, indeed, the negative effect of smoking in Crohn's disease (CD), could suggest a different immunological status of the competent cells in CD. By contrast, there is a link between vagotomy and subsequent CD, demonstrating the importance of VN integrity in CD prevention [18].

On the other hand, academic rather than clinical issues are those raised by questioning the way by which vagal terminals and intestinal macrophages come in contact. If the evidence is that vagal fibers do not "physically" contact intestinal immunocytes, the nature of these other cells is far from clear as well. Two theories, none of which currently prevail, argue that vagal fibers interact with special intestinal neuronic targets or that splenic sympathetic activation comes into play. Norepinephrine (NE), which binds to the two adrenergic receptors of splenic lymphocytes and releases ACh, is released from the distal end of the splenic nerve. ACh then prevents spleen macrophages from releasing TNF-α through α-7-nAchR [19]. The idea of a non-neural connection between the vagus and splenic sympathetic nerves was put forth by Martelli et al. [20]. They hypothesized that the essential α7-containing nicotinic receptor is placed not on the cell bodies but on the peripheral terminals of the splenic sympathetic nerves. These nerves produce NE in response to ACh from entering T-cells, which then inhibits the generation of TNF-α by splenic macrophages by acting on their β2 adrenergic receptors (Figure 2).

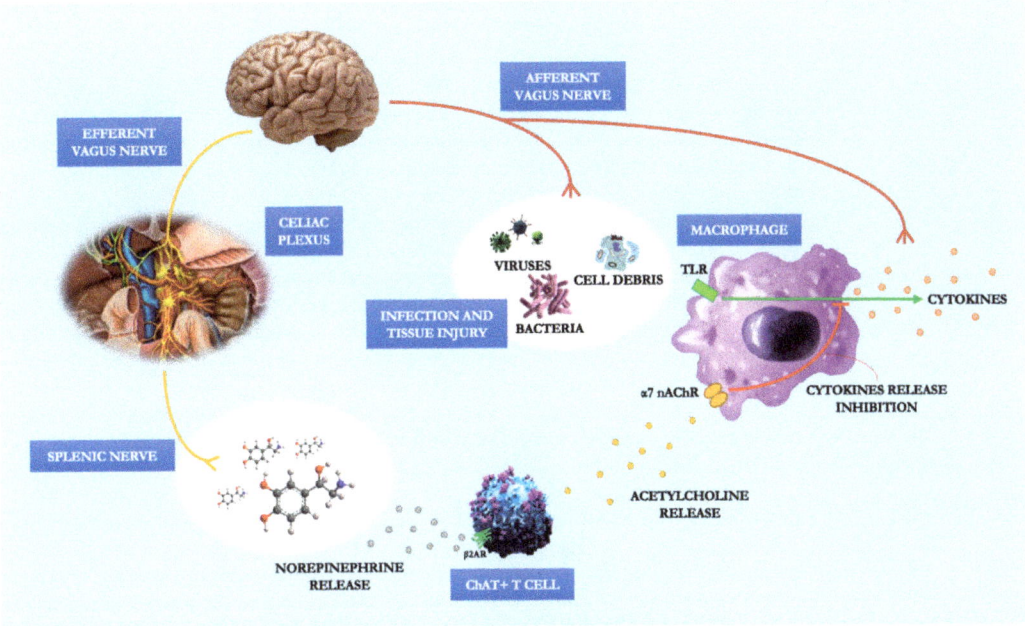

Figure 2. The anti-inflammatory cholinergic vagal pathway.

Intestinal macrophages are a diverse group of innate immune cells that not only play a significant part in host defense but also sustain the tissue in which they are found [21]. Depending on where they are located in the gut, tissue macrophages have varied roles, unique cell dynamics, and unique physical characteristics [22]. For instance, the lamina propria is home to the majority of the intestine's macrophages. These cells, which are identified by the expression of the CX3CR1 receptor, are situated close to the intestinal epithelium layer, where they monitor the environment, phagocytose potentially harmful antigens [23], and support epithelial cell renewal by secreting a number of mediators [24]. The lamina propria macrophages can also develop tolerance to food antigens and prevent excessive inflammation against safe commensal microorganisms, thanks to the production of anti-inflammatory cytokine receptors such as IL-10 [25,26]. In contrast to the lamina propria, the muscularis externa contains macrophages that are arranged in a complex network near the myenteric plexus. The latter represents the intrinsic innervation of the intestine, also known as the enteric neural system, along with the submucosal plexus. Intense reciprocal cross-talk is created by the near proximity of immune cells, particularly muscularis externa macrophages, to nerve fibers in the gut wall. This cross-talk is regulated by a complex combination of neurotransmitters, cytokines, and hormones [27,28]. In a mouse model of colitis, the severity of colitis was made worse by the adoptive transfer of macrophages from vagotomized mice into macrophage colony-stimulating factor 1 (MCSF 1)-deficient animals, indicating the crucial function of macrophages in the vagal anti-inflammatory effect [29].

Regarding the anti-TNF action of the VN, this effect of the VN is indirect, through contact with neuronal nitric oxide synthase (nNOS), choline O-acetyltransferase (ChAT), and vasoactive intestinal peptide (VIP) enteric neurons situated within the bowel muscularis mucosae; these neurons have nerve ends proximal to the resident macrophages [30]. T-cells that have been activated suppress macrophages systemically: additionally, they might move and reduce inflammation in regions that are not innervated by the VN [31].

By reducing intestinal permeability and modifying local immunity, the VN, through the CAIP, could modify the intestinal microbiota [8].

4. Possible Role of Vagus Nerve Stimulation in Chronic Inflammatory Bowel Disease

The demonstration that the vagal system affects inflammation regulation has endorsed exploratory attempts at therapeutics. Neuromodulation suggests using devices to control the nervous system's electrical activity in order to restore organ function and health, partially avoiding toxicity, collateral damage, and poor compliance [32]. Epileptic syndromes, depression, and chronic gastroenterological and rheumatological disorders were initially the main targeted fields. In the late 19th century, vagus nerve stimulation (VNS) was first employed to treat epilepsy. VNS is now authorized for the treatment of depression and refractory epilepsy. With rising efficacy of up to 10 years, VNS, used to treat drug-resistant epilepsy, drives a 50% reduction in seizure frequency and intensity in 40–60% of patients, demonstrating that this treatment is a slow-acting therapy [33].

In gastroenterology, clinicians have focused on inflammatory bowel disease (IBD). IBD is characterized by an imbalance of the autonomic nerve system, vagal dysfunction in UC [34], and sympathetic dysfunction in CD [35], which may contribute to its pathogenesis. High serum TNF-α levels and salivary cortisol levels were connected with low vagal tone in CD patients, supporting the idea that the HPA axis and the autonomic nervous system are out of balance [36].

Positive correlations between vagotomies and subsequent IBD have been found, and this is especially true for CD, which highlights the importance of VN integrity in the prevention of IBD [18]. Hence, it stands to reason that in those who are at risk, the degree of vagal tone is a good indicator of the emergence of an inflammatory illness. Vagal hypotonia, which, in turn, keeps this inflammatory state in place, can be caused by the systemic inflammation seen with IBD or other chronic inflammatory illnesses. Furthermore, due to its central effects, persistent inflammation can cause depression, which, in turn, might trigger an inflammatory flare-up of the illness [37,38].

In two early studies, Lindgren et al. measured the cardiac responses to tilt (acceleration and brake index) and deep breathing (E/I ratio) in 40 UC and 33 CD patients to assess autonomic nerve function. They discovered sympathetic dysfunction in CD and vagal dysfunction in UC [34,35]. An increasingly popular noninvasive test to evaluate autonomic function is heart rate variability (HRV). In 27 IBD patients who were in remission and 28 healthy controls, Mouzas et al. evaluated HRV. When compared to healthy controls, it was shown that UC and CD patients who were in remission appeared to have more vagal activity [39]. According to Ganguli et al. in 2007, patients with UC but not CD showed more sympathetic activity compared to controls [40]. In a recent study, CD patients in remission exhibited a considerably larger sympathetic–parasympathetic ratio, according to Zawadka-Kunikowska et al. [41].

Some vagal afferent fibers come into close touch with intestinal mucosal mast cells as they go to the tips of the jejunal villi. These findings offer the microanatomical foundation for mast cells in the gastrointestinal mucosa to communicate directly with the central nervous system [4]. It is interesting to note that the efferent VN interacts with enteric neurons instead of directly connecting to the gut's resident macrophages. Therefore, enteric neurons rather than vagal efferent fibers directly mediate the vagal regulation of these intestinal macrophages [27,30]. Pro-inflammatory cytokines that stimulate vagal afferents cause the activation of vagal efferents, which prevents tissue macrophages from releasing these cytokines, including TNF and other pro-inflammatory cytokines such as

IL-6 and IL-1β but not the anti-inflammatory cytokine IL-10 [42]. This is known as an inflammatory reflex.

4.1. Implantation of the Vagal Stimulator

The VNS maneuver requires the implantation of a device by a surgeon experienced in the specific field [43]. The maneuver takes about 1 h. An electrode is wrapped around the left VN neck area at the carotid artery, tunneled under the skin, and connected to a pulse generator implanted under the skin of the left chest. For the stimulation, the left VN is usually chosen because it is not involved in the regulation of heart rhythm [44]. The device is initially started at 0.25 mAmp, then progressively increased according to the patient's need and tolerance. Stimulation is intended as continuous but is alternated with ON–OFF phases. Direct VNS delivered by an implanted pulse generator is typically secure and well tolerated. Hoarseness, increased coughing, changes in voice/speech, discomfort, throat or larynx spasms, headache, sleeplessness, indigestion, and other adverse effects are possible with VNS used to treat epilepsy [43]. The most frequent of them, typically transient, are hoarseness, coughing, throat tickling, and shortness of breath.

The effectiveness of various therapies is significantly influenced by the frequency of stimulation for VN activation [45]. The most prevalent applications of high frequency (20–30 Hz) are in the treatment of epilepsy and depression. High frequency is traditionally thought to trigger vagal afferents. Lower frequency (1–10 Hz), on the other hand, is thought to activate vagal efferents, which have anti-inflammatory characteristics. The end point of neurostimulation therapy in IBD coincides with the activation of the cholinergic system/CAIP activator (see above) through low-frequency stimulation (1–10 Hz) of the efferent fibers. VNS likely activates both its afferent (which activates the HPA) and efferent (which activates the CAIP) fibers to exert its anti-inflammatory effects in IBD.

4.2. Clinical Data in Inflammatory Bowel Disease

An initial study of experimental 2,4,6-trinitrobenzene sulfonic acid (TNBS) colitis in rodents demonstrated that VNS was able to moderate inflammatory data and colic lesions [46].

A VNS study was recently performed in CD patients, for which the VNS was positioned in the therapeutic algorithm at the same level as an anti-TNF [47]. The majority of the patients (8/9) had active CD at the time of inclusion. Electrode Model 302 was implanted with bipolar pulse generator Model 102 (Cyberonics, Houston, TX, United States); 10 Hz, 500 s, 0.5 mA, 30 s ON, 5 min OFF, constantly were the stimulation parameters. Patients between the ages of 18 and 65 who had a Crohn's disease activity index (CDAI) score between 220 and 450 (i.e., moderate or severe CD), with small bowel (ileum) and/or colonic CD, C-reactive protein (CRP) > 5 mg/L and/or fecal calprotectin >100 µg/g, as well as a Crohn's disease endoscopic index of severity (CDEIS) score ≥ 7 (active) and had been diagnosed for more than 3 months, were treatment-naive, or had a stable treatment reference (two patients were failing azathioprine, while the remaining seven were treatment-naive) were included. At the time of inclusion, patients who were taking infliximab or another anti-TNF drug were ineligible. VNS was carried out constantly for a year. The first patient received an implant in April 2012 and the final one in March 2016. After three months of neurostimulation, due to a worsening of their condition, two individuals were taken out of the study, most likely as a result of the especially high inclusion scores for CDAI (>350), CDEIS (>14), and CRP (>88 mg/L), which implies that VNS is recommended for mild-to-moderate active CD due to its gradual effect, as seen for epilepsy [48]. The first patient got an ileo-cecal resection but decided to continue neurostimulation until the end of the research due to an initial positive result and drug treatment refusal; the second patient was excluded from the study after three months due to a deterioration of disease. Infliximab and azathioprine were used to treat the second patient, who likewise desired to continue using an active VNS. Five of the nine patients experienced a deep (clinical–biological–endoscopic) remission, with also restored vagal tone, after receiving VNS. Median CDAI passed from 264 to 88, median

CRP from 7 to 3 mg/L, median calprotectin from 847 to 61 µg/g, and median CDEIS from 8 to 0. They noticed that the VNS effect did not occur right away but rather took at least three months to manifest: in patients with significant flares, VNS should not be utilized alone, at least in the first months. Three more paradigmatic pro-inflammatory cytokines in CD, IL6, IL12, and IL23 were likewise decreased following a 12-month VNS. It is interesting to note that VNS decreases the perception of abdominal pain. Except for one patient who had an excessively high vagal tone, the majority of the CD patients studied here had low vagal tones upon inclusion that were restored to normal in all patients after a 12-month VNS. Although VNS might have a placebo effect, clinical remission following maintenance treatment ranged from 12% to 20% under placebo at 12 months in clinical trials using anti-TNF medicines in CD [49]. With the typical slight side effect of hoarseness as its main manifestation, VNS was well tolerated. According to the authors, these data indicate that VNS is feasible in IBD, but the study needs to be expanded to allow for interpretation.

In a second pilot trial, D'Haens et al. examined the effects of VNS over a period of 16 weeks in 16 patients who had colonic or small intestinal CD with biologic resistant disease [50]. Patients had CDAI 220–450, calprotectin >200 µg/g, an endoscopic score of activity (SES-CD: Simple Endoscopic Scale for Crohn's Disease) with a minimal ulcer score of 2 or 3 in at least one segment, a history of inadequate response and/or intolerance or adverse events to one or more TNF-α inhibitors (e.g., infliximab, adalimumab, or certolizumab pegol), and an 8-week washout of biologics (group 1) or concomitant biologic therapy (Group 2). One minute of daily stimulation was started two weeks after a VNS device was implanted; between weeks 4 and 6, this was extended to five minutes; in the event that CDAI remission was not reached by week 8, stimulation was increased to four times daily. CDAI decreased from 294 to 201, calprotectin 2974 to 590, and SED-CD from 22.3 to 17.5. Seven of the sixteen patients obtained a CDAI-70 response and four of the sixteen patients CDAI remission. In terms of side effects, one patient developed a postoperative infection due to the device.

In nine ileo-colonic CD patients, Kibleur et al. evaluated the effects of VNS on inflammation and brain activity. They found that 12 months of chronic VNS improved CDAI, fecal calprotectin, anxiety state, and vagal tone, which were associated with a decline in the electroencephalogram's α frequency band [51].

4.3. Possible Inclusion Criteria of Future Studies

- CD with extensive small bowel disease or less than 200 cm of small bowel due to surgery and refractory to all target therapies;
- CD with contraindications to target therapies (fragile patients, history of cancer, history of severe infections);
- Patients with CD who do not want to undergo target therapy or with a history of poor adherence to therapy;
- Steroid-dependent UC.

5. Conclusions

The vagal system can express a modulating action of inflammation through the afferent pathways of the hypothalamic–pituitary–adrenal axis as well as through the efferent pathways of the cholinergic CAIP complex. Attempts to exploit these properties by means of devices capable of stimulating the VN under controlled conditions have obviously turned, as a starting point, to the treatment of chronic colitis (IBD) and rheumatological diseases: in these pathologies, where patients are particularly afraid of the toxicity of prolonged immune therapies, the introduction of VNS in a dominant position is attractive. The data are encouraging, but they must come out of the anecdotal stage to arrive at controlled designs.

Author Contributions: Conceptualization, R.F., D.G.R. and G.C.A.; methodology, D.G.R.; software, G.P.C.; validation, D.P.; formal analysis, D.G.R. and G.C.A.; investigation, D.G.R. and G.C.A.; data curation, D.P.; writing—original draft preparation, D.G.R. and G.C.A.; writing—review and editing, R.F.; visualization, G.P.C.; supervision, G.P.C.; project administration, G.P.C. All authors have read and agreed to the published version of the manuscript.

Funding: This research received no external funding.

Institutional Review Board Statement: Not applicable.

Informed Consent Statement: Not applicable.

Data Availability Statement: Not applicable.

Acknowledgments: Fernanda Gilli's help was crucial in finalizing this paper.

Conflicts of Interest: The authors declare no conflict of interest.

References

1. Chang, J.T. Pathophysiology of Inflammatory Bowel Diseases. *N. Engl. J. Med.* **2020**, *383*, 2652–2664. [CrossRef]
2. Prechtl, J.C.; Powley, T.L. The Fiber Composition of the Abdominal Vagus of the Rat. *Anat. Embryol.* **1990**, *181*, 101–115. [CrossRef] [PubMed]
3. Furness, J.B.; Callaghan, B.P.; Rivera, L.R.; Cho, H.-J. The Enteric Nervous System and Gastrointestinal Innervation: Integrated Local and Central Control. *Adv. Exp. Med. Biol.* **2014**, *817*, 39–71. [CrossRef] [PubMed]
4. Williams, R.M.; Berthoud, H.R.; Stead, R.H. Vagal Afferent Nerve Fibres Contact Mast Cells in Rat Small Intestinal Mucosa. *Neuroimmunomodulation* **1997**, *4*, 266–270. [CrossRef] [PubMed]
5. Powley, T.L.; Jaffey, D.M.; McAdams, J.; Baronowsky, E.A.; Black, D.; Chesney, L.; Evans, C.; Phillips, R.J. Vagal Innervation of the Stomach Reassessed: Brain-Gut Connectome Uses Smart Terminals. *Ann. N. Y. Acad. Sci.* **2019**, *1454*, 14–30. [CrossRef]
6. Goehler, L.E.; Relton, J.K.; Dripps, D.; Kiechle, R.; Tartaglia, N.; Maier, S.F.; Watkins, L.R. Vagal Paraganglia Bind Biotinylated Interleukin-1 Receptor Antagonist: A Possible Mechanism for Immune-to-Brain Communication. *Brain Res. Bull.* **1997**, *43*, 357–364. [CrossRef]
7. Rivest, S.; Lacroix, S.; Vallières, L.; Nadeau, S.; Zhang, J.; Laflamme, N. How the Blood Talks to the Brain Parenchyma and the Paraventricular Nucleus of the Hypothalamus during Systemic Inflammatory and Infectious Stimuli. *Proc. Soc. Exp. Biol. Med.* **2000**, *223*, 22–38. [CrossRef]
8. Bonaz, B.; Bazin, T.; Pellissier, S. The Vagus Nerve at the Interface of the Microbiota-Gut-Brain Axis. *Front. Neurosci.* **2018**, *12*, 49. [CrossRef]
9. Cryan, J.F.; Dinan, T.G. Mind-Altering Microorganisms: The Impact of the Gut Microbiota on Brain and Behaviour. *Nat. Rev. Neurosci.* **2012**, *13*, 701–712. [CrossRef]
10. Cryan, J.F.; O'Riordan, K.J.; Cowan, C.S.M.; Sandhu, K.V.; Bastiaanssen, T.F.S.; Boehme, M.; Codagnone, M.G.; Cussotto, S.; Fulling, C.; Golubeva, A.V.; et al. The Microbiota-Gut-Brain Axis. *Physiol. Rev.* **2019**, *99*, 1877–2013. [CrossRef]
11. Ribaldone, D.G.; Caviglia, G.P.; Abdulle, A.; Pellicano, R.; Ditto, M.C.; Morino, M.; Fusaro, E.; Saracco, G.M.; Bugianesi, E.; Astegiano, M. Adalimumab Therapy Improves Intestinal Dysbiosis in Crohn's Disease. *J. Clin. Med.* **2019**, *8*, 1646. [CrossRef] [PubMed]
12. Raybould, H.E. Gut Chemosensing: Interactions between Gut Endocrine Cells and Visceral Afferents. *Auton. Neurosci.* **2010**, *153*, 41–46. [CrossRef] [PubMed]
13. Tanida, M.; Yamano, T.; Maeda, K.; Okumura, N.; Fukushima, Y.; Nagai, K. Effects of Intraduodenal Injection of Lactobacillus Johnsonii La1 on Renal Sympathetic Nerve Activity and Blood Pressure in Urethane-Anesthetized Rats. *Neurosci. Lett.* **2005**, *389*, 109–114. [CrossRef] [PubMed]
14. Bravo, J.A.; Forsythe, P.; Chew, M.V.; Escaravage, E.; Savignac, H.M.; Dinan, T.G.; Bienenstock, J.; Cryan, J.F. Ingestion of Lactobacillus Strain Regulates Emotional Behavior and Central GABA Receptor Expression in a Mouse via the Vagus Nerve. *Proc. Natl. Acad. Sci. USA* **2011**, *108*, 16050–16055. [CrossRef]
15. Wang, H.; Yu, M.; Ochani, M.; Amella, C.A.; Tanovic, M.; Susarla, S.; Li, J.H.; Wang, H.; Yang, H.; Ulloa, L.; et al. Nicotinic Acetylcholine Receptor Alpha7 Subunit Is an Essential Regulator of Inflammation. *Nature* **2003**, *421*, 384–388. [CrossRef] [PubMed]
16. Fornai, M.; van den Wijngaard, R.M.; Antonioli, L.; Pellegrini, C.; Blandizzi, C.; de Jonge, W.J. Neuronal Regulation of Intestinal Immune Functions in Health and Disease. *Neurogastroenterol. Motil.* **2018**, *30*, e13406. [CrossRef]
17. Cui, W.-Y.; Li, M.D. Nicotinic Modulation of Innate Immune Pathways via A7 Nicotinic Acetylcholine Receptor. *J. Neuroimmune Pharm.* **2010**, *5*, 479–488. [CrossRef]
18. Liu, B.; Wanders, A.; Wirdefeldt, K.; Sjölander, A.; Sachs, M.C.; Eberhardson, M.; Ye, W.; Ekbom, A.; Olén, O.; Ludvigsson, J.F. Vagotomy and Subsequent Risk of Inflammatory Bowel Disease: A Nationwide Register-Based Matched Cohort Study. *Aliment. Pharm.* **2020**, *51*, 1022–1030. [CrossRef]

19. Olofsson, P.S.; Katz, D.A.; Rosas-Ballina, M.; Levine, Y.A.; Ochani, M.; Valdés-Ferrer, S.I.; Pavlov, V.A.; Tracey, K.J.; Chavan, S.S. A7 Nicotinic Acetylcholine Receptor (A7nAChR) Expression in Bone Marrow-Derived Non-T Cells Is Required for the Inflammatory Reflex. *Mol. Med.* **2012**, *18*, 539–543. [CrossRef]
20. Martelli, D.; McKinley, M.J.; McAllen, R.M. The Cholinergic Anti-Inflammatory Pathway: A Critical Review. *Auton. Neurosci.* **2014**, *182*, 65–69. [CrossRef]
21. Okabe, Y.; Medzhitov, R. Tissue-Specific Signals Control Reversible Program of Localization and Functional Polarization of Macrophages. *Cell* **2014**, *157*, 832–844. [CrossRef] [PubMed]
22. Gabanyi, I.; Muller, P.A.; Feighery, L.; Oliveira, T.Y.; Costa-Pinto, F.A.; Mucida, D. Neuro-Immune Interactions Drive Tissue Programming in Intestinal Macrophages. *Cell* **2016**, *164*, 378–391. [CrossRef] [PubMed]
23. Niess, J.H.; Brand, S.; Gu, X.; Landsman, L.; Jung, S.; McCormick, B.A.; Vyas, J.M.; Boes, M.; Ploegh, H.L.; Fox, J.G.; et al. CX3CR1-Mediated Dendritic Cell Access to the Intestinal Lumen and Bacterial Clearance. *Science* **2005**, *307*, 254–258. [CrossRef] [PubMed]
24. Bain, C.C.; Mowat, A.M. Macrophages in Intestinal Homeostasis and Inflammation. *Immunol. Rev.* **2014**, *260*, 102–117. [CrossRef] [PubMed]
25. Hadis, U.; Wahl, B.; Schulz, O.; Hardtke-Wolenski, M.; Schippers, A.; Wagner, N.; Müller, W.; Sparwasser, T.; Förster, R.; Pabst, O. Intestinal Tolerance Requires Gut Homing and Expansion of FoxP3+ Regulatory T Cells in the Lamina Propria. *Immunity* **2011**, *34*, 237–246. [CrossRef]
26. Rivollier, A.; He, J.; Kole, A.; Valatas, V.; Kelsall, B.L. Inflammation Switches the Differentiation Program of Ly6Chi Monocytes from Antiinflammatory Macrophages to Inflammatory Dendritic Cells in the Colon. *J. Exp. Med.* **2012**, *209*, 139–155. [CrossRef]
27. Matteoli, G.; Gomez-Pinilla, P.J.; Nemethova, A.; Di Giovangiulio, M.; Cailotto, C.; van Bree, S.H.; Michel, K.; Tracey, K.J.; Schemann, M.; Boesmans, W.; et al. A Distinct Vagal Anti-Inflammatory Pathway Modulates Intestinal Muscularis Resident Macrophages Independent of the Spleen. *Gut* **2014**, *63*, 938–948. [CrossRef]
28. Muller, P.A.; Koscsó, B.; Rajani, G.M.; Stevanovic, K.; Berres, M.-L.; Hashimoto, D.; Mortha, A.; Leboeuf, M.; Li, X.-M.; Mucida, D.; et al. Crosstalk between Muscularis Macrophages and Enteric Neurons Regulates Gastrointestinal Motility. *Cell* **2014**, *158*, 1210. [CrossRef]
29. Ghia, J.-E.; Park, A.J.; Blennerhassett, P.; Khan, W.I.; Collins, S.M. Adoptive Transfer of Macrophage from Mice with Depression-like Behavior Enhances Susceptibility to Colitis. *Inflamm. Bowel. Dis.* **2011**, *17*, 1474–1489. [CrossRef]
30. Cailotto, C.; Gomez-Pinilla, P.J.; Costes, L.M.; van der Vliet, J.; Di Giovangiulio, M.; Némethova, A.; Matteoli, G.; Boeckxstaens, G.E. Neuro-Anatomical Evidence Indicating Indirect Modulation of Macrophages by Vagal Efferents in the Intestine but Not in the Spleen. *PLoS ONE* **2014**, *9*, e87785. [CrossRef]
31. Rosas-Ballina, M.; Olofsson, P.S.; Ochani, M.; Valdés-Ferrer, S.I.; Levine, Y.A.; Reardon, C.; Tusche, M.W.; Pavlov, V.A.; Andersson, U.; Chavan, S.; et al. Acetylcholine-Synthesizing T Cells Relay Neural Signals in a Vagus Nerve Circuit. *Science* **2011**, *334*, 98–101. [CrossRef]
32. Olofsson, P.S.; Tracey, K.J. Bioelectronic Medicine: Technology Targeting Molecular Mechanisms for Therapy. *J. Intern. Med.* **2017**, *282*, 3–4. [CrossRef] [PubMed]
33. Elliott, R.E.; Morsi, A.; Tanweer, O.; Grobelny, B.; Geller, E.; Carlson, C.; Devinsky, O.; Doyle, W.K. Efficacy of Vagus Nerve Stimulation over Time: Review of 65 Consecutive Patients with Treatment-Resistant Epilepsy Treated with VNS > 10 Years. *Epilepsy. Behav.* **2011**, *20*, 478–483. [CrossRef] [PubMed]
34. Lindgren, S.; Lilja, B.; Rosén, I.; Sundkvist, G. Disturbed Autonomic Nerve Function in Patients with Crohn's Disease. *Scand. J. Gastroenterol.* **1991**, *26*, 361–366. [CrossRef]
35. Lindgren, S.; Stewenius, J.; Sjölund, K.; Lilja, B.; Sundkvist, G. Autonomic Vagal Nerve Dysfunction in Patients with Ulcerative Colitis. *Scand. J. Gastroenterol.* **1993**, *28*, 638–642. [CrossRef] [PubMed]
36. Pellissier, S.; Dantzer, C.; Mondillon, L.; Trocme, C.; Gauchez, A.-S.; Ducros, V.; Mathieu, N.; Toussaint, B.; Fournier, A.; Canini, F.; et al. Relationship between Vagal Tone, Cortisol, TNF-Alpha, Epinephrine and Negative Affects in Crohn's Disease and Irritable Bowel Syndrome. *PLoS ONE* **2014**, *9*, e105328. [CrossRef] [PubMed]
37. Mikocka-Walus, A.; Knowles, S.R.; Keefer, L.; Graff, L. Controversies Revisited: A Systematic Review of the Comorbidity of Depression and Anxiety with Inflammatory Bowel Diseases. *Inflamm. Bowel. Dis.* **2016**, *22*, 752–762. [CrossRef]
38. Mikocka-Walus, A.; Pittet, V.; Rossel, J.-B.; von Känel, R. Swiss IBD Cohort Study Group Symptoms of Depression and Anxiety Are Independently Associated With Clinical Recurrence of Inflammatory Bowel Disease. *Clin. Gastroenterol. Hepatol.* **2016**, *14*, 829–835.e1. [CrossRef]
39. Mouzas, I.A.; Pallis, A.G.; Kochiadakis, G.E.; Marketou, M.; Chlouverakis, G.I.; Mellisas, J.; Vardas, P.E.; Kouroumalis, E.A. Autonomic Imbalance during the Day in Patients with Inflammatory Bowel Disease in Remission. Evidence from Spectral Analysis of Heart Rate Variability over 24 Hours. *Dig. Liver. Dis.* **2002**, *34*, 775–780. [CrossRef]
40. Ganguli, S.C.; Kamath, M.V.; Redmond, K.; Chen, Y.; Irvine, E.J.; Collins, S.M.; Tougas, G. A Comparison of Autonomic Function in Patients with Inflammatory Bowel Disease and in Healthy Controls. *Neurogastroenterol. Motil.* **2007**, *19*, 961–967. [CrossRef] [PubMed]
41. Zawadka-Kunikowska, M.; Słomko, J.; Kłopocka, M.; Liebert, A.; Tafil-Klawe, M.; Klawe, J.J.; Newton, J.L.; Zalewski, P. Cardiac and Autonomic Function in Patients with Crohn's Disease during Remission. *Adv. Med. Sci.* **2018**, *63*, 334–340. [CrossRef] [PubMed]

42. Borovikova, L.V.; Ivanova, S.; Nardi, D.; Zhang, M.; Yang, H.; Ombrellino, M.; Tracey, K.J. Role of Vagus Nerve Signaling in CNI-1493-Mediated Suppression of Acute Inflammation. *Auton. Neurosci.* **2000**, *85*, 141–147. [CrossRef]
43. Cheng, J.; Shen, H.; Chowdhury, R.; Abdi, T.; Selaru, F.; Chen, J.D.Z. Potential of Electrical Neuromodulation for Inflammatory Bowel Disease. *Inflamm. Bowel. Dis.* **2020**, *26*, 1119–1130. [CrossRef] [PubMed]
44. Bonaz, B.; Picq, C.; Sinniger, V.; Mayol, J.F.; Clarençon, D. Vagus Nerve Stimulation: From Epilepsy to the Cholinergic Anti-Inflammatory Pathway. *Neurogastroenterol. Motil.* **2013**, *25*, 208–221. [CrossRef] [PubMed]
45. Attenello, F.; Amar, A.P.; Liu, C.; Apuzzo, M.L.J. Theoretical Basis of Vagus Nerve Stimulation. *Prog. Neurol. Surg.* **2015**, *29*, 20–28. [CrossRef]
46. Payne, S.C.; Furness, J.B.; Burns, O.; Sedo, A.; Hyakumura, T.; Shepherd, R.K.; Fallon, J.B. Anti-Inflammatory Effects of Abdominal Vagus Nerve Stimulation on Experimental Intestinal Inflammation. *Front. Neurosci.* **2019**, *13*, 418. [CrossRef]
47. Sinniger, V.; Pellissier, S.; Fauvelle, F.; Trocmé, C.; Hoffmann, D.; Vercueil, L.; Cracowski, J.-L.; David, O.; Bonaz, B. A 12-Month Pilot Study Outcomes of Vagus Nerve Stimulation in Crohn's Disease. *Neurogastroenterol. Motil.* **2020**, *32*, e13911. [CrossRef]
48. Révész, D.; Fröjd, V.; Rydenhag, B.; Ben-Menachem, E. Estimating Long-Term Vagus Nerve Stimulation Effectiveness: Accounting for Antiepileptic Drug Treatment Changes. *Neuromodulation* **2018**, *21*, 797–804. [CrossRef]
49. Schreiber, S.; Reinisch, W.; Colombel, J.F.; Sandborn, W.J.; Hommes, D.W.; Robinson, A.M.; Huang, B.; Lomax, K.G.; Pollack, P.F. Subgroup Analysis of the Placebo-Controlled CHARM Trial: Increased Remission Rates through 3 Years for Adalimumab-Treated Patients with Early Crohn's Disease. *J. Crohns. Colitis* **2013**, *7*, 213–221. [CrossRef]
50. D'Haens, G.R.; Cabrijan, Z.; Eberhardson, M.; van den Berg, R.M.; Löwenberg, M.; Danese, S.; Fiorino, G.; Levine, Y.A.; Chernof, D.N. 367–Vagus Nerve Stimulation Reduces Disease Activity and Modulates Serum and Autonomic Biomarkers in Biologicrefractory Crohn's Disease. *Gastroenterology* **2019**, *156*, S-75. [CrossRef]
51. Kibleur, A.; Pellissier, S.; Sinniger, V.; Robert, J.; Gronlier, E.; Clarençon, D.; Vercueil, L.; Hoffmann, D.; Bonaz, B.; David, O. Electroencephalographic Correlates of Low-Frequency Vagus Nerve Stimulation Therapy for Crohn's Disease. *Clin. Neurophysiol.* **2018**, *129*, 1041–1046. [CrossRef] [PubMed]

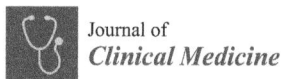

Case Report

Ruxolitinib as Adjunctive Therapy for Hemophagocytic LymPhohistiocytosis after Liver Transplantation: A Case Report and Literature Review

Kang He [1,2,3,†], Shanshan Xu [1,2,3,†], Lijing Shen [4], Xiaosong Chen [1,2,3], Qiang Xia [1,2,3,*] and Yongbing Qian [1,2,3,*]

1. Department of Liver Surgery, Renji Hospital, School of Medicine, Shanghai Jiao Tong University, Shanghai 200127, China
2. Shanghai Engineering Research Center of Transplantation and Immunology, Shanghai 200127, China
3. Shanghai Institute of Transplantation, Shanghai 200127, China
4. Department of Hematology, Renji Hospital, School of Medicine, Shanghai Jiao Tong University, Shanghai 200127, China
* Correspondence: xiaqiang@shsmu.edu.cn (Q.X.); qianyongbing@renji.com (Y.Q.)
† These authors contributed equally to this work.

Abstract: Hemophagocytic lymphohistiocytosis (HLH) is a rare but potentially fatal hyperinflammatory disorder characterized by dysfunctional cytotoxic T and natural killer cells. Liver transplantation is a predisposing factor for HLH. High mortality rates were reported in 40 cases of HLH following liver transplantation in adults and children. Herein, we describe a case of adult HLH triggered by cytomegalovirus (CMV) infection shortly after liver transplantation. The patient was successfully treated with ruxolitinib combined with a modified HLH-2004 treatment strategy. Our case is the first to report the successful use of ruxolitinib with a modified HLH-2004 strategy to treat HLH in a solid organ transplantation recipient.

Keywords: ruxolitinib; hemophagocytic lymphohistiocytosis; liver transplantation

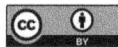

1. Introduction

Hemophagocytic lymphohistiocytosis (HLH), also known as hemophagocytic syndrome (HPS), is a rare but life-threatening disorder characterized by a high-grade fever, splenomegaly, cytopenia, and hyperferritinemia. It is believed that NK cell dysfunction, activated cytotoxic T-cell activity, and the cytokine storm constitute the underlying mechanism of HLH [1]. HLH can be divided into primary HLH and secondary HLH according to its cause. Primary HLH is considered to be genetic and often occurs in children with an underlying genetic defect. Bone marrow transplant is the only radical treatment for primary HLH [2]. In contrast, secondary HLH can occur at any age and is associated with infection, malignancy, autoimmune disease, transplantation, and drugs [1]. These factors may act as triggers or predisposing factors to the disease, or both. Viral infection is the most frequent trigger, and about 6% of cases are triggered by a cytomegalovirus (CMV) [1]. HLH is a rare disease, but has a very high mortality rate of around 41%, probably due to the nonspecific manifestations and delayed diagnosis [1].

After liver transplantation (LT), patients receive immunosuppression treatment and as a result are susceptible to infections and immune dysregulation. HLH after LT is often overlooked as a fever and cytopenia both of which are common after a liver transplant, and the initial manifestations of HLH are also similar to other complications, such as posttransplant lymphoproliferative disorders (PTLD), graft-versus-host disease (GVHD), autoimmune hemolytic anemia (AIHA), and sepsis [1,3]. To date, 21 pediatric cases (age ≤ 18 years) and 19 adult cases of HLH following liver transplantation (LT) have been reported in the literature, with a very high mortality rate of 55% (22/40) (Table 1). The high mortality rate may be attributed to a delayed diagnosis and a debatable treatment. The widely used HLH-2004 treatment protocol, including steroids (dexamethasone), immunosuppressive agents (cyclosporine A), and chemotherapy drugs (etoposide), was first proposed for pediatric patients with primary HLH. However, this protocol may not be appropriate for LT patients as they are already immunosuppressed [4].

Ruxolitinib is an inhibitor of JAK1/2 (the Janus family kinase 1 and 2) and can inhibit the release of cytokines. It is mainly used in the hematological field and also in COVID-19 patients [5]. There are case reports and pilot studies using ruxolitinib as a salvage therapy or first-line treatment for HLH patients showing good efficacy and safety [6–15]. However, it has never been used for post-transplant patients with HLH. In this study, we present one case of adult CMV-associated HLH following liver transplantation successfully treated by ruxolitinib and a modified HLH-2004 protocol. This report provides an alternative method for the treatment of HLH following LT.

Table 1. Cases of HLH after liver transplantation.

No	Author	Age (Years)	Dx	Donor Type	Time Post LT	IS regimen	Triggers	Treatment	Outcome
1	Chisuwa [16]	0.75	Biliary atresia	LRLT	15 d	Steroid, FK506	Unx	Steroid, IVIg, G-CSF, stopped IS	Died
2	Chisuwa [16]	1	Biliary atresia	LRLT	134 d	Steroid, FK506	Unx	G-CSF, stopped IS	Died
3	Karasu [17]	38	HBV/HDV	LRLT	131 d	Steroid, FK506	Unx	IVIg, G-CSF, PE, stopped IS	Alive
4	Lladó [18]	63	AIH	DDLT	75 d	CsA, basiliximab	Unx	Steroid, IVIg	Died
5	George [19]	10	Unx	Unx	6 y	FK506	EBV	Steroid, Stopped IS, etoposide	Alive
6	Tania [20]	37	Unx	LDLT	11 d	FK506	Unx	Steroid, IvIg, PE, CHDF	Died
7	Hardikar [21]	2.2	Unx	DDLT	15 d	Steroid, FK506, Aza	CMV	Stop IS, G-CSF, IVIg	Alive
8	Akamatsu [22]	59	HCV	LDLT	138 d	FK506	Aspergillus	Supportive	Died
9	Akamatsu [22]	49	PBC	LDLT	315 d	Steroid, FK506	CMV	Steroid, IVIg, PE, FK506 to CsA, 5x	Died
10	Akamatsu [22]	48	HCV	LDLT	50 d	Steroid, FK506, OKT3	HCV	G-CSF	Died
11	Yoshizumi [23]	63	HBV	LDLT	13 d		SFSS	Steroid, change IS, IVIg, G-CSF	Alive
12	Dharancy [24] L/K	49	Polycystic liver kidney disease	Combined Liver-kidney (CLK)	19 d	Steroid, CsA, MMF, basiliximab	HHV6	Supportive	Died
13	Zhang [25]	6	Unx	LRLT	8 d	Steroid, FK506	EBV	Steroid, IVIg, G-CSF, stopped IS, etoposide	Alive
14	Satapathy [26]	25	AIH	DDLT	6 m	Steroid, FK506, MMF	Still's disease	Steroid, anakinra	Alive
15	Somyama [27]	57	HCV/HCC	LDLT	32 d	Steroid, FK506	CMV/HCC	Steroid, IVIg, G-CSF	Died
16	Somyama [27]	63	HBV/HCC	LRLT	81 d	Steroid, FK506	Unx	Steroid, IVIg, G-CSF	Died
17	Rodriguez-Medina [28]	63	HCV	Unx	4 y	Steroid, CsA, Aza	TB	G-CSF	Died
18	Jha [29] 2015	2	Extrahepatic biliary atresia	LRLT	9 m		EBV	Reduced IS; rituximab	Alive
19	Vijgen [30]	66	Alcohol-related liver disease, HCC	DDLT	1 y	FK506, MMF	HHV8	Steroid, stopped IS, rituximab	Died
20	Iseda [31]	63	HBV	LDLT	12 d	Steroid, FK506, MMF	SFSS	Steroid, IVIg, G-CSF, stopped MMF, reduced FK506	Died
21	Cohen [32]	31	Drug-induced liver disease	DDLT	4 y	FK506	HHV8	Steroid, IVIg, rituximab, reduced FK506	Died

Table 1. Cont.

22	Jarchin [33]	18	Neonatal hepatitis	LRLT	17 y	FK506	Unx	Steroid, etoposide, stopped FK506	Died
23	Valenzuela [34]	48	AIH, PBC	DDLT	13 d	Steroid, FK506	EBV	Steroid, etoposide, IS switched to CsA	Died
24	Yamada [35]	2	Biliary atresia	Liver inteatinal transplantation	254 d	Steroid, FK506, everolimus	EBV	Steroid, etoposide, reduced IS, THP-COP	Died
25	Chesner [36]	58	AIH	Unx	16 y	Steroid, FK506, Aza	EBV	supportive	Died
26	Arikan [37]	1	Caroli disease	Unx	6 m	Steroid, FK506, sirolimus, MMF	CMV	Steroid, IVIg, rituximab	Died
27	Arikan [37]	2	Biliary atresia		8 m	Steroid, FK506, sirolimus	EBV	Steroid, IVIg, VP16, rituximab	Alive
28	Arikan [37]	1.5	Unx cholestasis		7 m	Steroid, FK506	HHV8	Steroid, IVIg, VP16	Alive
29	Arikan [37]	9	PFIC		4 m	Steroid, FK506, sirolimus	Acinetobacter	IVIg	Died
30	Arikan [37]	0.5	Biliary atresia		10 m	FK506	EBV	IVIg, VP16, rituximab	Alive
31	Arikan [37]	0.5	Unx cholestasis		7 m	Steroid, FK506	Klebsiella	Steroid, IVIg, VP16	Alive
32	Arikan [37]	0.67	Biliary atresia		9 m	Steroid, FK506	EBV	Steroid, IVIg, VP16, rituximab	Alive
33	Arikan [37]	0.67	Unx		5 m	Steroid, FK506, MMF	CMV, EBV	Steroid, IVIg, rituximab	Died
34	Arikan [37]	0.75	Unx cholestasis		6 m	Steroid, FK506	EBV	Steroid, IVIg, rituximab	Alive
35	Arikan [37]	2.1	PFIC		10 m	FK506	EBV	IVIg, VP16, rituximab	Alive
36	Arikan [37]	0.4	Unx cholestasis		8 m	FK506	EBV	Steroid, IVIg, rituximab	Alive
37	Arikan [37]	1	Bile salt synthesis defect		10 m	FK506, sirolimus	EBV	IVIg, rituximab	Alive
38	Gandotra [38]	47	HBV/HCV/HCC	LDLT	3 y	Steroid	TB	Steroid, IVIg	Alive
39	Nakajima [39]	2	EBV-LPD	LRLT	10 d	Steroid, FK506	EBV	Steroid, etoposide, HCT	Alive
40	Ferreira [40]	52	Cryptogenic cirrhosis	DDLT	2 m	Steroid, FK506, MMF	TB	Steroid, etoposide, stopped FK506	Died

AIH: autoimmune hepatitis, Aza: azathioprine, CMV: cytomegalovirus, CsA: cyclosporin A, d: days, DDLT: deceased donor liver transplantation, EBV: Epstein-Barr virus, EBV-G-CSF: granulocyte colony-stimulating factor, LPD: EBV associated T and NK cell lymphoproliferative disease, FK506: tacrolimus, HBV: hepatitis B virus, HCV: hepatitis C virus, HDV: hepatitis D virus, HCC: hepatocellular carcinoma, HCT: hematopoietic cell transplantation, HHV: human herpes virus, IVIg: intravenous immunoglobin, IS: immunosuppression, LDLT: living donor liver transplantation, LRLT: living related donor liver transplantation, m: months, MMF: mycophenolate mofetil, PBC: primary biliary cholangitis, PE: plasma exchange, PFIC: progressive familial intrahepatic cholestasis, SFSS: small-for-size syndrome, Sx: splenectomy, TB: tuberculosis, Unx: unknown, VP-16: etoposide, y: years.

2. Case Report

A 53-year-old male presented with fulminant hepatic failure, probable drug-induced liver injury and alcohol-induced hepatitis. Serologic tests for hepatitis A-D, Epstein-Barr virus (EBV), and tuberculosis were all negative. The autoimmune workup was normal. The CMV DNA was detected by PCR in peripheral blood with 4.64×10^4 copies/mL, with a positive cytomegalovirus (CMV) IgG and a negative IgM.

On admission, the patient's vitals were within normal ranges and his temperature was 36.5 °C. Initial examination showed normal hematological findings and an abnormal liver function and coagulopathy: total bilirubin 544.6 µmol/L, direct bilirubin 386.8 µmol/L, alanine aminotransferase (ALT) 537 U/L, aspartate aminotransferase (AST) 373 U/L, PT 24.1 s, INR 2.3, and fibrinogen 1.15 g/L.

On day 10 of admission, the patient underwent a deceased donor liver transplantation. The donor was a 50-year-old male with a height of 165 cm and weight of 55 kg (BMI 20.2 kg/m^2), diagnosed with brain death induced by intracranial hemorrhage. The donor was CMV-seronegative and had an identical blood type (type B) to the patient. The graft weight was 1515 g. The liver transplant took 6 h with 35 min of anhepatic time. During the surgery, 500 mg methylprednisolone was used for immunosuppression induction. The patient received a standard immunosuppression treatment with methylprednisolone tapering (tapering from 240 mg to 20 mg within one week), mycophenolate mofetil (720 mg/day), tacrolimus (4 mg/day), and basiliximab (20 mg on POD 0 and 4) after the surgery.

The post-transplant outcome is shown in Figure 1. On postoperative day (POD) 3, the patient developed a high-grade fever (above 38.5 °C), thrombocytopenia and anemia: WBC 4.97×10^9/L (neutrophil 4.36×10^9/L), hemoglobin 73 g/L, and platelets 43×10^9/L. Experimental anti-infection treatment was initiated with vancomycin and meropenem to treat the fever. Granulocyte colony-stimulating factor (G-CSF, 75 µg/day) was administered three times on POD 5, 9, and 17 to prevent white blood cell (WBC) count decline, but only temporary improvement was observed. A blood culture was immediately performed and repeated twice, revealing no bacterial infections. Next Generation Sequencing screening, bacterial culture of the intubation and drainage liquid, G test, GM test, TORCH test, respiratory virus test, and a chest X-ray were also all negative. On POD 8, the CMV DNA in peripheral blood increased to 4.64×10^6 copies/mL, and ganciclovir (400 mg/day) was initiated to treat the infection. Considering the normal hepatobiliary enzymes, bilirubin levels and normal daily ultrasonogram, immunosuppression therapy (tacrolimus, mycophenolate mofetil and methylprednisolone) was temporarily stopped in order to promote an immune response to overcome the infection.

Despite the use of ganciclovir, the patient's inflammatory factors, fever and pancytopenia showed no improvement. On POD 22, the WBC count declined to 1.21×10^9/L (neutrophil 1.09×10^9/L), and the patient exhibited a persistent high-grade fever. He was then tested for HCMV drug-resistant mutation, but the result was negative. Therefore, hemophagocytic lymphohistiocytosis (HLH) was strongly suspected even without a relevant family history. Bone marrow aspiration was performed on POD 23 and revealed hemophagocytosis (Figure 2). Laboratory findings: hemoglobin 58 g/L, platelets 72×10^9/L, WBC 1.65×10^9/L (neutrophils 1.54×10^9/L), ferritin 1592.5 ng/mL, fasting triglyceride 1.06 mmol/L, fibrinogen 2.78 g/L, sIL-2R 6150 U/mL, and low NK cell activity (2.1%). The patient met seven out of the eight HLH-2004 diagnostic criteria [4] and was diagnosed with HLH following LT. According to the HLH-2004 protocol, a combination of intravenous immunoglobulin (25 g/day), G-CSF (150 µg/d), steroids (methylprednisolone pulse 80 mg), and etoposide (100 mg/d) was immediately administered [4]. The JAK1/2 inhibitor ruxolitinib is a novel treatment for HLH and was started the next day after diagnosis in combination with dexamethasone. The dose of ruxolitinib was maintained at 5 mg/day until discharge, and dexamethasone was tapered from 20 mg/day to 5 mg/day over three weeks and maintained at 5 mg/day until discharge (POD 28 15 mg/day, POD 34 10 mg/day, POD38 7.5 mg/day, and POD 44 5 mg/day). The patient's fever improved rapidly following treatment initiation. On POD 25, the patient's temperature returned to normal. The inflammatory factors IL-6 and C-reactive protein declined rapidly after the treatment. Ferritin and sIL-2R are two reliable prognostic factors of HLH; sIL-2R showed a significant decline while ferritin showed a gradual decrease after treatment initiation [41]. The WBC, hemoglobin and platelet levels showed improvement after two weeks of HLH and supportive treatment. GSF and recombinant human interleukin-11 were given to improve the platelet level, and a therapeutic plasma exchange was performed to clear the excessive cytokines. On POD29, tacrolimus was resumed due to a slight increase in liver enzymes. On POD33, the patient tested positive for carbapenem-sensitive klebsiella pneumoniae (CSKP). Minocycline and meropenem were used. Dexamethasone was reduced to 10 mg/day the next day and then to 7.5 mg/day on POD38, which led to a significant improvement in neutropenia.

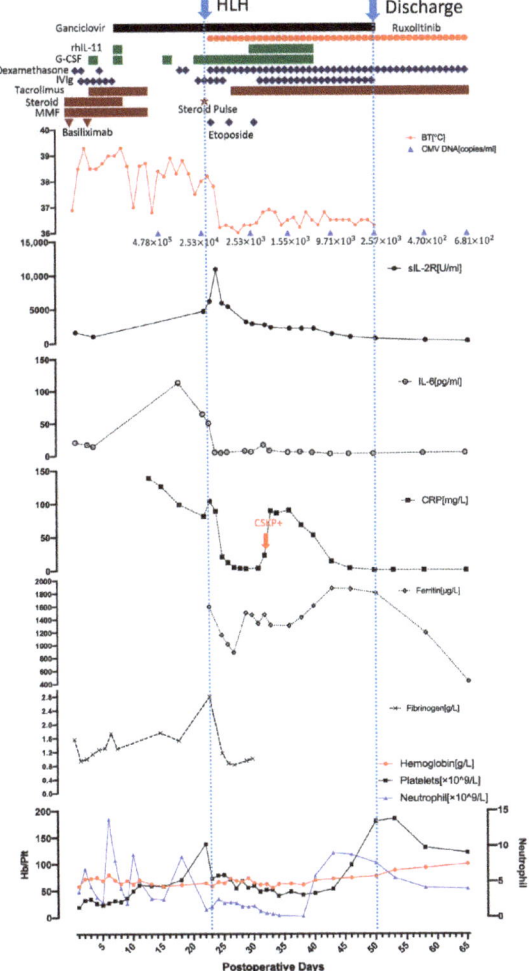

Figure 1. The posttransplant outcome of the patient. (BT: body temperature, CRP: C-reactive protein, CSKP: carbapenem-sensitive klebsiella pneumoniae, G-CSF: granulocyte colony-stimulating factor, Hb: hemoglobin, IL-6: interleukin-6, IVIg: intravenous immunoglobulin, MMF: mycophenolate mofetil, Plt: platelet, rhIL-11: recombinant human interleukin-11, sIL-2R: soluble interleukin-2 receptor).

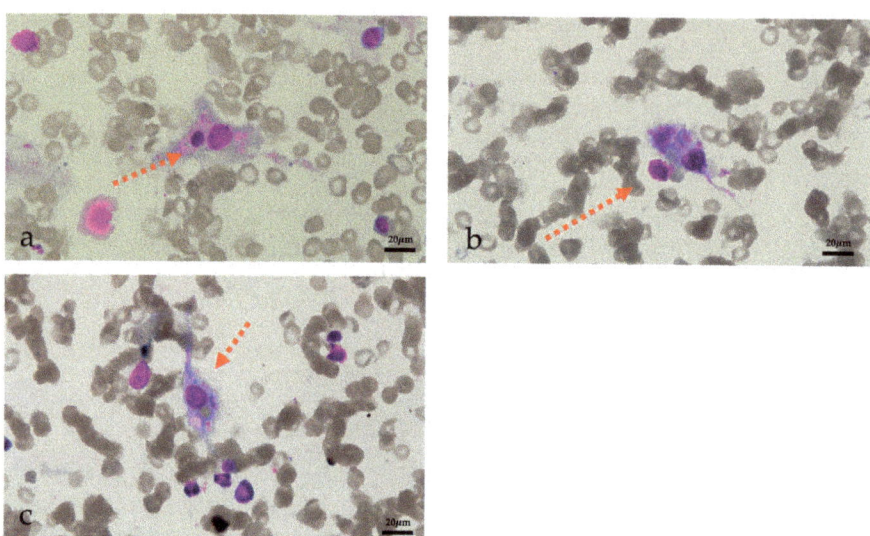

Figure 2. Image of bone marrow aspiration (**a**) phagocytic neutrophils (**b**) phagocytic platelets (**c**) erythrophagocytosis.

With a stable temperature and lab findings, the patient was discharged on POD 50. His maintenance treatment included ruxolitinib (5 mg/day), dexamethasone (4.5 mg/day), tacrolimus (1 mg/day), ganciclovir, and entecavir. Regular follow-ups were performed after discharge. Dexamethasone was reduced by one tablet (0.75 mg) per week forone1 month, which resulted in a rapid decline in WBC count, which was successfully treated by increasing ruxolitinib to 10 mg/day. On POD 71 (three weeks after discharge), the peripheral blood CMV DNA was undetectable, and ganciclovir was stopped. Three months after discharge, dexamethasone (2.25 mg/day) was changed to prednisone (5 mg/day), and ruxolitinib was stopped. The patient's temperature remained stable and the patient is doing well to date (12 months).

3. Discussion

HLH is hard to diagnose due to its non-specific symptoms. The patient's CMV DNA was 4.64×10^4 copies/mL before transplant. After liver transplantation, with the use of immunosuppression agents, the CMV DNA increased to 4.64×10^6 copies/mL on POD8. The initial symptoms were thought to be caused by CMV reactivation, and differential diagnoses such as HLH were only considered after failure of the initial treatment. Failure to treat CMV with ganciclovir in a timely manner was indeed one of the possible causes of secondary HLH in our case. Basiliximab, plus a delayed and low-dose immunosuppressive regimen of tacrolimus were intended to reduce further CMV flareups after the transplant. Bone marrow aspiration was performed to confirm the diagnosis, which is not a mandatory diagnostic criterion, but provides valuable information for differential diagnosis.

The HLH-2004 treatment protocol includes a combination of chemotherapy (etoposide), immunosuppressive therapy (cyclosporin A, CsA), glucocorticoid, and bone marrow transplantation, which has a 5-year survival rate of about 61% [4]. CsA is proven to be beneficial in pediatric and autoimmune cases and is recommended in the HLH-2004 protocol, while tacrolimus's efficacy has not been proved [1]. Hence, some clinicians choose to change the immunosuppression to CsA. It has been reported that tacrolimus has a stronger inhibitory effect on CD8 T cells and has shown efficacy in the treatment of HLH [42,43]. Thus, the need for switching tacrolimus to CsA is controversial (Table 1).

However, the HLH-2004 treatment protocol is a conflicting strategy for patients with HLH after transplantation, as these patients are already in an immunosuppressive state, which could also be a predisposing factor for HLH. Clinicians argued that CsA was ineffective in preventing HLH progression after solid organ transplantation [44]. The myelotoxicity, hepatotoxicity, and nephrotoxicity of etoposide may also have resulted in complications. Therefore, the immunosuppressants were stopped, and etoposide was given only three times during the early stages. Most importantly, the novel drug ruxolitinib was added to the treatment strategy.

Ruxolitinib is an oral JAK1/2 inhibitor and can inhibit the production of interferon-γ (IFN-γ) [6]. It has been approved to treat myelofibrosis, polycythemia, and steroid-refractory acute graft-versus-host disease (SR-aGVHD) by the US Food and Drug administration [45]. Considering the complexity of the cytokine storm in HLH, the pathogenesis is likely mediated by a network of cytokines rather than a single one. However, it is generally believed that the pathway involving STAT1 (signal transducer and activator of transcription 1), JAK1, JAK2, and IFN-γ is the common pathway of HLH [46–48]. Ruxolitinib has been reported to be effective in treating 61 secondary HLH patients, including 19 adults and 42 children. In nine cases, ruxolitinib was used as the first-line treatment, while in other cases it was used as a salvage therapy. However, ruxolitinib has never been reported to be used in HLH after solid organ transplantation.

In 2019, Ahmed et al. conducted a small pilot study that included seven patients, which had shown that ruxolitinib is an active and well-tolerated treatment for secondary HLH in adult patients and can be managed through an outpatient clinic [6]. Two of the patients' conditions were triggered by an autoimmune disorder, and three were idiopathic [6]. Among the seven patients, three of them achieved a complete response, and the others achieved a partial response with improved cytopenia within the first week [6]. The use of ruxolitinib allowed the reduction or discontinuation of corticosteroids [6]. All the patients were alive with a median follow-up of 490 days (range: 190-1075 days) [6]. However, one patient was diagnosed with primary HLH and suffered a relapse, while another patient experienced a drug-related adverse event (neuropathic foot pain) and stopped the treatment [6]. The only serious side effect of ruxolitinib was grade 4 febrile neutropenia without any drug-related death [6]. Currently, a multi-center phase 2 clinical trial is investigating the efficacy of ruxolitinib (NCT04551131). In addition, participants are being recruited for a phase 4 clinical trial focusing on malignancy-related HLH and the effect of ruxolitinib (NCT04999878).

Wang et al. conducted a clinical trial, which included 34 children with refractory/relapsed HLH [7]. Ruxolitinib was given as a salvage therapy after the HLH-94 regimen failure. Twenty five children responded to the therapy and five of them had complete remission. Leukopenia and thrombocytopenia were common side effects, but all the patients could tolerate them. At the end of the study, 15 patients died, and the median survival time was 22 weeks. The clinicians argued that ruxolitinib could alleviate the hyperinflammatory state but was not sufficiently potent. They suggested combining ruxolitinib with other treatment strategies to achieve better outcomes. A large-scale clinical trial is being conducted to validate the effectiveness of the DEP-ruxolitinib regimen (NCT03533790).

In 2019, Meng performed a single-center retrospective analysis evaluating 12 patients who developed SR-aGVHD after allogeneic hematopoietic stem cell transplantation (allo-HSCT), complicated by Epstein-Barr virus-associated HLH [8]. Among the 12 patients, seven achieved a complete response, three achieved a partial response, and two exhibited treatment failure. The side effects only included neutropenia (grade 3 to 4) and thrombocytopenia (grade 3 to 4). Ruxolitinib was apparently effective for patients with EBV-HLH combined with SR-aGVHD.

In 2020, Wei conducted a retrospective analysis of pediatric cases with refractory or recurrent HLH and found that ruxolitinib was effective as a salvage therapy [9]. Among the nine analyzed cases, five cases of HLH were secondary to EBV, one was secondary to an autoimmune disorder, two were familial HLH, and one was idiopathic. Before the use of ruxolitinib, all of them were treated according to the HLH-94 treatment strategy but did not show improvement. After receiving a continuous 28-day course of ruxolitinib, three of them achieved partial remission, five improved and one died.

Furthermore, six case reports argued that ruxolitinib is beneficial to refractory HLH both for children and adults. Slostad reported a case of histoplasmosis-related HLH treated with ruxolitinib as a first-line treatment, which achieved a rapid improvement [10]. Zandvakili presented a case of autoimmune disease-related HLH, also using ruxolitinib as a first-line therapy with a good outcome even after the patient developed sepsis [11]. Goldsmith reported two HLH cases, one autoimmune disorder-associated and the other EBV-related [12]. Ruxolitinib was used as a salvage therapy and led to a rapid symptom improvement. Zhao reported a pediatric case of EBV-associated HLH successfully treated with ruxolitinib as a bridge to allogeneic stem cell transplantation [13]. Brogile reported a pediatric case of idiopathic HLH receiving ruxolitinib after several failed treatments, including the biological treatment anakinra. The patient's fever subsided within 24 h of initiating ruxolitinib, and recovery was achieved without other treatments [14]. Ono successfully used ruxolitinib in a pediatric patient who developed HLH after hematopoietic cell transplantation [15].

The most commonly reported adverse effects of ruxolitinib were hematologic adverse reactions including thrombocytopenia and anemia [49,50]. Dizziness, headache, and infections are common nonhematologic adverse effects [45,49]. Hepatotoxicity is rare and only moderate liver toxicity was reported [51,52]. For patients with hepatic impairment, the dosage of ruxolitinib should be modified according to platelet counts [45]. Both tacrolimus and ruxolitinib are mainly metabolized through cytochrome P450 (CYP) 3A4 enzyme, but no drug interaction between them has been reported [53,54]. For ruxolitinib, dose reduction is only needed when a potent CYP3A4 inhibitor is concomitantly used [53]. However, tacrolimus has a narrow therapeutic index and is more likely to be influenced by other drugs that also metabolize through CYP3A4 [54]. So close monitoring of tacrolimus whole blood concentrations is recommended. Based on this information, we decided to lower the dose of ruxolitinib to 5 mg/day, in comparison to 20 mg twice daily for myelofibrosis patients [45]. The platelet count and liver function were closely monitored, and tacrolimus trough concentration was tested every day.

Our patient developed a high-grade fever shortly after the operation and only CMV infection was detected. However, no symptom improvement was observed following the initiation of ganciclovir. Furthermore, steroids and immunosuppression drugs, as the two major components of HLH-2004 treatment, had already been given for around two weeks. Hence, we considered that the patient was unresponsive to the HLH-2004 treatment protocol. In addition, a pilot study reported ruxolitinib as a first-line treatment for adult secondary HLH [6], and case reports described the use of ruxolitinib as a first-line therapy to treat Hematopoietic Cell Transplantation-associated HLH [10,11,15]. Moreover, some clinicians argued that ruxolitinib may exert a synergistic effect with HLH-2004 treatment [55]. Ruxolitinib was added to our treatment strategy and the dosage and frequency of etoposide were significantly reduced (100 mg three times instead of 150 mg ten times). Dexamethasone was tapered much more rapidly and was maintained at a low level (within three weeks instead of eight weeks according to HLH-2004 strategy).

Our case is the first to report the use of ruxolitinib as an initial therapy instead of a salvage therapy in HLH patients after solid organ transplantation. The patient's fever subsided within 24 h, with a rapid improvement in ferritin, and sIL-2R levels. However, ruxolitinib treatment resulted in a slow improvement in cytopenia, possibly due to the use of ganciclovir and tacrolimus or the adverse effect of ruxolitinib (neutropenia and thrombocytopenia). The neutropenia and thrombocytopenia spontaneously improved after a reduction in the dexamethasone dosage. The patient is now doing fine with a normal liver function and minimal immunosuppressants almost one year after liver transplantation.

In summary, we present an adult case of secondary HLH associated with CMV infection following a liver transplant successfully treated with a modified HLH-2004 treatment protocol, which included ruxolitinib. The rapid improvement and good prognosis indicate that ruxolitinib may be useful as an initial therapy for patients with HLH after solid organ transplantation.

Funding: This research received no external funding.

Institutional Review Board Statement: Not applicable.

Informed Consent Statement: Not applicable.

Data Availability Statement: Not applicable.

Conflicts of Interest: The authors declare no conflict of interest.

References

1. Ramos-Casals, M.; Brito-Zerón, P.; López-Guillermo, A.; A Khamashta, M.; Bosch, X. Adult haemophagocytic syndrome. *Lancet* **2014**, *383*, 1503–1516. [CrossRef]
2. Jordan, M.B.; Filipovich, A.H. Hematopoietic cell transplantation for hemophagocytic lymphohistiocytosis: A journey of a thousand miles begins with a single (big) step. *Bone Marrow Transpl.* **2008**, *42*, 433–437. [CrossRef] [PubMed]
3. Hara, H.; Ohdan, H.; Tashiro, H.; Itamoto, T.; Tanaka, Y.; Mizunuma, K.; Tokita, D.; Onoe, T.; Ito, R.; Asahara, T. Differential diagnosis between graft-versus-host disease and hemophagocytic syndrome after living-related liver transplantation by mixed lymphocyte reaction assay. *J. Investig. Surg.* **2004**, *17*, 197–202. [CrossRef] [PubMed]
4. Henter, J.-I.; Horne, A.; Aricó, M.; Egeler, R.M.; Filipovich, A.H.; Imashuku, S.; Ladisch, S.; McClain, K.; Webb, D.; Winiarski, J.; et al. HLH-2004: Diagnostic and therapeutic guidelines for hemophagocytic lymphohistiocytosis. *Pediatr. Blood Cancer* **2007**, *48*, 124–131. [CrossRef]
5. Di Lorenzo, G.; Di Trolio, R.; Kozlakidis, Z.; Busto, G.; Ingenito, C.; Buonerba, L.; Ferrara, C.; Libroia, A.; Ragone, G.; Ioio, C.D.; et al. COVID 19 therapies and anti-cancer drugs: A systematic review of recent literature. *Crit. Rev. Oncol.* **2020**, *152*, 102991. [CrossRef]
6. Ahmed, A.; A Merrill, S.; Alsawah, F.; Bockenstedt, P.; Campagnaro, E.; Devata, S.; Gitlin, S.D.; Kaminski, M.; Cusick, A.; Phillips, T.; et al. Ruxolitinib in adult patients with secondary haemophagocytic lymphohistiocytosis: An open-label, single-centre, pilot trial. *Lancet Haematol.* **2019**, *6*, e630–e637. [CrossRef]
7. Wang, J.; Wang, Y.; Wu, L.; Wang, X.; Jin, Z.; Gao, Z.; Wang, Z. Ruxolitinib for refractory/relapsed hemophagocytic lymphohistiocytosis. *Haematologica* **2019**, *105*, e210–e212. [CrossRef]
8. Meng, G.; Wang, J.; Wang, X.; Wang, Y.; Wang, Z. Ruxolitinib treatment for SR-aGVHD in patients with EBV-HLH undergoing allo-HSCT. *Ann. Hematol.* **2020**, *99*, 343–349. [CrossRef]
9. Wei, A.; Ma, H.; Li, Z.; Zhang, L.; Zhang, Q.; Wang, D.; Lian, H.; Zhang, R.; Wang, T. Short-term effectiveness of ruxolitinib in the treatment of recurrent or refractory hemophagocytic lymphohistiocytosis in children. *Int. J. Hematol.* **2020**, *112*, 568–576, Epub 20200714. [CrossRef]
10. Slostad, J.; Hoversten, P.; Haddox, C.L.; Cisak, K.; Paludo, J.; Tefferi, A. Ruxolitinib as first-line treatment in secondary hemophagocytic lymphohistiocytosis: A single patient experience. *Am. J. Hematol.* **2017**, *93*, E47–E49. [CrossRef]
11. Zandvakili, I.; Conboy, C.B.; Ayed, A.O.; Cathcart-Rake, E.J.; Tefferi, A. Ruxolitinib as first-line treatment in secondary hemophagocytic lymphohistiocytosis: A second experience. *Am. J. Hematol.* **2018**, *93*, E123–E125. [CrossRef] [PubMed]
12. Goldsmith, S.R.; Rehman, S.S.U.; Shirai, C.L.; Vij, K.; DiPersio, J.F. Resolution of secondary hemophagocytic lymphohistiocytosis after treatment with the JAK1/2 inhibitor ruxolitinib. *Blood Adv.* **2019**, *3*, 4131–4135. [CrossRef] [PubMed]
13. Zhao, Y.; Shi, J.; Li, X.; Wang, J.; Sun, J.; Zhou, Y.; Huang, H. Salvage therapy with dose-escalating ruxolitinib as a bridge to allogeneic stem cell transplantation for refractory hemophagocytic lymphohistiocytosis. *Bone Marrow Transplant.* **2020**, *55*, 824–826. [CrossRef] [PubMed]
14. Broglie, L.; Pommert, L.; Rao, S.; Thakar, M.; Phelan, R.; Margolis, D.; Talano, J.-A. Ruxolitinib for treatment of refractory hemophagocytic lymphohistiocytosis. *Blood Adv.* **2017**, *1*, 1533–1536. [CrossRef]
15. Ono, R.; Ashiarai, M.; Hirabayashi, S.; Mizuki, K.; Hosoya, Y.; Yoshihara, H.; Ohtake, J.; Mori, S.; Manabe, A.; Hasegawa, D. Ruxolitinib for hematopoietic cell transplantation-associated hemophagocytic lymphohistiocytosis. *Int. J. Hematol.* **2021**, *113*, 297–301. [CrossRef]
16. Chisuwa, H.; Hashikura, Y.; Nakazawa, Y.; Kamijo, T.; Nakazawa, K.; Nakayama, J.; Oh-Ishi, T.; Ikegami, T.; Terada, M.; Kawasaki, S. Fatal hemophagocytic syndrome after living-related liver transplantation: A report of two cases. *Transplantation* **2001**, *72*, 1843–1846. [CrossRef]
17. Karasu, Z.; Kilic, M.; Cagirgan, S.; Lebe, E.; Yilmaz, F.; Demirbas, T.; Tokat, Y. Hemophagocytic syndrome after living-related liver transplantation. *Transplant. Proc.* **2003**, *35*, 1482–1484. [CrossRef]
18. Lladó, L.; Figueras, J.; Comí, S.; Torras, J.; Serrano, T.; Castellote, J.; Motomura, T.; Mano, Y.; Itoh, S.; Harada, N.; et al. Haemophagocytic syndrome after liver transplantation in adults. *Transpl. Int.* **2004**, *17*, 221–223. [CrossRef]

19. George, T.I.; Jeng, M.; Berquist, W.; Cherry, A.M.; Link, M.P.; Arber, D.A. Epstein-Barr virus-associated peripheral T-cell lymphoma and hemophagocytic syndrome arising after liver transplantation: Case report and review of the literature. *Pediatr. Blood Cancer* **2005**, *44*, 270–276. [CrossRef]
20. Taniai, N.; Akimaru, K.; Kawano, Y.; Mizuguchi, Y.; Shimizu, T.; Takahashi, T.; Mamada, Y.; Yoshida, H.; Tajiri, T. Hemophagocytic syndrome after living-donor liver transplantation for fulminant liver failure: A case report. *Hepatogastroenterology* **2005**, *52*, 923–926.
21. Hardikar, W.; Pang, K.; Al-Hebbi, H.; Curtis, N.; Couper, R. Successful treatment of cytomegalovirus-associated haemophagocytic syndrome following paediatric orthotopic liver transplantation. *J Paediatr Child Health.* **2006**, *42*, 389–391. [CrossRef] [PubMed]
22. Akamatsu, N.; Sugawara, Y.; Tamura, S.; Matsui, Y.; Hasegawa, K.; Imamura, H.; Kokudo, N.; Makuuchi, M. Hemophagocytic syndrome after adult-to-adult living donor liver transplantation. *Transplant. Proc.* **2006**, *38*, 1425–1428. [CrossRef] [PubMed]
23. Yoshizumi, T.; Taketomi, A.; Kayashima, H.; Harada, N.; Uchiyama, H.; Yamashita, Y.-I.; Ikegami, T.; Soejima, Y.; Nishizaki, T.; Shimada, M.; et al. Successful treatment for a patient with hemophagocytic syndrome after a small-for-size graft liver transplantation. *Hepatogastroenterology* **2008**, *55*, 359–362. [PubMed]
24. Dharancy, S.; Crombe, V.; Copin, M.; Boleslawski, E.; Bocket, L.; Declerck, N.; Canva, V.; Dewilde, A.; Mathurin, P.; Pruvot, F. Fatal hemophagocytic syndrome related to human herpesvirus-6 reinfection following liver transplantation: A case report. *Transplant. Proc.* **2008**, *40*, 3791–3793. [CrossRef] [PubMed]
25. Zhang, M.; Guo, C.; Yan, L.; Pu, C.; Li, Y.; Kang, Q.; Ren, Z.; Jin, X. Successful treatment of Epstein-Barr Virus-associated haemophagocytic syndrome arising after living donor liver transplantation. *Hepatol. Res.* **2009**, *39*, 421–426. [CrossRef]
26. Satapathy, S.K.; Fiel, M.I.; Martin, J.D.R.; Aloman, C.; Schiano, T.D. Hemophagocytic syndrome occurring in an adult liver transplant recipient having Still's disease. *Hepatol. Int.* **2010**, *5*, 597–602. [CrossRef]
27. Soyama, A.; Eguchi, S.; Takatsuki, M.; Hidaka, M.; Tomonaga, T.; Yamanouchi, K.; Miyazaki, K.; Inokuma, T.; Tajima, Y.; Kanematsu, T. Hemophagocytic syndrome after liver transplantation: Report of two cases. *Surg. Today* **2011**, *41*, 1524–1530. [CrossRef]
28. Rodríguez-Medina, B.; Blanes, M.; Vinaixa, C.; Aguilera, V.; Rubín, A.; Prieto, M.; Berenguer, M. Haemophagocytic syndrome in a liver transplant patient during treatment with Telaprevir. *Ann. Hepatol.* **2013**, *12*, 974–978. [CrossRef]
29. Jha, B.; Mohan, N.; Gajendra, S.; Sachdev, R.; Goel, S.; Sahni, T.; Raina, V.; Soin, A. Prompt diagnosis and management of Epstein-Barr virus-associated post-transplant lymphoproliferative disorder and hemophagocytosis: A dreaded complication in a post-liver transplant child. *Pediatr. Transplant.* **2015**, *19*, E177–E180. [CrossRef] [PubMed]
30. Vijgen, S.; Wyss, C.; Meylan, P.R.; Bisig, B.; Letovanec, I.; Manuel, O.; Pascual, M.; de Leval, L. Fatal Outcome of Multiple Clinical Presentations of Human Herpesvirus 8-related Disease after Solid Organ Transplantation. *Transplantation* **2016**, *100*, 134–140. [CrossRef]
31. Iseda, N.; Yoshizumi, T.; Toshima, T.; Morinaga, A.; Tomiyama, T.; Takahashi, J.; Motomura, T.; Mano, Y.; Itoh, S.; Harada, N.; et al. Hemophagocytic syndrome after living donor liver transplantation: A case report with a review of the literature. *Surg. Case Rep.* **2018**, *4*, 101. [CrossRef] [PubMed]
32. Cohen, G.M.; Langer, A.L.; Sima, H.; Chang, C.; Troy, K.; Taimur, S. Hemophagocytic Lymphohistiocytosis Due to Primary HHV-8 Infection in a Liver Transplant Recipient. *Transplant. Direct* **2018**, *4*, e411. [CrossRef] [PubMed]
33. Jarchin, L.; Chu, J.; Januska, M.; Merola, P.; Arnon, R. Autoimmune hemolytic anemia: An unusual presentation of hemophagocytic lymphohistiocytosis in a pediatric post-liver transplant patient. *Pediatr. Transplant.* **2018**, *22*, e13281. [CrossRef]
34. Valenzuela, E.F.; García, A.C.; García-Pajares, F.; Tejada, J.T.; Muñoz, R.N.; Martín, C.M.; Delgado, L.S.; Martín, C.A.; Álvarez, C.A.; Fernández-Fontecha, E.; et al. Hemophagocytic Syndrome as Uncommon Cause of Severe Pancytopenia after Liver Transplantation. *Transplant. Proc.* **2020**, *52*, 1500–1502. [CrossRef]
35. Yamada, M.; Sakamoto, S.; Sakamoto, K.; Uchida, H.; Shimizu, S.; Osumi, T.; Kato, M.; Shoji, K.; Arai, K.; Miyazaki, O.; et al. Fatal Epstein-Barr virus-associated hemophagocytic lymphohistiocytosis with virus-infected T cells after pediatric multivisceral transplantation: A proof-of-concept case report. *Pediatr. Transplant.* **2021**, *25*, e13961. [CrossRef] [PubMed]
36. Chesner, J.; Schiano, T.D.; Fiel, M.I.; Crismale, J.F. Hemophagocytic lymphohistiocytosis occurring after liver transplantation: A case series and review of the literature. *Clin. Transplant.* **2021**, *35*, e14392. [CrossRef]
37. Arikan, C.; Erbey, F.; Ozdogan, E.; Akyildiz, M. Posttransplant Hemophagocytic Lymphohistiocytosis in Pediatric Liver Transplant Recipients. *Liver Transpl.* **2021**, *27*, 1061–1065. [CrossRef] [PubMed]
38. Gandotra, A.; Mehtani, R.; Premkumar, M.; Duseja, A.; De, A.; Mallik, N.; Durgadevi, S.; Das, A.; Kalra, N. Invasive Pulmonary Aspergillosis and Tuberculosis Complicated by Hemophagocytic Lymphohistiocytosis—Sequelae of COVID-19 in a Liver Transplant Recipient. *J. Clin. Exp. Hepatol.* **2022**, *12*, 1007–1011. [CrossRef] [PubMed]
39. Nakajima, K.; Hiejima, E.; Nihira, H.; Kato, K.; Honda, Y.; Izawa, K.; Kawabata, N.; Kato, I.; Ogawa, E.; Sonoda, M.; et al. Case Report: A Case of Epstein-Barr Virus-Associated Acute Liver Failure Requiring Hematopoietic Cell Transplantation after Emergent Liver Transplantation. *Front. Immunol.* **2022**, *13*, 825806. [CrossRef]
40. Ferreira, G.D.S.A.; Moreira, M.L.; Watanabe, A.L.C.; Trevizoli, N.C.; Murta, M.C.B.; Figueira, A.V.F.; Caja, G.O.N.; Ferreira, C.A.; Jorge, F.M.F.; Couto, C.D.F. Hemophagocytic Lymphohistiocytosis Secondary to Tuberculosis after Liver Transplantation: A Case Report. *Transplant. Proc.* **2022**, *54*, 1384–1387. [CrossRef]
41. Zhang, L.; Zhou, J.; Sokol, L. Hereditary and acquired hemophagocytic lymphohistiocytosis. *Cancer Control* **2014**, *21*, 301–312. [CrossRef] [PubMed]

42. Scott, L.J.; McKeage, K.; Keam, S.J.; Plosker, G.L. Tacrolimus: A further update of its use in the management of organ transplantation. *Drugs* **2003**, *63*, 1247–1297. [CrossRef] [PubMed]
43. Fukaya, S.; Yasuda, S.; Hashimoto, T.; Oku, K.; Kataoka, H.; Horita, T.; Atsumi, T.; Koike, T. Clinical features of haemophagocytic syndrome in patients with systemic autoimmune diseases: Analysis of 30 cases. *Rheumatology* **2008**, *47*, 1686–1691. [CrossRef] [PubMed]
44. Karras, A.; Thervet, E.; Legendre, C. Groupe Cooperatif de transplantation d'Ile de F. Hemophagocytic syndrome in renal transplant recipients: Report of 17 cases and review of literature. *Transplantation* **2004**, *77*, 238–243. [CrossRef]
45. Jakafi. Highlights of Prescribing Information. US Food and Drug Administration. 2020. Available online: https://www.jakafi.com/pdf/prescribing-information.pdf (accessed on 23 October 2022).
46. Jordan, M.B.; Hildeman, D.; Kappler, J.; Marrack, P. An animal model of hemophagocytic lymphohistiocytosis (HLH): CD8+ T cells and interferon gamma are essential for the disorder. *Blood* **2004**, *104*, 735–743. [CrossRef]
47. Schmid, J.P.; Ho, C.-H.; Chrétien, F.; Lefebvre, J.M.; Pivert, G.; Kosco-Vilbois, M.; Ferlin, W.; Geissmann, F.; Fischer, A.; Basile, G.D.S. Neutralization of IFNgamma defeats haemophagocytosis in LCMV-infected perforin- and Rab27a-deficient mice. *EMBO Mol. Med.* **2009**, *1*, 112–124. [CrossRef]
48. Das, R.; Guan, P.; Sprague, L.; Verbist, K.; Tedrick, P.; An, Q.A.; Cheng, C.; Kurachi, M.; Levine, R.; Wherry, E.J.; et al. Janus kinase inhibition lessens inflammation and ameliorates disease in murine models of hemophagocytic lymphohistiocytosis. *Blood* **2016**, *127*, 1666–1675. [CrossRef]
49. Verstovsek, S.; Mesa, R.A.; Gotlib, J.; Levy, R.S.; Gupta, V.; DiPersio, J.F.; Catalano, J.V.; Deininger, M.; Miller, C.; Silver, R.T.; et al. A double-blind, placebo-controlled trial of ruxolitinib for myelofibrosis. *N. Engl. J. Med.* **2012**, *366*, 799–807. [CrossRef]
50. Zeiser, R.; von Bubnoff, N.; Butler, J.; Mohty, M.; Niederwieser, D.; Or, R.; Szer, J.; Wagner, E.M.; Zuckerman, T.; Mahuzier, B.; et al. Ruxolitinib for Glucocorticoid-Refractory Acute Graft-versus-Host Disease. *N. Engl. J. Med.* **2020**, *382*, 1800–1810. [CrossRef]
51. Deyà-Martínez, A.; Rivière, J.G.; Roxo-Junior, P.; Ramakers, J.; Bloomfield, M.; Hernandez, P.G.; Lobo, P.B.; Abu Jamra, S.R.; Esteve-Sole, A.; Kanderova, V.; et al. Impact of JAK Inhibitors in Pediatric Patients with STAT1 Gain of Function (GOF) Mutations-10 Children and Review of the Literature. *J. Clin. Immunol.* **2022**, *42*, 1071–1082. [CrossRef]
52. Redondo, S.; Esquirol, A.; Novelli, S.; Caballero, A.C.; Garrido, A.; Oñate, G.; López, J.; Moreno, C.; Saavedra, S.-D.; Granell, M.; et al. Efficacy and Safety of Ruxolitinib in Steroid-Refractory/Dependent Chronic Graft-versus-Host Disease: Real-World Data and Challenges. *Transplant. Cell. Ther.* **2021**, *28*, 43.e1–43.e5. [CrossRef] [PubMed]
53. Shi, J.G.; Chen, X.; Emm, T.; Scherle, P.A.; McGee, R.F.; Lo, Y.; Landman, R.R.; McKeever, E.G.; Punwani, N.G.; Williams, W.V.; et al. The effect of CYP3A4 inhibition or induction on the pharmacokinetics and pharmacodynamics of orally administered ruxolitinib (INCB018424 phosphate) in healthy volunteers. *J. Clin. Pharmacol.* **2012**, *52*, 809–818. [CrossRef] [PubMed]
54. van Gelder, T. Drug interactions with tacrolimus. *Drug Saf.* **2002**, *25*, 707–712. [CrossRef] [PubMed]
55. Wang, H.; Gu, J.; Liang, X.; Mao, X.; Wang, Z.; Huang, W. Low dose ruxolitinib plus HLH-94 protocol: A potential choice for secondary HLH. *Semin. Hematol.* **2020**, *57*, 26–30. [CrossRef]

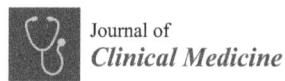

Article

Clinical Outcome of Resected Non-Ampullary Duodenal Adenocarcinoma: A Single Center Experience

Soo Yeun Lim [1,†], Dong Il Chung [2,†], Hye Jeong Jeong [1], Hyun Jeong Jeon [1], So Jeong Yoon [1], Hongbeom Kim [1], In Woong Han [1], Jin Seok Heo [1] and Sang Hyun Shin [1,*]

[1] Division of Hepatobiliary-Pancreatic Surgery, Department of Surgery, Samsung Medical Center, Sungkyunkwan University School of Medicine, Seoul 06351, Republic of Korea
[2] Department of Medicine, Sungkyunkwan University School of Medicine, Suwon 16419, Republic of Korea
* Correspondence: surgeonssh@skku.edu; Tel.: +82-2-3410-6980
† These authors equally contributed to this work.

Abstract: (1) Background: This study identified the clinical outcome and prognostic factors of resected non-ampullary duodenal adenocarcinoma (NADA) in a single tertiary cancer center. (2) Methods: The medical records of 109 patients with NADA who underwent curative surgery between 2000 and 2018 were reviewed retrospectively. (3) Results: The mean age was 62.4 years with a male predominance (70.6%). The majority of tumors were located at the 2nd portion (58.7%). Fifty-seven patients (52.3%) had symptoms at diagnosis. CA19-9 was elevated in 32 patients (29.4%). Of this cohort, most patients were diagnosed as stage III (64.2%). The median overall survival was 92.9 months, and the 1-, 3-, and 5-year survival rates were 84.4%, 71.6%, and 53.7%, respectively. In univariate and multivariate analysis, age, symptoms, CA19-9, and margin status were associated with overall survival and symptoms, CA19-9 and margin status were also associated with recurrence. When correlating symptoms with stages, patients with symptoms at diagnosis had more advanced stages (all $p < 0.001$). (4) Conclusion: Old age, elevated CA19-9, symptoms, and margin status were independent prognostic factors of NADA, and the patients with symptoms at diagnosis tend to have more advanced stages and a poor prognosis.

Keywords: duodenal cancer; non-ampullary duodenal cancer; clinical outcome

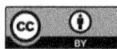

1. Introduction

Tumors arising in the non-ampullary parts of the duodenum are considered genuine duodenal cancer. These non-ampullary duodenal adenocarcinomas (NADA) are uncommon, representing less than 0.5% of gastrointestinal malignancies and constitute approximately 45% of small bowel adenocarcinomas (SBA) [1]. The analysis of NADA is frequently combined with other periampullary cancers originating from pancreatic, small bowel, and distal bile duct cancers, which leads to the absence of studies concerning the sole clinicopathologic characteristics and incidence of NADA [2]. In addition, various pathological factors such as lymph node metastasis, the positive resection margin, and cellular differentiation have been known to be prognostic factors; however, results are inconsistent throughout various studies likely due to small sample size, different standards, and misclassifications [3].

Recently, a study in Japan has observed a rising prevalence and a higher risk of NADA in Asia than in western countries, implying a high clinical relevance of this cancer as a potentially important area for research [4]. Approximately 40–60% of NADA are asymptomatic which leads to late detection. Therefore, duodenal cancers are detected at a far-advanced stage, making it the poorest prognosis among all small intestine cancers [5]. However, early detection through endoscopy and endoscopic mucosal resection of superficial non-ampullary duodenal epithelial tumor (early stage of NADA) has led to favorable outcomes indicating the importance of surveillance by esophagogastroduodenoscopies during routine checkups [6]. Identification of the risk factors associated with NADA, especially among South Koreans, will provide a framework for risk stratification that can be used in screening tests [7].

This single center retrospective study was conducted to determine the natural history of patients with operatively managed NADA. The study attempts to identify the clinical course and prognostic factors of NADA.

2. Materials and Methods

2.1. Study Design and Population

This retrospective study included patients who underwent surgery for NADA, with a curative intention, at the Samsung Medical Center (Seoul, South Korea) between January 2000 and December 2019. The inclusion criteria were defined as follows: (1) histologically diagnosed as adenocarcinoma by surgical biopsy; (2) tumor located at non-ampullary duodenum; and (3) no distant organ metastasis. This study protocol was approved by the Institutional Review Board of the Samsung Medical Center Sungkyunkwan University School of Medicine, Seoul, Korea, for clinical research [Registration No.: 2022-06-157-001]. This study was conducted in accordance with the ethical principles of the Declaration of Helsinki (1989).

Medical records including clinicopathologic, postoperative, and survival data were investigated retrospectively and outcomes of patients with survival and recurrence were also reviewed from the Samsung Medical Center Hepatobiliary-pancreas database in Seoul, South Korea. The following clinicopathologic parameters were collected: patient characteristics: gender, age, comorbidity (cardiovascular, pulmonary, and endocrine disease), presenting with symptoms at diagnosis, preoperative tumor markers (carcinoembryonic antigen [CEA], and carbohydrate antigen 19-9 [CA19-9]); pathologic findings: T stage, N stage, TNM stage according to the AJCC 8th edition, cellular differentiation, primary location, margin status, lympho-vascular invasion, perineural invasion; perioperative findings: operation name and adjuvant therapy; postoperative complication: a complication as defined by the Clavien–Dindo classification system [8], surgical site infection, intraabdominal abscess, pneumonia, acute kidney injury, biliary fistula, chylous ascites, postoperative pancreatic fistula (POPF), delayed gastric emptying (DGE), and postoperative hemorrhage. The follow-up duration was measured from the time of surgery until death or the last visit to the outpatient department.

2.2. Statistical Analysis

The student's t test was used to compare continuous variables. The x^2 test and Fisher's exact were used to compare categorical variables. All continuous variables are summarized as median (SD) and all categorical variables are reported as frequencies (percentages). Overall survival (OS) and disease free survival (DFS) were estimated by the Kaplan–Meier method and the log-rank test was used for univariable survival analysis. Multivariable analysis of independent prognostic factors for OS and DFS was identified by using the Cox proportional hazard model. All tests were two-sided and a p-value under 0.1 was considered statistically significant. All statistical analyses were performed using the SPSS 27 version (IBM, New York, NY, USA).

3. Results

3.1. Demographic and Clinicopathologic Characteristics

Tables 1 and 2 summarize the demographic and clinicopathological characteristics of patients. Of the 109 patients, the mean age was 62.4 ± 10 years with a male predominance (70.6%). The presence of symptoms at diagnosis, found in 57 patients (52.3%), included: weight loss, jaundice, projectile vomiting, abdominal pain, melena, and hematochezia. CA19-9 was elevated in 32 patients (29.4%). The 2nd portion of the duodenum was the most common location of NADA (57.7%), followed by the 1st portion (11%). The mean tumor diameter was 3.7 ± 1.8 cm. Pancreatoduodenectomy (PD) or pylorus preserving pancreatoduodenectomy (PPPD) was performed in 96 patients (88.1%), duodenal segmental resection in five patients (4.6%), and a subtotal gastrectomy in seven patients (6.4%). Only one patient underwent a total pancreatectomy due to severe pancreatitis. The pathologic depth of the tumors was: T1 in 11 patients (10.1%), T2 in six patients (5.5%), T3 in 46 patients (42.2%), and T4 in 46 patients (42.2%). Seventy patients (69.7%) had lymph node metastasis. More than half of the patients were diagnosed with TNM stage III (64.2%). The majority of patients underwent R0 resection (94.5%) and 48 patients (44%) received adjuvant therapy following surgery. The Figure 1 shows illustration of duodenal adenocarcinoma.

Table 1. Demographic and clinical characteristics ($n = 109$).

Characteristics		N (%) or Mean (±SD)
Age		62.4 (±10.7)
Sex	Male	77 (70.6)
	Female	32 (29.4)
Comorbidity		
Cardiovascular	No	77 (70.6)
	Yes	32 (29.4)
Pulmonary	No	103 (94.5)
	Yes	6 (5.5)
Endocrine	No	90 (82.6)
	Yes	19 (17.4)
Symptom [†]	Asymptomatic	52 (47.7)
	Symptomatic	57 (52.3)
Preoperative Lab		
CEA	Normal	80 (73.4)
	Elevated	12 (11.0)
	NA	17 (15.6)
CA19-9	Normal	67 (61.5)
	Elevated	32 (29.4)
	NA	10 (9.2)
Location	1st portion	12 (11.0)
	1st–2nd portion	9 (8.3)
	2nd portion	64 (58.7)
	2nd–3rd portion	9 (8.3)
	3rd portion	10 (9.2)
	3rd–4th portion	3 (2.8)
	4th portion	2 (1.8)
Tumor size		3.7 (±1.8)
Operation name	PD/PPPD	96 (88.1)
	Duodenum Segmental resection	5 (4.6)
	Subtotal gastrectomy	7 (6.4)
	Total pancreatectomy	1 (0.9)
Combined organ resection	No	93 (85.3)
	Yes	16 (14.7)
Adjuvant therapy	No	61 (56.0)
	Yes	48 (44.0)

[†] Symptoms include jaundice, weight loss, abdominal pain, and projectile vomiting. SD, standard deviation; NA, not available; PD/PPPD, pancreaticoduodenectomy/pylorus-preserving pancreaticoduodenectomy.

3.2. Survival and Recurrence Pattern of NADA

The survival and recurrence rates by Kaplan–Meier survival curves are shown in Figure 2. The median overall survival after surgery was 92.9 months. Overall survival rates at 1-, 2-, and 5-years were 84.4%, 71.6%, and 53.7% respectively. Recurrence developed in 55 patients (50.5%) during follow-up and the median DFS was 20.9 months. The estimated 1-, 2-, and 5-years DFS rates were 57.5%, 47.4%, and 42.7%, respectively. Figure 3 shows survival comparisons according to TNM stage, symptoms at diagnosis, and level of CA19-9. Stage I showed the best prognosis with statistical significance ($p = 0.04$ for I versus IIA, 0.009 for I versus IIIA, and 0.002 for I versus IIIB in Figure 3A). Patients with symptoms (Figure 3B) and elevated CA19-9 (Figure 3C) showed poorer survival ($p = 0.001$ and <0.001, respectively).

Table 2. Pathological characteristics ($n = 109$).

Characteristics		N (%) or Mean (±SD)
T stage	T1a	3 (2.8)
	T1b	8 (7.3)
	T2	6 (5.5)
	T3	46 (42.2)
	T4	46 (42.2)
N stage	N0	39 (35.8)
	N1	37 (33.9)
	N2	33 (30.3)
TNM staging	I	14 (12.8)
	IIA	16 (14.7)
	IIB	9 (8.3)
	IIIA	37 (33.9)
	IIIB	33 (30.3)
Differentiation	Well	18 (16.5)
	Moderate	66 (60.6)
	Poor	25 (22.9)
Margin status	R0	103 (94.5)
	R1	6 (5.5)
Lymphovascular invasion	No	17 (15.6)
	Yes	30 (27.5)
	NA	62 (56.9)
Perineural invasion	No	18 (16.5)
	Yes	22 (20.2)
	NA	69 (63.3)

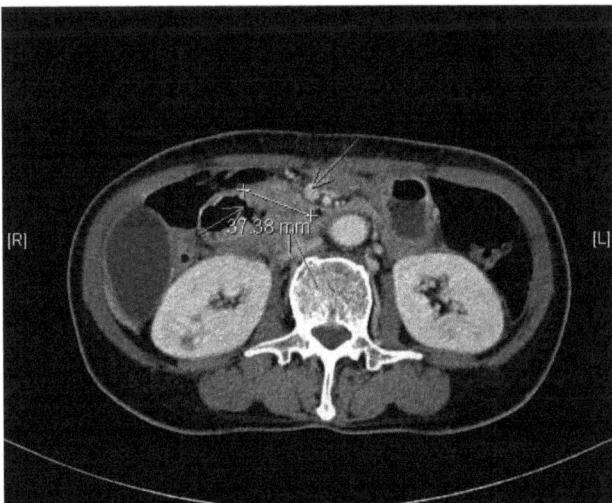

Figure 1. Illustration of non-ampullary duodenal adenocarcinoma. The green arrows indicate the duodenal adenocarcinoma from a 57 years old female patient, about 37 mm size tumor.

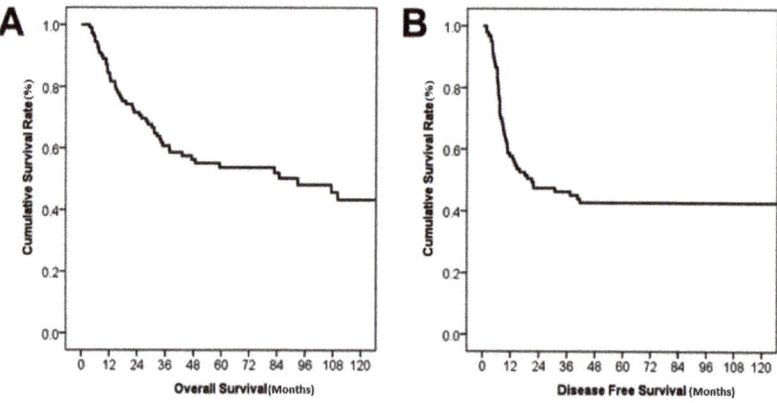

Figure 2. Kaplan–Meier survival curves of overall survival and disease free survival (n = 109). (**A**) The median overall survival was 92.9 months, and the estimated 1-, 2-, and 5-year survival rates were 84.4%, 71.6%, and 53.7%, respectively. (**B**) The median disease free survival was 20.9 months, and the estimated 1-, 2-, and 5-year disease free survival rates were 57.7%, 47.4%, and 42.7%, respectively.

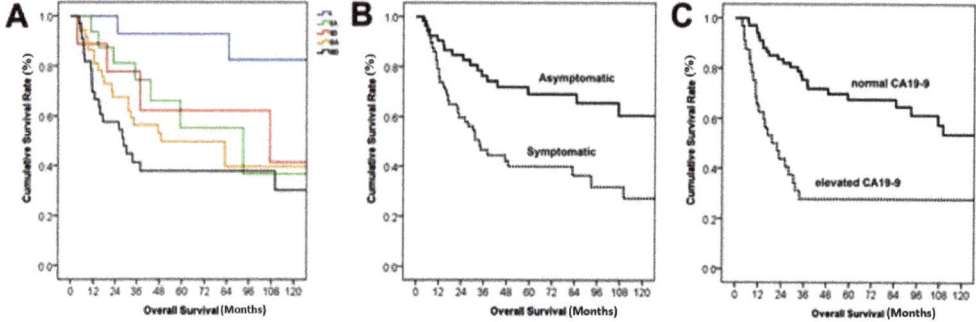

Figure 3. Kaplan–Meier survival curves of survival comparison according to TNM staging, symptoms, and levels of CA19-9. (**A**) In survival comparison according to the American Joint Committee of Cancer staging system, p values were 0.04 for I versus IIA, 0.009 for I versus IIIA, and 0.002 for I versus IIIB. The others were not statistically significant. (**B**) The median survival was not reached in asymptomatic patients (n = 52), and the median survival of symptomatic patients (n = 57) was 33.7 months (p = 0.001). (**C**) The median survival was not reached in patients with normal CA19-9, and the median survival of patients with elevated CA19-9 was 19.1 months (p < 0.001).

3.3. Uni- and Multivariate Analysis Affecting Survival

A multivariate analysis also showed that symptoms at diagnosis (hazard ratio [HR] 2.354, 95% confidence interval [CI] 1.236 to 4.486) and elevated CA19-9 (HR 2.821, 95% CI 1.555 to 5.117) were independent prognosis factors (Table 3). In addition, old age and margin status were other prognosis factors used in the multivariate analysis (HR 1.048, 95% CI 1.016 to 1.082 and HR 2.763, 95% CI 1.049 to 7.279, respectively). Moreover, a multivariate analysis for patients' recurrence showed that symptoms at diagnosis in Table 4 (HR 3.720, 95% CI 1.807 to 7.657), elevated CA19-9 (HR 3.166, 95% CI 1.761 to 5.692), and Margin status (HR 3.447, 95% CI 1.174 to 10.124) were also independent prognostic factors.

Table 3. Uni- and multivariate analysis identifying factors affecting patients' survival (n = 109).

Factors		Median Survival (mo)	Univariate Analysis Hazard Ratio	p	Multivariate Analysis Hazard Ratio	p
Age			1.029 (1.002–1.058)	0.035	1.048 (1.016–1.082)	0.003
Sex	Male	107.3	Reference			
	Female	48.8	1.115 (0.620–2.006)	0.716		
Symptoms [†]	Asymptomatic	Not reached	Reference		Reference	
	Symptomatic	33.7	2.577 (1.443–4.603)	0.001	2.354 (1.236–4.486)	0.009
CEA	Normal	92.9	Reference			
	Elevated	Not reached	0.979 (0.385–2.489)	0.965		
CA19-9	Normal	Not reached	Reference		Reference	
	Elevated	19.1	3.298 (1.850–5.879)	<0.001	2.821 (1.555–5.117)	0.001
TNM Stage	I	Not reached	Reference		Reference	
	IIA	92.9	3.984 (0.825–19.247)	0.085	3.003 (0.568–15.879)	0.196
	IIB	107.3	4.357 (0.797–23.823)	0.090	5.140 (0.902–29.284)	0.065
	IIIA	48.8	5.541 (1.283–23.934)	0.022	1.433 (0.259–7.918)	0.680
	IIIB	28.7	7.692 (1.798–32.905)	0.006	2.409 (0.467–12.440)	0.294
Tumor size			1.033 (0.894–1.194)	0.661		
Combined resection	No	107.3	Reference			
	Yes	31.3	1.623 (0.835–3.158)	0.153		
Location	1st–2nd portion	82.9	Reference			
	3rd–4th portion	92.9	0.842 (0.422–1.679)	0.625		
Margin status	R0	107.3	Reference		Reference	
	R1	7.0	3.966 (1.562–10.073)	0.004	2.763 (1.049–7.279)	0.040
Differentiation	Well	Not reached	Reference		Reference	
	Moderate	59.2	2.510 (0.978–6.440)	0.056	1.483 (0.404–5.436)	0.553
	Poor	34.9	2.679 (0.964–7.447)	0.059	2.825 (0.714–11.174)	0.139
Adjuvant therapy	No	85.0	Reference			
	Yes	Not reached	0.885 (0.508–1.541)	0.666		

[†] Symptoms include jaundice, weight loss, abdominal pain, and projectile vomiting.

Table 4. Uni- and multivariate analysis identifying factors affecting patients' recurrence (n = 109).

Factors		Median DFS (mo)	Univariate Analysis Hazard Ratio	p	Multivariate Analysis Hazard Ratio	p
Age			1.005 (0.979–1.031)	0.719		
Sex	Male	19.1	Reference			
	Female	20.9	0.906 (0.519–1.579)	0.727		
Symptoms [†]	Asymptomatic	Not reached	Reference		Reference	
	Symptomatic	8.7	5.684 (2.972–10.870)	<0.001	3.720 (1.807–7.657)	<0.001
CEA	Normal	30.8	Reference			
	Elevated	6.2	1.152 (0.454–2.922)	0.965		
CA19-9	Normal	Not reached	Reference		Reference	
	Elevated	6.7	3.089 (1.764–5.410)	<0.001	3.166 (1.761–5.692)	<0.001
TNM Stage	I	Not reached	Reference			
	IIA	41.4	8.773 (1.096–70.200)	0.041		
	IIB	Not reached	3.955 (0.358–43.648)	0.262		
	IIIA	10.5	14.469 (1.950–107.357)	0.009		
	IIIB	8.9	19.378 (2.601–144.347)	0.004		
Tumor size			1.077 (0.941–1.233)	0.279		
Combined resection	No	20.9	Reference			

Table 4. Cont.

Factors		Median DFS (mo)	Univariate Analysis		Multivariate Analysis	
			Hazard Ratio	p	Hazard Ratio	p
Location	Yes	18.0	1.174 (0.555–2.486)	0.674		
	1st–2nd portion	18.0	Reference			
	3rd–4th portion	41.4	0.724 (0.426–1.596)	0.566		
Margin status	R0	21.6	Reference		Reference	
	R1	4.2	4.003 (1.439–11.132)	0.008	3.447 (1.174–10.124)	0.024
Differentiation	Well	Not reached	Reference		Reference	
	Moderate	10.7	4.952 (1.523–16.102)	0.008	1.761 (0.482–6.442)	0.392
	Poor	14.0	5.376 (1.555–18.591)	0.008	2.264 (0.592–8.649)	0.232
Adjuvant therapy	No	Not reached	Reference			
	Yes	11.6	1.539 (0.900–2.632)	0.115		

[†] Symptoms include jaundice, weight loss, abdominal pain, and projectile vomiting.

3.4. Postoperative Outcomes

In terms of postoperative outcomes (Table 5), the median hospital stay was 15.9 days, ranging from 9 to 105 days. Major complications, with a Clavien–Dindo grade over 3, account for 11.0% of patients. Forty-seven patients had POPF (43.1%), 17 patients had a DGE (15.6%), and six patients had a postoperative hemorrhage (5.5%).

Table 5. Postoperative outcomes.

Factors	N (%) or Mean (±SD)
Hospital stay	15.9 (±12.4)
Complication [†]	
Major complication [‡]	12 (11.0)
Surgical site infection	2 (1.8)
Intraabdominal abscess	2 (1.8)
Pneumonia	2 (1.8)
Acute kidney injury	1 (0.9)
Biliary fistula	1 (0.9)
Chylous ascites	9 (8.3)
POPF	47 (43.1)
Delayed gastric emptying	17 (15.6)
Postoperative hemorrhage	6 (5.5)

[†] Complication cases are duplicated. [‡] Major complication indicated Clavien–Dindo grade ≥ 3. SD, standard deviation; POPF, postoperative pancreatic fistula.

3.5. Relationship between Symptoms at Diagnosis and Tumor Stages

Table 6 shows the relationship between the presence of symptoms at diagnosis and tumor stages. The symptomatic group showed a higher T stage ($p < 0.001$) and N stage ($p < 0.001$) with statistical significance. Consequently, the TNM stage was also higher in the symptomatic group ($p < 0.001$).

Table 6. Correlations between symptoms and tumor stages ($n = 109$).

Factors	Asymptomatic (%)	Symptomatic (%)	p
T stage			<0.001
T1a	3 (5.8)	0 (0.0)	
T1b	8 (15.4)	0 (0.0)	
T2	6 (11.5)	0 (0.0)	
T3	19 (36.5)	27 (47.4)	
T4	16 (30.8)	30 (52.6)	
N stage			<0.001
N0	34 (65.4)	5 (8.8)	
N1	8 (15.4)	29 (50.9)	
N2	10 (19.2)	23 (40.4)	
TNM stage			<0.001
I	14 (26.9)	0 (0.0)	
IIA	11 (21.2)	5 (8.8)	
IIB	9 (17.3)	0 (0.0)	
IIIA	8 (15.4)	29 (50.9)	
IIIB	10 (19.2)	23 (40.4)	

4. Discussion

In this single center, retrospective study, we enrolled more than 100 duodenal adenocarcinoma patients that received curative surgery over the course of 20 years and investigated these cases in detail. Although there have been several large-scale multi-center studies involving data from the registered database, most previous studies suffer from selection bias as they choose not to distinguish between non-ampullary duodenal adenocarcinomas and periampullary cancers such as pancreatic, small bowel, and distal bile duct cancers [2]. Most non-ampullary duodenal cancer remains asymptomatic until a far-advanced stage, leading to its poor prognosis and high clinical relevance. Moreover, the fact that previous studies show that early detection through surveillance using esophagogastroduodenoscopies and endoscopic mucosal resection leads to favorable outcomes, implies the necessity of specified research [6,9–11]. We expect our single center study to have a lower risk of selection bias and our findings to likely reflect the sole clinicopathologic characteristics of non-ampullary duodenal adenocarcinomas and present the associated risk factors that may indicate the need for screening tests.

This study revealed that old age, CA19-9, and symptoms at diagnosis were prognostic factors for the survival of NADA after surgery. Previous retrospective studies reported various possible prognostic factors including CA19-9, gross appearance, tumor size, tumor invasion, lymph node metastases, TNM stage, lymphovascular invasion, perineural invasion, positive margin, poor differentiation, tumor markers (CEA and CA19-9), high lactate dehydrogenase, symptoms at diagnosis, and old age [10–13]. Our study results were similar to previous reports, however our findings also identified the tendency to have advanced T, N, and TNM stages when patients have symptoms at diagnosis, although these parameters were not found to be independent risk factors.

4.1. Incidence and Current Treatment of NADA

NADA, though it accounts for half of all SBA, showed a rate of 3.7 to 5.4 cases per 1 million persons per year, which is relatively rare [1]. The etiology of SBA including NADA is unknown. There are several theories, among which the theory that digestive contents cause irritation to the mucosa while passing through the intestine corresponds to both the facts that 2/3 of SBA occurs in duodenum and the SBA is rare compared to the large intestine [14]. NADA is a more common disease in men, accounting for a 2.4 times higher rate than females in this study. The difference in the ratio between men and women shows similar results to those of a study published in Japan, which showed a 1.7 times higher occurrence in males [4,10,14]. However, racial difference should also be considered as a study from a European population, little difference was observed between the male and female population and the occurrence of NADA. Regardless of race, the development of NADA was a common risk factor in the over 60s, at approximately 55%, and an increase in incidence with age was also observed in the multi-analysis results from this study. Hirashita et al. (2018) reported that 56% of tumors are most commonly located in the descending portion of the duodenum. This study showed a similar result, that 58.7% of the tumors were located in the 2nd portion of the duodenum [10]. The curative surgical procedures for NADA are various and depend on the tumor location. As shown in the previous results, the 2nd portion of the duodenum accounts for the largest proportion, therefore PPPD is the main surgical treatment [2,13]. The choice of surgical procedure for NADA occurring in the 3rd and 4th portion of the duodenum, is a controversial matter. Based on previous findings that lymph node metastasis and lymphovascular invasion are possible prognostic factors of disease recurrence and survival, some reports suggest that segmental resection could be an unsuitable treatment modality as it results in insufficient lymph node dissection compared to PPPD. Several studies found that for the early stage of NADA, local resection offered less morbidity, less mortality, and had a similar oncological benefit compared to PPPD [1,3,13,15,16]. From this study, it was not possible to make any conclusion regarding the links between significant survival benefits and tumor location, since only 15 patients had a tumor located in the 3rd and 4th portion. It is difficult to draw conclusions as to which operative procedure is the safest, most effective, and still provides an adequate surgical margin and minimal invasiveness. Therefore, further study is needed.

Even after surgery, there is a lack of a well-established adjuvant chemotherapy regimen and protocol. Haan et al. (2012) reported that SBA has a similar immunophenotypic pattern, molecular characteristics, and genome-wide DNA copy number aberrations with colorectal cancer. Consequently, many clinicians have applied the chemotherapy regimen used for colorectal cancer, to SBA, including NADA [2,17]. A combination of fluoropyrimidine and oxaliplatin (FOLFOX or CAPOX) is commonly utilized as an effective first line chemotherapy regimen for SBA, followed by an alternative front line combination of 5-FU and cisplatin or fluoropyrimidine and irinotecan (FLOFIRI) [2]. Adjuvant therapy, received by 44% of the total patients in this study was not a statistically significant factor for OS. This result was contradictory to the results of previous studies [2,5]. Due to its rarity, a large-scale investigation focusing on adjuvant therapy and its survival outcome will be a necessity in the future. As the lack of established principle of adjuvant therapy and prevention, periodic regular checkup is inevitably more emphasized as a prevention for NADA.

4.2. CA19-9 as a Prognostic Factor

Serum CA19-9 is a carbohydrate antigen expressed in tissue as a monosialoganglioside and a mucous protein. It is widely used as a biomarker for biliopancreatic malignancies, treatment response monitoring, and a marker of recurrence for pancreatic cancer. Elevated CA19-9 can be found not only in the detection of cancer, but also in a number of benign diseases including pancreatitis, cholestasis, acute hepatitis, chronic liver disease, diabetes mellitus, intestinal pulmonary disease, and even collagen vascular disease. Ventrucci et al. (2009) reported a possible mechanism for the elevation of serum CA19-9 with various benign diseases, especially those related to obstructive jaundice. In obstructive jaundice, CA19-9 can be overproduced by irritated bile duct cells and inflammatory proliferation of epithelial cells. Even accumulation of CA19-9 in the biliary tract can exacerbate the reflux of blood and bile into the circulation. Therefore, clearance of the biliary mucin decreases, making both the hepatic function and the ability to degrade the antigen decreased sequentially [9,18,19]. An elevated level of CA19-9 is associated with low survival of NADA, indicating that as the severity of the disease increases, NADA could cause obstructive jaundice by forming a mass effect that compresses the surrounding tissues.

4.3. Correlation with Symptoms and Tumor Stages in NADA

This study discovered that symptomatic patients had advanced stage NADA compared to non-symptomatic patients. Sakae et al. (2017) presented the common symptoms of small bowel cancer as stenosis-related such as abdominal pain or vomiting, and bleeding related such as melena or hematemesis [5]. The symptoms reported in this study are also consistent with these previous findings, including the presence of jaundice. Another study reported that early SBA patients rarely have stenosis-related symptoms because the products in the small intestine are mostly liquid [14,17]. We discovered that tumors with an advanced TNM stage result in the presentation of symptoms at diagnosis. Because many cases are asymptomatic until they reach the advanced stages of disease, early detection is delayed which results in a poorer disease prognosis. Therefore, this study emphasizes the importance of the early detection of asymptomatic NADA patients. A health checkup through esophagogastroduodenoscopy, which is already applied to adults over the age of 40, is a possible screening method, though there is a limit that the range of screening can only include up to 1st and 2nd portions of the duodenum. In addition, computerized tomography may be used as a screening method, however, considering the low incidence of disease and the cost values involved, discussion is inevitable regarding its use.

4.4. Limitation

Further limitations regarding this study include; first, this study is designed to be a retrospective study which has low statistical power. Second, almost half of the patients were presenting with symptoms at the first diagnosis. Additionally, the incidence of advanced TNM stage in patients was 64.2% of the total patients. Since the study was conducted at a large tertiary hospital, it is possible that the proportion of severely ill patients was high. Despite the several limitations, the strength of this study is that it confirmed the current clinical status for NADA, which is a rare but relatively common in Asia, and addressed the importance of early detection and appropriate surgical resection including the extent of lymph node dissection.

5. Conclusions

In conclusion, our study conducted a solitary data analysis of NADA clinical outcome and discovered that symptoms at diagnosis, aging, high CA19-9, and resection margin positive are independent prognostic factors for NADA. Patients with symptoms at diagnosis show an advanced TNM stage of NADA.

Author Contributions: Conceptualization, S.Y.L., D.I.C. and S.H.S.; methodology, S.Y.L., D.I.C. and S.H.S.; software, S.Y.L., D.I.C. and S.H.S.; validation, S.Y.L., D.I.C., H.J.J. (Hye Jeong Jeong), H.J.J. (Hyun Jeong Jeon), S.J.Y., H.K., I.W.H., J.S.H. and S.H.S.; formal analysis, S.Y.L., D.IC. and S.H.S.; investigation, S.Y.L., D.I.C., H.J.J. (Hye Jeong Jeong), H.J.J. (Hyun Jeong Jeon), S.J.Y. and S.H.S.; resources, S.Y.L., D.I.C., H.J.J. (Hye Jeong Jeong), H.J.J. (Hyun Jeong Jeon), S.J.Y., H.K., I.W.H., J.S.H. and S.H.S.; data curation, S.Y.L., D.I.C., H.J.J. (Hye Jeong Jeong), H.J.J. (Hyun Jeong Jeon), S.J.Y. and S.H.S.; writing—original draft preparation, S.Y.L., D.I.C. and S.H.S.; writing—review and editing, S.Y.L., D.I.C., H.J.J. (Hye Jeong Jeong), H.J.J. (Hyun Jeong Jeon), S.J.Y., H.K., I.W.H., J.S.H. and S.H.S.; visualization, S.Y.L., D.I.C. and S.H.S.; supervision, S.Y.L., D.I.C. and S.H.S.; project administration, S.Y.L., D.I.C. and S.H.S.; All authors have read and agreed to the published version of the manuscript.

Funding: This research received no external funding.

Institutional Review Board Statement: The study was conducted in accordance with the Declaration of Helsinki, and approved by the Institutional Review Board of the Samsung Medical Center Sungkyunkwan University School of Medicine, Seoul, Korea (Registration No.: 2022-06-157-001, 7 July 2022).

Informed Consent Statement: Not applicable.

Data Availability Statement: Not applicable.

Conflicts of Interest: The authors declare no conflict of interest.

References

1. Struck, A.; Howard, T.; Chiorean, E.G.; Clarke, J.M.; Riffenburgh, R.; Cardenes, H.R. Non-ampullary duodenal adenocarcinoma: Factors important for relapse and survival. *J. Surg. Oncol.* **2009**, *100*, 144–148. [CrossRef] [PubMed]
2. Moati, E.; Overman, M.J.; Zaanan, A. Therapeutic Strategies for Patients with Advanced Small Bowel Adenocarcinoma: Current Knowledge and Perspectives. *Cancers* **2022**, *14*, 1137. [CrossRef] [PubMed]
3. Sun, H.; Liu, Y.; Lv, L.; Li, J.; Liao, X.; Gong, W. Prognostic Factors and Clinical Characteristics of Duodenal Adenocarcinoma With Survival: A Retrospective Study. *Front. Oncol.* **2021**, *11*, 795891. [CrossRef] [PubMed]
4. Yoshida, M.; Yabuuchi, Y.; Kakushima, N.; Kato, M.; Iguchi, M.; Yamamoto, Y.; Kanetaka, K.; Uraoka, T.; Fujishiro, M.; Sho, M. The incidence of non-ampullary duodenal cancer in Japan: The first analysis of a national cancer registry. *J. Gastroenterol. Hepatol.* **2021**, *36*, 1216–1221. [CrossRef] [PubMed]
5. Sakae, H.; Kanzaki, H.; Nasu, J.; Akimoto, Y.; Matsueda, K.; Yoshioka, M.; Nakagawa, M.; Hori, S.; Inoue, M.; Inaba, T. The characteristics and outcomes of small bowel adenocarcinoma: A multicentre retrospective observational study. *Br. J. Cancer* **2017**, *117*, 1607–1613. [CrossRef] [PubMed]
6. Hara, Y.; Goda, K.; Dobashi, A.; Ohya, T.R.; Kato, M.; Sumiyama, K.; Mitsuishi, T.; Hirooka, S.; Ikegami, M.; Tajiri, H. Short-and long-term outcomes of endoscopically treated superficial non-ampullary duodenal epithelial tumors. *World J. Gastroenterol.* **2019**, *25*, 707. [CrossRef] [PubMed]
7. Yabuuchi, Y.; Yoshida, M.; Kakushima, N.; Kato, M.; Iguchi, M.; Yamamoto, Y.; Kanetaka, K.; Uraoka, T.; Fujishiro, M.; Sho, M. Risk factors for non-ampullary duodenal adenocarcinoma: A systematic review. *Dig. Dis.* **2022**, *40*, 147–155. [CrossRef] [PubMed]
8. Clavien, P.A.; Barkun, J.; De Oliveira, M.L.; Vauthey, J.N.; Dindo, D.; Schulick, R.D.; De Santibañes, E.; Pekolj, J.; Slankamenac, K.; Bassi, C. The Clavien-Dindo classification of surgical complications: Five-year experience. *Ann. Surg.* **2009**, *250*, 187–196. [CrossRef] [PubMed]
9. Ventrucci, M.; Pozzato, P.; Cipolla, A.; Uomo, G. Persistent elevation of serum CA 19-9 with no evidence of malignant disease. *Dig. Liver Dis.* **2009**, *41*, 357–363. [CrossRef] [PubMed]
10. Hirashita, T.; Ohta, M.; Tada, K.; Saga, K.; Takayama, H.; Endo, Y.; Uchida, H.; Iwashita, Y.; Inomata, M. Prognostic factors of non-ampullary duodenal adenocarcinoma. *Jpn. J. Clin. Oncol.* **2018**, *48*, 743–747. [CrossRef] [PubMed]
11. Bakaeen, F.G.; Murr, M.M.; Sarr, M.G.; Thompson, G.B.; Farnell, M.B.; Nagorney, D.M.; Farley, D.R.; Van Heerden, J.A.; Wiersema, L.M.; Schleck, C.D. What prognostic factors are important in duodenal adenocarcinoma? *Arch. Surg.* **2000**, *135*, 635–642. [CrossRef] [PubMed]
12. Lee, H.G.; You, D.D.; Paik, K.Y.; Heo, J.S.; Choi, S.H.; Choi, D.W. Prognostic factors for primary duodenal adenocarcinoma. *World J. Surg.* **2008**, *32*, 2246–2252. [CrossRef] [PubMed]
13. Solaini, L.; Jamieson, N.; Metcalfe, M.; Abu Hilal, M.; Soonawalla, Z.; Davidson, B.; McKay, C.; Kocher, H.; UK Duodenal Cancer Study Group. Outcome after surgical resection for duodenal adenocarcinoma in the UK. *J. Br. Surg.* **2015**, *102*, 676–681. [CrossRef] [PubMed]
14. Talamonti, M.S.; Goetz, L.H.; Rao, S.; Joehl, R.J. Primary cancers of the small bowel: Analysis of prognostic factors and results of surgical management. *Arch. Surg.* **2002**, *137*, 564–571. [CrossRef] [PubMed]
15. Cloyd, J.M.; George, E.; Visser, B.C. Duodenal adenocarcinoma: Advances in diagnosis and surgical management. *World J. Gastrointest. Surg.* **2016**, *8*, 212. [CrossRef] [PubMed]
16. Kaklamanos, I.G.; Bathe, O.F.; Franceschi, D.; Camarda, C.; Levi, J.; Livingstone, A.S. Extent of resection in the management of duodenal adenocarcinoma. *Am. J. Surg.* **2000**, *179*, 37–41. [CrossRef] [PubMed]
17. Raghav, K.; Overman, M.J. Small bowel adenocarcinomas—Evolving paradigms and therapy options. *Nature Rev. Clin. Oncol.* **2013**, *10*, 534. [CrossRef]
18. Mann, D.; Edwards, R.; Ho, S.; Lau, W.; Glazer, G. Elevated tumour marker CA19-9: Clinical interpretation and influence of obstructive jaundice. *Eur. J. Surg. Oncol.* **2000**, *26*, 474–479. [CrossRef] [PubMed]
19. Marrelli, D.; Caruso, S.; Pedrazzani, C.; Neri, A.; Fernandes, E.; Marini, M.; Pinto, E.; Roviello, F. CA19-9 serum levels in obstructive jaundice: Clinical value in benign and malignant conditions. *Am. J. Surg.* **2009**, *198*, 333–339. [CrossRef] [PubMed]

Disclaimer/Publisher's Note: The statements, opinions and data contained in all publications are solely those of the individual author(s) and contributor(s) and not of MDPI and/or the editor(s). MDPI and/or the editor(s) disclaim responsibility for any injury to people or property resulting from any ideas, methods, instructions or products referred to in the content.

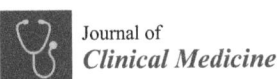

Article

Epidemiology of Inflammatory Bowel Diseases: A Population Study in a Healthcare District of North-West Italy

Gian Paolo Caviglia [1], Angela Garrone [2], Chiara Bertolino [2], Riccardo Vanni [3], Elisabetta Bretto [1], Anxhela Poshnjari [1], Elisa Tribocco [1], Simone Frara [1], Angelo Armandi [1], Marco Astegiano [4], Giorgio Maria Saracco [1], Luciano Bertolusso [2] and Davide Giuseppe Ribaldone [1,*]

[1] Department of Medical Sciences, University of Turin, 10126 Turin, Italy
[2] A.S.L. CN2 Alba-Bra, 12051 Alba (CN), Italy
[3] Unit of Gastroenterology and Digestive Endoscopy, Michele e Pietro Ferrero Hospital, 12060 Verduno, Italy
[4] Unit of Gastroenterology, A.O.U. Città della Salute e della Scienza di Torino—Molinette Hospital, 10126 Turin, Italy
* Correspondence: davidegiuseppe.ribaldone@unito.it; Tel.: +39-11-633-3710

Abstract: The burden of inflammatory bowel diseases (IBD), including Crohn's disease (CD) and ulcerative colitis (UC), is increasing worldwide. The aim of the present study was to investigate the clinical characteristics and the changing in epidemiology of IBD in the Healthcare District Bra, an area of North-West Italy accounting for 57,615 inhabitants as of 31 December 2021. Clinical and demographic data were retrieved from administrative databases and the medical records of general practitioners (n = 39) at Verduno Hospital. Prevalence and incidence rates were calculated for the time span 2016–2021 and compared to the 2001–2006 period. IBD prevalence was 321.2 per 100,000 population in 2021 and, compared with 2006 (200 per 100,000 population), the prevalence has increased at a rate of +46%. Similarly, the average incidence has increased from the period 2001–2006 (6.7 per 100,000 population/year) to the period 2016–2021 (18.0 per 100,000 population/year) at a rate of +169%; such an increase was greater for CD than UC. In the 2016–2021 period, the mean age at diagnosis was 42.0 ± 17.4 years and 30.9% required at least one hospitalization, while 10.9% of patients underwent at least one surgery. In conclusion, the prevalence and incidence of IBD distinctly increased over a two decade period in the Healthcare District Bra paralleling the results of previous surveys from other Italian regions. These data warrant specific interventions to improve patients' management and resources' allocation.

Keywords: burden; incidence; Crohn's disease; prevalence; ulcerative colitis

1. Introduction

Inflammatory bowel diseases (IBD) are chronic inflammatory conditions with a multifactorial etiopathogenesis that affect the gastrointestinal system. The two main entities are Crohn's disease (CD) and ulcerative colitis (UC) [1]. The epidemiology of IBD is rapidly changing worldwide; the estimated prevalence (>0.3%) continues to rise in Western countries, with a high burden of IBD in North America, Oceania, and Europe [2]. The prevalence is also growing in newly industrialized countries in Africa, Asia, and South America mirroring the growing incidence of IBD observed in the 1990s in Western countries occurring with urbanization and the rapid socioeconomic development [3].

In Italy, the Global Burden of Diseases (GBD) estimated an IBD prevalence of 80.9 per 100,000 population in 1990 (56,469 cases) that increased to 93.8 per 100,000 population in 2017 (76,581 cases) (age-standardized percentage change: 16.0%), with a death rate over the study period increasing from 0.4 per 100,000 population in 1990 to 0.8 per 100,000 population in 2017 (age-standardized percentage change: 99.0%) [4]. However, local studies published in the last 10 years reported a significantly higher order of magnitude of IBD

Citation: Caviglia, G.P.; Garrone, A.; Bertolino, C.; Vanni, R.; Bretto, E.; Poshnjari, A.; Tribocco, E.; Frara, S.; Armandi, A.; Astegiano, M.; et al. Epidemiology of Inflammatory Bowel Diseases: A Population Study in a Healthcare District of North-West Italy. *J. Clin. Med.* **2023**, *12*, 641. https://doi.org/10.3390/jcm12020641

Academic Editor: John Mayberry

Received: 26 December 2022
Revised: 9 January 2023
Accepted: 11 January 2023
Published: 13 January 2023

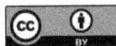

Copyright: © 2023 by the authors. Licensee MDPI, Basel, Switzerland. This article is an open access article distributed under the terms and conditions of the Creative Commons Attribution (CC BY) license (https:// creativecommons.org/licenses/by/ 4.0/).

cases in Italy. The prevalence of IBD ranges from 442 per 100,000 population in the district of Milan (North Italy) to 187 per 100,000 population in Sardinia [5,6], with a lower prevalence of CD compared with UC in the whole country [5–9]. Incidence rates of CD varies from 6.1 to 17.9 per 100,000 population/year for CD and from 12.2 to 15.3 per 100,000 population/year for UC [5–9].

Considering the clinical relapsing course and the high probability of complications [10–12], in spite of a marginal reduction of life expectancy [13], IBD leads to a substantial socio-economic burden on the health-care system, in terms of hospitalization and pharmacologic treatments, and on society in terms of working productivity. Therefore, a correct estimation of the current epidemiological scenario is crucial for planning health-care policy and resource allocation.

The aim of the present study was to evaluate the clinical characteristics and the change in the epidemiology of IBD in a Healthcare District in the North-West of Italy.

2. Materials and Methods

2.1. Study Design

Data for the present retrospective, observational study were retrieved from an administrative database (resident population) and medical records of general practitioners (all general practitioners who are in charge of the entire population residing in the district were involved, total number of general practitioners = 39) and hospital service (Michele and Pietro Ferrero Hospital–Verduno) of A.S.L. CN2 from the Healthcare District of Bra (Cuneo, North–West Italy) that includes the municipalities of Bra, Cherasco, Sommariva del Bosco, Sommariva Perno, La Morra, Verduno, Sanfrè, Ceresole d'Alba, S.Vittoria d'Alba, Pocapaglia, and Narzole. In particular, data on the resident population of the district were retrieved from the official site of the Piedmont Region "PISTA", which reports socio-demographic and economic information, including data on the structure and movements of the resident population according to province, municipality, sex, and age, health data, foreign residents, and censuses of general population [14].

We collected data from subjects with age ≥ 14 years (general practitioners and not pediatricians of free choice were involved) with a diagnosis of IBD (CD, UC, or IBD unclassified (IBDU)) within the time span 2016–2021. Patients were classified as IBDU in case of endoscopic, radiographic, and histologic evidence of chronic inflammatory bowel disease confined to the colon, but without fulfillment of diagnostic criteria for UC and CD. In detail, the following data (from IBD diagnosis to last follow-up visit) were retrieved, and recorded in a specific database: demographic features, data concerning the diagnosis of the disease (year of diagnosis, type, and location [15]), family history, hospitalization, and surgery for IBD, occurrence of neoplasms (intestinal and extra-intestinal), current and previous IBD therapy, death, and cause of death. Patients included had unique identifiers that ensured that there were no duplicate patient entries within the study period; in case of data retrieved from both the hospital service and general practitioner, medical records were reviewed and used to double-check the general practitioner data. Epidemiologic data estimated in the time span 2016–2021 were compared to those estimated in the same district in the time span 2001–2006 (the method of involvement of all general practitioners in the district was the same in the 2 periods [16]). Patients who had not died in the meantime or who had not changed residence were also included in the 2016–2021 analysis. Incidence and prevalence were computed both annually and as averages for 2016–2021, while as an average only for 2001–2006.

2.2. Statistical Analysis

The characteristics of the study cohort were reported as mean and standard deviation (SD) for continuous, normally distributed variables, and as absolute numbers (n) and percentages (%) for categorical data. Continuous variables were compared between groups by Students' t test, while categorical data were analyzed by chi-squared (χ^2) test. Standardized prevalence and incidence were reported as rates per 100,000 population. For all the analyses, we considered significant a p value < 0.05. Statistics were performed by MedCalc software v.20.104 (MedCalc Software Ltd., Ostend, Belgium).

3. Results

On 31 December 2021, the population in the Healthcare District of Bra area was 57,615 inhabitants. The total number of patients affected by IBD was 186, of whom 103 were males (M) and 83 were females (F) (Table 1); 70 patients had a diagnosis of CD (35 M and 35 F); 81 had a diagnosis of UC (47 M and 34 F); and 24 were affected by IBDU (13 M and 11 F). Concerning the remaining 11 patients (eight M and three F), we were unable to retrieve any data since they underwent instrumental investigations at the Verduno Hospital but were followed-up for their disease by other centers outside the Health Care District of Bra. These patients were included in the calculation of IBD incidence and prevalence, but were excluded from CD, UC, and IBDU subgroup analysis.

Table 1. Patients affected by IBD in the Healthcare District of Bra.

Municipality	Population (n)	IBD (n)	CD (n)	UC (n)	IBDU (n)	IBD Witout Clinical Data (n)
Bra	25,996	87 M = 48; F = 39	31 M = 14; F = 17	39 M = 24; F = 15	12 M = 7; F = 5	5 M = 3; F = 2
Ceresole d'Alba	1791	3 M = 1; F = 2	2 M = 0; F = 2	1 M = 1; F = 0	0	0
Cherasco	8098	18 M = 9; F = 9	11 M = 6; F = 5	4 M = 1; F = 3	3 M = 2; F = 1	0
Santa Vittoria d'Alba	2504	11 M = 7; F = 4	3 M = 3; F = 0	6 M = 3; F = 3	2 M = 1; F = 1	0
La Morra	2379	5 M = 3; F = 2	2 M = 1; F = 1	1 M = 1; F = 0	1 M = 0; F = 1	1 M = 1; F = 0
Narzole	3014	6 M = 5; F = 1	1 M = 1; F = 0	4 M = 3; F = 1	1 M = 1; F = 0	0
Pocapaglia	2848	9 M = 5; F = 4	4 M = 3; F = 1	2 M = 1; F = 1	2 M = 0; F = 2	1 M = 1; F = 0
Sanfrè	2632	9 M = 5; F = 4	2 M = 1; F = 1	6 M = 4; F = 2	0	1 M = 0, F = 1
Sommariva Del Bosco	5473	18 M = 11; F = 7	6 M = 3; F = 3	8 M = 5; F = 3	1 M = 0; F = 1	3 M = 3; F = 0
Sommariva Perno	2388	18 M = 8; F = 10	8 M = 3; F = 5	9 M = 4; F = 5	1 M = 1; F = 0	0
Verduno	492	2 M = 1; F = 1	0	1 M = 0; F = 1	1 M = 1; F = 0	0
Healthcare Disctric of Bra	57,615	186 M = 103; F = 83	70 M = 35; F = 35	81 M = 47; F = 34	24 M = 13; F = 11	11 M = 8; F = 3

Population with age ≥ 14 years on 31 December 2021. Abbreviations: CD, Crohn's disease; F, female; IBD, inflammatory bowel disease; IBDU, IBD unclassified; M, male; n, number; UC, ulcerative colitis.

The mean age at diagnosis was 42.0 ± 17.4 years for the whole IBD population (Figure 1). The mean age for CD, UC, and IBDU was 41.0 ± 17.2 years, 42.0 ± 16.8 years, and 50.0 ± 19.0 years, respectively. The M-to-F ratio was 1.2:1 for IBD, 1:1 for CD, 1.4:1 for UC, and 1.2:1 for IBDU. Immigrants born abroad comprised 20 out of 175 (11.4%) patients with IBD, 10 from East–Europe (Romania, Russia, and Balkan Countries) and 10 from Africa. Patients' mean follow-up was 12.5 ± 10.3 years. No deaths occurred within the study period.

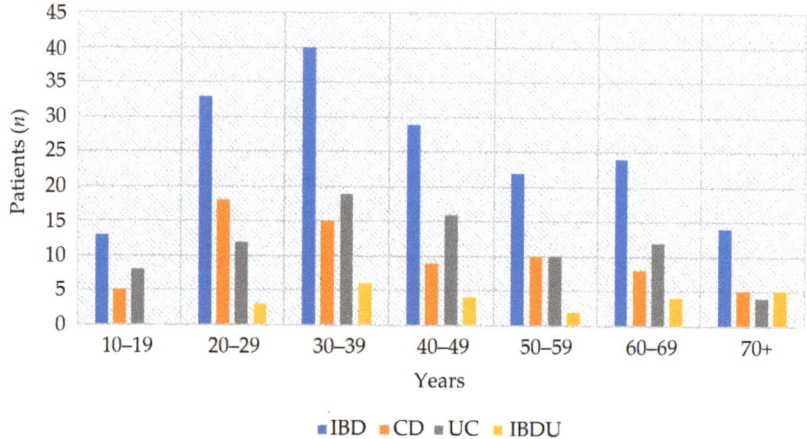

Figure 1. Distribution of IBD diagnosis according to age groups. Abbreviations: CD, Crohn's disease; IBD, inflammatory bowel disease; IBDU, IBD unclassified; UC, ulcerative colitis.

3.1. Clinical Characteristics

The diagnosis of IBD was mainly achieved by endoscopy (colonoscopy, video capsule, esophagogastroduodenoscopy) associated to a histological examination of bioptic samples (167 out of 175; 95.4%). In seven (4.0%) patients, the final diagnosis was achieved after a surgical procedure, while in one (0.6%) patient, IBD was diagnosed by imaging alone.

Among UC patients (n = 81), 16 (19.8%) had ulcerative proctitis (E1), five (6.2%) had left–side colitis (E2), and 60 (74.1%) had extensive (E3). Among CD patients (n = 70), the disease was confined to the ileum in 15 (21.4%) patients (L1), to the colon in 22 (31.4%) patients (L2), while 33 (47.1%) patients had an ileocolonic location (L3). Finally, in IBDU patients, the main localization of disease was in the colon alone (n = 7; 29.2%), followed by colon and rectum (n = 7; 29.2%), rectum alone (n = 5; 20.8%), ileum alone (n = 3; 12.5%), ileum and colon (n = 1; 4.2%), and rectum and anus (n = 1; 4.2%).

Overall, 54 out of 175 (30.9%) IBD patients required at least one hospitalization; patients with CD required hospitalization more frequently than those with UC (30 (42.9%) vs. 17 (21.0%); p = 0.004). Regarding surgical procedures, 19 (10.9%) IBD patients underwent at least one surgery; patients with CD underwent surgery more frequently than those with UC (17 (24.3%) vs. 2 (2.9%); p < 0.001). In the whole IBD population, 11 out of 19 (57.9%) patients underwent surgery within 5 years from diagnosis.

Neoplasm occurred in 14 (8.0%) patients; six patients developed an intestinal neoplasm (all adenomas with mild dysplasia), while eight patients developed a miscellanea of extra-intestinal neoplasm, including pancreatic, uterine, upper lip carcinoma, laryngeal, skin, bladder, prostate, and breast cancer. No difference was observed in neoplasm incidence according to IBD type.

During the analyzed period, azathioprine or methotrexate was prescribed in 29 (16.6%) IBD patients (13 out of 70 (18.6%) CD patients, 14 out of 81 (17.3%) UC patients, two out of 24 (8.3%) IBDU patients). Biologic therapy and/or small molecule drugs were prescribed at least once in 34 out of 175 (19.4%) IBD patients (19 out of 70 (27.1%) CD patients and 15 out of 81 (18.5%) UC patients). Among the overall number of biologic therapy and/or small molecule prescriptions (n = 49), adalimumab accounted for the 53.1% (n = 26) of total prescriptions, followed by infliximab (n = 10; 20.4%), vedolizumab (n = 6; 12.2%), ustekinumab (n = 3; 6.1%), and tofacitinib (n = 3; 6.1%).

3.2. Prevalence

IBD prevalence in the Healthcare District of Bra on 31 December 2021 was 321.2 per 100,000 population. The municipality with the lowest prevalence was Ceresole d'Alba (167.5 per 100,000 population), while the municipality with the highest prevalence was Sommariva Perno (753.8 per 100,000 population). Compared with 2006 (146 IBD diagnosis) [16], IBD prevalence grew by 46% ($p = 0.001$) in 2021 (220 per 100,000 population vs. 321.2 per 100,000 population). The municipality with the greatest increase was Pocapaglia (+351%), followed by Sommariva Perno (+202%), and La Morra (+200%). Conversely, in the municipalities of Ceresole d'Alba and Sanfrè, we observed a decrease in IBD prevalence as there was a percentage decrease of −42% and −2%, respectively (Table 2). As per IBD type, CD prevalence increased significantly by 76% ($p = 0.003$), while no significant variation was observed for UC (+15%; $p = 0.352$) and IBDU (+39%; $p = 0.352$).

Table 2. IBD prevalence in the Healthcare District of Bra according to time-period.

Municipality	IBD Prevalence (2021)	IBD Prevalence (2006)	Variation (%) 2006–2021	CD Prevalence (2021)	UC Prevalence (2021)	IBDU Prevalence (2021)
Bra	334.4	250	+34%	119.2	150.0	46.0
Ceresole d'Alba	167.5	290	−42%	111.7	55.8	0
Cherasco	222.2	160	+39%	135.8	49.4	37.0
Santa Vittoria d'Alba	439.3	270	+63%	119.8	239.6	79.9
La Morra	210.2	70	+200%	84.2	42.0	42.0
Narzole	199.1	150	+33%	33.2	132.7	33.2
Pocapaglia	315.9	70	+351%	140.4	70.2	70.2
Sanfrè	342.0	350	−2%	76.0	228.0	0
Sommariva Del Bosco	310.7	250	+24%	109.6	128.0	18.3
Sommariva Perno	753.8	250	+202%	335.0	376.9	41.9
Verduno	406.6	380	+7%	0	203.3	203.3
Health Care Disctric of Bra	321.2	220	+46%	121.5	138.9	41.7

Prevalence is reported per 100,000 population. Abbreviations: CD, Crohn's disease; IBD, inflammatory bowel disease; IBDU, IBD unclassified; UC, ulcerative colitis.

CD showed a lower prevalence than UC (121.5 per 100,000 vs. 138.9 per 100,000). The lowest CD prevalence was recorded in Verduno (no CD cases), while the highest was in Sommariva Perno (335.0 per 100,000 population). The lowest UC prevalence was recorded in La Morra (42.0 per 100,000 population), while the highest was in Sommariva Perno (376.9 per 100,000 population). Most of the municipalities recorded a higher prevalence for UC compared with CD, except for Ceresole d'Alba, Cherasco, La Morra, and Pocapaglia. IBDU showed a prevalence of 41.7 per 100,000 inhabitants, ranging from a minimum of 0 in Sanfrè and Ceresole D'Alba to a maximum of 203.3 per 100,000 population in Verduno.

3.3. Incidence

The average IBD incidence rate in the Healthcare District of Bra in the time span 2016–2021 was 18.0 per 100,000 population/year. The average IBD incidence increase from 2001–2006 to 2016–2021 was 169%. The incidence rate estimated in the time span 2016–2021 was similar among CD and UC, while in the time-span 2001–2006 was higher for UC, with a percentage increase of 121% in CD and 73% in UC (Table 3 and Figure 2).

Table 3. IBD incidence in the Healthcare District of Bra according to time-period.

	2016	2017	2018	2019	2020	2021	2016–2021 (Mean ± SD)	2001–2006 (Mean)	Variation (%) 2006–2021
IBD	5.3	13.9	17.4	26.1	15.7	29.5	18.0 ± 8.0	6.7	169%
CD	1.8	5.2	3.5	12.2	3.5	12.1	6.4 ± 4.2	2.9	121%
UC	3.5	8.7	12.2	3.5	7.0	3.5	6.4 ± 3.3	3.7	73%
IBDU	0	0	1.7	10.4	5.2	13.9	5.2 ± 5.3	N/A	

Incidence is reported per 100,000 population/year. Abbreviations: CD, Crohn's disease; IBD, inflammatory bowel disease; IBDU, IBD unclassified; N/A, not available; SD, standard deviation; UC, ulcerative colitis.

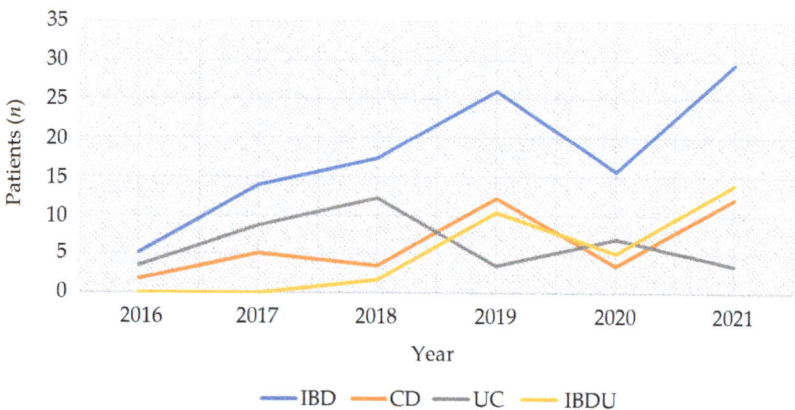

Figure 2. IBD incidence in the Healthcare District of Bra in the time span 2016–2021. Abbreviations: CD, Crohn's disease; IBD, inflammatory bowel disease; IBDU, IBD unclassified; UC, ulcerative colitis.

4. Discussion

The prevalence of IBDs has undergone an important phase of growth during the 21st century. This increase entails new organizational needs for the Healthcare System in order to improve patients' management and to allow costs' reduction. In the present study, we investigated the clinical features and the epidemiologic scenario of IBD in a Healthcare District of North-West Italy. As the main findings, we observed that IBD prevalence in the Healthcare District of Bra was 321.2 per 100,000 population in 2021, compared with 2006 (200 per 100,000 population), the prevalence has increased at a rate of +46%. Similarly, the average incidence has increased from the period 2001–2006 (6.7 per 100,000 population/year) to the period 2016–2021 (18.0 per 100,000 population/year) at a rate of +169%; such an increase was greater for CD than UC.

Despite some degree of variability, our data are in agreement with the results of previous epidemiologic studies carried out in Italy [5–9]. In particular, a previous Italian epidemiologic study carried out in the Barletta-Andria-Trani Province of the Apulia region, found an IBD prevalence of 187.2/100,000 (95% CI: 160.6–217.0) and an incidence of 16.2/100,000 (95% CI 12.5–20.7) per year [17]; taking into account that these data were published in 2013, they are consistent with our findings of an increase in IBD prevalence and incidence. Concerning CD and UC, we observed a prevalence of 121.5 per 100,000 population and 138.9 per 100,000 population, respectively. These data are lower than those reported from Northern Europe (CD: 143.0 per 100,000 population and UC: 297.9 per 100,000 population), but higher than those estimated in Asia (CD: 27.1 per 100,000 population and UC: 55.4 per 100,000 population) and Africa (CD: 19.0 per 100,000 population and UC: 10.6 per 100,000 population) [2]. Conversely, the incidence of CD observed in our study was similar to that reported in Northern Europe (6.4 per 100,000 population/year vs. 5.7 per 100,000 population/year, respectively), while the incidence of UC was distinctly lower (6.4 per 100,000 population/year vs. 29.8 per 100,000 population/year, respectively). As compared to data from Asia (CD: 4.2 per 100,000 population/year and UC: 3.3 per 100,000 population/year) and Africa (CD: 5.9 per 100,000 population/year and UC: 3.3 per 100,000 population/year), the incidence of both CD and UC was higher in our population [2]. There was a decline of new diagnoses of IBD in 2020, probably caused by a delay in the first visits due to the concomitant presence of the SARS-CoV-2 pandemic; these diagnoses, which in the absence of a pandemic would have occurred in 2020, presumably were performed in 2021, creating an overestimation in that year. This is confirmed by an international survey, which found that 85% of endoscopy units have reduced the volume of procedures by more than 50% due to the pandemic [18].

From a clinical point of view, the average age at diagnosis was about 40 years which, having also excluded patients <14 years of age, confirms that IBD arises at a young age and remains a condition for the patient's entire life [19]. The rate of hospitalizations, but above all that of surgical interventions, although confirmed to be higher for CD (about 25%) than for UC (about 3%), is lower than that reported in the literature (about 60% in CD, about 10% in UC) [20]. This probably derives from the fact that our study was not based on a population of a tertiary care center but collected data from the entire population affected by IBD living in a given territory, and therefore more closely reflects the disease trend in the general IBD population. With regard to the use of advanced therapies (biological drugs and small molecules), a greater use is confirmed in CD (about 30%) compared with UC (about 20%); moreover, the percentage of the use of advanced therapies does not differ from the literature data (more than 30% in CD, more than 10% in UC) [21]. Our figure would perhaps have been even higher if we had also included the pediatric population [22].

The main strengths of this study are represented by involving all the general practitioners operating in the district in which we analyzed the prevalence and incidence of IBD and having checked these data with those of the only hospital in the district. The main limitations consist in the fact that the data on the characteristics of the IBD were collected by the medical records of the general practitioners of the patients and that the second check with the data present in the medical records of the district hospital could only be done for the patients by a specialist of that hospital.

5. Conclusions

In conclusion, the prevalence of IBD as of 31 December 2021 in the Health Care District of Bra was 321.2 per 100,000 inhabitants, with a significant increase of 46% compared with 2006 (220 per 100,000 inhabitants); the average incidence of IBD in the period 2016–2021 was 18 per 100,000 inhabitants/year, with an increase of 169% compared with the period 2001–2006 (6.7 per 100,000 inhabitants/year) and the increase was greater for CD than for UC. The incidence and prevalence values that emerged from our study were lower than the values that emerged from other studies conducted in Italy, but comparable to the values estimated for Europe.

These data are essential for understanding the epidemiological trend and for planning health resources for these patients.

Author Contributions: Conceptualization, M.A. and L.B.; methodology, L.B.; software, G.P.C.; validation, E.B., A.P., E.T., S.F. and A.A.; formal analysis, A.G.; investigation, A.G. and C.B.; resources, G.M.S. and R.V.; data curation, A.G. and C.B.; writing—original draft preparation, G.P.C.; writing—review and editing, D.G.R.; visualization, E.B., A.P., E.T., S.F. and A.A.; supervision, D.G.R. and G.M.S.; project administration, G.M.S. All authors have read and agreed to the published version of the manuscript.

Funding: This research received no external funding.

Institutional Review Board Statement: The study was conducted in accordance with the Declaration of Helsinki, and ethical review and approval were waived for this study due to the fact that all data was collected anonymously on the territory.

Informed Consent Statement: Each general practitioner has obtained the consent of his patients to process his data anonymously.

Data Availability Statement: The data presented in this study are available upon request from the corresponding author.

Conflicts of Interest: The authors declare no conflict of interest.

References

1. Actis, G.C.; Pellicano, R.; Fagoonee, S.; Ribaldone, D.G. History of Inflammatory Bowel Diseases. *J. Clin. Med.* **2019**, *8*, 1970. [CrossRef] [PubMed]
2. Ng, S.C.; Shi, H.Y.; Hamidi, N.; Underwood, F.E.; Tang, W.; Benchimol, E.I.; Panaccione, R.; Ghosh, S.; Wu, J.C.Y.; Chan, F.K.L.; et al. Worldwide incidence and prevalence of inflammatory bowel disease in the 21st century: A systematic review of population-based studies. *Lancet* **2017**, *390*, 2769–2778. [CrossRef] [PubMed]

3. Kaplan, G.G.; Ng, S.C. Globalisation of inflammatory bowel disease: Perspectives from the evolution of inflammatory bowel disease in the UK and China. *Lancet Gastroenterol. Hepatol.* **2016**, *1*, 307–316. [CrossRef] [PubMed]
4. GBD 2017 Inflammatory Bowel Disease Collaborators. The global, regional, and national burden of inflammatory bowel disease in 195 countries and territories, 1990–2017: A systematic analysis for the Global Burden of Disease Study 2017. *Lancet Gastroenterol. Hepatol.* **2020**, *5*, 17–30. [CrossRef] [PubMed]
5. Crocetti, E.; Bergamaschi, W.; Russo, A.G. Population-based incidence and prevalence of inflammatory bowel diseases in Milan (Northern Italy), and estimates for Italy. *Eur. J. Gastroenterol. Hepatol.* **2021**, *33*, e383–e389. [CrossRef]
6. Macaluso, F.S.; Mocci, G.; Orlando, A.; Scondotto, S.; Fantaci, G.; Antonelli, A.; Leone, S.; Previtali, E.; Cabras, F.; Cottone, M.; et al. Prevalence and incidence of inflammatory bowel disease in two Italian islands, Sicily and Sardinia: A report based on health information systems. *Dig. Liver Dis.* **2019**, *51*, 1270–1274. [CrossRef] [PubMed]
7. Di Domenicantonio, R.; Cappai, G.; Arcà, M.; Agabiti, N.; Kohn, A.; Vernia, P.; Biancone, L.; Armuzzi, A.; Papi, C.; Davoli, M. Occurrence of inflammatory bowel disease in central Italy: A study based on health information systems. *Dig. Liver Dis.* **2014**, *46*, 777–782. [CrossRef] [PubMed]
8. Valpiani, D.; Manzi, I.; Mercuriali, M.; Giuliani, O.; Ravaioli, A.; Colamartini, A.; Bucchi, L.; Falcini, F.; Ricci, E. A model of an inflammatory bowel disease population-based registry: The Forlì experience (1993–2013). *Dig. Liver Dis.* **2018**, *50*, 32–36. [CrossRef] [PubMed]
9. Piscaglia, A.C.; Lopetuso, L.R.; Laterza, L.; Gerardi, V.; Sacchini, E.; Leoncini, E.; Boccia, S.; Stefanelli, M.L.; Gasbarrini, A.; Armuzzi, A. Epidemiology of inflammatory bowel disease in the Republic of San Marino: The "EPIMICI-San Marino" study. *Dig. Liver Dis.* **2019**, *51*, 218–225. [CrossRef] [PubMed]
10. Caviglia, G.P.; Rosso, C.; Stalla, F.; Rizzo, M.; Massano, A.; Abate, M.L.; Olivero, A.; Armandi, A.; Vanni, E.; Younes, R.; et al. On-Treatment Decrease of Serum Interleukin-6 as a Predictor of Clinical Response to Biologic Therapy in Patients with Inflammatory Bowel Diseases. *J. Clin. Med.* **2020**, *9*, 800. [CrossRef] [PubMed]
11. Carli, E.; Caviglia, G.P.; Pellicano, R.; Fagoonee, S.; Rizza, S.; Astegiano, M.; Saracco, G.M.; Ribaldone, D.G. Incidence of Prostate Cancer in Inflammatory Bowel Disease: A Meta-Analysis. *Medicina* **2020**, *56*, 85. [CrossRef] [PubMed]
12. Ribaldone, D.G.; Pellicano, R.; Actis, G.C. The gut and the inflammatory bowel diseases inside-out: Extra-intestinal manifestations. *Minerva Gastroenterol. Dietol.* **2019**, *65*, 309–318. [CrossRef] [PubMed]
13. Kuenzig, M.E.; Manuel, D.G.; Donelle, J.; Benchimol, E.I. Life expectancy and health-adjusted life expectancy in people with inflammatory bowel disease. *CMAJ* **2020**, *192*, E1394–E1402. [CrossRef] [PubMed]
14. Available online: https://servizi.regione.piemonte.it/catalogo/pista-piemonte-statistica-bdde (accessed on 15 July 2022).
15. Silverberg, M.S.; Satsangi, J.; Ahmad, T.; Arnott, I.D.; Bernstein, C.N.; Brant, S.R.; Caprilli, R.; Colombel, J.F.; Gasche, C.; Geboes, K.; et al. Toward an integrated clinical, molecular and serological classification of inflammatory bowel disease: Report of a working party of the 2005 Montreal world congress of gastroenterology. *Can. J. Gastroenterol.* **2005**, *19*, 5–36. [CrossRef] [PubMed]
16. Vanni, R. Epidemiological study of inflammatory bowel disease in Bra, Piemonte, Italy: Methodological problems. In Proceedings of the FISMAD Conference, Palermo, Italy, 29 September–3 October 2007.
17. Tursi, A.; Elisei, W.; Picchio, M. Incidence and prevalence of inflammatory bowel diseases in gastroenterology primary care setting. *Eur. J. Intern. Med.* **2013**, *24*, 852–856. [CrossRef] [PubMed]
18. Alboraie, M.; Piscoya, A.; Tran, Q.T.; Mendelsohn, R.B.; Butt, A.S.; Lenz, L.; Alavinejad, P.; Emara, M.H.; Samlani, Z.; Altonbary, A.; et al. The global impact of COVID-19 on gastrointestinal endoscopy units: An international survey of endoscopists. *Arab. J. Gastroenterol.* **2020**, *21*, 156–161. [CrossRef] [PubMed]
19. Agrawal, M.; Jess, T. Implications of the changing epidemiology of inflammatory bowel disease in a changing world. *United Eur. Gastroenterol J.* **2022**, *10*, 1113–1120. [CrossRef] [PubMed]
20. Annese, V.; Duricova, D.; Gower-Rousseau, C.; Jess, T.; Langholz, E. Impact of New Treatments on Hospitalisation, Surgery, Infection, and Mortality in IBD: A Focus Paper by the Epidemiology Committee of ECCO. *J. Crohns Colitis* **2016**, *10*, 216–225. [CrossRef] [PubMed]
21. Candido, F.D.; Fiorino, G.; Spadaccini, M.; Danese, S.; Spinelli, A. Are Surgical Rates Decreasing in the Biological Era In IBD? *Curr Drug Targets* **2019**, *20*, 1356–1362. [CrossRef] [PubMed]
22. Burgess, C.J.; Jackson, R.; Chalmers, I.; Russell, R.K.; Hansen, R.; Scott, G.; Henderson, P.; Wilson, D.C. The inexorable increase of biologic exposure in paediatric inflammatory bowel disease: A Scottish, population-based, longitudinal study. *Aliment. Pharmacol. Ther.* **2022**, *56*, 1453–1459. [CrossRef] [PubMed]

Disclaimer/Publisher's Note: The statements, opinions and data contained in all publications are solely those of the individual author(s) and contributor(s) and not of MDPI and/or the editor(s). MDPI and/or the editor(s) disclaim responsibility for any injury to people or property resulting from any ideas, methods, instructions or products referred to in the content.

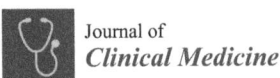

Brief Report

Effect of Long-Term Proton Pump Inhibitor Use on Blood Vitamins and Minerals: A Primary Care Setting Study

Giuseppe Losurdo [1,2,*], Natale Lino Bruno Caccavo [3], Giuseppe Indellicati [1], Francesca Celiberto [1,2], Enzo Ierardi [1], Michele Barone [1] and Alfredo Di Leo [1]

[1] Section of Gastroenterology, Department of Precision Medicine and Jonic Area, University "Aldo Moro" of Bari, 70124 Bari, Italy
[2] Ph.D. Course in Organs and Tissues Transplantation and Cellular Therapies, Department of Precision Medicine Jonic Area, University "Aldo Moro" of Bari, 70124 Bari, Italy
[3] College of General Practitionners, ASL BA, 70056 Molfetta, Italy
* Correspondence: giuseppelos@alice.it

Abstract: Background and objectives. Long-term proton pump inhibitor (PPI) use is frequently encountered in primary care. Its effect on micronutrient absorption is known, as vitamin B12, calcium or vitamin D insufficiency may occur in such patients. Materials and methods. We recruited patients using a PPI (pantoprazole) for >12 months. The control group was represented by subjects attending the general practitioner not taking any PPI in the last 12 months. We excluded subjects using nutritional supplements or with diseases interfering with micronutrient blood levels. All subjects underwent blood sampling with full blood count, iron, ferritin, vitamin D, calcium, sodium, potassium, phosphate, zinc and folate. Results. We recruited 66 subjects: 30 in the PPI group and 36 in the control group. Long-term pantoprazole users had lower red blood cell count but similar hemoglobin. We did not find any significant difference in blood iron, ferritin, vitamin B12 and folate. Vitamin D deficit was observed more frequently in the PPI group (100%) than in controls (30%, $p < 0.001$), with blood levels lower in pantoprazole consumers. No differences in calcium, sodium and magnesium were observed. Pantoprazole users had lower phosphate levels than controls. Finally, a non-significant trend for zinc deficiency was found in PPI users. Conclusions. Our study confirms that chronic PPI users may encounter alterations in some micronutrients involved in bone mineral homeostasis. The effect on zinc levels deserves further investigation.

Keywords: proton pump inhibitors; vitamin B12; vitamin D; *Helicobacter pylori*

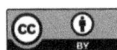

1. Introduction

Proton Pump Inhibitors (PPIs) are a class of widely used medications with different indications. In Italy, they are currently approved by the "Agenzia Italiana del Farmaco" (AIFA, i.e., the Italian drug administration agency) for the management of peptic ulcer disease, esophageal reflux disease with or without esophagitis, Zollinger–Ellison Syndrome, non-ulcerative dyspepsia, as well as for the prevention of gastrointestinal ulcers in conditions, such as chronic non-steroidal anti-inflammatory drug (NSAID) administration [1]. PPIs are also crucial in treating *Helicobacter pylori* infection in association with antibiotics [2]. Their mechanism of action is the inhibition of the H+,K+ ATPase located in gastric parietal cells [3].

Long-term use of these medications has become extremely common, and some adverse effects have been observed linked to their chronic use [4]. These adverse effects can be divided into: (i) infective, (ii) related to hypergastrinemia and (iii) absorption deficiencies due to hypochlorhydria [5]. Infections recognize the increase in gastric pH as a possible mechanism, i.e., the reduction in a first-line barrier against bacteria introduced with food [5]. The most common infections associated with PPI chronic use are C. difficile infection and non-typhoid Salmonella and Campylobacter enteric infections; studies have shown conflicting results for other infections, such as spontaneous bacterial peritonitis, encephalopathy in cirrhotic patients and community-acquired pneumonia [5]. The most important effects related to hypergastrinemia are gastric hyperplasia/metaplasia and rebound acid hypersecretion [5]. The most-studied absorption deficiencies associated with chronic PPI administration are vitamin B12 and iron deficiency (anemia), hypomagnesemia and alterations in vitamin D and calcium metabolism, with some studies showing an increased bone fracture risk [5,6]; in particular, a meta-analysis of 18 studies showed that PPI use could moderately increase the risk of hip fracture with an RR = 1.26 [7]. Other potential adverse effects with weaker evidence are dementia and renal disease [6].

Several studies [8–11] assessed the importance of gastric acid secretion in vitamin and mineral absorption. For example, gastric pH contributes to reducing ferric ion into its ferrous form, which is more soluble, thus avoiding the formation of ferric complexes that reduce absorption and bioavailability [9]. Given that defective intestinal calcium absorption has been reported in patients with gastric achlorhydria, it is thought that the pH-dependent ionization of calcium salts from ingested foods is a prerequisite for its absorption [10]. Regarding vitamin B12, several factors are involved in its absorption. First, peptic enzymes and the gastric acidic environment contribute to the release of B12 from food; then, the gastric pH favors the binding between vitamin B12 and Haptocorrin (HC), a protein secreted by the salivary glands [12]. This prevents vitamin B12 hydrolysis by gastric acid and reduces degradation by intestinal microbiota [12]. In the duodenum, pH elevation decreases the affinity between vitamin B12 and HC, promoting B12 binding to another protein, the intrinsic factor (IF) [12]. IF is secreted by gastric mucosa and helps B12 absorption through the intestinal wall in the distal ileum by the binding to Cubulin, the receptor of complex B12-IF [12].

It is evident that gastric acid has a role in absorption mechanisms and, thus, PPIs, by blocking acid gastric secretion, which may likely interfere with these absorption mechanisms. In this prospective case–control study, we aimed to investigate possible alterations in micronutrients in chronic PPI users in a general practitioner setting.

2. Materials and Methods

The study was planned as a transversal case–control study. We recruited, in the period January–December 2020, patients using PPIs (pantoprazole) for at least 12 months attending the general practitioner. Control group was represented by subjects not taking any PPI in the last 12 months, recruited in the same setting. We excluded subjects < 18 years old. We excluded subjects taking oral or parenteral nutritional supplements containing iron, folate, vitamin B12 or D, or taking other medications (such as corticosteroids), which could influence vitamin and micronutrient levels. Additionally, we ruled out subjects with diseases (atrophic gastritis, celiac disease, inflammatory bowel disease, and hematological disease) that could cause alterations in micronutrient blood levels. All subjects underwent blood sampling with full blood count, iron, ferritin, vitamin D, calcium, sodium, potassium, phosphate, zinc and folate. The study was carried out in accordance with the Declaration of Helsinki and approved by the Internal Gastroenterology Institutional Review Board of our unit. Written informed consent was obtained from all subjects involved in the study. All laboratory analyses were performed according to the local best-practice rule. Considering the prevalence of vitamin D deficiency, by estimating a difference in prevalence of 35% between the two groups (which is much less than what we found, i.e., 75%), an alpha error of 0.05 and a statistical power of 80%, the total sample size would be 60 patients (30 per group).

Student's t test and Fisher's exact test were used for statistical comparison for continuous and dichotomous variables, respectively. Correlation analysis was performed via Spearman r coefficient. A multivariate binomial regression analysis was used to assess odds ratios (ORs) and relative 95% confidence intervals (95% CIs). The statistical software programs GraphPad Prism version 5 (San Diego, CA, USA) and SPSS 23 were used.

3. Results

We recruited 66 subjects: 32 males and 34 females; there were 30 in the PPI group and 36 in the control group. In detail, all patients assumed pantoprazole at a dose of 40 mg/day. Patients in the PPI group were older than controls (75.6 ± 9.6 versus 63.2 ± 16.4 years, $p < 0.001$). Regarding comorbidities, the most common ones in the PPI group were hypertension (n = 26) and diabetes (n = 6).

Long-term PPI users had lower red blood cell count (4.26 ± 0.52 versus 4.86 ± 0.36 × 10^6, $p < 0.001$) but similar hemoglobin and mean cell volume values. We did not find any significant difference in blood iron (85.9 ± 22.3 versus 83.4 ± 32.3, $p = 0.71$), ferritin (170.0 ± 271.0 versus 364.5 ± 677.1, $p = 0.14$), vitamin B12 (441.2 ± 195.5 versus 419.4 ± 227.3, $p = 0.68$) and folate (8.5 ± 3.5 versus 8.6 ± 2.9, $p = 0.92$).

Vitamin D deficiency was observed more frequently in the PPI group (100%) than in controls (25%, $p < 0.001$), with blood levels lower in PPI consumers (15.5 ± 6.8 versus 36.6 ± 21.2, $p < 0.001$). No differences in calcium and magnesium levels were observed. PPI users had lower phosphate (3.44 ± 0.60 versus 3.98 ± 0.73, $p = 0.002$).

Regarding other minerals, potassium levels were lower than controls (4.18 ± 0.47 versus 4.49 ± 0.54, $p = 0.02$). Finally, a non-significant trend for zinc deficiency was found in PPI users (81.2 ± 13.9 versus 87.0 ± 12.7, $p = 0.08$) and also a borderline significant trend for lower sodium levels in PPI users (139.8 ± 3.8 versus 141.8 ± 4.6, $p = 0.05$).

The overall results are summarized in Table 1.

Table 1. Characteristics and laboratory values of the studied population (mean ± SD or percentage).

Variables	PPI Group (n = 30)	Controls (n = 36)	p Value
Age (y)	75.6 ± 9.6	63.2 ± 16.4	<0.001
RBC (×10^6/mm^3)	4.26 ± 0.52	4.86 ± 0.36	<0.001
Hb (g/dL)	12.6 ± 1.9	13.2 ± 2.3	0.28
Mean corpuscolar volume (fL)	88.8 ± 6.3	86.8 ± 1.8	0.28
WBC (×10^3/mm^3)	6.39 ± 2.02	7.27 ± 2.25	0.99
Iron (µg/dL)	85.9 ± 22.3	83.4 ± 32.3	0.71
Ferritin (µg/L)	170.0 ± 271.0	364.5 ± 677.1	0.14
Vitamin D (ng/mL)	15.5 ± 6.8	36.6 ± 21.2	<0.001
Vitamin D deficit	30 (100%)	9 (25%)	<0.001
Calcium (mg/dL)	8.7 ± 2.2	9.2 ± 0.4	0.25
Magnesium (mg/dL)	2.09 ± 0.33	2.05 ± 0.28	0.58
Phosphate (mg/dL)	3.44 ± 0.60	3.98 ± 0.73	0.002
Zinc (µg/dL)	81.2 ± 13.9	87.0 ± 12.7	0.08
Sodium (mEq/L)	139.8 ± 3.8	141.8 ± 4.6	0.05
Potassium (mEq/L)	4.18 ± 0.47	4.49 ± 0.54	0.02
Gastrin (pg/mL)	28.9 ± 37.9	39.6 ± 108.5	0.61
APCA positivity	4 (13.3%)	6 (16.7%)	0.74
Vitamin B12 (pg/mL)	441.2 ± 195.5	419.4 ± 227.3	0.68
Vitamin B12 deficit	0 (0%)	4 (11.1%)	0.12
Folate (ng/mL)	8.5 ± 3.5	8.6 ± 2.9	0.92
Folate deficit	2 (6.7%)	2 (5.5%)	1
TSH (mU/L)	2.08 ± 0.86	2.36 ± 0.95	0.21
TPO (UI/mL)	7.09 ± 96.3	96.3 ± 346.4	0.16

To exclude the effect of age as a confounding factor for vitamins and minerals involved in bone metabolism, we correlated age with such micronutrients and found no correlation with vitamin D (r = 0.08, p = 0.64), calcium (r = 0.25, p = 0.18), phosphate (r = −0.22, p = 0.23) and zinc (r = −0.23, p = 0.21).

Furthermore, a multivariate analysis aiming to explore the possible associated and confounding factors for vitamin D deficiency, reported in Table 2, did not find any variable associated with such a deficit.

Table 2. Multivariate analysis of factors associated with vitamin D deficiency.

	OR	95% CI	p Value
Calcium	0.012	0–∞	0.971
Magnesium	0.021	0–∞	0.967
Phosphate	2577	0.314–639	0.999
Age	0.154	0–∞	0.960
Sex	254.21	0.236–36685	0.964
Hypertension	815.33	0–∞	1
Diabetes	0.031	0–∞	0.981

4. Discussion

Several studies investigated the link between chronic administration of PPIs and vitamins and mineral absorption. According to our results, the most important studies, which evaluated long-term use of PPIs on B12 absorption [13–16], concluded that there were no significant alterations in vitamin B12 levels during long-term PPI therapy, except in the case of Zollinger–Ellison syndrome patients, which were completely achlorhydric due to heavy PPI treatment, with a consequent decrease in vitamin B12 blood levels [14]. However, the literature is quite heterogeneous when dealing with PPI-induced adverse events. For example, we added a study that found that PPI consumers had slightly higher vitamin B12 [17], which is in full disagreement with another that did not find any effect on folate, B12, calcium and vitamin D [18].

There are some case reports [19] and a review [20] that correlate the chronic use of PPIs to hypomagnesemia, with a pooled relative risk of hypomagnesemia in patients with PPIs of 1.43 (95% CI, 1.08–1.88) [18]. The proposed mechanism [21] involves an increase in the pH in the intestinal lumen caused by PPI chronic administration, which reduces the affinity between the Mg+ ion and its transporter, Transient Receptor Potential Melastatin 6/7 (TRPM 6/7). This reduction in binding between Mg+ ion and its transporter may trigger mRNA transcription of TRPM 6 in most individuals, but epigenetic modifications may explain why hypomagnesemia occurs only in a few individuals [21]. In our study, there was no significant difference in magnesium levels between the two groups (Table 1), maybe due to the small sample size.

The acidic pH of gastric juice could affect the bioavailability of vitamin D, despite the fact that there are no available data on the susceptibility of major dietary forms of vitamin D to gastrointestinal pH conditions [22]. Another mechanism that could explain the influence of PPIs on vitamin D homeostasis is through hypomagnesemia because several steps in vitamin D metabolism depend on magnesium as a cofactor, such as vitamin D binding to vitamin D binding protein, 25(OH)D synthesis, 1,25 (OH)2D synthesis, 25-hydroxylase synthesis and vitamin D receptor expression for cellular effects [23]. Sharara et al. [24] analyzed the effect of PPIs on bone metabolism, including vitamin D. Most of the study participants had hypovitaminosis D at baseline, but vitamin D increased in both the PPI and control groups after 3 months of treatment without statistically significative difference between the two groups (p = 0.971). In another study, by Hinson et al. [25], which evaluated the hyperparathyroidism associated with PPI therapy, the differences in vitamin D levels in patients taking PPIs for at least 6 months and in patients without PPIs were not statistically significant, independently from bisphosphonate co-administration. These findings do not seem to agree with our findings: significantly lower vitamin D levels in PPI consumers

($p < 0.001$). This could be explained by the fact that the PPI-user sample is significantly older ($p < 0.001$) than the non-PPI-user group in our study, as advanced age is a factor associated with suboptimal vitamin D levels [26]. Other factors that could explain our result could be the fact that body mass index was not considered in this evaluation, since 25 (OH) vitamin D, which is fat-soluble, can be sequestered in the adipose tissue [27]. Additionally, specific interfering drugs were not considered in our study design (for example, bile acid sequestrants, anti-epileptic drugs) [28]. Finally, we selected subjects taking pantoprazole for >12 months, a longer time from the 6 months of Hinson.

Theoretically, an acidic environment in the stomach facilitates the release of ionized calcium from insoluble calcium salts such as calcium carbonate [29]. In fact, in achlorhydric patients, the absorption of insoluble calcium salts such as calcium carbonate taken under fasting conditions virtually does not occur, while soluble calcium salts such as calcium citrate are still normally absorbed [29]. Despite these results, a review by Insogna et al. [30] analyzed several studies about the influence of PPIs on calcium absorption, finding conflicting results. Moreover, most of the analyzed studies were on patients with comorbidities that could influence calcium metabolism (chronic kidney disease or achlorhydria). Thus, it is not possible to state the effective role of PPIs on calcium intestinal absorption. On the other hand, it has been demonstrated that PPIs can also inhibit osteoclast proton pumps, reducing bone calcium phosphate reabsorption, thus decreasing calcium blood levels [31]. Our study did not show any significant differences between calcium levels in PPIs users versus controls (Table 1). In this regard, the American Gastroenterology Association guidelines [32] do not support either the routine supplementation of calcium intake in chronic PPI users, unless it is below the recommended daily allowance, independently of PPI administration, or the routine evaluation of bone mass density in such patients.

Termanini et al. [15], in his study on patients with Zollinger–Ellison syndrome, investigated, apart from B12 levels, folate levels and complete blood counts yearly for a mean of 4.5 years. He did not find any significant decrease in these parameters. Another study, by Attwood et al. [33], who evaluated the safety of long-term pantoprazole therapy by comparing the results of the LOTUS and the SOPRAN studies (two studies that compared PPI therapy vs. surgery in GERD), demonstrated that folate levels did not vary significantly in time in both groups (those receiving PPI therapy and those receiving surgery). These findings are coherent with our findings on folate levels.

Gastric acid facilitates the absorption of non-heme iron by reducing ferric iron to the more soluble ferrous form and also enhances iron salt dissociation from ingested food and allows for the formation of complexes with amines and sugars that also increase absorption [4]. Thus, it is expected that PPIs, by reducing gastric acid secretion, can potentially cause iron malabsorption. Two relatively recent case–control studies [34,35] investigated the link between chronic PPI administration and iron deficiency, finding a positive association between the two conditions, with a stronger association for higher daily doses (>1.5 vs. <0.75 PPI pills/d; p value interaction = 0.004), and decreased after medication discontinuation (p-trend < 0.001) [34]. Despite these results, a review by Priyanka et al. [36] concluded that "clinically significant iron deficiency is less likely to occur with the long-term use of PPIs in normal subjects although it may happen". However, PPI use may be associated with difficulty in achieving adequate iron store repletion in iron-deficient subjects. In our study, there was no significant difference in blood iron between subjects taking PPIs and the control group (Table 1).

Finally, we found a non-significant trend for zinc deficiency in PPI users ($p = 0.08$) (Table 1). A study by Farrell et al. [37] evaluated the effect of PPIs on zinc absorption and storage; they found significantly lower levels of blood zinc in chronic PPI users vs. controls, despite the low numerosity in the samples (75 ± 3 mcg/dL vs. 91 ± 3 mcg/dL, $p = 0.004$). Surprisingly, this issue has not been investigated extensively in the literature; therefore, our paper might have merit to have shed new light on the topic, deserving further investigation.

Our study suffers from some limitations, such as the small sample and the missed evaluation of potentially confounding factors including eating habits. However, this was a pilot study performed on a few patients under the care of a single physician; therefore, larger samples are necessary. Furthermore, our study did not evaluate baseline levels of micronutrients, and a study with a follow-up before and after long-term use of PPIs could have been more proper and provided more interesting results. Some imbalances in group composition could be another limitation; for example, the age in the PPI group was higher than in controls. However, the fact that PPI-taking subjects were older than controls may be explained by the fact that these drugs are mostly needed by elderly patients in the long term. However, we found that age did not correlate with any of the levels of micronutrients involved in bone metabolism (Vitamin D, Ca, Zn and P), as shown in Figure 1. This could provide evidence that the use of PPIs could play a role in the deficiency of such molecules more than the age itself [38]. The primary care context is, however, a field in which chronic PPI effects on micronutrients have been poorly explored so far. Sarzynski et al. [39] performed a similar case–control study in an academic outpatient population, but it was retrospective and evaluated only blood markers related to iron deficiency (hemoglobin, hematocrit, mean corpuscular volume). Qorraj-Bytyqi et al. [40] prospectively analyzed vitamin B12, homocysteine and ferritin levels in a population of patients with osteoarthritis undergoing 12 months of PPI therapy associated with NSAIDs at baseline and after 12 months. Thus, other existing studies have some differences from our study, and we did not find other similar studies in general practitioner settings. Moreover, the several existing studies come to different conclusions, and the most recent guidelines [32] do not recommend routine screening or monitoring of bone mineral density, serum creatinine, magnesium or vitamin B12. Moreover, the results of our study and the evidence from the literature should be interpreted with wit, and, when PPI indication is evidence-based, there is no reason for PPI withdrawal because of fear of side effects [41,42]. Of note, ten patients showed APCA positivity, which did not reflect the presence of atrophy at gastric biopsy; such patients could be considered as potential autoimmune gastritis cases [43], but the absence of atrophy warrants that impaired absorption is secondary to pantoprazole and not atrophic gastritis.

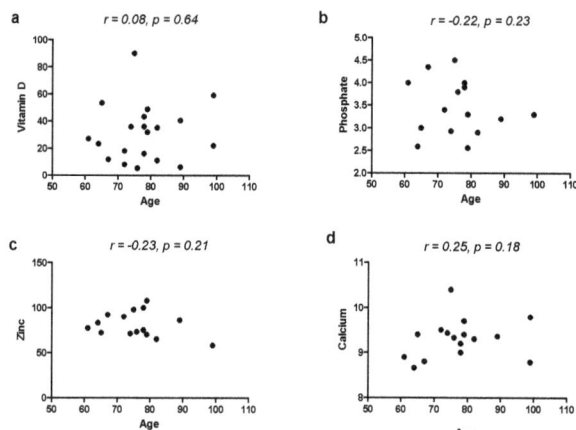

Figure 1. Correlation between age and blood levels of vitamin D (**a**), phosphate (**b**), zinc (**c**) and calcium (**d**).

5. Conclusions

Despite the above-cited limitations, our study seems to confirm that chronic pantoprazole use may engender alterations in micronutrients involved in bone mineral homeostasis, while other element absorption, such as iron and B12, seem not to be affected. Interestingly, the effect on zinc levels is an interesting finding, which requires further investigation.

Author Contributions: Conceptualization, G.L., M.B. and A.D.L.; methodology, G.L., E.I., F.C.; software G.I., N.L.B.C.; formal analysis, G.L., F.C.; investigation, N.L.B.C., G.I.; resources, E.I., G.I.; data curation, A.D.L.; writing—original draft preparation, G.I.; writing—review and editing, G.L., E.I., F.C., M.B. All authors have read and agreed to the published version of the manuscript.

Funding: This research received no external funding.

Institutional Review Board Statement: The study was conducted in accordance with the Declaration of Helsinki and approved by the Internal Gastroenterology Institutional Review Board.

Informed Consent Statement: Informed consent was obtained from all subjects involved in the study.

Data Availability Statement: Not applicable.

Conflicts of Interest: The authors declare no conflict of interest.

References

1. Tosetti, C.; Ubaldi, E.; Grattagliano, I.; Scoglio, R.; Mastronuzzi, T.; Belvedere, A.; Bertolusso, L.; Bozzani, A.; Discafani, G.; Napoli, L. La prescrizione degli inibitori di pompa protonica: Un decalogo per la Medicina Generale. *Riv. Soc. Ital. Med. Gen.* **2018**, *25*, 36–42.
2. Ierardi, E.; Losurdo, G.; Fortezza, R.F.; Principi, M.; Barone, M.; Di Leo, A. Optimizing proton pump inhibitors in *Helicobacter pylori* treatment: Old and new tricks to improve effectiveness. *World J. Gastroenterol.* **2019**, *25*, 5097–5104. [CrossRef] [PubMed]
3. Sachs, G. Improving on PPI-based therapy of GORD. *Eur. J. Gastroenterol. Hepatol.* **2001**, *13*, S35–S42.
4. Sheen, E.; Triadafilopoulos, G. Adverse effects of long-term proton pump inhibitor therapy. *Dig. Dis. Sci.* **2010**, *56*, 931–950. [CrossRef]
5. Haastrup, P.F.; Thompson, W.; Søndergaard, J.; Jarbøl, D.E. Side Effects of Long-Term Proton Pump Inhibitor Use: A Review. *Basic Clin. Pharmacol. Toxicol.* **2018**, *123*, 114–121. [CrossRef]
6. Eusebi, L.H.; Rabitti, S.; Artesiani, M.L.; Gelli, D.; Montagnani, M.; Zagari, R.M.; Bazzoli, F. Proton pump inhibitors: Risks of long-term use. *J. Gastroenterol. Hepatol.* **2017**, *32*, 1295–1302. [CrossRef]
7. Zhou, B.; Huang, Y.; Li, H.; Sun, W.; Liu, J. Proton-pump inhibitors and risk of fractures: An update meta-analysis. *Osteoporos. Int.* **2016**, *27*, 339–347. [CrossRef]
8. Jacobs, A.; Miles, P.M. Role of gastric secretion in iron absorption. *Gut* **1969**, *10*, 226–229. [CrossRef] [PubMed]
9. Miret, S.; Simpson, R.J.; McKie, A.T. Physiology and molecular biology of dietary iron absorption. *Ann. Rev. Nutr.* **2003**, *23*, 283–301. [CrossRef] [PubMed]
10. Graziani, G.; Como, G.; Badalamenti, S.; Finazzi, S.; Malesci, A.; Gallieni, M.; Brancaccio, D.; Ponticelli, C. Effect of gastric acid secretion on intestinal phosphate and calcium absorption in normal subjects. *Nephrol. Dial. Transplant.* **1995**, *10*, 1376–1380.
11. Saltzman, J.R.; Kemp, J.A.; Golner, B.B.; Pedrosa, M.C.; Dallal, G.E.; Russell, R.M. Effect of hypochlorhydria due to omeprazole treatment or atrophic gastritis on protein-bound vitamin B12 absorption. *J. Am. Coll. Nutr.* **1994**, *13*, 584–591. [CrossRef]
12. Petrus, A.; Fairchild, T.; Doyle, R. Traveling the Vitamin B12 Pathway: Oral Delivery of Protein and Peptide Drugs. *Angew. Chem. Int. Ed.* **2009**, *48*, 1022–1028. [CrossRef] [PubMed]
13. Koop, H. Review article: Metabolic consequences of long-term inhibition of acid secretion by omeprazole. *Aliment. Pharmacol. Ther.* **1992**, *6*, 399–406. [CrossRef] [PubMed]
14. Koop, H.; Bachem, M.G. Serum iron, ferritin, and vitamin B12 during prolonged omeprazole therapy. *J. Clin. Gastroenterol.* **1992**, *14*, 288–292. [CrossRef]
15. Termanini, B.; Gibril, F.; Sutliff, V.E.; Yu, F.; Venzon, D.J.; Jensen, R.T. Effect of long-term gastric acid suppressive therapy on serum vitamin B12 levels in patients with Zollinger-Ellison syndrome. *Am. J. Med.* **1998**, *104*, 422–430. [CrossRef]
16. Howden, C.W. Vitamin B12 levels during prolonged treatment with proton pump inhibitors. *J. Clin. Gastroenterol.* **2000**, *30*, 29–33. [CrossRef]
17. Lerman, T.T.; Cohen, E.; Sochat, T.; Goldberg, E.; Goldberg, I.; Krause, I. Proton pump inhibitor use and its effect on vitamin B12 and homocysteine levels among men and women: A large cross-sectional study. *Am. J. Med. Sci.* **2022**, *364*, 746–751. [CrossRef]
18. Hatemi, İ.; Esatoğlu, S.N. What is the long term acid inhibitor treatment in gastroesophageal reflux disease? What are the potential problems related to long term acid inhibitor treatment in gastroesophageal reflux disease? How should these cases be followed? *Turk. J. Gastroenterol.* **2017**, *28* (Suppl. S1), S57–S60. [CrossRef] [PubMed]
19. Epstein, M.; McGrath, S.; Law, F. Proton-pump inhibitors and hypomagnesemic hypoparathyroidism. *N. Engl. J. Med.* **2006**, *355*, 1834–1836. [CrossRef]
20. Cheungpasitporn, W.; Thongprayoon, C.; Kittanamongkolchai, W.; Srivali, N.; Edmonds, P.J.; Ungprasert, P.; Erickson, S.B. Proton pump inhibitors linked to hypomagnesemia: A systematic review and meta-analysis of observational studies. *Ren. Fail.* **2015**, *37*, 1237–1241. [CrossRef]
21. William, J.H.; Danziger, J. Proton-pump inhibitor-induced hypomagnesemia: Current research and proposed mechanisms. *World J. Nephrol.* **2016**, *5*, 152–157. [CrossRef] [PubMed]

22. Maurya, V.K.; Aggarwal, M. Factors influencing the absorption of vitamin D in GIT: An overview. *J. Food Sci. Technol.* **2017**, *54*, 3753–3765. [CrossRef]
23. Pramod, R.; Edwards, L.R. Magnesium Supplementation in Vitamin D Deficiency. *Am. J. Ther.* **2019**, *26*, e124–e132.
24. Sharara, A.I.; El-Halabi, M.M.; Ghaith, O.A.; Habib, R.H.; Mansour, N.M.; Malli, A.; El Hajj-Fuleihan, G. Proton pump inhibitors have no measurable effect on calcium and bone metabolism in healthy young males: A prospective matched controlled study. *Metabolism* **2013**, *62*, 518–526. [CrossRef] [PubMed]
25. Hinson, A.M.; Wilkerson, B.M.; Rothman-Fitts, I.; Riggs, A.T.; Stack, B.C.; Bodenner, D.L. Hyperparathyroidism associated with long-term proton pump inhibitors independent of concurrent bisphosphonate therapy in elderly adults. *J. Am. Geriatr. Soc.* **2015**, *63*, 2070–2073. [CrossRef]
26. Dawson-Hughes, B.; Harris, S.S.; Dallal, G.E. Plasma calcidiol, season, and serum parathyroid hormone concentrations in healthy elderly men and women. *Am. J. Clin. Nutr.* **1997**, *65*, 67–71. [CrossRef] [PubMed]
27. Wortsman, J.; Matsuoka, L.Y.; Chen, T.C.; Lu, Z.; Holick, M.F. Decreased bioavailability of vitamin D in obesity. *Am. J. Clin. Nutr.* **2000**, *72*, 690–693. [CrossRef]
28. Robien, K.; Oppeneer, S.J.; Kelly, J.A.; Hamilton-Reeves, J.M. Drug-vitamin D interactions: A systematic review of the literature. *Nutr. Clin. Pract.* **2013**, *28*, 194–208. [CrossRef] [PubMed]
29. Yang, Y.X. Chronic Proton Pump Inihibitor Therapy and Calcium Metabolism. *Curr. Gastroenterol. Rep.* **2012**, *14*, 473–479. [CrossRef]
30. Insogna, K.L. MD The Effect of Proton Pump-Inhibiting Drugs on Mineral Metabolism. *Am. J. Gastroenterol.* **2009**, *104*, S2–S4.
31. Farina, C.; Gagliardi, S. Selective inhibition of osteoclast vacuolar H+-ATPase. *Curr. Pharm. Des.* **2002**, *8*, 2033–2048. [CrossRef]
32. Freedberg, D.E.; Kim, L.S.; Yang, Y.X. The Risks and Benefits of Long-term Use of Proton Pump Inhibitors: Expert Review and Best Practice Advice from the American Gastroenterological Association. *Gastroenterology* **2017**, *152*, 706–715. [CrossRef]
33. Attwood, S.E.; Ell, C.; Galmiche, P.J.; Fiocca, R.; Hatlebakk, J.G.; Hasselgren, B.; Langstrom, G.; Jahreskog, M.; Eklund, S.; Lind, T.; et al. Long-term safety of proton pump inhibitor therapy assessed under controlled, randomised clinical trial conditions: Data from the SOPRAN and LOTUS studies. *Aliment. Pharmacol. Ther.* **2015**, *41*, 1162–1174. [CrossRef]
34. Tran-Du, A.; Connel, N.J.; Vanmolkt, F.H.; Souverein, P.C.; de Wit, N.J.; Stehouwer, C.D.A.; Hoes, A.W.; de Vries, F.; de Boer, A. Use of proton pump inhibitors and risk of iron deficiency: A population-based case–control study. *J. Ontern. Med.* **2019**, *285*, 205–214. [CrossRef] [PubMed]
35. Lam, J.R.; Schneider, J.L.; Quesenberry, C.P.; Corley, D.A. Proton pump inhibitor and histamine-2 receptor antagonist use and iron deficiency. *Gastroenterology* **2017**, *152*, 821–829. [CrossRef] [PubMed]
36. Priyanka, P.; Sofka, S.; Reynolds, G. Effect of Long—Term Proton Pump Inhibitor Use on Iron Absorption: A Systematic Review. *Am. J. Gastroenterol.* **2018**, *113*, S702–S704. [CrossRef]
37. Farrell, C.P.; Morgan, M.; Rudolph, D.S.; Hwang, A.; Albert, N.E.; Valenzano, M.C.; Wang, X.; Mercogliano, G.; Mullin, J.M. Proton Pump Inhibitors Interfere with Zinc Absorption and Zinc Body Stores. *Gastroenterol. Res.* **2011**, *4*, 243–251. [CrossRef] [PubMed]
38. Sahota, O. Understanding vitamin D deficiency. *Age Ageing* **2014**, *43*, 589–591. [CrossRef] [PubMed]
39. Sarzynski, E.; Puttarajappa, C.; Xie, Y.; Grover, M.; Laird-Fick, H. Association Between Proton Pump Inhibitor Use and Anemia: A Retrospective Cohort Study. *Dig. Dis. Sci.* **2011**, *56*, 2349–2353. [CrossRef]
40. Qorraj-Bytyqi, H.; Hoxha, R.; Sadiku, S.; Bajraktari, I.H.; Sopjani, M.; Thaçi, K.; Thaçi, S.; Bahtiri, E. Proton Pump Inhibitors Intake and Iron and Vitamin B12 Status: A Prospective Comparative Study with a Follow up of 12 Months. *Open Access Maced. J. Med. Sci.* **2018**, *12*, 442–446. [CrossRef]
41. Losurdo, G.; Di Leo, A.; Leandro, G. What Is the Optimal Follow-up Time to Ascertain the Safety of Proton Pump Inhibitors? *Gastroenterology* **2020**, *158*, 1175. [CrossRef] [PubMed]
42. Helgadottir, H.; Bjornsson, E.S. Problems Associated with Deprescribing of Proton Pump Inhibitors. *Int. J. Mol. Sci.* **2019**, *20*, 5469. [CrossRef] [PubMed]
43. Lenti, M.V.; Miceli, E.; Vanoli, A.; Klersy, C.; Corazza, G.R.; Di Sabatino, A. Time course and risk factors of evolution from potential to overt autoimmune gastritis. *Dig. Liver Dis.* **2022**, *54*, 642–644. [CrossRef] [PubMed]

Disclaimer/Publisher's Note: The statements, opinions and data contained in all publications are solely those of the individual author(s) and contributor(s) and not of MDPI and/or the editor(s). MDPI and/or the editor(s) disclaim responsibility for any injury to people or property resulting from any ideas, methods, instructions or products referred to in the content.

MDPI
St. Alban-Anlage 66
4052 Basel
Switzerland
www.mdpi.com

Journal of Clinical Medicine Editorial Office
E-mail: jcm@mdpi.com
www.mdpi.com/journal/jcm

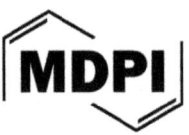

Disclaimer/Publisher's Note: The statements, opinions and data contained in all publications are solely those of the individual author(s) and contributor(s) and not of MDPI and/or the editor(s). MDPI and/or the editor(s) disclaim responsibility for any injury to people or property resulting from any ideas, methods, instructions or products referred to in the content.